Manual of Pain Management

Second Edition

Manual of Pain Management

Second Edition

Edited by

Carol A. Warfield, M.D.

Edward Lowenstein Professor of Anaesthesia
Harvard Medical School
Chairman, Department of Anesthesia and Critical Care
Beth Israel Deaconess Medical Center
Boston, Massachusetts

Hilary J. Fausett, M.D.

Director, Pain Management Center
Department of Anesthesia
Kaiser Permanente, Los Angeles Medical Center
Los Angeles, California

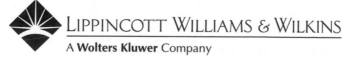

LIPPINCOTT WILLIAMS & WILKINS
A **Wolters Kluwer** Company
Philadelphia • Baltimore • New York • London
Buenos Aires • Hong Kong • Sydney • Tokyo

Acquisitions Editor: Craig Percy
Developmental Editor: Kerry B. Barrett
Production Editor: Jonathan Geffner
Manufacturing Manager: Colin Warnock
Cover Designer: Mark Lerner
Compositor: Lippincott Williams & Wilkins Desktop Divison
Printer: Maple Press

Library of Congress Cataloging-in-Publication Data

Manual of pain management / edited by Carol A. Warfield, Hilary J. Fausett.—2nd ed.
     p. ; cm.
   Includes bibliographical references and index.
   ISBN 0-7817-2313-2
     1. Pain—Treatment—Handbooks, manuals, etc.   I. Warfield, Carol A.   II. Fausett, Hilary J.
   [DNLM: 1. Pain—therapy. WL 704 M294 2001]
   RB127.M3842001
   616'.0472—dc21

                                                                                2001041363

Care has been taken to confirm the accuracy of the information presented and to describe generally accepted practices. However, the authors, editors, and publisher are not responsible for errors or omissions or for any consequences from application of the information in this book and make no warranty, expressed or implied, with respect to the currency, completeness, or accuracy of the contents of the publication. Application of this information in a particular situation remains the professional responsibility of the practitioner.

The authors, editors, and publisher have exerted every effort to ensure that drug selection and dosage set forth in this text are in accordance with current recommendations and practice at the time of publication. However, in view of ongoing research, changes in government regulations, and the constant flow of information relating to drug therapy and drug reactions, the reader is urged to check the package insert for each drug for any change in indications and dosage and for added warnings and precautions. This is particularly important when the recommended agent is a new or infrequently employed drug.

Some drugs and medical devices presented in this publication have Food and Drug Administration (FDA) clearance for limited use in restricted research settings. It is the responsibility of the health care provider to ascertain the FDA status of each drug or device planned for use in their clinical practice.

10 9 8 7 6 5 4 3 2 1

To my children, Rick, Chris, and Alex
(C.A.W.)

To my children, Asher and Ellie
(H.J.F.)

Contents

III. Common Painful Syndromes

IV. Pain Management

Medications

Injection Therapies

Contributing Authors

Vijayasree Arvind, M.D.
Anesthesiologist
Beth Israel Deconess Medical Center
Boston, Massachusetts
Anesthesiologist
Anesthesiology Methodist Medical Center
Dallas, Texas

George K. Asdourian, M.D.
Professor
Department of Surgery/Ophthalmology
University of Massachusetts Medical School
Chief
Department of Ophthalmology
University of Massachusetts Memorial Health
 Care/Hahneman Campus
Worcester, Massachusetts

Joseph F. Audette, M.A., M.D.
Instructor
Department of Physical Medicine &
 Rehabilitation
Harvard Medical School
Spaulding Rehabilitation Hospital
Attending Staff
Department of Anesthesia
Beth Israel Deaconess Medical Center
Boston, Massachusetts

Zahid H. Bajwa, M.D.
Assistant Professor
Department of Anesthesia and Neurology
Harvard Medical School
Director, Clinical Pain Research
Department of Anesthesia
Beth Israel Deaconess Medical Center
Boston, Massachusetts

Benjamin S. Battino, M.D.
Chief Resident
Division of Urology
University of Cincinnati and
University Hospital
Cincinnati, Ohio

Michael P. Biber, M.D.
Clinical Instructor
Department of Neurology
Harvard Medical School
Senior Associate Neurologist
Beth Israel Deaconess Medical Center
Boston, Massachusetts

Loren J. Borud, M.D.
Instructor in Surgery
Division of Plastic Surgery
Harvard Medical School
Attending Physician
Department of Surgery
Beth Israel Deaconess Medical Center
Boston, Massachusetts

Roy J. Braganza, M.D.
Assistant Chief
Department of Anesthesia
Kaiser Permanente
Los Angeles Medical Center
Los Angeles, California

Harsimran S. Brara, M.D.
Staff Neurosurgeon
Department of Neurosurgery
Kaiser Permanente Medical Group and
 Kaiser Permanente Foundation Hospital
Los Angeles, California

Margaret A. Caudill-Slosberg, M.D., Ph.D.
Adjunct Associate Professor
Department of Anesthesiology
Dartmouth Medical School
Hanover, New Hampshire

David S. Chapin, M.D.
Assistant Professor
Department of Obstetrics, Gynecology, and
 Reproductive Biology
Harvard Medical School
Director of Gynecology
Department of Obstetrics and Gynecology
Beth Israel Deaconess Medical Center
Boston, Massachusetts

Barry R. Chi, M.D.
Associate Clinical Professor
Department of Internal Medicine
University of California at Los Angeles
Interventional Pain Physiatrist
Chronic Pain Program and
Department of Physical Medicine
Kaiser Permanente Hospital–Los Angeles
Los Angeles, California

Jong M. Choe, M.D.
Assistant Professor
Department of Surgery
Division of Urology
University of Cincinnati College of
   Medicine
Director of Continence Program
Department of Surgery
Division of Urology
University of Cincinnati Medical Center
Cincinnati, Ohio

Liane Clamen Glazer, M.D.
Ophthalmology Resident
Department of Ophthalmology
Massachusetts Eye and Ear Infirmary
Harvard Medical School
Boston, Massachusetts

Robert I. Cohen, M.D.
Instructor
Department of Anesthesia and
   Critical Care
Harvard Medical School
Anesthesiologist
Department of Anesthesia and
   Critical Care
Beth Israel Deaconess Medical Center
Boston, Massachusetts

Kirsten E. Colton, OTR/L, M.B.A.
Occupational Therapist III
Occupational Therapy Team Leader
Inpatient Services
Department of Rehabilitation
Beth Israel Deaconess Medical Center
Boston, Massachusetts

Stephanie Cooper Kochhar, M.D.
Staff Physician
Department of Anesthesiology
O'Connor Hospital
San José, California

Kimberly A. Cox, M.D.
Clinical Fellow in Pain Management
Department of Anesthesia
Harvard University
Pain Fellow
Department of Anesthesia
Beth Israel Deaconess Medical Center
Boston, Massachusetts

Frederic J. Curlin, IV, M.D.
Director, Pain Management
Department of Anesthesiology
Kaiser Foundation Medical Center, Fontana
Fontana, California

David A. Danforth, Ph.D.
Instructor in Psychology
Department of Psychiatry
Harvard Medical School
Affiliated Attending Medical Psychologist
Department of Psychiatry
Beth Israel Deaconess Medical Center
Boston, Massachusetts

Ralph J. Di Libero, M.D.
Orthopedic Surgeon
Los Angeles Medical Center
Southern California Permanente Medical Group
Los Angeles, California

Lena E. Dohlman, M.D, M.P.H.
Instructor in Anesthesia
Department of Anesthesia and Critical Care
Harvard Medical School
Assistant in Anesthesia
Massachusetts General Hospital
Boston, Massachusetts

Joel L. Dunsky, D.D.S.
Assistant Clinical Professor
Department of Endodontics
Harvard School of Dental Medicine
Staff Associate
Department of Clinical Sciences
The Forsyth Institute
Boston, Massachusetts

Eric M. Emont, M.D.
Assistant Clinical Professor
Department of Internal Medicine
University of California at Los Angeles
Physician
Department of Geriatrics/Continuing Care
Kaiser Permanente
Los Angeles, California

Hilary J. Fausett, M.D.
Director
Pain Management Center
Department of Anesthesia
Kaiser Permanente, Los Angeles Medical Center
Los Angeles, California

Jillian B. Frank, Ph.D.
Instructor in Psychology
Department of Psychiatry
Harvard Medical School
Leader of the Mind/Body Cancer Program
Harvard Vanguard Medical Associates
Supervising Psychologist
Arnold Pain Management Center
Beth Israel Deaconess Medical Center
Boston, Massachusetts

Tobin N. Gerhart, M.D.
Clinical Assistant Professor
Department of Orthopedic Surgery
Harvard Medical School
Attending Orthopedic Surgeon
Department of Orthopedics
Beth Israel Deaconess Medical Center
Boston, Massachusetts

Richard L. Gilbert, M.D.
Chief
Department of Anesthesiology
Carolinas Medical Center
Charlotte, North Carolina

Paul A. Glazer, M.D.
Clinical Instructor
Combined Harvard Orthopedic Program
Boston Orthopedic Group
Brookline, Massachusetts

David B. Golden, M.D.
Assistant in Surgery
Department of Orthopedic Surgery
Harvard Medical School
Fellow in Sports Medicine
Department of Orthopedic Surgery
Massachusetts General Hospital
Boston, Massachusetts

Kenneth R. Goldschneider, M.D.
Assistant Professor
Department of Anesthesia
University of Cincinnati
Director, Division of Pain Management
Department of Anesthesia
Children's Hospital Medical Center
Cincinnati, Ohio

Dan P. Gray, M.D.
Clinical and Research Fellow
Department of Anesthesia and Critical Care
Beth Israel Deaconess Medical Center
Boston, Massachusetts

Sanjay Gupta, M.D.
Director
Einstein Pain Center
Albert Einstein Health Care Network
Philadelphia, Pennsylvania

José M. Hernández-García
Department of Anesthesiology
Harvard Medical School
Fellow in Pain Management
Department of Anesthesiology
Beth Israel and Deaconess Medical Center
Boston, Massachusetts

Charles C. Ho, M.D.
Clinical Instructor
Department of Anesthesiology
Harvard Medical School and
Beth Israel Deaconess Medical Center
Boston, Massachusetts

Stephen A. Houser, M.D.
Anesthesiologist
Department of Anesthesiology
Lunkenau Hospital
Wynnewood, Pennsylvania

Cynthia H. Kahn
Lahey Clinic
Burlington, Massachusetts

Joseph P. Kannam, M.D.
Assistant Professor
Division of Cardiology
Harvard Medical School
Beth Israel Deaconess Medical Center
Boston, Massachusetts

Carol P. Keck, OTR/L
Clinical Services Manager
Department of Rehabilitation Services
Beth Israel Deaconess Medical Center
Boston, Massachusetts

Dhanalakshmi Koyyalagunta, M.D.
Assistant Professor
Department of Anesthesiology
University of Texas Medical Branch
Galveston, Texas

David Cheng-chih Lai, M.D.
Instructor in Anesthesia
Department of Anesthesiology
Harvard Medical School
Coordinator of Resident Curriculum
Department of Anesthesia and
*   Critical Care*
Beth Israel Deaconess Medical Center
Boston, Massachusetts

John C. Makrides, M.D.
Staff Anesthesiologist
Department of Anesthesia
Maine Medical Center
Portland, Maine

James Mann, DPM
Chestnut Hill, Massachusetts

Keira P. Mason, M.D.
Instructor of Anesthesia (Radiology)
Department of Anesthesia
Harvard Medical School
Director of Radiology Anesthesia
Department of Anesthesia
Children's Hospital
Boston, Massachusetts

Eran D. Metzger, M.D.
Instructor
Department of Psychiatry
Harvard Medical School
Boston, Massachusetts
Associate Director of Geropsychiatry
Department of Medicine
Hebrew Rehabilitation Center for Aged
Roslindale, Massachusetts

Edward Michna M.D.
Instructor
Department of Anesthesia
Harvard Medical School
Anesthesiologist
Department of Anesthesia
Brigham and Women's Hospital
Boston, Massachusetts

Anne Miller, M.D.
Instructor in Anesthesia
Department of Anesthesia
Beth Israel Deaconess
*   Medical Center*
Boston, Massachusetts

Kyung Won Park, M.D.
Assistant Professor
Department of Anesthesia
Harvard Medical School
Director, Vascular Anesthesia
Department of Anesthesia and Critical Care
Beth Israel Deaconess Medical Center
Boston, Massachusetts

Jagruti Patel, M.D.
Resident in Plastic and Reconstructive
*   Surgery*
Rhode Island Hospital
Brown University School of Medicine
Providence, Rhode Island

Christine Peeters-Asdourian, M.D.
Instructor
Department of Anesthesia
Harvard Medical School
Director, Arnold Pain Management Center
Department of Anesthesiology and
*   Critical Care*
Beth Israel Deaconess Medical Center
Boston, Massachusetts

Donald T. Reilly, M.D., Ph.D.
Assistant Professor
Harvard University Medical School
Orthopedic Surgeon
New England Baptist Hospital
Boston, Massachusetts

Deborah L. Rochman, M.S., OTR/L
Lecturer
Boston School of Occupational Therapy
Tufts University
Medford, Massachusetts
Clinical Instructor
Gelb Orofacial Pain Center
Tufts University School of Dental Medicine
Boston, Massachusetts

Seward B. Rutkove, M.D.
Assistant Professor
Department of Neurology
Harvard Medical School
Associate Neurologist
Department of Neurology
Beth Israel Deaconess Medical Center
Boston, Massachusetts

Naveed Sami, M.D.
Research Fellow
Harvard Medical School
Boston, Massachusetts

Mukesh C. Sarna, M.D.
Instructor in Anesthesia
Department of Anesthesia
Beth Israel Deaconess Medical Center
Boston, Massachusetts

John Sharp, M.D.
Instructor
Department of Psychiatry
Harvard Medical School
Associate Director, Inpatient Services
Medical Student Educator
Department of Psychiatry
Beth Israel Deaconess Medical Center
Boston, Massachusetts

Kathleen E. Shillue, P.T., O.C.S.
Program Coordinator
Department of Rehabilitation Services
Beth Israel Deaconess Medical Center
Boston, Massachusetts

Adam J. Silk, M.D.
Clinical Instructor
Department of Psychiatry
Harvard Medical School
Boston, Massachusetts
Psychiatrist
Department of Mental Health
Massachusetts Institute of Technology
Cambridge, Massachusetts

Anna G. A. Sottile, M.D.
Associate Professor
Department of Anesthesia
Roger Williams Medical Center
Assistant Director of Pain Management
Staff Anesthesiologist
Department of Anesthesia/SNAPA
Roger Williams Medical Center
Providence, Rhode Island

David D. Staskin, M.D.
Assistant Professor
Department of Urology
Harvard Medical School
Department of Urology
Beth Israel Deaconess Medical Center
Boston, Massachusetts

Alicja Soczewko Steiner, M.D.
Instructor in Anesthesia
Department of Anesthesia and Critical Care
Harvard Medical School
Attending Physician
Department of Anesthesia and Critical Care
Beth Israel Deaconess Medical Center
Boston, Massachusetts

Danielle S. Stranc, M.D.
Staff Anesthesiologist
Department of Anesthesiology
Kaiser Permanente Los Angeles
Medical Center
Los Angeles, California

Andrew M. Strassman, Ph.D.
Assistant Professor
Department of Anesthesia
Harvard Medical School
Department of Anesthesia and
Critical Care
Beth Israel Deaconess Medical Center
Boston, Massachusetts

Praveen K. Suchdev, M.D.
Medical Director
Pain Solutions Pllc.
Southern New Hampshire Medical Center
Nashua, New Hampshire

Michael L. Tran, M.D.
Instructor of Anesthesiology
Department of Anesthesia
Harvard Medical School
Instructor of Anesthesiology
Department of Anesthesia
Beth Israel Deaconess Medical Center
Boston, Massachusetts

Joseph Upton, M.D.
Associate Clinical Professor
Department of Surgery
Harvard Medical School
Senior Associate
Department of Surgery
Children's Hospital
Boston, Massachusetts

David M. Vernick, M.D.
Assistant Professor
Department of Otology and Laryngology
Harvard Medical School
Chief of Otolaryngology
Department of Surgery
Beth Israel Deaconess Medical Center
Boston, Massachusetts

Carol A. Warfield, M.D.
Edward Lowenstein Professor of Anesthesia
Harvard Medical School
Chairman
Department of Anesthesia and Critical Care
Beth Israel Deaconess Medical Center
Boston, Massachusetts

Wilma Wasco, Ph.D.
Assistant Professor
Department of Neurology
Harvard Medical School
Assistant Professor
Department of Neurology
Massachusetts General Hospital
Charleston, Massachusetts

Aida B. Won, M.D.
Instructor of Medicine
Department of Internal Medicine
Division of Aging
Harvard Medical School
Geriatrician
Department of Internal Medicine
Hebrew Rehabilitation Center for Aged
Boston, Massachusetts

Joshua Wootton, M.Div., Ph.D.
Instructor in Psychology
Department of Psychiatry
Harvard Medical School
Director of Pain Psychology
Arnold Pain Management Center
Department of Anesthesia and Critical Care
Beth Israel Deaconess Medical Center
Boston, Massachusetts

Jeffrey L. Zilberfarb, M.D.
Clinical Instructor
Department of Orthopaedic Surgery
Harvard Medical School
Staff Surgeon
Department of Orthopaedic Surgery
Beth Israel Deaconess Medical Center
Boston, Massachusetts

Introduction

The revised edition of *Manual of Pain Management* reflects the changes that have occurred in medicine over the past decade. While keeping the same easy-to-use format of self-contained chapters, the new edition also provides a basic framework of the study of pain management. The first section describes the basic physiologic concepts and some of the requisite testing needed for proper diagnosis. The majority of the book is a description of the most common pain syndromes as classified anatomically—the ways in which patients present and physicians approach a "chief complaint." The next section focuses on medications, procedures, and therapies commonly used for patients with pain complaints, including complementary therapies.

This edition recognizes the importance of pediatric-pain management and also the unique issues that arise when treating the elderly population. The chapter on treating the pain of human immunodeficiency virus (HIV)/acquired immunodeficiency syndrome (AIDS) addresses the challenges of treating the pain, whether from the disease itself or from the side effects of a potentially life-saving drug. *Manual of Pain Management* also addresses the difficulty of providing good medical care to the patient with addiction. In addition, there is a chapter on the legal issues that face all clinicians, with special emphasis on the quandaries the pain clinician might face.

This updated edition employs a true collaborative and multidisciplinary approach. Each chapter is written by an expert in a particular area. The book as a whole reflects the balance achieved when different disciplines work collaboratively to address the needs of the patient with pain.

This edition of *Manual of Pain Management* is published at the beginning of a new millennium. The past decade has wrought tremendous change in the medical fields and specifically in the area of pain management. The changes have not only been clinical and scientific, as would be predicted; there have also been tremendous social and political changes in the management of pain. Perhaps the biggest impact on the treatment of patients with pain will be from the implementation of new standards for practice by the Joint Commission on Accreditation of Healthcare Organizations (JCAHO).

PATIENTS HAVE THE RIGHT TO APPROPRIATE ASSESSMENT AND MANAGEMENT OF PAIN

The JCAHO has established new pain assessment and management standards, and those standards will first be scored in 2001. Under the new standards, healthcare providers are expected to be knowledgeable about pain assessment and management, and facilities are expected to develop policies and procedures supporting the appropriate assessment of pain and the use of analgesics and other pain control interventions. Some key concepts include:

1. Recognize the right of patients to appropriate assessment and management of pain. Assess the existence of pain and, if it does in fact exist, the nature and intensity of pain in all patients.
2. Record the results of the assessment in a way that facilitates regular reassessment and follow-up.
3. Determine and assure staff competency in pain assessment and management, and address pain assessment and management in the orientation of all new staff.
4. Establish policies and procedures that support the appropriate prescription or ordering of effective pain medications.
5. Educate patients and their families about effective pain management, and address patient needs for symptom management in the discharge planning process.

In terms of pain measurement, the standards include the following statement: An organization selects pain-intensity measures to ensure consistency across departments, for example, the 0–10 scale, the Wong–Baker FACES pain rating scale (smile–frown), and the verbal descriptor scale. Adult patients are encouraged to use the 0–10 scale. If they cannot understand or are unwilling to use it, the smile–frown or the verbal scale is used. The smile–frown scale is especially helpful in patients who do not understand English and in the pediatric population.

PAIN: THE FIFTH VITAL SIGN

The American Pain Society (APS) has created the phrase "Pain: The Fifth Vital Sign" to elevate awareness of pain treatment among healthcare professionals. The slogan was developed to remind health practitioners of the importance of monitoring and treating patients with pain.

With its new standards, JCAHO has sent a clear message that pain is indeed now considered the "fifth" vital sign and is to be assessed during all patient encounters. Healthcare facilities are required to provide educational materials and document that patients and their families are informed of the intent to provide effective pain relief as an integral aspect of their care. Patients should expect information regarding appropriate options for enhanced pain relief and participate in the decision regarding treatment of their symptoms. The pain initiative will be applied to all patient populations. JCAHO stipulates that infants, children, and impaired patients will require special assessment tools based on developmental stage, chronological age, function status, and cognitive abilities.

Patients expect to receive state-of-the-art pain management, and the advent of the Internet and the technology to allow access to the world-wide web has dramatically altered the role of the physician/educator. Healthcare providers are able to learn about new techniques and conduct reviews of the literature from their own offices. And patients are able to access the Internet to learn as well. The beauty of the Internet is that it provides a "printing press" for anyone to disseminate information. The problem is that the content of the Internet is unregulated and not peer-reviewed. Thus, there is no way of assessing the accuracy or validity of any claim made on a web site.

Many physicians and educators have become alarmed at the potential for medical fraud and direct harm to individuals that exists due to the unregulated nature of the web. The World Health Organization (WHO) has proposed the creation of a separate hosting site for medical literature that has been validated and peer reviewed. As of this writing, such a concept has been held over by the Internet Corporation for Assigned Names and Numbers as premature. Only time will tell if the decision not to create a distinct hosting site (".health") will have a detrimental effect on the ability of physicians to provide good care and the right of patients to stay free from medical charlatans. "Snake oil" is available for sale on several web sites.

However, even more web sites provide quick access to medical literature. All of the major medical associations sponsor a web site, as do all of the major medical journals. Many of these sites restrict some of the access to their content to members only; other sites have free access. A number of search engines exist which allow individuals to search the Internet for web sites that address specific topics. Entering the words "pain" and "management" will turn up thousands of web sites, all with some content related to the management of pain.

The American Medical Association has a web site, *http://www.ama-assn.org*, which offers a number of functions. Physicians can search journals or learn more about ethical issues and public-health issues. Information about continuing medical education and educational opportunities also exists.

The APS has a web site, *http://www.ampainsoc.org*, which provides some content and also links to other sites. Pain management clinics can have their site listed there.

The web site of the JCAHO, *http://www.jcaho.org*, publishes the latest standards and also has a search function, links to complementary sites, and the ability to pose questions and receive answers from hospital surveyors.

There are a number of for-profit sites such as Pain.com, Paindoc.com, Painmed.com, and Painspecialist.com. These are all sites sponsored by particular institutions and, like all web sites that are designed as commercial endeavors, are accessible for the lay person. These sites seek to profit from those who access the site.

In contrast, Fibromyalgia.com is an information resource site for patients with "The Fibro Five," as defined by the site to be: fibromyalgia, interstitial cystitis, chronic fatigue, migraine headache, and irritable bowel. Such a site might provide a patient with valuable information.

The Internet provides a wonderful opportunity for the quick dissemination of information, albeit with the obvious pitfall that rumor and innuendo can be couched in respectability by appearing as printed speech. The savvy healthcare provider will ask the patient where such information was gleaned. It may be wise to search the sites and provide some reputable web sites for the interested patient.

Our hope is that this text will provide the interested physician, student, and healthcare provider with a starting point for future study. The book is arranged in the same successful format as the first edition, as a pathway from the basic science to the clinical diagnosis to the basic treatment strategies for the most common pain complaints. This edition pays close attention to the importance of providing resources for those interested in learning more, and each chapter ends with a "selected readings" section: our suggestions of where to look for further information. Each chapter stands on its own, so that *Manual of Pain Management* can serve as a rapid reference tool for the clinician who has little time between patients. *Manual of Pain Management* is designed to be the ideal reference guide for anesthesia residents who need to learn about pain management as a requirement of the residency. The first edition of the book was widely used in pain-management-fellowship training programs, and this edition should also be a good first text for those readers intent on further study

The new millennium brings many challenges to the healthcare provider. It is our hope that the information in this edition of *Manual of Pain Management* provides the support needed to successfully meet the challenge of providing good pain management care.

Carol A. Warfield, M.D.
Hilary J. Fausett, M.D.

Illustration Credits

The following figures are reproduced from *Hospital Practice* (Maclean Hunter Medical Communications Group, Inc.), with permission. Figures and illustrators' names (in parentheses) are followed by articles' authors and titles, and volume, issue, and page numbers:

2.1, 2.2, 2.3, 2.4 (Kevin Somerville): Dwarakanath GH, Warfield CA. The pathophysiology of acute pain; 21(4):64*g*, 64*h*, 64*l*.

7.1 (Nancy Lou Makris): Biber MP, Warfield CA. Headache; 19(10):41.

8.2 (Pauline Thomas): Vernick DM, Warfield CA. Diagnosis and treatment of otalgia; 22(3):171, 175.

9.2 (Pauline Thomas): Kohrman BD, Warfield CA. Eye pain; 22(12):35.

12.1 (Susan Tilberry): Gerhart T, Dohlman L, Warfield CA. Clinical diagnosis of shoulder pain; 20(9):136.

19.1, 19.2, 19.3, 19.4 (Nancy Lou Makris): Trnka Y, Warfield CA. Chronic abdominal pain; 19(3):202, 203, 207, 208.

21.2 (Pauline Thomas): Uppington J, Warfield CA. Pain in the perineum, groin and genitalia; 23(7):38.

25.2, 25.3 (Pauline Thomas): Kine GD, Warfield CA. Myofascial pain syndrome; 21(9):194c, 194g.

28.1 (Susan Tilberry): Stabile MJ, Warfield CA. The pain of peripheral vascular disease; 23(3):100.

31.1 (Nancy Lou Makris): Nuzzo J, Warfield CA. Thalamic pain syndrome; 20(8):32c.

33.1 (Susan Tilberry): Sandrock NJG, Warfield CA. Managing the pain of herpes; 21 (11A):86.

50.1, 50.3 (Susan Tilberry):Warfield CA. Facet synd and the relief of low back pain; 23(10A):41, 47.

51.1, 51.4 (Pauline Thomas): Warfield CA. Nerve blocks for pain management; 23(4):35, 40.

59.2 (Susan Tilberry): Dubuisson D, Warfield CA. Neurosurgical procedures for nonmalignant pain; 21(1):118.

59.4, 59.5, 59.6, 59.7 (Susan Tilberry): Dubuisson D, Warfield CA. Neurosurgery for the pain of malignancy; 23(6):43, 53, 54, 58.

PART I

Understanding Pain

CHAPTER 1

History of Pain Relief

David Cheng-chih Lai

Mankind has undoubtedly experienced pain since the beginning of time. From prehistoric bones to artifacts of ancient civilizations, evidence of pain and attempts at its relief has been found throughout history. Present-day agents and techniques have been modified from and improved upon those of the past.

Wine, the opium poppy, the coca plant, and the willow tree all have modern-day pharmaceutical counterparts. Further developments upon the needle and syringe, along with innovative regional anesthesia techniques, have allowed us to deliver those drugs in new and promising ways. The discovery of x-rays has led to their applications in the diagnosis and treatment of pain, as well as an adjunct to increasingly invasive pain-treatment procedures. Modern pain management, while moving forward, recognizes and embraces older therapies such as treating the psyche, distraction and relaxation techniques, biofeedback, acupuncture, physical therapy, and even electrical stimulation.

Early man attributed pain to demons, evil humors, and dead spirits. Accordingly, treatment of pain entailed discouraging their entrance into the body, blocking their entry, or once inside, drawing, transferring, or removing them from the body. Later, pain was felt to be a punishment from the gods. The word "pain" comes from the Latin *poena*, for punishment.

Finding the source of pain is an ongoing mystery that still challenges us today. Aristotle (384 to 322 B.C.) coined the term *sensorium commune* for this elusive seat of pain. Even by the 18th century, there still were two schools of thought on the location of pain perception: heart versus brain.

Ancient Egyptians had no knowledge of a nervous system. During the embalming process in preparation for the afterlife, the brain was the one organ destroyed or discarded. On the other hand, the heart was the most exalted organ, and in it rested the center of pain.

People of ancient India had knowledge of a nervous system, but it was mistakenly centered on the heart. Hindus believed the heart was the seat of all pain. Going away from a specific anatomical location, Buddhism in the fifth century B.C. linked pain to the frustration of desires.

Mesopotamia was the area between the Euphrates and Tigris rivers. This "Cradle of Civilization" designated the heart as the seat of intelligence, and still regarded pain as a punishment from the gods demanding sacrifice and prayer. Exploration of alternative treatments was hampered by the Code of Hammurabi: "If a surgeon has opened an eye infection with a bronze instrument and so saved the man's eye, he shall take ten shekels. If a surgeon has opened an eye infection with a bronze instrument and thereby destroyed the man's eye, they shall cut off his hand."

In ancient China, pain involved an imbalance between the Yin and the Yang. The heart was the most important organ, while the brain was simply the marrow of the skull. Acupuncture practice today still strives to adjust the balance of these energies in one's Chi.

The first great medical figure in ancient Greece was Alcmaeon (c. 500 B.C.), a disciple of Pythagoras (566 to 497 B.C.). Although he postulated the brain as the center of sensation, later Greek theory would not concur. Like the ancient Chinese, Hippocrates (c. 460 to 370 B.C.) felt pain was a manifestation of conditions disturbing the natural balance of the body. Both Democritus (460 to 362 B.C.) and Plato (427 to 347 B.C.) attributed pain to the intrusion of particles into the soul. Aristotle believed that the brain controlled the temperature of the heart, and that vital heat in the heart determined pain.

In ancient Alexandria, two men returned the seat of pain to the brain: Herophilus (315 to 280 B.C.) and later Erasistratus (310 to 250 B.C.). Unfortunately, their original work has not survived the ravages of time and only exists today in piecemeal accounts.

During the first century A.D. in Rome, Celsus made his famous observations on the classic signs of inflammation (tumor, rubor, and calor) and their relationship to dolor (pain). Galen (A.D. 130 to 200) postulated that the brain was the center of sensation and pain. William Harvey, who discovered the circulation of blood in 1628, still believed that the heart was the seat of pain. His contemporary, Descartes, postulated that the brain was the center of sensation. This concept of the pain pathway with delicate threads was posthumously published in 1664, and resurfaced over 300 years later in Melzack and Wall's famous 1965 article in *Science*.

The opium poppy (*Papaver somniferum*) is the source of morphine. In Sumerian texts from 4,000 B.C., it was known as hul gil, the plant of joy. Given the Christian belief that God is the source of pain on earth, it is only fitting that God provide an effective treatment when prayer alone does not suffice. Thomas Sydenham (1624 to 1689) wrote "Among the remedies which it has pleased Almighty God to give to man to relieve his sufferings, none is so universal and so efficacious as opium." Sir William Osler (1849 to 1919) felt morphine was "God's own medicine"; from this came the acronym "G.O.M." God also could provide the cure for morphine addiction. Early 20th century missionaries in China distributed antiopium pills that became known as "Jesus opium." Not surprisingly, their active ingredient was morphine.

Friedrich Wilhelm Adam Sertuerner (1783 to 1841) became an apothecary's assistant in 1803. Experimenting with crude opium, he discovered morphine in 1804. His findings first were announced in a journal letter (1805), then in a journal paper (1806), and finally in a later, definitive paper (1817). Opioids now were widely available as either the crude opium form, or as morphine, which E. Merck & Company of Darmstadt, Germany began commercially manufacturing in 1827.

Local anesthetics often are generically referred to as "Novocain," which is the proprietary name for procaine, discovered in 1904 by Alfred Einhorn (1856 to 1917). This was in response to the need for a less toxic agent than cocaine. Albert Niemann isolated the alkaloid in 1860 from erythroxylon coca, and Karl Koller first used it clinically in 1884.

In 1533 when Francesco Pizarro found the coca leaf being chewed in Peru, it had long been a part of Incan culture. In fact, its use probably predated the legend that the children of the sun had presented the Incas with the coca leaf to "satisfy the hungry, provide the weary and fainting with new vigor, and cause the unhappy to forget their miseries."

During Nazi-occupied Denmark during World War II, cocaine provided another type of escape. Trying to prevent Jews from escaping to Sweden, the Gestapo boarded ships with police dogs to hunt them down. On the behest of the anesthesiologist Dr. Trier Moerch, the Danes provided their sailors with handkerchiefs laced with cocaine powder and dried blood. The sailors carefully discharged the secret contents near the dogs. The dogs sniffed the mixture from the decks and, needless to say, never caught a single fugitive.

One of the recent advances in pain treatment has been the discovery of COX-2 (cyclooxygenase-2) inhibitors: celecoxib, rofecoxib, and parecoxib. Their pharmaceutical heritage derives from nonsteroidal antiinflammatory drugs (NSAIDs) and from acetylsalicylic acid (ASA), also known as aspirin. Besides being rediscovered as the all-purpose wonder drug, aspirin has made fortunes for Bayer, and has won John Vane a knighthood and the 1982 Nobel Prize in Medicine for his elucidation of its prostaglandin synthetase inhibitory properties.

The willow tree is perhaps the best known of the natural aspirin remedies; several other plants also contain salicin, the active compound. Ancient Egyptians used myrtle leaves (*Myrtus communis*), while Hippocrates favored white willow bark (*Salix alba*). Meadowsweet (*Filipendula ulmaria*), held sacred by the Druids, was mentioned by Chaucer in his *Canterbury Tales*. Closely related methyl salicylate is found in two additional plants: sweet birch (*Betula lenta*) and wintergreen (*Gaultheria procumbens*), commonly known as "oil of wintergreen" or "oil of Gaultheria".

Salicin compounds were effective, but hard on the stomach. Felix Hoffman, wishing to improve upon sodium salicylate, resurrected an old formula for acetylsalicylic acid, and the rest, as they say, is history. But how did the name "aspirin" come about?

The original source of the salicin used to make Bayer Aspirin (trademarked in Germany March 6, 1899) was the meadowsweet plant (*Filipendula ulmaria*). Its former botanical name, however, was *Spirea ulmaria*. The suffix "-in" was, and still is, a common ending for drugs (e.g., digoxin, heparin, and coumarin). Aspirin is short for acetyl (a), spirea (spir) and (in). Another Bayer acetyl product was diacetyl morphine, marketed as Heroin. Both of these trademarks were given up in 1919 at the Treaty of Versailles as part of Germany's war reparations, reducing them to generic drugs.

The first multidisciplinary pain clinic may have been at the temple of Aesculapius, the Greek god of medicine. Patients in pain came to sleep at the temple. During the night, Aesculapius, priests, and physicians effected a cure through magic potions (nepenthe), bandages, medical and physical procedures, as well as mystical and transcendental energies.

E. A. Rovenstine, in 1948 with E. M. Papper, wrote, "events in the changing medical world have made it imperative that we accept the challenge of pain occurring outside the surgical amphitheater. Such a concept fully justifies an anesthesia clinic on the therapy of pain." E. M. Papper later wrote, "attention to individuality by the romantic poets, essayists, and philosophers was crucial to preparing the way for change in clinical medicine designed to relieve pain and suffering and to prevent it where possible."

In 1944, the young anesthesiologist John Bonica (1917 to 1994) was assigned to oversee pain control at Madigan Army Hospital in Washington. Based on the success of an informal collaboration with an orthopedist, a neurosurgeon, and a psychiatrist, Bonica established a multidisciplinary pain clinic at Tacoma General Hospital in 1947. At the same time, William K. Livingston started his "Pain Project" at the University of Oregon. Bonica later brought his pain clinic to the University of Washington in 1960.

With the exception of the acquired immune deficiency syndrome (AIDS), there have been very few new diseases to plague modern man. We are living longer as a result of continual advances in medicine, surgery, and anesthesia. On the other hand, increasing life expectancies put us at increased risk for the development of chronic pain secondary to trauma, cancer, and old age itself. Although it is possible to treat 90% of postsurgical, posttrauma, and cancer pain, in reality less than 50% get relief worldwide. Of more concern, less than 10% of chronic, noncancer pain is relieved. This is the same figure that was *possible* 20 years ago. Today the potential relief rate of chronic, noncancer pain is 70% to 80%.

Severe chronic pain is a massive medical, economic, and societal problem. Cousins has called it a silent epidemic, the disease of the 21st century. We must continue to work to alleviate pain for the benefit of mankind.

POSTSCRIPT

Francis Rynd, who used a cannula and trocar in 1844 to introduce morphine for the treatment of trigeminal nerve pain, died in 1861 of an apparent heart attack. How amazed would he be to know the advances in pain treatment since then?

Symptoms of angina might prompt immediate administration of aspirin and morphine. If a course of surgical treatment with coronary artery bypass grafting were planned, preoperative benzodiazepines likely would be given. An opioid-based technique might help ensure a smooth surgical course. Alternatively, intrathecal opioids might be chosen to facilitate "fast-tracking." If immediate surgical revascularization was not favorable, then a thoracic epidural or a spinal-cord stimulator for refractory angina might be offered. One can only hope for advances of this magnitude for the future of pain relief.

SELECTED READINGS

Bergman NA. Early intravenous anesthesia: an eyewitness account. *Anesthesiology* 1990;72:185–186.

Bonica JJ. History of pain concepts and therapies. In: Bonica JJ, ed. *The Management of Pain*, 2nd ed. Malvern, PA: Lea & Febiger, 1990:2–17.

Caton D. "The poem in the pain" The social significance of pain in Western civilization. *Anesthesiology* 1994;81:1044–1052.

Caton D. The secularization of pain. *Anesthesiology* 1985;62:493–501.

Cousins MJ. Pain: the past, present, and future of anesthesiology? The E. A. Rovenstine Memorial Lecture. *Anesthesiology* 1999;91:538–551.

Dewick PM. *Medicinal Natural Products — A Biosynthetic Approach*. Chichester, England: John Wiley & Sons Ltd., 1997

Faulconer A Jr, Keys TE. *Foundations of Anesthesiology*. Park Ridge, IL: Wood Library–Museum of Anesthesiology, 1993.

Fink BR. History of neural blockade. In: Cousins MJ, Bridenbaugh P, eds. *Neural Blockade in Clinical Anesthesia and Management of Pain*, 2nd ed. Philadelphia: J. B. Lippincott Company, 1988:3–21.

Fink BR. Leaves and needles: the introduction of surgical local anesthesia. *Anesthesiology* 1985;63:77–83.

Papper EM. *Pain, suffering and anesthesia in the romantic era*. PhD thesis, University of Miami, 1990.

Raj PP. Historical aspects of regional anesthesia. In: Raj PP, ed. *Clinical Practice of Regional Anesthesia*. New York: Churchill Livingstone, 1991: 3–9.

Raj PP. History of pain management. In: Raj PP, ed. *Practical Management of Pain*. Chicago: Year Book Medical Publishers, Inc., 1986:3–13.

Todd EM. Pain: historical perspectives. In: Warfield C, ed. *Principles and Practice of Pain Management*. New York: McGraw–Hill, Inc., 1993:1–9.

Vandam LD, Fink BR. *The History of Anesthesiology, Volume 28, Pain: Perspectives & Trends*. Park Ridge, IL: Wood Library–Museum of Anesthesiology, 1998.

http://www.library.ucla.edu/libraries/biomed/his/PainExhibit/

CHAPTER 2

Pathophysiology of Pain

Praveen K. Suchdev

Pain is a common experience to all of us. Its complexities go well beyond the mere transmission of a signal from the periphery to the brain. Interplay from society, upbringing, culture, past experiences, and motivations all play a critical factor in the way pain is expressed to the outside world. Pain is as much an objective phenomenon as it is a subjective one — something that cannot be measured independent of the person experiencing it. In 1994, the International Association for the Study of Pain defined pain as an *"unpleasant sensory and emotional experience associated with actual or potential tissue damage or described in terms of such damage."* This definition, although very broad, ties together sensory and emotional factors, i.e., suffering; it talks about actual and potential tissue damage and makes it difficult to separate that which is observable from that which is not. Although this definition is very broad in its scope, it stands today as the benchmark definition attesting to the complexity of pain. J. D. Loeser in 1980 broke pain down into a more practical description, coming up with four dimensions of pain. The four dimensions included nociception, perception of pain, suffering, and pain behavior. Understanding all four of these components, not just nociception, allows providers to better manage and treat suffering from pain.

SOCIETAL IMPACT

Substantial portions of the working-age population in industrialized countries suffer from chronic pain. Cousins estimated that the healthcare costs of chronic pain exceeded the combined costs of coronary artery disease, cancer, and acquired immune deficiency syndrome (AIDS). Bonica, in 1987, estimated that 30% of the population of developed countries suffered from chronic pain. He estimated that 70 million Americans report chronic pain, of which, more than 50 million are totally disabled from a few days to weeks or months. Tollison nicely summarized the impact of chronic pain on society.

Chronic low-back pain impacts 31 million Americans with over 8 million office visits per year and 89 million workdays lost per year. Six percent of all Americans will suffer a back injury during their lives that will disable them for 6 months or more, as low-back pain is the second leading cause of physician office visits and is the third leading cause of hospital admissions. Seventy percent to 80% of the population suffers from headaches at least once per month, causing over 157 million workdays to be lost. Arthritis afflicts 20 to 50 million Americans. There are over 600,000 newly diagnosed cases each year, and over 108 million workdays lost each year as a result of arthritis. Chronic pain really is the hidden epidemic.

NOCICEPTION

Nociception is purely about the biochemical and neural changes that occur in response to a noxious stimuli. This response is relatively consistent from one individual to the next even though the entire process of "pain" is unique to the person experiencing it. The process of nociception can be divided into the following four separate processes: transduction, transmission, modulation, and perception. Perception, the fourth process, has a tremendous influence on modulation of pain.

Transduction

Transduction is the conversion of tissue injury and a biochemical response to a neural response. Tissue damage caused by any form of injury or inflammation releases local pain-producing substances or algesic substances into the local milieu of the extracellular fluid surrounding the injury. The sources of these substances are quite variable, but they include K+, H+ prostaglandins and other inflammatory mediators of the arachidonic cascade. Histamines are released from mast cells, platelets, and basophils, and serotonin is released from mast cells and platelets. Other substances such as leukotrienes, bradykinins, substance P, and slow-reacting substance of anaphylaxis (SRS-A) also can be released with tissue damage. Many of these substances are products of the arachidonic acid cascade, which are formed via enzymatic conversion by cyclooxygenase and lipoxygenase. Cyclooxygenase can be inhibited by agents such as aspirin, indomethacin, ibuprofen, and most recently, more highly selective cyclooxygenase inhibitors such as celecoxib and rofecoxib. Substance P, which has been the focus of intense research over the past decade, is released from the unmyelinated nociceptive nerve terminals themselves. Substance P is produced in the cell bodies of the spinal and gasserian ganglia with four times as much substance P released into the peripheral nervous system as into the central nervous system. Both somatic and visceral nervous systems possess stores of substance P. Although the role of substance P is pain is still being defined, substance P, a vasodilator, is believed to cause local microdilation and changes in vascular permeability along with recruitment of other local nociceptor fibers. Thus, it is believed that substance P may cause local tissue edema and lower the threshold of surrounding nociceptive fibers increasing both the field of local response and the intensity. Considerable amount of focus on depletion of substance P has been made. In fact, capsaicin, the active ingredient in chili peppers is believed to deplete substance P from peripheral nerve terminals when applied locally.

Although the exact method in which these substances convert injury into a painful impulse is not known, it most likely represents a multifactorial response, involving both direct and indirect mediation. Local chemicals such as bradykinins, and K+ may directly activate the nociceptive fibers. Chemicals such as prostaglandins may indirectly sensitize the nervous system to physical and chemical stimulation and algesic chemicals such as substance P, which cause local microedema and recruitment of other nociceptive fibers.

Transmission

Nociceptors

Injury and inflammation activate distinct peripheral nerves that process and transmit painful stimulation to the central nervous system. These nerves are called nociceptors. Two types of nociceptors (C fibers and A-δ fibers), along with subcategories of each, are present as free nerve endings in the periphery and viscera. C fibers are unmyelinated fibers that are activated by chemical, thermal, mechanical, and cold noxious stimulation. A-δ fibers, which are myelinated fibers, transmit at rates of 10 to 25 times the speed of C fibers, and are activated by both mechanical and thermal noxious stimulation. They have subcategories with different threshold levels. Somatic structures, such as the skin, and deep structures, such as muscles and joints, are rich with both C and A-δ fibers. Visceral structures are rich in C fibers, along with some A-δ fibers. A-δ fibers can transmit noxious stimuli to the central nervous system at faster rates, defining precise location of injury. These fibers may allow the organism to remove itself or the effected area from the source of injury in a timely fashion to prevent further damage. C fibers, transmitting at a significantly slower rate, rich in the visceral nervous system, and not so clearly defined in the somatic system, may allow for continued transmission of pain, ill-defined, to continue for a time after injury, thus possibly causing the organism to seek shelter (or treatment, in the case of humans) after the injury to help promote healing (Table 1).

Sensitization

Unlike other fibers that transmit sensory information such as touch and proprioception, nociceptors are unusual in that repeated stimulation results in enhanced sensitivity, lowered threshold, and longer response, versus fatigue and higher threshold levels for other fibers. Both peripheral and central sensitization has been demonstrated. Peripheral sensitization can occur with the release of local algesic substances such as substance P and the direct lowering of thresholds of nociceptors by repeated pain stimuli. The central nervous system, and more specifically, the dorsal horn, has been shown to undergo changes in its morphological makeup with repeated noxious stimuli. This "rewiring" that takes place most recently has been coined as the term, *neuroplasticity*. Neuroplastic changes that take place to repeated painful stimuli also contribute to the sensitization process. If fact, much research has been focused on these

TABLE 2.1. *Characteristics of Nerve Fibers*

Type	Function	Diameter (μm)	Conduction velocity (m/sec)
C	Pain, mechanical stimuli	1	0.2–1.5
B	Preganglionic, autonomic	1	3–14
A-δ	Pain, mechanical, and thermal stimulation	1	5–15
A-γ	Touch, muscle tone	4	15–40
A-β	Touch, proprioception	8	40–70
A-α	Motor	13	70–120

neuroplastic changes and in methods to prevent these changes from occurring. Use of neuraxial anesthesia such as epidurals or spinals prior to surgery or amputations have been shown to preempt these changes, thus preventing sensitization. Hyperalgesia, allodynia, and spontaneous pain along with an increased field of pain may characterize sensitization.

Central Nervous System

Dorsal Horn

Afferent neurons of the spinal nerves, and cranial nerves transmit both sensory and nociceptive stimulation via the dorsal-root ganglia to the dorsal horn of the spinal cord. The dorsal horn was once thought of as a simple connection between first- and second-order neurons, and as a relay station. Large amounts of research and focus over the past two to three decades have revealed complex circuitry, along with multiple synaptic and biochemical interactions resulting not only in a simple relay but in considerable amounts of signal processing, summation, and selection. Signals from the periphery converge at the dorsal horn and are acted upon by inhibitory and excitatory influences from local interneurons, higher central nervous system structures, and from local biochemistry prior to the transmission to higher spinal cord and brain levels. The dorsal horn anatomically has been divided into laminae, with lamina I being the most lateral and superficial of the layers. A-δ fibers and C fibers converge to form the second-order synapses largely in laminae I, Iii, Iio (substantia

gelatinosa), and V. These neurons also are somatotypically arranged in lamina I. Larger, more heavily myelinated A fibers that transmit light touch, proprioception, and muscle tone, synapse to a large degree in laminae Iii, III, IV, and V. Lamina V also appears to have a high concentration of wide-dynamic neurons (WDNs). WDNs appear to receive input from both nociceptive and non-nociceptive sensory fibers, and inputs from visceral and somatic structures. Because WDNs receive input from both visceral and somatic structures, it is believed that the possibility of referred visceral pain may be influenced from these neurons. Other important phenomena such as override stimulation (i.e., rubbing an injured area to help alleviate pain) may be influenced through WDNs. Multiple interneurons such as stalk cells, thought to be excitatory, are largely located in lamina IIo, and islet cells, thought to be inhibitory, are located in lamina Iii. Multiple neurotransmitters have been localized in the dorsal horn, such as the excitatory transmitters glutamate and aspartate, and others such as somatostatin, cholecystokinin, vasoactive intestinal polypeptide, and substance P (Figs. 2.1 and 2.2).

Gate Control Theory

In the 1960s, Melzack and Wall developed the gate-control theory of pain. Their hypothesis stipulated that both non-nociceptive transmission via large myelinated fibers and nociceptive fibers via A-δ and C fibers entered the dorsal horn and the substantia gelatinosa and then the dorsal column and T cells that mediated transfer of signal to the

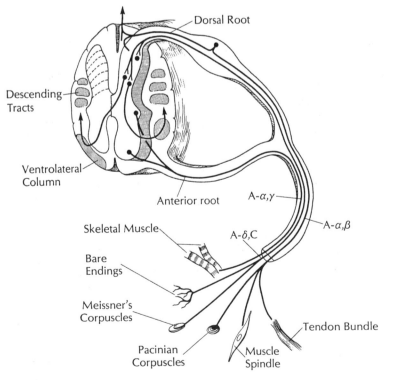

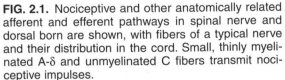

FIG. 2.1. Nociceptive and other anatomically related afferent and efferent pathways in spinal nerve and dorsal born are shown, with fibers of a typical nerve and their distribution in the cord. Small, thinly myelinated A-δ and unmyelinated C fibers transmit nociceptive impulses.

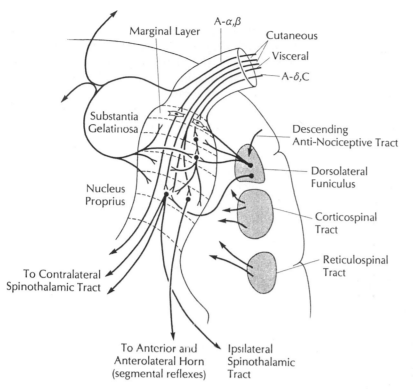

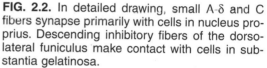

FIG. 2.2. In detailed drawing, small A-δ and C fibers synapse primarily with cells in nucleus proprius. Descending inhibitory fibers of the dorsolateral funiculus make contact with cells in substantia gelatinosa.

brain. According to the gate-control theory, the transfer of information to the T cells and subsequently the brain is influenced by the relative amount of activity of large-diameter somatosensory fibers and small-diameter nociceptive fibers. If the activity of the larger fibers were greater than the transmission of pain, impulses would be inhibited and the gate closed. If the influences from pain fibers were greater than those of other sensory fibers, the pain signal would be allowed to propagate to higher central nervous system structures. Descending influences from the brain that play a role in the ease at which the gate would be opened or closed also influences the T cells (Fig. 2.3).

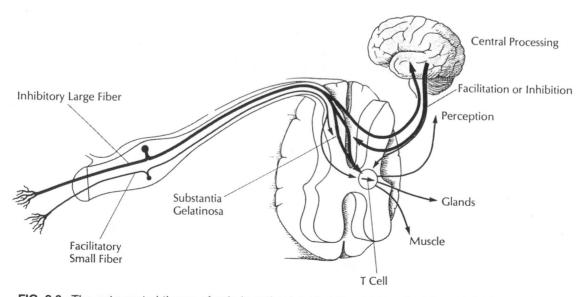

FIG. 2.3. The gate-control theory of pain hypothesizes that impulses evoked by peripheral stimulation are transmitted to cells in the substantia gelatinosa, the dorsal column fibers that project toward the brain, and the spinal column T cells that mediate transfer of information to the brain. Opening and closing of the gate in dorsal born is determined by the relative amount of activity in small- and large-diameter fibers. Spinal-gating mechanism also is influenced by neural impulses from the brain.

Ascending Pain Transmission

After modulation and interneuron influence, second-order neurons pass to the anterior and anterolateral aspect of the contralateral side of the spinal cord. The predominant spinal-pain tracts are made up of the spinothalamic tract, the spinoreticular tract, and the spinomesencephalic tract. The ascending spinal-pain tracts can further be divided into two distinct tracts, the first one being the neospinothalamic (new) tract, which is composed of the lateral aspect of the spinothalamic tract. The second is the paleospinothalamic (old) tract, which is composed of the medial aspects of the spinothalamic tract, the spinoreticular tract, and the spinomesencephalic tract. Pain transmission from the head and neck has similar anatomic and physiologic distribution via the trigeminal nerve, forming

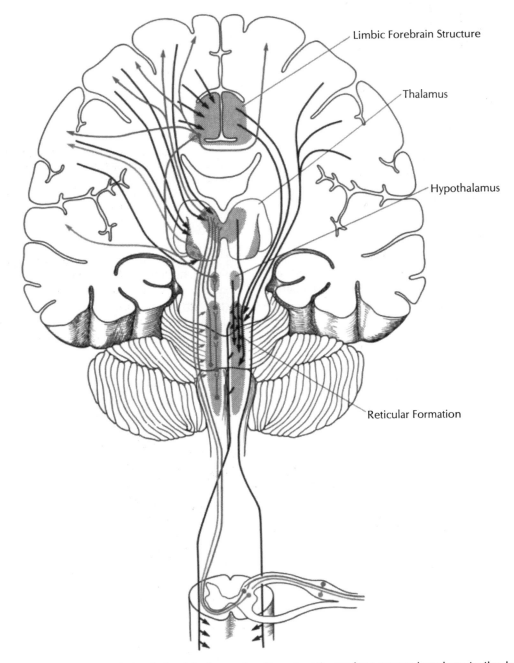

Limbic Forebrain Structure

Thalamus

Hypothalamus

Reticular Formation

FIG. 2.4. Lateral spinothalamic tract is the main afferent pathway for sensory impulses to the brain. Anatomically and physiologically, it is divided into neospinothalamic and paleospinothalamic pathways. Descending pathways from cerebral cortex through dorsolateral funiculus make connections at different levels of the spinal cord.

the neotrigeminothalamic tract and the paleotrigemino-thalamic tract. The neospinothalamic tract is composed of large myelinated fibers that propagate toward the brain to form a third-order synapse within the ventral, posterior, and lateral aspects of the thalamus. From there, tracts extend third-order neurons to the somatosensory cortex distributed anatomically in a somatotopical manner. The neospinothalamic tract makes very few synapses along the way and is much larger in humans than in other species. The paleospinothalamic tract is composed of both long and short fibers and is not as richly myelinated as the neospinothalamic tract. This tract makes various synapses along the way to deep-brain structures, such as the periaqueductal gray, hypothalamus, and to the medial aspect of the thalamus. From there, further projection may be made in a diffuse manner to the limbic system and frontal cortex.

The anatomy of the neospinothalamic tract, with very few synapses and quick transmission to the somatosensory cortex, may imply that this tract transmits information about the injury, location, and severity so that action can be taken to remove the organism from the source. The paleospinothalamic tract has a relatively slow transmission time, makes multiple synapses, and projects to deep-brain structures that influence emotions and memory. This tract may play a role in increasing the level of arousal; either to prevent such injuries from occurring in the future or promoting behavior to protect the injured area so that healing can take place (Fig. 2.4).

Descending Pathways

Considerable research has focused on descending pathways both for the understanding of the pathophysiology of pain and for the development of new treatment modalities. Descending systems pass to areas of the spinal cord via the dorsolateral funiculus to synapse at laminae I, IIo, and V, and are inhibitory using serotonergic and possibly norepinephrine neurotransmitters. The activity of antidepressants, mainly tricyclic antidepressants, has been presumed to influence these descending pathways, enhancing modulation by these pathways. Input also occurs into the descending system from higher brain structures such as cortical and diencephalic systems, the medulla, periaquaductal gray, and periventricular gray area.

Perception of Pain, Suffering, and Pain Behavior

Pain is more than just transmission of a signal from the periphery to the cerebral cortex. It is a multidimensional process involving past experiences, emotions, cultural background, motivations, and family and societal dynamics. We know that the hypothalamus, the medial thalamus, and limbic system are involved in motivational and emo-tional experiences, and readily synapse with the paleospinothalamic tract. These systems also influence other brain structures such as the hypothalamus and forebrain, which may activate autonomic reflexes that influence features such as respiratory rate and blood pressure. Influences from the reticular formation create the drive to move the injured organism into action away from the noxious stimuli. Emotional and motivational states also have a great influence via the limbic, hypothalamic, and frontal cortex on descending inhibitory systems, which allow higher brain function to influence pain processing via these pathways.

ACUTE AND CHRONIC PAIN

Acute pain is one of the basic adaptations that most species have to warn the organism of internal or external stimuli potentially harmful to the well-being of that organism. It usually increases as the severity of the injury or disease increases, although the painful sensation may be present after the injury. Continued noxious stimulation also can lead to increased sensitivity, sensitization, and severe pain even to a weak, painful stimuli. Acute pain promotes healing by telling the organism to seek shelter, and in the case of humans, seek medical care. The sensitization process can take place in both the peripheral as well as the central nervous system. As the healing process takes place, acute pain tends to subside.

Chronic pain exists when pain symptoms are prolonged past the natural course of the disease process or a disease process is protracted over the course of many months to years. In most instances, chronic pain serves no vital importance to the organism suffering from it, and in fact can become a detriment to the organism survival and well-being. Multiple physiological theories exist as to why this state develops. These theories include sensitization both in the periphery and central nervous system; spontaneous activity and discharges in axons subject to injury; demyelination resulting from chronic irritation and development of interactions between bare neurons; and balances between the lateral and the medial thalamus and the influences of deep-brain structures such as reticular formation, which influences emotional states of people in stress. Emotional, social, financial, cultural, and motivational states immensely influence those who suffer from chronic pain. The toll of chronic pain on the mental states of sufferers makes treatment of chronic pain patients difficult, at best. Treatment requires immense determination by both the patient and the providers. Treatment plans frequently require input from multiple specialties, such as physical medicine, rehabilitation, and psychiatry, along with medical and surgical support teams. Only when providers from these multiple teams work in unison does the likelihood of success increase.

SELECTED READINGS

Bonica JJ. Importance of the problem. In: Anderson S, Bond M, Mehta M, et al., eds. *Chronic Non-cancer*. Lanchaster, UK: MTP Press Limited, 1987:13.

Cousins MJ. Forward: back pain in the workplace. In: *Management of Disability in Nonspecific Conditions*. Seattle: IASP Press, 1995:ix.

Fordyce WE. The problem: back pain in the workplace. In: *Management of Disability in Nonspecific Conditions*. Seattle: IASP Press, 1995:5–9.

Loeser JD. Perspectives on pain. In: Turner P, ed. *Proceeding of First World Conference on Clinical Pharmacology and Therapeutics*. London: Macmillan, 1980:316–326.

Raj PP. Pain mechanisms. In: *Pain Medicine*. St. Louis: Mosby–Year Book, 1996:12–25.

Tollison CD. Pain and its magnitude. In: *Pain In Perspective*. CRC Press, 1998:3–25.

CHAPTER 3

Endogenous Opioids

Danielle S. Stranc

Since the initial description, the concept of endogenous opiates has stimulated the interest of the layperson and the scientist alike. *Endorphins* are released by the body as a defense against pain or during physical exercise, deep relaxation, sexual activity, crying, and laughing.

The term endorphin is used to characterize a group of endogenous peptides whose pharmacologic action mimics that of opium and its analogs. The endogenous opioid system is complex with a multiplicity of functions. There exist about two dozen known endogenous opioids that belong to one of three endogenous opioid systems: (a) the endorphin system, (b) the enkephalins, and (c) the dynorphin system.

The pituitary gland and hypothalamus of vertebrates produce endorphins. They lower the perception of pain by reducing the transmission of signals between nerve cells. Endogenous opiates are released as part of the general response to stress, so that low levels of stimulation are pleasant while high levels may be numbing. The endogenous opiates released by inescapable stress lead to analgesia. Such stress, however, also may contribute to depression, and learned helplessness.

Endorphins not only regulate pain, but they also modulate the hunger response and are involved in the release of sex hormones from the pituitary gland. Opiates act in a similar way to endorphins but are not rapidly degraded by the body, as natural endorphins are, and thus have a long-lasting effect on pain perception and mood. Endorphin release is also stimulated by exercise.

ENDOGENOUS OPIATE PEPTIDES

The endogenous opioids are peptides. A peptide is a biologically active substance composed of amino acids that are produced in neurons. The opioid peptides are considered to be a distinct and separate group of psychoactive substances in the brain.

Three types of endogenous opioid peptides have been identified, including the β-*endorphins*, the enkephalins (*met- and leu-enkephalin*), and the dynorphins (*dynorphin and α-neoendorphin*) (Table 3.1).

These endorphins are formed from larger proendorphin peptides:

- Proopio-melanocortin (POMC): β-endorphin precursor
- Proenkephalin A: met- and leu-enkephalin precursor
- Proenkephalin B (Prodynorphin): dynorphin and α-neoendorphin precursor

The POMC gene is expressed in the anterior and intermediate lobes of the pituitary gland. The POMC gene gives rise to both the adrenocorticotrophic hormone (ACTH), which plays an important role in mediating the body's corticosteroid stress response, and the endorphin precursors.

All proendorphins are synthesized in the nucleus and transported to the nerve terminal by microtubule transport. At the nerve terminal, they are cleaved by specific proteases. These proteases recognize the double basic

TABLE 3.1. *The Most Prevalent Opioid Receptor Types and Their Common Agonists and Antagonists*

Receptor Type	Endogenous Ligand	Agonist	Antagonist
μ	enkephalins β-endorphin	morphine sufentanil DAGO DAMGO	naloxone naltrexone β-FNA
δ	enkephalins β-endorphins	DADLE DSLET DPDPE	ICI 174864 naltrindole
κ	dynorphins	EKC bremazocine trifluadom	nor-BNI

DAGO, Tyr-Ala-Gly-Mephe-NH(CH$_2$)$_2$-OH (also DAMGO); DADLE, d-Ala2-dLeu5-enkephalin; DSLET, Tyr-d-Ser-Gly-Phe-Leu-Thr; DPDPE, d-Pen2-d-Pen5-enkephalin; EKC, [3 H]-ethylketocyclazocine; nor-BNI, nor-binaltorphimine. β-FNA is an affinity label.

13

TABLE 3.2. *Clinical Effects of Opiate Ligands Mediated via Receptor Subtypes*

Property	Receptor subtype		
	μ/δ	κ	σ
Analgesia	supraspinal/spinal	spinal	none
Behavioral effects	euphoria	dysphoria	dysphoria++
Physical dependence	++	+	none
Respiratory depression	++	+	none
Effect on pupil	constriction	none	dilation
Gastrointestinal motility	reduced	none	none
Smooth muscle spasm	++	none	none

++, strong effect; +, some effect.

amino-acid sequences positioned just before and after the opioid peptide. The peptides are released when the nerve fires and bind to postsynaptic receptors, stimulating second messenger systems. The action of opioid peptides is terminated by membrane-bound proteases, which cleave the terminal Gly-3-Tyr-4 bonds.

ENDOGENOUS OPIATE RECEPTORS

Analgesic activity is mediated by opiate receptors in the central nervous system (CNS). Five major categories of opioid receptors have been identified and cloned. There are known as: *mu* (μ), *kappa* (κ), *sigma* (σ), *delta* (δ), and *epsilon* (ε).

The opiate medications used clinically occupy the same receptors as endogenous opioid peptides—enkephalins or endorphins—which are described in more detail below. Both the endogenous agonist and the opiate analgesics may alter the central release of specific neurotransmitters from afferent nerves sensitive to noxious stimuli.

The actions of the opiate analgesics commercially available can be defined by their activity at three of the specific opiate receptor types: mu (μ), kappa (κ), and delta (δ). The opiate analgesics are classified pharmacologically in reference to their specific activity at the opioid receptor. As explained in detail in Chapter 45, the opiate analgesics are classified as agonists, mixed agonist–antagonists, or partial agonists.

The μ receptors are of primary interest to clinicians, as they mediate the analgesic effects of the opioids. Activation of the μ receptor may also produce euphoria, respiratory and physical depression, miosis, and reduced gastrointestinal motility (see Table 3.2). These receptors have been further subtyped as μ-1, which mediate analgesia and are located in the supraspinal regions of the CNS; and μ-2, which mediate respiratory depression.

Both enkephalins and endorphins are endogenous ligands for these receptors, and morphine is the classic exogenous ligand. The μ-1 receptor is morphine-selective.

The δ receptors mediate both spinal and supraspinal analgesia and also appear to be responsible for the dysphoria and psychotomimetic effects (e.g., hallucinations) of many of the commercially available opiate medications. Enkephalins are the endogenous ligand for these

receptors, and morphine is an exogenous ligand. These receptors have been subtyped as δ-1 and δ-2; however, this scientific distinction appears to be relatively unimportant in terms of analgesia.

The κ receptors mediate pentazocinelike analgesia at the spinal level. In addition, the prominent sedating effect of the opiates is a κ-mediated effect, as is respiratory depression and dysphoria.

Dynorphins are endogenous ligands at these receptors and morphine functions as an exogenous ligand. These receptors have been further subtyped as κ-1, which mediates spinal analgesia; κ-3, which mediates supraspinal analgesia; and κ-2, whose function is unknown. These receptors are proposed to mediate a sedating analgesia with reduced addiction liability. There is a great deal of interest in creating medications that mimic the effects of the dynorphins.

The σ sites have been implicated in psychomimetic and dysphoric side-effects of the opiates. Dilation of the pupil may possibly be a σ-mediated effect.

CONCLUSION

The clinical effects of the opioids are widespread. There is scientific interest in the interaction between the opioid agonists and the immune system. Any alteration in immune function could have profound implications for patients with cancer or infected with the human immunodeficiency virus (HIV) There is also interest in whether opioid peptides may have a cardioprotective effect and the ability to limit the extent of cellular damage caused by ischemia. Certainly, the synthesis of clinically useful specific opioid agonists will have many uses.

SELECTED READINGS

Drolet G, Dumont EC, Gosselin I, et al. Role of endogenous opioid system in the regulation of the stress response. *Prog Neuropsychopharmacol Biol Psychiatry* 2001;25:729–741.

Horvath G. Endomorphin-1 and endomorphin-2: pharmacology of the selective endogenous mu-opioid receptor agonists. *Pharmacol Ther* 2000; 88:437–463.

LaForge KS, Yuferov V, Kreek MJ. Opioid receptor and peptide gene polymorphisms: potential implications for addictions. *Eur J Pharmacol* 2000;410:249–268.

Stefano GB, Goumon Y, Casares F, et al. Endogenous morphine. *Trends Neurosci* 2000;23:436–442.

Vaccarino AL, Kastin AJ. Endogenous opiates: 1999. *Peptides* 2000;21: 1975–2034.

CHAPTER 4

Neurotransmitters

Andrew M. Strassman

The body possesses a sensory system that is specialized for the detection of intense, potentially tissue-damaging stimuli (nociception). This system is responsible for evoking the perception of pain as well as the somatic, autonomic, and endocrine responses that often accompany pain. The neural system for pain may be divided into (a) the peripheral sensory apparatus for detecting noxious stimuli and transmitting this information to the central nervous system; (b) the multisynaptic central ascending pathways that subserve the reflexive, behavioral, and perceptual responses evoked by such stimuli; and (c) the central neural systems responsible for pain modulation, both excitatory and inhibitory. The nociceptive system also can be strongly modulated by the sensory systems that detect non-noxious thermal and mechanical stimuli. As a result of the multiple modulatory influences exerted on the system, as well as the sustained alterations in intrinsic neuronal properties that can be induced by injurious stimuli, the relationship between stimulus intensity and pain is highly variable. This chapter will give an overview of the current state of knowledge of the neurotransmitters involved in the transmission and modulation of nociceptive information. The focus will be on mechanisms at the level of the spinal–dorsal horn, which has received the most study. More detailed reviews with extensive references to the primary literature can be found in the suggested readings.

ANATOMICAL ORGANIZATION OF THE DORSAL HORN

Primary afferent nociceptors have small to medium-sized cell bodies located in the dorsal root and trigeminal (Gasserian) ganglia and mostly possess small, myelinated (A-δ fiber) or unmyelinated (C fiber) axons. The main central termination site of primary afferent nociceptors is the spinal–dorsal horn and its trigeminal equivalent, the trigeminal subnucleus caudalis (medullary–dorsal horn).

Nociceptive primary afferents terminate most heavily in the superficial part of the dorsal horn, laminae I and II (marginal zone and substantia gelatinosa, respectively), as well as in lamina V. Additional terminals also are found in lamina X, the area around the central canal.

Central terminals of small-diameter, primary afferents in the dorsal horn form synaptic contacts on the cell bodies and dendrites of projection neurons whose axons ascend to specific regions of the brainstem and thalamus, as well as on local interneurons whose axons remain within the dorsal horn. Dorsal-horn interneurons form synaptic contacts on the cell bodies and dendrites of other dorsal-horn neurons, as well as on the axonal terminals of primary afferent neurons. Nociceptive projection neurons are most heavily concentrated in laminae I and V, while lamina II contains primarily local interneurons. In addition to the axonal projections from primary afferents and local interneurons, dorsal-horn neurons also receive descending axonal projections from brainstem regions such as the nucleus raphe magnus that exert modulatory influences on nociceptive transmission. These brainstem projections descend in part via the dorsolateral funiculus of the spinal cord and terminate heavily in laminae I, II, and V.

PRIMARY AFFERENT TRANSMITTERS/MODULATORS

Stimulation of small-diameter, primary afferent fibers evokes excitatory postsynaptic potentials (EPSPs) in dorsal-horn neurons that exhibit two kinetically and pharmacologically distinct components: a fast, brief excitation resulting from release of glutamate, and a slower, more prolonged excitation resulting from the release of the neuropeptide substance P. Glutamate and substance P are colocalized in many small-diameter, primary afferents and are thought to be coreleased from their central terminals. The postsynaptic actions of glutamate are mediated by two classes of receptors: ionotropic, which are directly coupled to membrane ion channels, and metabotropic, which exert their effects by coupling via G proteins to intracellular second messenger systems. The fast excitation evoked by glutamate in dorsal-horn neurons is mediated by ionotropic receptors, of which there are three subtypes: NMDA (*N*-methyl-D-aspartate), kainate, and AMPA. The ionotropic glutamate receptors all act by opening a Na^+/Ca^{++} cation channel, although the NMDA receptor has a relatively greater permeability to Ca^{++}, which is important in the phenomenon of NMDA-mediated central sensitization (see NMDA Receptors and Central Sensitization, below). The slower excitation produced by substance P and the related peptide neurokinin A is mediated by the neurokinin receptors NK1 and NK2, and results from a decrease in K^+ conductance. It is thought that the excitation produced by a brief, acute noxious stimulus is mediated primarily by the non-NMDA (kainate and AMPA) ionotropic glutamate receptors, whereas activation of NMDA and neurokinin receptors occurs with more prolonged noxious stimuli.

A number of other neuropeptides are contained in small-diameter, primary afferent neurons, including calcitonin gene-related peptide (CGRP), somatostatin, vasoactive intestinal polypeptide (VIP), cholecystokinin, galanin, and dynorphin. More than one peptide may be present in the same cell. For example, most substance P-containing cells also colocalize CGRP, and CGRP appears to enhance the effects of substance P. The peptide content of primary afferents can be altered following inflammation or nerve injury, and such changes may contribute to hyperalgesia and chronic pain conditions. For example, substance P, which normally is expressed primarily in small-diameter, primary afferent neurons, shows increased levels of expression in large-diameter, presumably non-nociceptive, primary afferent neurons following inflammation, which may contribute to exaggerated neuronal and behavioral responses to tactile stimuli.

Depolarization can evoke the release of neuropeptides from the peripheral as well as the central terminals of small-diameter, primary afferent neurons. The release of neuropeptides from peripheral nerve endings can evoke inflammatory changes in the innervated tissue, including vasodilation and plasma extravasation, which are collectively referred to as neurogenic inflammation. The role of neurogenic inflammation in clinical pain states is uncertain, although it has been hypothesized to contribute to the pathogenesis of conditions such as arthritis and migraine.

NMDA RECEPTORS AND CENTRAL SENSITIZATION

At resting membrane potentials, ion flow through the NMDA receptor/ion channel is blocked by Mg^{++} ions. This Mg^{++} block is voltage-dependent and is removed by depolarization. Thus, glutamate binding to the receptors produces no ion flow unless the cell is already depolarized, such as by co-release of substance P. Once the cell has been depolarized, opening of the channel results in influx of both Na^{++} and Ca^{++}, which produces further depolarization, and in turn causes further Ca^{++} inflow due to opening of voltage-dependent Ca^{++} channels. The resulting elevation in intracellular Ca^{++} results in activation of protein kinase C and phosphorylation of the NMDA receptor. Phosphorylation of the receptor partially removes the Mg^{++} block, so that glutamate binding produces ion flow even at resting membrane potentials. The phosphorylation-induced increase in glutamate sensitivity results in an increased state of neuronal excitability, such that previously subthreshold inputs are capable of generating action potentials. This increased excitability in central neurons is termed central sensitization and is thought to contribute to hyperalgesia.

TRANSMITTERS IN DORSAL HORN NEURONS

Whereas the direct actions of primary afferents on dorsal-horn neurons are primarily excitatory, dorsal-horn interneurons may be either excitatory or inhibitory in the effects they exert on their target neurons within the dorsal horn. As a result, primary afferent stimulation typically evokes a mixture of excitatory and inhibitory effects on dorsal-horn neurons. In addition to their direct postsynaptic effects on dorsal-horn neurons, interneurons also can influence sensory transmission by exerting "presynaptic" modulatory effects on the release of transmitter from primary afferent terminals.

The most abundant inhibitory transmitter in dorsal-horn interneurons is GABA (γ-amino-butyric acid), which is present in roughly 30% of neurons in the superficial dorsal horn. About half of the GABA-containing cells also contain the inhibitory transmitter glycine. Both GABA, through an action at the $GABA_A$ receptor, and glycine produce inhibition by opening of chloride channels. Acetylcholine, which also exerts inhibitory actions, is present in a subset of the GABAergic neurons that do not contain glycine. Antagonism of spinal glycine, GABA, or cholinergic receptors by intrathecal administration of strychnine, bicuculline, or atropine, respectively, can produce hypersensitivity and aversive behavioral responses to non-noxious, mechanical stimuli. Strychnine and bicuculline also reduce the myelinated afferent-induced inhibition of nociceptive dorsal-horn neurons. From these observations, it appears that myelinated afferents activate GABA- and glycinergic-inhibitory interneurons, which in turn attenuate the responses of nociceptive projection neurons to non-noxious stimulation.

The opioid-peptide enkephalin also is present in a subset of dorsal-horn interneurons. Enkephalin has a hyperpolarizing (inhibitory) effect on dorsal-horn neurons mediated by μ-opiate receptors. μ Agonists produce a selective inhibition of nociceptive responses. δ-Opiate receptors also are present in the dorsal horn but are located predominantly on axons, where they are thought to mediate presynaptic inhibition. A separate subset of dorsal-horn neurons contains dynorphin, the endogenous ligand for the κ-opiate receptor. The number of dynorphin-containing neurons in the dorsal horn is greatly increased following peripheral inflammation or nerve injury, although the role this may play in the development of hyperalgesia is uncertain.

The majority of neurons in the dorsal horn do not contain inhibitory transmitters or peptides and are thought to be excitatory. Glutamate is thought to be the primary excitatory transmitter of both interneurons and projection neurons in the dorsal horn. In addition, a number of peptides have been found in a small percentage of projection neurons (spinothalamic, spinomesencephalic, or spinobulbar), including cholecystokinin, somatostatin, substance P, VIP, and dynorphin.

TRANSMITTERS IN DESCENDING PROJECTIONS FROM BRAINSTEM

Brainstem neurons that contain the biogenic amines serotonin (5-HT) and noradrenaline (NA) give rise to major descending projections to the spinal–dorsal horn. Activation of these descending projections by electrical stimulation or morphine microinjection strongly inhibits spinal nociceptive transmission. Descending 5-HT projections originate entirely from a subset of neurons in the nucleus raphe magnus, which is located in the rostral ventromedial medulla (RVM). Spinal-projecting NA neurons are distributed in specific cell groups of the dorsolateral pontomesencephalic tegmentum (DLPT), including the locus coeruleus and the A7 region. Spinal actions of NA on dorsal-horn, nociceptive transmission are mediated by α-2 receptors and are inhibitory. 5-HT actions in the dorsal horn are mediated by several receptor subtypes, including 5-HT$_{1A}$, 5-HT$_2$, and 5-HT$_3$, and include both facilitory and inhibitory effects. In addition to the biogenic amines, a number of other transmitters and neuromodulators have been localized in populations of spinal-projecting brainstem neurons, including enkephalin, substance P, and GABA.

SELECTED READINGS

Coggeshall RE, Carlton SM. Receptor localization in the mammalian dorsal horn and primary afferent neurons. *Brain Res Rev* 1997;24:28–66.

Fields HL, Basbaum AI. Central nervous system mechanisms of pain modulation. In: Wall PD, Melzack R, eds. *Textbook of Pain*. New York: Churchill Livingstone, 1994.

Levine J, Fields HL, Basbaum, AI. Peptides and the primary afferent nociceptor. *J Neurosci* 1993;13:2273–2286.

Millan MJ. The induction of pain: an integrative review. *Prog Neurobiol* 1999;57:1–164.

Todd AJ, Spike RC. The localization of classical transmitters and neuropeptides within neurons in laminae I-III of the mammalian spinal dorsal horn. *Prog Neurobiol* 1993;41:609–645.

Woolf, CJ. Windup and central sensitization are not equivalent. *Pain* 1996;66:105–108.

Yaksh TL, Malmberg AB. Central pharmacology of nociceptive transmission. In: Wall PD, Melzack R, eds. *Textbook of Pain*. New York: Churchill Livingstone, 1994.

CHAPTER 5

Nerve Conduction Studies and Electromyography in Pain Management

Seward B. Rutkove

Unlike radiologic studies, electromyography (EMG) and nerve conduction studies (NCSs) are poorly understood by many clinicians, including neurologists. This is likely true for two reasons. First, rather than providing straightforward images of pathology within the neuraxis, they give functional information that then must be interpreted. Moreover, the actual techniques involved are obscure to most nonelectromyographers.

NERVE CONDUCTION STUDIES

NCSs are almost always performed as part of a standard EMG. Unlike the EMG, which generally provides more qualitative information, NCSs give quantitative information.

In the arms, the nerves that are commonly studied include the median, radial, and ulnar, and in the legs, the posterior tibial, deep peroneal, and sural. These nerves are easily accessible to stimulation and are involved frequently in neurogenic illness.

Motor Nerve Conduction Studies

When performing motor studies, an active recording electrode is placed over a muscle belly and a referential recording electrode is placed over the tendon insertion of that muscle. The nerve is then stimulated at a fixed distance from the muscle. In median nerve studies, for example, recording is made over the abductor pollicis brevis muscle in the hand, and stimulation is performed 7 cm proximally at the wrist (Fig. 5.1). The electrical response represents the depolarization of the muscle beneath the active electrode relative to the referential electrode (Fig. 5.2). Stimulus intensity is increased gradually until the motor response [the compound motor action potential (CMAP)] no longer increases in ampli-

tude. This is called a supramaximal response and suggests that all motor axons are participating. Supramaximal stimulation then is performed at a second, more proximal, site such as in the antecubital fossa in the case of the median nerve.

Latencies and amplitudes are identified for each stimulation site. By subtracting the latency of the distal site from that of the proximal stimulation site and dividing by the distance between these two sites, a conduction velocity for that nerve segment can be obtained. A conduction velocity for the distal segment cannot be obtained because of the delays inherent to the neuromuscular junction and the depolarization of the muscle fibers.

F-responses also are recorded during motor studies. F-responses are after-discharges that occur normally in most motor neurons. When the nerve is supramaximally stimulated, as described above, depolarization of the axon

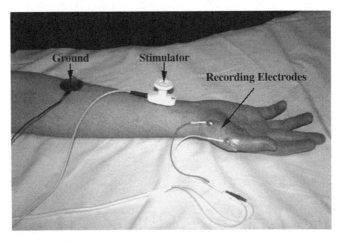

FIG. 5.1. Standard set-up for median motor nerve conduction study, with stimulator at the wrist and recording electrodes over abductor pollicis brevis.

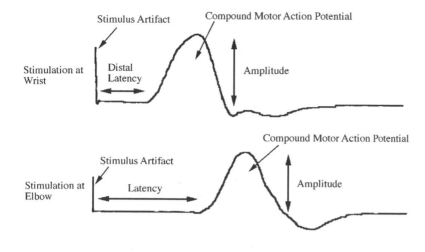

FIG. 5.2. Median motor responses recording from both wrist and elbow.

actually progresses both distally and proximally. The distal depolarization produces the motor response (CMAP) described above. The proximal depolarization, meanwhile, reaches the spinal cord and the cell bodies of the motor neurons in that nerve. At this point, a backfiring of a limited number of motor neurons occurs and a new descending depolarization results. Eventually, this small, second nerve depolarization reaches the muscle and causes a very small depolarization there. This is the F-response. F-responses allow for the integrity of the entire nerve to be studied.

A similar study called the H-reflex also is performed. Unlike the F-response, which is present in most muscles, H-reflexes can be obtained in only a few muscles in the adult. The soleus muscle in the leg is usually the only muscle on which H-reflex testing is performed routinely. When obtaining an H-reflex, submaximal stimulation is used to depolarize selectively the large 1A afferent fibers at the level of the popliteal fossa. The depolarization spreads proximally to the dorsal horn of the spinal cord, which, in turn, produces a depolarization of the motor neurons through one synapse. This depolarization then travels down the nerve to the muscle, producing a contraction. In some sense, the H-reflex is very similar, although not identical, to the ankle jerk.

Sensory Nerve Conduction Studies

When performing sensory studies, active and reference recording electrodes are placed over the nerve to be tested. The nerve then may be stimulated at a fixed distance proximal to the recording electrodes (antidromic recordings). Alternatively, the distal portion of the nerve may be stimulated with recording electrodes placed proximally (orthodromic recording). Antidromic recordings generally are preferred as they provide larger amplitude responses and are less painful for the patient. In antidromic median sensory studies, for example, record-

ing is made over digit 2, and stimulation is performed 13 cm proximally at the wrist (Fig. 5.3). The electrical response represents the depolarization of the nerve fibers beneath the active electrode relative to the referential electrode (Fig. 5.4). Similar to motor recordings, stimulation intensity is increased gradually until the sensory response [sensory nerve action potential (SNAP)] amplitude no longer increases in size. Unlike the motor studies, stimulation at a second site usually is not performed, as a distal conduction velocity can be calculated from the first site alone.

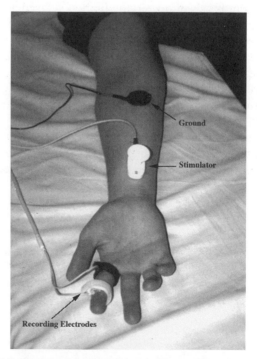

FIG. 5.3. Standard set-up for median antidromic, sensory conduction study, with stimulator at the wrist and recording electrodes on digit 2.

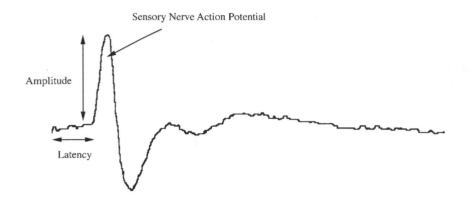

Sensory Nerve Action Potential

Amplitude

Latency

FIG. 5.4. Antidromic median sensory response recording from digit 2.

ELECTROMYOGRAPHY

After NCSs are completed, needle electromyography is performed. The needles are electrodes, with an active recording surface at the tip and the entire barrel making up the reference (so-called concentric needle electrodes). Standard needles are small, corresponding to a 27- or 29-gauge, blood-drawing needle. The needle is attached through a wire to an oscilloscope with an amplifier. Both by observing the waveforms on the screen and listening to the characteristics of their sound, information can be obtained about the functioning of the muscle fibers closest to the needle.

There are two basic parts to electromyography: evaluation of spontaneous activity and evaluation of the motor unit action potentials. To evaluate spontaneous activity, the patient is asked to keep the limb as relaxed as possible. The neurologist then makes small movements with the needle to examine insertional activity. Normal muscle should remain unexcitable after needle movement. If the muscle fiber membrane is unstable for any reason, fibrillations or positive sharp waves may be present (Fig. 5.5). Occasionally, other abnormal discharges may be identified as well.

After evaluating for spontaneous activity, the patient is asked to perform an isometric muscle contraction. The electromyographer observes and listens to the electrical signals from motor units (groups of muscle fibers innervated by a single motor axon). Abnormally enlarged motor units suggest chronic neurogenic disease, while small ones most frequently suggest a primary muscle disorder (Fig. 5.6). In addition to these basic abnormalities, the electromyographer evaluates the "recruitment" of motor units. In normal individuals, with increasing effort, more and more motor units are incorporated into the contraction until the oscilloscope screen fills up with dozens of motor units all firing simultaneously (Fig. 5.7). In patients with neurogenic disease, fewer motor units are present, so that with increasing effort, the functioning units fire faster than normal, compensating for their missing counterparts. This pattern is described as reduced recruitment. In extreme cases, only one motor unit may remain, firing up to five times as fast as normal. In patients with a primary muscle disease, the opposite occurs, as the number of motor units is relatively normal, but their size is reduced as a result of muscle-fiber loss. Hence, with only minimal effort, many motor units fire, producing a full-interference pattern.

Finally, activation also is examined. Activation is the term used to describe the central nervous system drive involved in contracting a muscle. Central drive, whether reduced by a cortical stroke, spinal cord trauma, or simply poor effort, will look identical on EMG. In a patient with poor activation, a few motor units fire no matter how

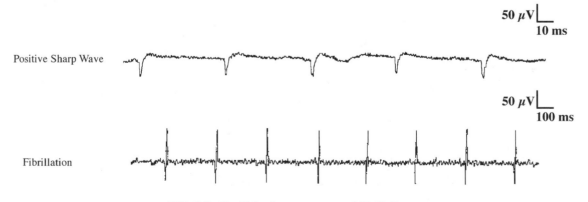

50 μV
10 ms

Positive Sharp Wave

50 μV
100 ms

Fibrillation

FIG. 5.5. Positive sharp waves and fibrillations.

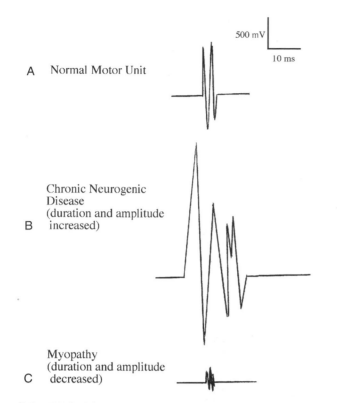

500 mV

10 ms

A   Normal Motor Unit

Chronic Neurogenic
Disease
(duration and amplitude
B   increased)

Myopathy
(duration and amplitude
C   decreased)

FIG. 5.6. Motor unit action potential (MUAP) morphology. **A:** Normal MUAP. **B:** Loss of neighboring motor neurons as a result of neurogenic injury has resulted in the remaining MUAPs to increase in size over normal, with increased amplitude, duration, and phases. **C:** Loss and injury to muscle fibers in a myopathy produces MUAPs with reduced amplitude, duration, and increased phases.

A   Normal Recruitment
Pattern

B   Reduced Recruitment
(neurogenic injury)

C   Early Recruitment
(myopathy)

FIG. 5.7. Recruitment of MUAPs. **A:** Normal recruitment. **B:** Reduced recruitment, as seen in neurogenic injury. As fewer motor units are present, to produce a muscle contraction with the greatest force, the remaining motor units muscle fire more rapidly. In this case, two motor units remain. **C:** Early recruitment. In this example, the patient is minimally contracting, yet many small-motor units are brought into the contraction to produce some force.

hard the patient seems to try. Unlike reduced recruitment, however, the firing rate does not increase above "normal" levels, as each unit fires no more than about 10 Hz.

INTERPRETATION OF THE FINDINGS

There are essentially two types of abnormalities that may be identified on NCSs: axon-loss lesions and demyelinative lesions. Reductions in motor or sensory response amplitude suggest an axon-loss lesion, while prolongations of latency or reduction in conduction velocity suggest a demyelinative lesion. For example, in a generalized polyneuropathy secondary to alcohol abuse in which axon loss is the predominant abnormality, motor and sensory response amplitudes will be reduced diffusely, although the leg may show the most marked abnormalities. Carpal tunnel syndrome, which is the result of a predominantly demyelinative lesion, produces prolonged median-nerve motor and sensory latencies. Similarly in patients with Guillain–Barré syndrome, which is a demyelinative motor polyneuropathy, motor conduction velocities will be reduced and F-response latencies prolonged. In many situations, however, a combination of both axon loss and myelin damage is present. For example, in severe carpal tunnel syndrome, in addition to prolonged motor and sensory latencies, response amplitude is decreased. Likewise, many polyneuropathies, including that of diabetes mellitus, often have components of both axon and myelin damage.

Another aspect to the interpretation of NCSs is that in radiculopathies, sensory response amplitudes are preserved. Unlike polyneuropathies, entrapment neuropathies, or plexopathies, radiculopathies generally occur proximal to the dorsal-root ganglion, where the cell body of the neuron is located. Hence, even if a complete transection of sensory fibers occurs at the root level, the integrity of the distal sensory nerve remains, producing a normal sensory response with stimulation.

Based on the abnormalities identified on NCSs and the nature of the referral, a variety of muscles are studied during EMG. The electromyographer attempts to discern if there is a pattern to the abnormalities identified. For example, abnormalities in tibialis anterior, tibialis posterior, extensor hallucis longus, short-head biceps femoris, and gluteus medius would suggest an L5 radiculopathy. A normal, superficial, peroneal sensory response would help support such a diagnosis. Alternatively, in a patient with slowing of ulnar conduction velocity across the elbow, several forearm muscles are examined to confirm that abnormalities are present only in those innervated by the ulnar nerve.

Generally, when trying to localize any lesion, muscles from several different root levels and nerves are studied in an attempt to "frame" the lesion.

In Table 5.1, the common patterns of different types of neurogenic lesions are summarized. Table 5.2 reviews the value of EMG in varied pain syndromes.

TABLE 5.1. *Common Diagnostic Problems: NCS/EMG Abnormalities*

	Motor studies	F and H responses	Sensory studies	EMG
Mononeuropathy	Focal conduction velocity slowing across affected segment if mild; reduction in amplitude if severe	Mild prolongation in F responses	Slowing of conduction velocity across affected segment; reduction in amplitude if severe	Reinnervation and PSWs and fibrillations in muscles supplied by that nerve
Radiculopathy	Usually normal; occasional reduction in amplitude if severe and muscle studied is derived from affected root	Mild to moderate prolongation of F and H response latencies	Normal	Reinnervation and PSWs/fibrillations in muscles supplied by that root
Plexopathy	Reduced amplitude in muscles supplied by affected fibers	Mild to moderate prolongation of F and H response latencies	Reduced amplitude in sensory nerves traversing affected part of plexus	Reinnervation and PSWs/fibrillations in muscles supplied by affected fibers
Axonal polyneuropathy	Reduced amplitude in muscles of feet	Mild to moderate prolongation of F and H responses	Reduced amplitude of distal nerves (e.g., sural)	Reinnervation and PSWs/fibrillations in distal muscles
Demyelinating polyneuropathy	Variable amplitude reduction;severe slowing of conduction velocity, prolongation of distal latency	Severe prolongation/ absence of F and H responses from multiple nerves	Reduced amplitude and conduction velocity	Variable degrees of chronic reinnervation and fibrillations/PSWs. Reduced recruitment of motor units
Mononeuropathy multiplex	Focal "axonal" lesions of multiple nerves with markedly decreased amplitude	Mild prolongation or absence of F and H responses	Reduced or absent responses in affected nerves	Marked abnormalities in muscles supplied by affected nerve
Myopathy	Amplitude reduced	Normal	Generally normal	Small motor units; fibrillations and PSWs often present

EMG, electromyography; NCS, nerve conduction study; PSW, positive sharp wave.

TABLE 5.2. *Pain Problems: NCS/EMG Abnormalities*

Problem	Possible testing	Utility
Regional complaints		
Muscle stiffness/pain	Can evaluate for several disorders (stiff-person syndrome, benign fasciculations) with EMG and NCS	Generally helpful
Facial pain	Tests of trigeminal and facial nerves	Occasionally helpful; normal in trigeminal neuralgia
Thoracic/abdominal pain	Limited EMG/NCS possible	Usually unhelpful
Perineal region pain	Pudendal nerve/bulbocavernosus reflex testing; low sacral paraspinals can be studied	Occasionally helpful
Specific problems		
Thoracic outlet syndrome	Evaluation for lower trunk brachial plexopathy	If "neurogenic," clear abnormalities may be identified; if "vascular," study will be normal
Herpes zoster	Sensory (and occasionally motor) conductions will show reduced amplitudes, if affecting a limb rather than trunk	May be helpful in diagnosis
Reflex sympathetic dystrophy	No specific tests available. Standard sensory and motor nerve conductions can be performed.	Usually unhelpful; concomitant nerve injury may be identified
Fibromyalgia myofascial pain syndrome	No consistent abnormalities	Helpful in excluding true myopathy
Polymyalgia rheumatica	EMG of proximal musculature	Unless a concomitant myopathy is present, studies are generally normal.

DISCOMFORT

As with most procedures, discomfort is inevitable. Generally, patients tolerate the NCSs well. Needle EMG is clearly more unpleasant. However, in experienced hands, the duration of each needle insertion can be reduced to the point that the study is well tolerated. In addition, patients often come to the EMG laboratory prepared for the worst. In one study of 100 patients who underwent EMG, over 80% admitted the procedure was not as uncomfortable as they had expected.

LIMITATIONS OF ELECTROMYOGRAPHY/NERVE CONDUCTION STUDIES

Like any test, EMG/NCS results can be affected by a number of factors that can decrease its sensitivity and specificity. The following are some of these factors:

1. Hyperacute injuries are difficult to interpret. In cases of proximal nerve damage (e.g., at the root level), it may be several days to 1 week before NCSs show an abnormality. It may be as long as 3 weeks before fibrillations and positive sharp waves appear. With more distal lesions, fibrillations will develop sooner and if the nerve can be stimulated proximal to the site of the lesion, evidence of acute conduction block can be demonstrated. Finally, recruitment abnormalities may be present on EMG immediately after the injury. In short, contrary to generally stated rules, EMGs can provide useful information immediately after an nerve injury. However, the study may be relatively limited or indeterminate.

2. Superimposed processes may make interpretation difficult. For example, making a firm diagnosis of radiculopathy in a patient with diabetic polyneuropathy may be difficult.

3. Many technical factors can play into the accuracy and legitimacy of a study. If a patient's limbs are cool when performing a study, conduction velocity will slow and response amplitude will increase. For example, a patient may be inadvertently diagnosed with carpal tunnel syndrome if the hand is cool. Normal values for NCSs have not been firmly established in older populations, and some variability in interpretation in this set of people is inevitable. Obesity may make certain tests more difficult to perform. Electrical interference or other hardware/software problems also can interfere with results.

4. An EMG/NCS can only evaluate large, myelinated neurons. Yet, many diseases, especially those that are painful, affect smaller myelinated or unmyelinated nerve fibers. In such situations, an EMG/NCS may be entirely normal. In short, just because there is no electrophysiologic evidence for a polyneuropathy does not mean that one does not exist.

5. The quality of the study may vary considerably. For one, this may depend on how well the patient tolerates and cooperates with the test. No matter how kind an electromyographer may be, the test still hurts and occasionally patients can simply not complete it. Unfortunately, however, the quality of the study also may be suboptimal because of the electromyographer. Some people who perform EMG/NCS have limited training or may perform studies infrequently. Usually, such physicians have little difficulty identifying straightforward problems, such as carpal-tunnel syndrome or radiculopathy. But when faced with a more complex situation, the likelihood of an accurate diagnosis is much lower. Generally, physicians who perform EMG/NCSs on a regular basis should have passed either the American Board of Electrodiagnostic Medicine (ABEM) or the Added Qualification in Clinical Neurophysiology Examination (a subspecialty board within neurology) with at least 6 months of full-time EMG training prior to practice.

6. Not all clinical disorders have EMG correlates. For example, vascular thoracic outlet syndrome, reflex sympathetic dystrophy, and fibromyalgia/myofascial-pain syndrome, have no definite associated EMG abnormalities (Table 5.2). Regardless of the validity of these clinical disorders, the likelihood that electrophysiologic findings will support any of these syndromes is relatively low. It is useful to keep this in mind before sending a patient with one of these possible diagnoses for testing.

7. Finally, the EMG/NCS is only a test, with false negatives and positives. A negative result does not exclude the possibility that the disease exists (very mild carpal-tunnel syndrome, mild radiculopathies, polyneuropathy). At the same time, a positive result may have nothing to do with the patient's symptoms. An EMG does not simply provide "*the* answer" to the patient's problem, but rather must be interpreted in the context of an individual patient's history and examination.

SELECTED READINGS

Albers JW. Clinical neurophysiology of generalized polyneuropathy. *J Clin Neurophys* 1993;10:149–166.

Albers JW, Kelly JJ. Acquired inflammatory demyelinating polyneuropathies: clinical and electrodiagnostic features. *Muscle Nerve* 1989;12: 435–451.

Brown WF, Bolton CF. *Clinical Electromyography*, 2nd ed. Boston: Butterworth-Heinemann, 1993.

Cornblath DR. Electrophysiology in Guillain–Barré syndrome. *Ann Neurol* 1997;27(suppl):S17–S20.

Ferrante MA, Wilbourn AJ. The utility of various sensory nerve conduction responses in assessing brachial plexopathies. *Muscle Nerve* 1995;18: 878–879.

Kimura J. *Electrodiagnosis in Diseases of Nerve and Muscles: Principles and Practice.* 2nd ed. Philadelphia: FA Davis, 1989.

Kincaid JC. AAEM minimonograph #31: the electrodiagnosis of ulnar neuropathy at the elbow. *Muscle Nerve* 1988;11:1005–1015.

Liguori R, Fuglsang-Frederiksen A, Nix W, et al. Electromyography in myopathy. *Neurophysiol Clin* 1997;27:200–203.

Oh SJ. *Clinical Electromyography: Nerve Conduction Studies,* 2nd ed. Baltimore: Williams & Wilkins, 1993.

Preston DC, Shapiro BE. *Electromyography and Neuromuscular Disorders.* Boston: Butterworth-Heinemann, 1998.

Stevens JC. AAEM minimonograph #26: the electrodiagnosis of carpal tunnel syndrome. *Muscle Nerve* 1997;20:1477–1486.

Wilbourn AJ, Aminoff MJ. AAEM minimonograph #32: the electrophysiologic examination in patients with radiculopathy. *Muscle Nerve* 1988;11: 1099–1114.

CHAPTER 6

Psychological Evaluation of Chronic Pain

Joshua Wootton

When asked to see a psychologist or to respond to a questionnaire or self-report psychological instrument, like the MMPI-2, many patients respond defensively, as though their integrity is being challenged. The idea that their pain might somehow be influenced by psychological factors is bound with their anxiety that their pain may be perceived by others as psychogenic. How the physician approaches the patient, therefore, becomes a critical step in discerning the comprehensive picture of his or her chronic pain and utilizing that picture both to assess prognosis and to develop the best possible plan for treatment.

It is frequently useful to remind patients with chronic pain that, in all likelihood, their pain itself constitutes the most severe and distressing problem in their lives and that it would be surprising if such a stressor did not affect them emotionally and interfere with their usual ways of coping. While the origin of pain may not be psychological, how one *responds* to it *is*. Even the most well-adjusted individual may encounter symptoms of anxiety and depression, in the wake of severe or enduring pain, and find that his or her basic assumptions about relationships and indeed the way the whole world works suddenly are called into question.

THE QUESTION OF PAIN OR DISABILITY

Why some individuals develop chronic pain, while others, with seemingly the same injuries, extent of tissue damage, and quality of medical care, do not, remains a difficult conundrum. While nociceptive or purely physiological factors appear to instigate the initial report of pain, behavioral and psychosocial factors tend to complicate this simple picture over time, often resulting in the exacerbation or maintenance of pain well beyond its organic usefulness and the subsequent development of physical and psychological disability.

In this larger, more complex picture of chronic pain, the question of disability becomes more than one of simple injury and tissue damage. It incorporates the whole of the individual's response to pain — including temperament, personality traits, and a prevailing explanatory model, all of which dispose the individual to make sense of his or her pain in a particular way — and environmental factors that influence the relative success or failure with which the individual attempts to cope with chronic pain, long after the identified cause has been assuaged or resolved.

There are few objective clinical or laboratory measures with any predictive validity, where the development and duration of disability are concerned. Physical examinations often are notoriously at variance with patients' reports of their own experience. Even the use of Waddell's signs for nonorganic pain — frequently misused by insurance companies as an acid test for malingering or factitious disorder — is just as frequently skewed by the patient's endorsement of contradictory symptoms and sensations in an attempt to draw attention to his or her plight and have his or her chronic pain taken seriously.

This failure to find a reliable and predictive relationship between the patient's self-report of pain and either clinical or empirical evidence of pathology has historically led to speculation that chronic pain may be the result, principally or entirely, of psychological factors or even a particular type of personality. But the search for the "pain-prone personality" never yielded a satisfying or useful unified theory or model. The possible expressions of the combination of temperament with the range of personality traits, the variety of environmental factors, the spectrum of psychopathology, and the individuality of personal explanatory models are so overwhelming as to be expressed uniquely in each patient. If "profiling" cannot reliably help us to distinguish pain-prone individuals, then how can we identify those who are at greatest risk for the development of chronic pain?

PSYCHOSOCIAL RISK FACTORS

Of far greater usefulness is the comparatively recent trend of identifying those psychosocial factors that are highly statistically correlated with the development of chronic-pain syndromes, pain disorders, and disability. A considerable research effort, much of which has occurred within the last decade, has resulted in the identification of a number of largely independent risk factors that tend to be associated with poor recovery from injury and acute pain and predispose the individual toward the development of chronic pain and disability. When these risk factors are present premorbidly or when they develop comorbidly, they tend to complicate the pain picture, often moving the patient toward a state of learned helplessness, with disability being the end result.

The first of these factors, *(a) pain duration*, is better considered a comorbid influence: the longer the pain endures, the more likely that a chronic pain syndrome and disability have developed. Two years of pain, accompanied by multiple, invasive procedures and courses of treatment, sometimes is cited as the decisive threshold; but when a successful return to work is the decisive criterion, an even shorter period becomes significant. After 6 months of unemployment resulting from chronic pain, there is only a 50% likelihood that a patient will return to his or her job. After 1 year, the likelihood drops to only 10%.

Two risk factors that may be considered either premorbid or comorbid include *(b) a history of major psychopathology* and *(c) a history of substance abuse or dependence*. The presence of premorbid mood disorder, anxiety disorder, thought disorder, or personality disorder certainly places the burden of greater risk upon the patient with pain, but mood disorder, anxiety disorder, and adjustment disorder also can represent comorbid developments, where chronic pain is concerned, contributing in their own right to the pain–stress cycle and disability. Similarly, problems with substance abuse and dependence can exist as predisposing factors or develop from the injudicious use of prescription medications, principally opioids and anxiolytics/hypnotics.

The remaining risk factors all are generally considered premorbid influences and include *(d) job dissatisfaction; (e) a history of prolonged recovery from previous experiences of pain; (f) a history of psychological or physical trauma; (g) a history of psychological, physical, or sexual abuse; (h) a pattern of reduced activity, coupled with excessive pain behaviors, supported by family and other social contacts who are either too solicitous or inconsistent or too harsh and punitive in their responses;* and *(i) negative or anxiety-provoking beliefs about the meaning of pain*. Most of these require little elaboration, but the last usually is construed to mean maladaptive beliefs about chronic pain that may not be physiologically accurate or psychologically realistic—"If it hurts, I must be aggravating the injury " or "I'll never be able to walk with this pain."

A final predisposing factor that has received increasing attention in the past few years concerns the patient's *(j) explanatory model* of pain: how does the individual make sense of his or her pain in the context of his or her relationship to the world or to God? There is a growing body of evidence to suggest that affirming beliefs and an essentially optimistic philosophy can make a critical contribution to recovery from illness and the restoration of health. Patients who feel pessimistic about their pain or who feel that they are being persecuted or punished or victimized by forces beyond their control clearly have a more difficult path to recovery and often tend to contribute to the poor tractability of their situations with passive attitudes toward pain management and lack of compliance with treatment.

In addition to these ten predisposing factors, five risk factors have been identified as predictors of negative outcome in the treatment of chronic pain. These include three of the ones already mentioned — *job dissatisfaction; reduced activity, coupled with excessive pain behaviors;* and *negative or anxiety-provoking beliefs* — along with a *sustained attitude of hostility, anger, and alienation* and a reliance upon *maladaptive coping strategies*. The more these predictors of negative outcome are represented in the lives of chronic-pain sufferers, the more likely will their treatment be characterized by frustration, iatrogenic stress, and ultimately, failure. Evaluating which risk factors may be operative in the lives of patients, as well as the degree to which each is influential, is critical in the development of effective treatment plans and essential to shaping interventions to fit the individual. There are two principal means of gathering this data: (a) the clinical interview of the patient and, if possible, one or more family members, and (b) the psychometric assessment of the patient through one or more self-report psychological instruments.

THE CLINICAL INTERVIEW

The pain physician, like the psychologist, uses the clinical interview not only in the service of diagnosing physical pathology but also to learn about the patient and his or her response to illness and pain. Evidence of one or more of the previously mentioned risk factors is usually grounds for a more comprehensive, psychosocially based clinical interview. In pain-management centers and group and hospital-based practices, this often is undertaken by a psychologist, psychiatrist, or clinical social worker, but many pain physicians are familiar with and comfortable administering such clinical interviews, when time allows and a team or multidisciplinary approach is not possible. To allay the patient's initial fears and any defensiveness, it frequently is helpful to begin by stating that the purpose of the interview is to find out more about the impact of the patient's pain upon his or her life — how the pain has affected his or her work and family, financial status, and personal goals — as well as what seems to exacerbate or to soothe the pain.

Few structured interviews have been adapted specifically for use with the pain patient, but one that has received much attention is the Psychosocial Pain Inventory (PSPI). The PSPI is designed to evaluate patients according to psychosocial factors that tend to sustain or exacerbate the experience of chronic pain. The interviewer collects responses to 25 questions, each representing a psychosocial category or dimension in which chronic pain may be influential, including items that explore the patient's previous exposure to familial models of chronic pain and illness, the patient's major stressful life events, and social reinforcement of the patient's pain behaviors. Each category is awarded a numerical score, with the total reportedly having a high interrater reliability, as well as a high predictive validity for poor response to medical treatment.

While not developed specifically to evaluate patients with chronic pain, structured and semistructured psychiatric interviews also have been used in pain clinics and chronic-pain research, having both proven their adaptability and established their durability in assessing the psychosocial histories and symptomatological profiles of patients. Two often-cited formats for the psychiatric interview are based on the current edition of the *Diagnostic and Statistical Manual of Mental Disorders* (DSM-IV). The National Institute of Mental Health Diagnostic Interview Schedule for DSM-IV (DIS-IV) and the Structured Clinical Interview for DSM-IV (SCID) assess not only current psychiatric symptoms and disorders, but also lifetime histories of psychiatric diagnoses. Both require a brief course of training to administer properly, but the SCID offers clinicians greater latitude to supplement the structured interview with spontaneous questions for clarification and challenges to inconsistent responses. Because of their essentially structured formats, both the DIS-IV and the SCID also are offered in computerized versions.

Offering even greater latitude and more direct applicability to patients with chronic pain is the generic psychiatric interview adapted to the situation of chronic pain. There is no established structure for the basic psychiatric interview, but it generally is acknowledged to consist of the following elements: presenting problem, history of presenting problem, psychiatric history, substance abuse history, medical history, developmental and social history, and mental status examination. Each of these broad sections can include questions relevant to the patient's experience of pain, but the entire format can be revised to focus on the presenting problem of pain. Table 6.1 presents an example of how the general format of the psychiatric interview can be altered and expanded to provide a background against which the problem of pain can be portrayed in its psychosocial context and with reference to the influence of psychosocial risk factors.

The flexibility inherent in this example over more structured approaches is critical to the clinical investigation of a broad range of psychosocial issues with special meaning in the context of chronic pain. Exploring possible sources of reinforcement for pain and disability, as well as models of pain and illness behaviors available to the patient, is essential to understanding the patient's expression of pain and how he or she has adjusted to the situation of chronic pain. Even questions about caffeine and nicotine use—stimulants whose effects are frequently overlooked or discounted —take on particular relevance in the context of pain because of the effect of these substances on autonomic arousal and the patient's resulting subjective experience of pain.

Assessing the presence and degree of trauma also is critical because of the possible relationship between chronic pain and a history of emotional, physical, or sexual abuse. The high prevalence of posttraumatic stress disorder (PTSD) and posttraumatic stress-type symptoms among patients with chronic pain is well documented, and understanding whether and how the connection may exist in a patient's life becomes crucial to understanding and treating his or her pain. Questions directed toward assessing the patient's willingness to accept some measure of personal responsibility for managing his or her pain also will provide important prognostic clues, as well as indications about where to begin with treatment. In a psychosocially based clinical pain interview, the clinician has the opportunity to develop his or her lines of inquiry sequentially in a purposeful manner, tailoring each successive question to the individual's immediate verbal and affective responses. What might be termed an organic or *process* approach to understanding the patient's pain becomes the guiding principle of the evaluation.

TABLE 6.1. *A Concise Guide to the Psychosocially Based Clinical Pain Interview*

- **Presenting Pain Complaint.** What is the origin, nature, and duration of the pain? What previous attempts have been made at treating the pain? Are there current medications and ongoing treatments and therapies? What exacerbates and what tends to relieve the pain? What are the patient's beliefs about his or her pain, including why it continues? Why does the patient come for treatment, here and now, and with what expectations?

- **Current Level of Functioning.** How has the pain changed the patient's life, including changes of status at work, socially, and within the family? What is the patient's current level of activity? Does he or she need assistance with activities of daily living (ADLs), like bathing, dressing, and household chores? Has his or her pain interfered with sexual intimacy? Has the patient had to give up activities, pastimes, and recreational pursuits?

- **Current Identifiable Stressors.** What related and unrelated problems, worries, anxieties, and conflicts is the patient aware of, including stressors at work and at home? Has the patient's financial status or ability to provide for his or her family been affected? Has he or she applied for worker's compensation or disability, and, if so, what has the process been like? Has litigation been considered or undertaken around the original source of injury?

- **Medical History.** Has the patient experienced previous episodes of chronic pain, work-related injuries, or extended illnesses? Are there concurrent or previous unrelated medical problems? Is the patient taking medications for any other symptoms or problems? Does he or she have any surgical history or history of hospital admissions for other reasons? Who is his or her primary-care physician and for how long? Does the patient exercise or take any over-the-counter (OTC) remedies, vitamins, homeopathic or herbal remedies? How does the patient describe his or her diet, eating behaviors, and attitudes toward nutrition? Is there a family history of significant illness or chronic pain?

- **Psychiatric History.** Has the patient ever consulted with a psychologist, psychiatrist, or psychotherapist, and is he or she currently in any form of psychiatric treatment? Has he or she ever taken psychotropic medications or been admitted to a psychiatric facility or hospital for any reason? Are there psychological symptoms or problems for which he or she would now like consultation or treatment (e.g., family or marital conflicts, sleep disturbance, anxiety, or depression)? Is there any family psychiatric history?

- **Substance Abuse History.** Has the patient ever been treated for substance abuse or been referred to a detox or 12-step program? Does he or she have any experience with "recreational" substances, other than alcohol? Have substances, including alcohol, ever proved to be a problem or to cause problems in his or her work or social life? What is his or her current level of consumption of alcohol, caffeine, and nicotine? Is he or she aware of the effects of stimulants and depressants on his or her body and mental status? Has the patient ever had problems modulating the use of prescribed medications, especially opioids and anxiolytics? Is there any family history of substance abuse?

- **Developmental and Social History.** Where was the patient raised, and what were his or her family's circumstances? How would he or she characterize his or her childhood and adolescence, schooling, and relationships with parents and siblings? Has the patient suffered important losses through death, estrangement, or loss of contact? Is there a history of emotional, physical, or sexual abuse? Is there a history of other emotional or physical trauma? What is the patient's significant relational history, including his or her relationships with spouse and children? What is his or her sexual history, and how would he or she characterize his or her current sexual relationship? What is the patient's education and work history; military and legal history? What are his or her interests and pursuits outside of work? Does he or she have a network of friends and social supports? To whom does the patient turn when he or she needs to discuss problems, needs a favor, or has to ask for help?

- **Mental Status Examination.** Questions included in this section are meant to enhance and systematize the clinician's observations about the patient's appearance, attitude, and behavior—especially the presence or absence of pain behaviors—as well as his or her affect, mood, speech, perception, quality of thinking and reality testing, judgment, and cognitive and intellectual functioning. It also may be helpful to ask about the effects of chronic pain on his or her mental status. Has he or she ever felt suicidal or felt moved to violence toward another because of the pain? How does the pain affect his or her mood and what was it like, before the onset of pain? How has the patient's medication regimen affected his or her mental status? How has the burden of treatment affected his or her mental status?

- **Psychological Testing.** If the results of psychological testing are available, it often is helpful to review them, in brief, with the patient. When the results are at variance with the patient's interview, it is frequently a good idea to point this out and to see what sense the patient is able to make of it. Patients sometimes will deny feeling depressed during the interview, for example, but may have indicated considerable mood and neurovegetative disturbance on the Beck Depression Inventory (BDI) or the Minnesota Multiphasic Personality Inventory (MMPI-2).

- **Patient's Questions and Goals for Treatment.** Is there anything the patient has not talked about that he or she feels is important for the interviewer to know? Does he or she come, today, with specific expectations or questions about what can be done for his or her pain? Does the patient think that the physician who referred him or her had any specific recommendations in mind? Is he or she open to learning new ways of managing his or her pain, apart from procedures and medications? Does the patient feel that he or she has a role in helping to control his or her pain? What are the patient's goals for treatment, and how does he or she envision the next month of treatment? The next 6 months?

CROSS-VALIDATION THROUGH PSYCHOMETRIC ASSESSMENT

While the clinical interview remains the most efficient method for gathering the most information about the patient, the process of developing impressions about his or her pain and how best to treat it, based solely on the patient's verbal self-report, is sometimes a problematic enterprise. Anyone is capable of forgetting, editorializing, and censoring him or herself, whether consciously or unconsciously, in presenting his or her story to medical providers. One way to improve the fidelity—or, in some cases, test the veracity—of the patient's self-report is to cross-validate it with other resources. Examining the available medical records and referral data, interviewing spouses and other family members when possible, and administering one or more psychometric instruments are all methods of cross-validating the data from the clinical interview and improving the likelihood of arriving at an accurate formulation of the patient's difficulties.

When a patient's report of his situation and circumstances is at variance with that of his or her spouse or the medical record, inconsistencies can be identified easily and, in most cases, can be reconciled. When they cannot be reconciled, that, too, is useful information—as in the case of the patient who is reluctant to admit his or her lack of compliance with recommendations and treatment. Where psychometric instruments are concerned, patients frequently react differently to the situation of taking a pencil-and-paper or computerized test or inventory than they do in the presence of physicians and psychologists. When a patient endorses an item on a questionnaire or psychological inventory suggesting that he or she is suicidal but denies any suicidal ideation or feelings of hopelessness to his or her physician, this is an inconsistency worth investigating. Nor is the point of questions on psychological measures always immediately discernible to patients, which sometimes results in a less-guarded response. If we are to use our experience as clinicians to the best advantage, having an actuarial or statistically meaningful basis for interpreting and cross-validating a patient's responses also becomes an invaluable tool.

Measures Developed for Use in Chronic Pain and Chronic Illness

There are hundreds of psychometric instruments developed for use with chronic-pain and chronic-illness populations or applied clinically or in quantitative or qualitative studies to some aspect of the pain patient's experience. Many instruments, like verbal-rating scales (VRSs), visual-analog scales (VASs), graphic-rating scales (GRSs), and pain drawings are used only to assess the intensity and location of pain. These provide quantitative estimates of the patient's pain, as well as a basis for longitudinal comparison; but they do not offer a valid basis for comparison between patients; and, in the case of the scales, there is an underlying assumption that pain is unidimensional, with intensity as the most important qualifier. The McGill Pain Questionnaire (MPQ), by contrast, presents 20 subclasses or groupings of pain-related adjectives to patients, who—through their endorsement of the word most accurately describing their pain in each category—give a multidimensional picture of their pain according to a scale of intensity and three psychological dimensions of pain: sensory, affective, and evaluative. The MPQ is the most often used and cited measure of the experience of pain in clinical practice and research, and the availability of a short form of the instrument makes it even more versatile.

Another category of psychometric measures is geared toward assessing the functional capacity and psychosocial context of patients with chronic illness or pain. These instruments are therefore less concerned with describing pain than they are with portraying and quantifying disability. This group includes the West Haven–Yale Multidimensional Pain Inventory (WHYMPI or, simply, MPI), the Pain Disability Index (PDI), the Sickness Impact Profile (SIP), the Short-Form Health Survey (SF-36), the Chronic Illness Problem Inventory (CIPI), the Illness Behavior Inventory (IBI), the Illness Behavior Questionnaire (IBQ), and the Waddell Disability Instrument (WDI). Evaluating the psychosocial context of the patient with chronic pain is achieved with two basic approaches: assessing the degree to which illness-related and pain behaviors are present (IBI, IBQ, WDI, and CIPI) and assessing the degree to which healthy activity is impaired (MPI, PDI, SIP, SF-36, and CIPI).

While most of these instruments can be useful as screening devices and outcome measures, those based on the latter approach tend to have a wider circulation in pain clinics and, of these, the MPI is perhaps the most successful in clinical utility and applications to research. The most frequently administered version contains 52 items and requires 15 to 20 minutes to complete. A psychosocial section yields scores on five scales: pain severity, interference with activity, perceived control of pain upon life, emotional distress, and perceived level of support and concern from others. Two behavioral sections present scores on how the patient sees and interprets the responses of his or her spouse or significant other to his or her pain and level of functional impairment and how impaired the patient is according to 18 common daily activities. From the pattern of scores generated across sections, patients can be classified according to four types, each with implications for treatment: adaptive copers, dysfunctional, interpersonally distressed, or hybrid.

A third category of psychometric measures related to chronic pain consists of those instruments that purport to assess or characterize patients' pain attitudes, coping strategies, maladaptive pain beliefs, or self-efficacy. What a patient believes about his or her pain is an influential variable in treatment outcome. Unrealistic or negative thoughts and fantasies can increase distress, decrease functioning, and render pain less tractable, just as a poor coping style will result in maladjustment. The Coping Strategies Questionnaire (CSQ), the Vanderbilt Pain Management Inventory (VPMI), the Ways of Coping Questionnaire (WOC), the Pain Management Inventory (PMI), the Survey of Pain Attitudes (SOPA), the Inventory of Negative Thoughts in Response to Pain (INTRP), the Pain Beliefs Questionnaire (PBQ), the Pain Information and Beliefs Questionnaire (PIBQ), the Pain and Impairment Relationship Scales (PAIRS), the Pain Beliefs and Perception Inventory (PBAPI), and the Pain Cognitions Questionnaire (PCQ) all attempt to delineate the contribution of negative beliefs and maladaptive coping strategies to poor outcome in treatment.

A comparatively recent development in the psychometric assessment of patients with chronic pain is an instrument designed to evaluate the individual's readiness to adopt a self-management approach to his or her pain. The Pain Stages of Change Questionnaire (PSOCQ) applies the transtheoretical model of behavioral change linked to a cognitive-behavioral perspective on chronic pain in a 30-item format. According to the transtheoretical model, individuals progress through a series of specific stages in the process of change and successful adjustment. The PSOCQ characterizes the patient's stage of readiness on a continuum of four scales: precontemplation, contemplation, action, and maintenance. The relevance and importance of assessing patients' readiness for change is discussed in Chapter 57; however, the application becomes readily apparent, when faced with compliance issues and choices about how to proceed with treatment. The value of an instrument that can cross-validate a patient's simple profession of his or her level of motivation and readiness to adopt new, more adaptive beliefs and coping strategies cannot be overestimated in clinical practice.

Measures of Psychopathology Applied to Chronic Pain

Most patients with chronic pain do not have histories of premorbid psychopathology, but assessing psychopathology and its potential influence on the development and maintenance of chronic pain and disability is important for three reasons. First, chronic pain is greatly overrepresented in psychiatric populations; second, the likelihood of patients developing comorbid psychiatric symptoms is high; and, third, major psychopathology is indicative of a poor prognosis in the treatment of chronic pain and disability. The psychometric instruments most frequently used in the evaluation of patients with chronic pain include the Beck Depression Inventory (BDI), the Symptom Checklist 90, Revised (SCL-90R), the Spielberger State/Trait Anxiety Inventory (STAI), the Beck Anxiety Inventory (BAI), the Millon Behavioral Health Inventory (MBHI), and the Minnesota Multiphasic Personality Inventory (MMPI-2). The Illness Behavior Questionnaire (IBQ) and the MPI, previously mentioned as measures of functional capacity, also are useful tools in the assessment of psychopathology.

The BDI, SCL-90R, BAI, and STAI are all essentially inventories of symptoms. The BDI is a 21-item questionnaire designed to assess the mood and neurovegetative aspects of depression. The latter sometimes can be overestimated, given that sleep disturbance and diminished sexual appetite both can occur with pain in the absence of depression, but the BDI remains one of the better instruments for tracking changes in the level of depression over time. The STAI and BAI both assess levels of anxiety; but most of the BAI's 21 items tend to focus on autonomic and physiological symptoms, while the STAI's 40-item format measures anxiety both as a character trait (i.e., how anxious the individual is generally) and according to current functioning (i.e., how anxious the individual feels at present). The SCL-90R assesses the general level of the individual's emotional distress, as well as his or her functioning across nine scales of psychopathology, including somatization, obsessiveness, interpersonal sensitivity, depression, anxiety, hostility, phobic anxiety, paranoid ideation, and psychoticism.

The MBHI is a 150-item inventory that was developed to evaluate the psychological functioning specifically of medical patients. Linked to an empirically validated theory of personality, the MBHI yields scores on 20 clinical scales. Eight of these measure basic coping styles (e.g., introversive, inhibitive, cooperative, sociable, confident, forceful, respectful, and sensitive), which are suggestive of patients' styles of relating to their providers. Six assess psychosocial attitudes, such as chronic tension, recent stress, premorbid pessimism, future despair, social alienation, and somatic anxiety; and three depict probable responses to illness, including allergic inclination, gastrointestinal susceptibility, and cardiovascular tendency. Three final scales purport to characterize prognostic indices, like pain-treatment responsivity, life-threat reactivity, and emotional vulnerability. The MBHI is more directly relevant to pain than any of the other major personality inventories, and its face validity as an assessment tool for medical patients generally results in a friendlier, less-guarded administration for patients with chronic pain.

The MMPI and its successor the MMPI-2 are, by a considerable margin, the most widely used psychometric instruments in the assessment of chronic pain. The MMPI-2's 567 true–false items are distributed across seven validity scales, assessing individuals' attitudes toward responding to the test, and ten principal clinical scales, each measuring a construct of psychopathology. The ten principal clinical scales are hypochondriasis, depression, hysteria, psychopathic deviate, masculinity–femininity, paranoia, psychasthenia, schizophrenia, mania, and social introversion. In addition, there are many supplementary scales with robust applications to the chronic-pain population. Although some clinicians and many patients find the MMPI-2 daunting because of its length and the obviously psychiatric tenor of many of its items, it has demonstrated in a large body of studies its capacity to derive and portray distinct profiles of patients affected with chronic pain. Some of these patterns have been shown to be predictive of response to surgical intervention and likelihood of returning to work. Of all the measures of psychopathology applied to chronic pain, the MMPI-2 is the most effective at delineating psychiatric disorders and symptomatology, despite the problem of not being able to distinguish premorbid from comorbid expressions. Several short forms and a computerized administration of the instrument are available.

That so many measures have been developed to assist physicians and psychologists to understand chronic pain and disability is ample evidence of the complexity of the problem. No one method or instrument can depict all that we need to know about a patient's experience of pain, and certainly no one avenue of evaluation will tell us unfailingly how to proceed with treatment. Employing multiple measures, therefore, in an attempt to get the best cross-validation of the most detailed and comprehensive understanding of the patient's experience is the only way to ensure the greatest likelihood of a successful outcome.

SELECTED READINGS

Abram SE, Haddox JD, eds. *The Pain Clinic Manual*. Philadelphia: Lippincott Williams & Wilkins, 2000.

Eimer BN, Freeman A. *Pain Management Psychotherapy: A Practical Guide*. New York: John Wiley & Sons, 1998.

Jamison RN. *Mastering Chronic Pain: A Professional's Guide to Behavioral Treatment*. Sarasota, FL: Professional Resource Press, 1996.

Keller LS, Butcher JN. *Assessment of Chronic Pain Patients with the MMPI-2*. Minneapolis, University of Minnesota, 1991.

Kerns RD, Rosenberg R, Jamison RN, et al. Readiness to adopt a self-management approach to chronic pain: the pain stages of change questionnaire (PSOCQ). *Pain* 1997;72:227–234.

Skevington SM. *The Psychology of Pain*. Chichester: John Wiley & Sons, 1995.

Turk DC, Melzack R, eds. *Handbook of Pain Assessment*. New York: Guilford, 1992.

PART II

Pain by Anatomic Location

CHAPTER 7

Headache

Michael P. Biber

In considering the diagnosis of headache, it is helpful to know the pain-sensitive structures of the head and their innervation. Blood vessels, dural and arachnoid membranes, skin, muscles, aponeuroses, periosteum, upper-cervical spinal roots, joints, eyes, ears, paranasal sinuses, and turbinates are sensitive to pain (Fig. 7.1). Most, if not all, of the brain is not a pain-sensitive structure. The upper three cervical–spinal roots, with contributions from the ninth and tenth cranial nerves, innervate most of the ipsilateral posterior fossa. Contents of the anterior and middle fossae are innervated by the ipsilateral trigeminal nerve. Stimulation of the C1 root has been reported to cause ipsilateral frontal and eye pain.

HEADACHES THAT MAY REQUIRE URGENT AND SPECIFIC TREATMENT

The clinician first should consider the possibility that headache may be the result of a cause that requires urgent treatment. Often, careful history taking provides the most important diagnostic clues. Most patients with headache have no relevant signs on elementary physical examination. However, sometimes even subtle anisocoria, strabismus, papilledema, a retinal or subhyaloid hemorrhage, a tender, firm temporal artery, an intracranial bruit, a scalp infection, hemiparesis, and other signs may help secure a diagnosis requiring urgent diagnosis and treatment.

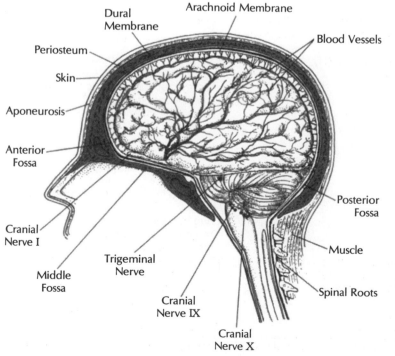

FIG 7.1 Blood vessels, dural and arachnoid membranes, skin, muscles, aponeurosis, periosteum, spinal roots, joints, eyes, ears, parinasal sinuses, and turbinates are sensitive to pain; the brain, for the most part, is not. Most of the posterior fossa on one side is innervated by the ipsilateral upper three cervical roots, with contributions from the ninth and tenth cranial nerves. Contents of the anterior and middle fossae are innervated by the ipsilateral trigeminal nerve. Stimulation of the first cervical–spinal root has been reported to cause ipsilateral frontal and eye pain.

The abrupt onset of severe headache, often accompanied by photophobia, nausea, and vomiting, is highly suggestive of subarachnoid hemorrhage from a ruptured intracranial aneurysm or arteriovenous malformation. Neurologic signs may include neck rigidity, decreased level of consciousness, retinal or subhyaloid hemorrhages, third or sixth cranial nerve dysfunction, papilledema, leg weakness, abulia, or focal signs from ischemia secondary to spasm of cerebral arteries (Table 7.1). Seizures may occur. The diagnosis of nontraumatic, subarachnoid hemorrhage is even more likely if the pain began during straining or coitus. When a patient's presentation suggests a nontraumatic, subarachnoid hemorrhage, then immediate work-up and treatment are mandatory. A computed tomogram (CT) should be obtained.

If, despite a high index of suspicion, the CT does not document evidence of subarachnoid blood, then, assuming that there is no strong contraindication, a lumbar puncture (LP) should be done. If the CT or LP documents evidence of subarachnoid blood, then a magnetic resonance arteriogram (MRA) of the head should be obtained promptly. If no aneurysm or arteriovenous malformation (AVM) is seen but the history and signs strongly suggest a subarachnoid hemorrhage, then conventional cerebral arteriography should be considered. If an intracerebral aneurysm or AVM is found, then immediate neurosurgery and, when indicated, an interventional neuroradiology consultation should be obtained.

Twenty percent to 50% of patients who have subarachnoid hemorrhages have abrupt-onset, severe, minutes- to hours-long headaches weeks or months before they hemorrhage. Though often overlooked, these warning or "sentinel" headaches require the same full and immediate diagnostic work-up as the more full-blown symptoms and signs of subarachnoid hemorrhage.

The same constellation of symptoms and signs suggestive of nontraumatic subarachnoid hemorrhage may denote an intracerebral hemorrhage. Hypertension is a critical pre-

TABLE 7.1. *Differential Diagnosis and Treatment of Headache*

Cause	Diagnosis	Treatment
Subarachnoid hemorrhage Aneurysm; arteriovenous malformation	CT then LP if CT does not show hemorrhage; MRA or angiogram when indicated	Surgery, interventional radiologic procedure, or radiosurgery, when indicated
Intracerebral hemorrhage Aneurysm; arteriovenous malformation; dural-venous sinus thrombosis; cavernous angioma; amylid angiopathy; venous angioma; vasculitis; brain tumor; infarct; cocaine or alcohol abuse	CT; MRA, MRI, or angiogram when indicated	Surgery, interventional radiologic procedure, or radiosurgery, when indicated
Infection Meningitis/encephalitis	Urgent LP; consider immediate MRI or radionucleide brain scan when herpes simplex is suspected;	Specific antibiotics, when indicated
Sinusitis	History; physical exam; CT, when indicated	Warm, hypertonic-saline nasal douching; corticosteroid nasal sprays, antibiotics, when indicated
Malignant hypertension	Increased BP; papilloedema	i.v. antihypertensives
Temporal arteritis	Increased erythrocyte sedimentation rate; temporal artery biopsy, when indicated	Corticosteroids
Increased intracranial pressure Intracranial mass	MRI or CT	Surgery or radiosurgery, when indicated;
Pseudotumor cerebri	MRI or CT	Decrease intracranial pressure
Neurovascular headache Migraine	History	Drug treatment,
Cluster	History	Oxygen; drug treatment,
Chornic paroxysmal hemicrania	History	Indomethacin
Cervical headache	History; physical examination	Collar; greater occipital nerve block
"Tension" headache	History; physical examination	Stress reduction
Posttraumatic headache	History; physical examination	Local injection, when indicated
Spinal headache	History	Recumbency; hydration; analgesics; blood patch, when indicated
Drug-related headache	History	Discontinuation of the offending drug

BP, blood pressure; CT, computed tomography; i.v., intravenous; LP, lumbar puncture; MRA, magnetic resonance arteriogram; MRI, magnetic resonance imaging

disposing factor. In addition to intracranial aneurysms and arteriovenous malformations, other vascular abnormalities, including amyloid angiopathy, cavernous angiomas, venous angiomas, dural vein thromboses, and vasculitis all increase the risk of intracerebral hemorrhage. Each of these has a distinctive time course, typical extent, prevalence, and risk of recurrence. Brain tumors and infarcts sometimes bleed. Cocaine and alcohol use may cause bleeding within the brain. Anticoagulants and antiplatelet agents promote hemorrhage. In patients who may have intracranial hemorrhages, nonsteroidal, antiinflammatory drugs must be avoided until hemorrhage is ruled out.

When symptoms and signs suggestive of intracranial hemorrhage evolve gradually over hours and days, and usually in association with fever, then an infectious cause such as pyogenic meningitis, subdural empyema, or viral encephalitis should be suspected. Severe headache and meningismus may come on very rapidly in cases of meningitis caused by rupture of an abscess or tuberculoma or when the infecting organism is *Neisseria meningitides.*

When meningismus is of acute onset, then spinal fluid must be examined emergently. In general, even if a bacterial cause is suspected, antibiotic treatment should be deferred until spinal fluid is obtained for cell count and culture. If meningococcal meningitis is strongly suspected because of an evolving ecchymotic rash, autonomic collapse, or exposure to others proven or suspected to have this infection, then it may be appropriate to treat with antibiotics before spinal puncture. Whenever symptoms and signs suggest an intracranial mass in patients presenting with meningismus, then brain CT or magnetic resonance imaging (MRI) should precede lumbar puncture, unless obtaining these neuroimages would cause a potentially dangerous delay. The priority of CT or MRI versus lumbar puncture must be individualized.

Tuberculous and fungal meningitis may present important diagnostic and treatment challenges. They often have a subacute presentation. Cerebrospinal fluid (CSF) culture results may be delayed and microscopic inspection of spinal fluid sediment may be nondiagnostic. When available, polymerase chain reaction tests can identify infecting pathogens quickly. However, once CSF is obtained for analysis, the best approach often is to begin appropriate antibiotic treatment immediately to minimize the risk of such catastrophic complications as brain infarcts, hydrocephalus, or infectious masses.

Dissection of a craniocervical artery may cause neck or ipsilateral head pain. When there is sufficient associated ischemia, the affected brain regions often are transiently dysfunctional or infarcted. Often, internal carotid dissections cause burning or pulsatile pain in the ipsilateral neck or the periorbital, nose, jaw, or frontal regions of the head. Most patients have an ipsilateral Horner's syndrome. Usually, pain from a vertebral artery dissection is in the neck or occiput. High-velocity, rotational manipulation of the neck may trigger vertebral-artery dis-

sections. When dissections of the internal carotid or vertebral arteries are suspected, then an MRA, or if that is inadequate or unavailable, conventional arteriography, is warranted. If a dissection is documented, then initial treatment includes anticoagulation and cautious normalization of blood pressure.

Malignant hypertension with papilledema may be associated with severe headache and warrants immediate treatment. However, it should be emphasized that moderate hypertension is a very unlikely cause of headache and other etiologies should be sought.

Acute angle-closure glaucoma can cause intense eye pain of rapid onset. Carbon monoxide poisoning is associated with headache. Pseudotumor cerebri often presents with chronic or recurrent head pain. Thromboses of intracranial venous sinuses and also brain infarcts resulting from arterial occlusion can cause head pain and, sometimes, associated hemorrhage.

Temporal arteritis causes bilateral or unilateral temporal or generalized dull headache in elderly and sometimes younger patients. Claudication of masticatory muscles is an important symptom. Patients often complain of a painful, tender face or scalp. In some cases, there is knobby thickening, firmness, and/or tenderness of the temporal artery on one or both sides. The low-grade fever and muscle and joint pain of polymyalgia rheumatica often are associated with temporal arteritis. Usually, the laboratory work-up is benign except for, in most cases, a substantially elevated erythrocyte sedimentation rate. When temporal arteritis is suspected, treatment with steroids should be initiated quickly because it can prevent incipient retinal infarction. Once steroids are administered, temporal artery biopsy can be carried out. However, this biopsy should be deferred until testing has documented that the temporal artery to be biopsied does not supply the brain, as may occur when there is significant occlusion of the ipsilateral internal carotid. Treatment with steroids usually continues for months or longer. The dose is tapered by using head pain and the sedimentation rate as guides.

In most instances, headaches do not require urgent diagnostic tests. In patients with chronic head pain, associated symptoms and the temporal pattern of recurrences are the most important diagnostic clues.

HEADACHES DUE TO INCREASED INTRACRANIAL PRESSURE

Headache is most likely to occur when there is an increased pressure gradient between intracranial compartments. Such gradients may stretch or distort pain-sensitive structures such as the dura, arachnoid, blood vessels, and/or nerves. This occurs most commonly when an intracerebral mass lesion such as a tumor; subdural, epidural, or intraparenchymal hemorrhage; abscess; or parameningeal infection is present. Other symptoms depend on the specific brain structures that are affected. For example, a posterior fossa mass may compress the cerebral aqueduct, causing hydrocephalus. Consequent symptoms may include a decreased level of consciousness, apathy, and akinetic mutism. Direct compression of the brainstem and/or cerebellum may cause compounding nausea, vomiting, and ataxia. The headache from an intracerebral mass lesion may worsen abruptly with bending over and may awaken the patient from sleep during the night.

Headache also may result from apparently generalized increased intracranial pressure. The best example is idiopathic intracranial hypertension (IIH), also called pseudotumor cerebri or benign intracranial hypertension, in which intracranial pressure may be markedly increased. Seventy-five percent of patients with IIH have headaches. IIH occurs most frequently in obese young women. Eight women are affected for every man. In some cases, IIH is associated with menstrual irregularity, pregnancy, use of oral contraceptives, weight gain, excessive intake of vitamin A, withdrawal from corticosteroids, or treatment with tetracycline, nitrofurantoin, or nalidixic acid. In a minority of patients, there may be a history of prior head injury or meningitis. Common symptoms may include headache, pulsatile tinnitus, or less frequently, diplopia. Neurologic signs may include papilledema, and rarely, dysfunction of the sixth cranial nerve, and even less frequently, the third, fifth, or seventh cranial nerves. CT or MRI of the head may document small slitlike ventricles and, sometimes, an empty sella. A spinal tap quantifies increased pressure, above 250 mm of H_2O, with normal CSF cell counts and chemistries, while at the same time, serving as a means of pressure reduction. When obese patients with pseudotumor lose weight, their CSF pressure may normalize and their symptoms may resolve. If the patient is taking a nonessential hormone, such as an estrogen-containing birth-control pill or another causative medication, then its discontinuation should be the first priority. If CSF pressure remains elevated, then serial lumbar punctures, sometimes combined with diuretic treatment, are warranted. Acetazolamide is often the diuretic of choice. If those measures are insufficient, then dexamethasone treatment may reduce pressure. In the most refractory cases, a lumbar-peritoneal or ventriculo-peritoneal shunt can be installed. It is important to be aware that tonsillar herniation is a rare complication of lumbar-peritoneal shunting in adults but substantially more common in children. In most children, the herniation is asymptomatic, but serious consequences requiring surgical intervention occur in a small minority. In children, serial MRIs to look for tonsillar herniation may be warranted. In IIH, a reduction in CSF pressure is important because long-term elevations can result in permanent impairment of vision in 4% to 12% of cases.

The possibility of subdural hematoma must not be neglected. A history of trauma followed by unilateral headache, hemiparesis, and drowsiness is powerfully suggestive. However, the causative trauma may be remote, minimal, or there may be no history of trauma at all. Patients taking medications with anticoagulant or antiplatelet effects, the latter including all nonsteroidal analgesics, are at much increased risk for developing subdural hematomas. Lateralizing signs may be absent. CT is an important diagnostic aid, but bilateral, subdural collections often are missed if the patient is sufficiently anemic or if the CT is obtained during the interval (1 to 6 weeks) when the collections may be isodense with adjacent brain tissue.

HEADACHES DUE TO DECREASED INTRACRANIAL PRESSURE

Cerebrospinal hypotension may follow diagnostic lumbar puncture, myelography, or spinal anesthesia. Low intracranial pressure can cause headaches elicited by sitting or upright posture and relieved when the patient lies flat. Perhaps, the most common cause is the headache that occurs in 13% to 40% of patients who undergo lumbar puncture. Once it develops, usually during the hours following the procedure, the headache typically recurs when the patient assumes the upright position and markedly diminishes within minutes after lying flat. Nausea, vomiting, and, rarely, a sixth cranial nerve paresis may occur. Remaining recumbent for hours after the procedure does not reduce the incidence of headache. The larger the caliber of the needle used to puncture the dura, the higher the probability of a spinal headache. Only 2.5% of patients whose spinal tap was done using a needle with a conical tip and side aperture developed postlumbar puncture headaches. Most often, headaches caused by spinal taps last days or weeks. Treatment includes hydration and bedrest. In refractory cases, epidural injection, at the level of the spinal tap, of a patient's own nonanticoagulated blood relieves the spinal headache in most cases.

Any cause of leakage of CSF resulting from head trauma, erosion of the meninges by an invasive tumor, dural tear, or avulsion of a spinal root can cause intracranial hypotension. Also, it can result from infections of the meninges or brain, dehydration, hyperventilation, uremia, or intravenous infusion of hypertonic solutions. In addition, intracranial hypotension can be idiopathic. As with postlumbar puncture headaches, others caused by reduced intracranial pressure are postural. CSF pressure tends to be below 60 mm H_2O. MRI may document downward "sagging" of the cerebellum and brainstem. With gadolinium injection, there may be enhancement of the meninges.

MIGRAINE

The province of migraine is difficult to determine because the diagnostic criteria of the International

Headache Society do not distinguish it from the cervical headache. Migraines tend to begin in adolescence, sometimes preceded by related symptoms such as bouts of vomiting and/or abdominal pain, increased susceptibility to motion sickness, and vertigo during childhood. In adults, women are affected three times as often as men, while in children, the male to female ratio is approximately 1:1. Pregnancy may be associated with a relative remission of common migraine, whereas the use of birth-control pills may exacerbate preexistent migraine or precipitate an initial attack. By middle age, migraines may cease to occur or change their quality. A more than chance association between migraine and hypertension, myocardial infarction, and stroke has been described. Usually, migraine is familial.

Estimates of the prevalence of migraine vary according to the method of epidemiologic analysis, the population studied, and definitions used. In two large studies, in America and France, respectively, the prevalence of migraine was 18% in women and 6% in men. High-income patients report migraine more frequently, but epidemiologic studies have not confirmed a relationship between migraine prevalence and intelligence or social class. Migraine and epilepsy are comorbid.

Historically, migrainous aura and headaches were ascribed to constriction and then dilation of cerebral and extracranial arteries, respectively. However, there has not been convincing evidence that these arteries are more dilated during headaches compared with headache-free periods.

The nerve terminals on pain-sensitive cranial arteries contain neurotransmitters. Most of these terminals arise from neurons in the trigeminal ganglia that contain substance P and calcitonin gene-related peptide. In rats, stimulation of these trigeminal neurons terminating on dural blood vessels triggered extravasation of plasma with release of substance P and other vasoactive peptides. It has been suggested that substance P may mediate local neuroinflammatory changes in the trigeminal nerve or its branches that underlie vascular head pain, supporting a theory of peripheral nervous system mechanisms in the genesis of migraines. However, a substance P inhibitor did not abort migraines. Furthermore, it does not appear that substance P is released during migraine attacks. There is substantial evidence of brain-centered mechanisms of migraine that a peripheral theory alone cannot explain. The pathophysiology of migraine and its triggers remain only partially defined.

Administration of prostaglandin A_1, a vasodilator, can elicit a headache in nonmigraineurs.

Experimental evidence and clinical experience support the role of serotonin in migraine. Migraine treatment has long relied on drugs that mimic or block serotonin. Agonists of 1B and 1D 5-hydroxytryptamine ($5HT_{1B}$ and $5HT_{1D}$) receptors have been used widely to abort incipient migraines. Some migraine prophylactic drugs, such as pro-

pranolol, block $5HT_{2B}$ receptors. These receptors may be involved in release of nitric oxide, which can, in turn, trigger a migraine. Platelets of migraineurs aggregate more readily than those of controls, and platelets contain most of the serotonin present in blood. Retinal and cerebral symptoms of migrainous aurae may be from platelet clumping and vasoconstriction resulting from serotonin release.

Brain factors clearly play a role in migraine. Stress, attention, expectation, anxiety, and mood affect these headaches. Treatments that induce relaxation can provide relief. Depressed patients are more likely to develop migraines. Depression intensifies pain. Conversely, patients with severe migraines are more likely to be depressed. Migraine also is associated with an increased prevalence of bipolar disorder and anxiety.

The similarity between the clinical manifestations of migraine and the narcotic abstinence syndrome prompted investigation of the endogenous opiate receptor systems in migraineurs. A decreased level of CSF opiates during migraine attack (when elevated levels would be expected) and hypersensitivity of receptors to 5-hydroxytryptamine may suggest that an abnormality in the opiate and other neurotransmitter-binding sites occurs in individuals prone to migraine. Continued emotional stress results in release of endogenous opiates, and the sudden cessation of tension may cause an abrupt drop in endogenous opiate levels. This may account for the common occurrence of migraine on weekends and when vacations begin. There are decreased peripheral blood mononuclear cell β-endorphin concentrations in both patients whose migraines occur with and without aura. When children with migraine were treated with either acupuncture or sham acupuncture, the degree of relief experienced was proportionate to the rise in plasma panopioid and β-endorphin levels. Matched children without migraines had higher levels of panopioids than migraineurs.

Migraine is genetically complex. Studies of monozygotic and dizygotic twins have supported a genetic contribution to migraine. When the parents of patients with migraine without aura were interviewed directly, 91% of the patients had one or both parents with migraines. This finding suggests an autosomal-dominant transmission. The rare syndrome of mitochondrial encephalomyopathy, lactic acidosis, and strokelike episodes (MELAS), has been attributed to a mutation of mitochondrial DNA. More recently, familial hemiplegic migraine (FHM) was linked to a mutation of chromosome 19 in 55% of FHM families. Later, FHM in 15% of families was linked to chromosome 1. In the remaining 30% of FHM families, there was no linkage to either chromosome 1 or 19, supporting a yet-to-be defined heterogeneity. It is not clear whether common forms of migraine are linked to mutations on chromosomes 1 or 19.

In a minority of patients, behavioral symptoms occur during the day before a migraine. Euphoria, irritability, depression, hunger, thirst, and drowsiness are common.

The nature of these symptoms is consistent with a locus of dysfunction within the brain, possibly involving the hypothalamus and limbic system.

In classic migraine, an aura, possibly caused by cerebral ischemia, precedes the headache. A zone of reduced cerebral blood flow spreads at the rate of approximately 2 to 3 mm per minute across the cortex and the spread of sensory symptoms across limbs takes place at a corresponding rate. Often, visual symptoms herald an attack. They may include scotomata and even hemianopsia, light or dark floaters, shimmering vision, defocusing, or alterations in visual perception such as micropsia. Other symptoms attributable to transient dysfunction of brain structures supplied by the vertebrobasilar circulation may precede the headache. These may include vertigo, partial ophthalmoplegia (especially affecting the oculomotor nerve), transient amnesia, paresthesias, or weakness. Aphasia or other signs of insufficient anterior circulation may constitute the aura. The headaches of classic migraine vary in duration but usually last several hours. There may be a throbbing quality to the pain. Frequently, the headache is unilateral.

Common migraines lack the aura of classic migraines. However, photophobia and hyperacusis often are present. Often, patients awaken with the headache. Sleep, even a nap, may reduce the pain intensity and duration. Anorexia, nausea, and/or vomiting may be present. Individual migraineurs report that certain foods, such as fermented cheeses, red wine, and the additive monosodium glutamate, may precipitate their headaches. The common migraine, like the classical type, tends to be unilateral. Usually, if many headaches have occurred, each side of the head has been affected at one time or another. If recurrent headaches are always on the same side, then a vascular malformation, tumor, and other lesions of the head and neck should be considered.

In both classic and common migraine, patients prefer to remain recumbent in a dark, quiet environment. This distinguishes them from patients with some other recurrent headaches, such as cluster headaches, that may be characterized by motoric restlessness. Often, if they fall asleep during a migraine, patients awaken with reduced or absent pain.

The symptoms and signs of migrainous prodrome are more often because of transient dysfunction within the distribution of the posterior rather than anterior circulation. If brainstem structures innervating the extraocular muscles are affected, then ophthalmoplegic migraine may result. Similarly, if the corticospinal system is affected, then hemiplegic migraine is manifest. Aphasia can occur as an expression of migraine. If the neurologic deficits from migraine persist for more than 24 hours, complicated migraine is diagnosed. When migraine presents with an objective neurologic deficit, a prior history compatible with migraine may help to distinguish migraine from stroke or hemorrhage.

Often, migraine can be relieved by sleep induced in a dark, quiet environment. When necessary, sleep onset can be hastened with hypnotic or sedating anxiolytic drug treatment.

No single analgesic is predictably superior for treatment of migraine. All tend to be most effective if begun early during the headache. Often, acetaminophen, acetylsalicylic acid, and combinations of the two with or without added caffeine provide sufficient relief for mild to moderate headaches. Combinations of a barbiturate, caffeine, and either aspirin or acetaminophen are commonly prescribed for mild to moderate pain and have been reported to relieve severe migrainous pain in some patients. Nonsteroidal antiinflammatory drugs (NSAIDs) also can be helpful. All of these can cause dyspepsia or, when taken repeatedly, gastritis or ulceration. When the patient is nauseated or vomiting, indomethacin rectal suppositories can be effective while oral treatment is precluded.

Overuse of analgesics, and especially combinations of acetaminophen or acetylsalicylic acid with a barbiturate and caffeine, may perpetuate headaches. Barbiturate-containing medications can be addictive. Special caution should be exercised when the patient has a history of prior substance dependency, including smoking or overuse of alcohol.

Often, nausea and vomiting are important migraine symptoms. Metoclopramide, if the patient is not too nauseated to tolerate pills, can be helpful. Prochlorperazine also can be effective and is available as a suppository. Triptan medications, used for aborting migraines, also can reduce nausea.

A combination of metoclopramide (10 mg) and lysine acetylsalicylic acid (900 mg) has been reported to be as effective as 100 mg of oral sumatriptan in aborting a first attack of migraine. However, the effectiveness of the drug combination decreased during a second attack while sumatriptan continued to be effective.

In addition to NSAIDs, other nonopiate analgesics can reduce migraine pain. Tramadol is effective for some migraines. Gabapentin, carbamazepine, lamotrigine, divalproex, and topiramate, all anticonvulsants, may reduce pain. They are taken chronically rather than on an as-needed basis.

The availability of sumatriptan, a $5HT_1$ agonist, revolutionized the treatment of migraine. Sumatriptan does not affect the migrainous aura and it is recommended that it not be given until the aura resolves because it is more likely to reduce the subsequent headache if it is administered after the aura. Seventy percent of patients who take sumatriptan report clinical improvement within 4 hours of the onset of their migraine. Eighty-six percent report improvement within 2 hours after subcutaneous injection of sumatriptan. The FDA-approved triptan armamentarium recently has enlarged to include rizatriptan, zolmitriptan, and naratriptan. When there is nausea, then intranasal sumatriptan or sublingual rizatriptan or zolmitriptan, like intramuscular sumatriptan, may be preferred alternatives to oral triptans. As yet, there are no published head-to-head comparison studies of the various triptans. Sometimes, patients whose migraines fail to respond to one triptan, respond adequately to another.

Before the triptans became available, when nonnarcotic analgesics failed to control migraine pain, then serotonin antagonists, such as ergot, could be helpful. Nausea was a frequent side effect of ergot. It could be prevented in some patients if metoclopramide was taken approximately 1/2 hour before the ergot. If ergot was taken too frequently, the headache might reappear when an attempt was made to withdraw from it. Excessive doses caused peripheral vasoconstriction. Because of its vasoconstrictive properties, ergot was contraindicated when coronary-artery disease was suspected and in pregnant women. With triptans and many alternative analgesics available, the role of ergot treatment is diminished. However, intranasal dihydroergotamine (DHE) can be effective and well tolerated in some patients who respond inadequately to triptan treatment.

Opiates rarely are indicated in the treatment of migraine. However, when severe migraines are infrequent and other measures noted above have failed, and there are no contraindications such as a history of substance abuse, then abortive treatment for migraines with opiates can be reasonable. For mild to moderate pain, combinations of acetaminophen and codeine or oxycodone are reasonable. Alternatively, slow-release oxycodone can be prescribed. For rare, very severe migraines, hydromorphone may be appropriate. Butorphanol, an opiate agonist/antagonist, can provide pain relief. However, it is expensive and provides no therapeutic benefit relative to opiate analgesics.

In general, if there is good communication between patient and physician, then emergency room treatment should be required very rarely for treatment of migraines. Often, in the emergency room, physicians with neurologic expertise are not immediately available. Treatment often is delayed. The emergency room environment may exacerbate the patient's anxiety and this may intensify the head pain. However, in those uncommon instances when a very severe migraine continues despite nonnarcotic analgesics, triptans, or serotonin antagonists, then more aggressive treatment requiring parenteral treatment may need to be considered. In adults without excessive vulnerability to hypotension or heart failure, intravenous hydration with injection of 7.5 mg of chlorpromazine up to a net dose of 30 mg can be effective. During the infusion, blood pressure and electrocardiogram must be monitored carefully. An alternative approach is the intravenous administration of 10 mg of metoclopramide followed 10 minutes later by 1 mg of DHE. From 0.5 to 1 mg of DHE may be infused hourly as needed as long as the cumulative dose does not exceed 3 mg in 1 day or 6 mg in 1 week. DHE should not be used in patients who may have cardiac or cerebral ischemia. Parenteral opioids combined with an antiemetic or steroids are sometimes required if other approaches are contraindicated or insufficient.

If headaches are severe or frequent, then prophylactic medication may be warranted. β-Blockers, tricyclic antidepressants, trazodone, verapamil, and divalproex can be helpful. β-Blockers are contraindicated when there is a question of asthma or idiopathic hypertrophic subaortic stenosis, and, should only be considered with caution if there is a history of possible depression. Trazodone and tricyclics can cause a morning hangover, and, the latter more than the former, anticholinergic side effects and weight gain. Divalproex can cause weight gain, especially in women. Cyproheptadine and monoamine-inhibitor antidepressants provide less-predictable migraine prophylaxis. Newer anticonvulsants such as gabapentin, lamotrigine, and topiramate may reduce the intensity of pain. If these fail, then prophylaxis with methysergide, a serotonin blocker, can be considered. After every 3 months of treatment, it must be stopped for 4 weeks to reduce the risk of retroperitoneal fibrosis or other serious connective-tissue dysfunction. Methysergide is contraindicated in patients with ischemic heart disease, severe hypertension, peripheral vascular disease, phlebitis, peptic ulcer, hepatic or renal failure, valvular heart disease, or collagen disease.

Taking high-estrogen, oral contraceptive pills exacerbates migraines. Low-dose estrogen oral contraceptives may not increase the intensity or frequency of migraines. Use of estrogen for contraception may increase the risk of brain infarction.

In 60% of premenopausal women migraineurs, migraines recur or intensify during the days before menstruation. This corresponds with the nadir of plasma estradiol and progesterone. Progesterone supplementation did not delay the onset of migraines in women with menstrual migraines but estradiol supplementation did. In many women with catamenial migraines, prophylaxis can be achieved by preventing the drop in estrogen that occurs before menstruation. Application of an estrogen patch 2 days before the onset of menstruation prevented migraines in 18 of 26 women compared with one of seven placebo-treated controls. Daily treatment with 2.5 mg of bromocriptine reduced migraine frequency in 75% of women.

Most women migraineurs have relief from migraines during pregnancy, and this is independent of the sex of the fetus. Women with a history of catamenial migraines are substantially more likely to go through pregnancy without migraines compared with women whose migraines are not coupled to their menstrual cycles.

OTHER UNLATERAL HEADACHES WITH AUTONOMIC FEATURES

Cluster headaches are much less common than migraines and affect men five to nine times more frequently than women. The pain, most often in and around an eye, may radiate to adjacent upper and lower face regions innervated by the ophthalmic and maxillary divisions, and less commonly, the mandibular division of the trigeminal nerve. Typically, the pain is excruciating and a dull remnant often persists between attacks. Most patients' pain is on the same side each time. Commonly, cluster headaches interrupt sleep. In most cases, the headaches last 15 to 90 minutes. Unlike migraineurs who seek to remain recumbent and immobile during headaches, many cluster headache patients walk about. Some apply pressure to the affected eye or the ipsilateral superficial temporal artery. Ipsilateral lacrimation, coryza, conjunctival injection, nausea, ptosis and miosis, photophobia, facial flushing or pallor, temporal artery tenderness, and hyperalgesia of the face and scalp can precede or accompany the pain. Usually, the headaches occur repeatedly, one to three times per day, over a period of 4 to 8 weeks and then remit for months or years before another severe bout supervenes. Roughly one fifth of patients have chronic cluster headaches that recur frequently without any prolonged headache-free intervals over months or years.

The same triptan medications that abort migraines in a majority of patients are effective for some patients with cluster headaches. Alternatively, or in addition, inhalation of 100% oxygen for up to 20 minutes relieves up to 90% of cluster headaches. Sublingual or inhaled ergotamine tartrate, 1 mg initially with up to two repeat doses over 15 minutes, can be effective alone or in combination with oxygen. In some cases, application of 4% lidocaine solution to the sphenopalatine fossa to anesthetize the sphenopalatine ganglion can promptly relieve cluster headaches. The solution can be dripped along the lateral aspect of the nasal septum ipsilateral to the pain, or a cotton swab saturated in the solution can be inserted into the nostril and applied to the sphenopalatine fossa.

During a cluster of attacks, prophylactic treatment to prevent recurrent headaches usually is essential. Verapamil is the drug of choice. The dose is increased stepwise, with cautious monitoring for side effects, to as high as 480 mg per day, if ultimately required. Side effects may include hypotension, intolerable constipation, or dependent edema. Alternatively, lithium, ergotamine, or methysergide may provide prophylaxis. Prompt suppression of recurrent cluster headaches also may be achieved using prednisone, begun at a dose of 30 to 40 mg per day and then tapered over 2 to 3 weeks. β-blockers and tricyclic drugs usually are not effective.

Attacks of chronic paroxysmal hemicrania (CPH), often agonizing, resemble cluster headaches and the associated autonomic symptoms and signs. However, they tend to last 10 to 20 minutes, recurring repeatedly 10 to 15 times during the day and night. Typically they are chronic rather than clustered. Uniquely, indomethacin usually affords dramatic relief.

Frequent 15 to 60 seconds duration unilateral headaches with cluster features that recur five to 30 times per hour have been termed short-lasting unilateral neuralgiform headache attacks with conjunctival injection and tearing (SUNCT) syndrome. These headaches are reported to be refractory to treatment with indomethacin or carbamazepine.

CERVICAL HEADACHES

One insufficiently recognized cause of headaches is irritation of one or more of the upper three cervical–spinal roots or their branches. Sjaastad and his colleagues described strict diagnostic criteria for what they term cervicogenic headache. Unfortunately, in the view of this writer, the entity they have defined represents a very small proportion of headaches attributable to injury or irritation of upper-cervical spinal roots or their branches. An alternative label proposed for neck-caused head pain is cervical headache or upper-cervical syndrome.

Headaches caused by upper-cervical spinal root irritation can be occipital, temporal, parietal, frontal, or orbital. The pain can be a pressure, aching, steady, or like a constricting band around the head. Sometimes, a lancinating pain compounds the more steady pain. At times, the pain can be throbbing. Uncommonly, there are compounding migrainous features such as photophobia or nausea. Retroauricular pain and, sometimes, ipsilateral paresthesias of the lateral face are described. Rarely, there can be odd sensations of liquid dribbling or formication. Car riding, straining the neck, extreme range-of-motion movements, and sleeping sitting up all may trigger or exacerbate these headaches. Not infrequently, there is a history of recent or remote neck injury, maintenance of an awkward sitting posture sitting for hours per day at a workstation, or a recent involvement in vigorous, often jarring, exercise. Neurologic exam may reveal signs of cervical spondylosis or myelopathy. Often, there are paresthesias or pain in one or both arms attributable to associated involvement of lower cervical spinal roots.

Tenderness of the greater occipital nerve at the base of the skull can be a hallmark of upper-cervical root irritation. Headache caused by upper-cervical radiculopathy can awaken patients from sleep. Frequently, headaches are present on awakening, sometimes associated with an unrefreshed feeling, possibly resulting from multiple pain-related arousals during the preceding sleep periods. Nocturnal predilection may be related to excessive neck movements during sleep irritating inflamed edematous cervical roots. Furthermore, during recumbency, venous pressure in neck veins is increased, possibly compounding compression of irritated spinal roots. Excessive neck movement during sleep may account for the increased prevalence of headache reported by some authors in patients with obstructive sleep-apnea syndrome. Cervical–spinal root irritation also may play a role in migraine, because upper-cervical spinal roots innervate intracranial pain-sensitive arteries. (See also Chapter 11.)

Usually, laboratory tests including plain films, CTs, and MRIs are of little use in the diagnosis of cervical headache. Unless there is reason to suspect tumor, fracture, skeletal anomaly, or a mechanical problem such as subluxation, cervical-spine films can be deferred as long as the pain or associated symptoms do not worsen during a 2 week or more trial of conservative treatment. The duration should depend on the intensity of the pain and the degree of suspicion for underlying causes that might require more aggressive treatment. If the initial trial of treatment fails, then MRI of the neck may be warranted. Cervical radiculopathy may occur in a young person with normal MRI films of the cervical spine just as it may be absent in an elderly individual with predictable changes of cervical osteoarthritis.

Treatment of headache from cervical radiculopathy is directed to the putatively inflamed roots and their painful branches. In this writer's opinion, a restrictive cervical collar to maintain the neck in a neutral position is most helpful. Many clinicians discount the value of collars. In fact, the standard soft foam collars most often prescribed do not limit, more than minimally, neck range of motion. Also, as usually applied, standard collars maintain the neck in extension, an unfavorable position for patients with cervical–spinal root irritation. Many physicians do not instruct or convince patients to wear their collars 24 hours per day, including during sleep. In this author's experience, wearing a relatively firm custom-fitted collar for 24 hours, except for showers and driving, usually shortens the recovery time. When the pain begins to diminish, use of the collar may be reduced. Use during sleep should be maintained as a last residual of treatment until the pain resolves completely. In theory, if root dysfunction is mainly the result of edema, then pain may decrease over a period of a few days or 1 week. If root demyelination underlies the dysfunction, then pain may persist for several weeks or longer. Injection of a local anesthetic and methylprednisolone in a fan pattern across the greater occipital nerve at the base of the skull can alleviate the pain of occipital neuralgia and may lead to long-term relief. In a very small percentage of cases, when conservative treatment fails, cervical epidural steroid injection or operative foraminotomy or other decompressive operations can be considered.

Conditioning exercises can play an important role in the treatment of chronic pain. However, in the case of cervical radiculopathy, exercises that involve extreme movements of the neck (e.g., freestyle swimming and neck rolls), bouncing (e.g., jogging and high-impact aerobics), or straining (e.g., weight training with isometric contraction of neck muscles) may trigger or exacerbate pain and should be avoided until the pain resolves.

TENSION HEADACHE

Tension or muscle-contraction headache may be diagnosed more frequently than other varieties. Unfortunately, there is no sufficient evidence for a specific pathophysiology. While some patients are purported to have excessive tone of jaw and scalp muscles, it is not clear whether this is a cause of the headaches. Furthermore, treatment is nonspecific, generally consisting of analgesics, especially NSAIDs. There may be considerable overlap with other kinds of chronic headache. For example, cervical headaches, as noted above, may be exacerbated when stress or anxiety triggers excessively restless sleep, which, in turn, may increase cervical–spinal root irritation. Resolution of the underlying stress may be very therapeutic for the headache. Mild analgesics and reassurance can be sufficient therapy in some cases. Antidepressants and transcutaneous electrical stimulation also are sometimes useful along with biofeedback and other forms of relaxation therapy. Recent reports of uncontrolled studies suggest that injection of botulinum toxin A into cranial muscles provided relief of head pain attributed to tension-type headaches and migraines.

POSTTRAUMATIC HEADACHE

Chronic posttraumatic headache is defined as headache persisting for more than 2 months following an injury. As noted above, since a subdural hematoma can cause persisting or chronic recurring head pain, it must be considered. It may be difficult to assess the contribution of psychogenic factors. Personality and environment must be correlated with physical exam findings and headache pattern. Customary prolonged delays in the settlement of injury-related workmen's compensation claims and lawsuits may contribute to persisting pain. A well-localized area of scalp tenderness usually associated with hyperesthesia or hypoesthesia may result from nerve entrapment in scar or neuroma formation and may respond to 1- to 2-mL injections of a half-and-half mixture of 1% lidocaine and methylprednisolone acetate. Sometimes, a single injection may provide sustained relief. At other times, several repeated injections at weekly intervals may be required.

DRUG-RELATED HEADACHE

Some prescription drugs, including nitrates, dipyridamole, trazodone, indomethacin, cimetidine, ranitidine, gemfibrozil, simvastatin, primidone, modafinil, hydralazine, and cyclosporine can trigger headaches. Patients taking monoamine-oxidase–inhibiting drugs develop severe headaches when they eat tyramine-containing foods. Rarely, NSAID use can cause aseptic meningitis.

Chronic use, or withdrawal from chronic use, of nicotine, caffeine, ergot, triptans, anxiolytics, and analgesics can precipitate headaches. (See Chronic Daily Headaches, below.) Heavy consumption of alcohol results in hangover headaches. These may be a result of cervical–spinal root irritation precipitated by excessive neck movement during sleep associated with alcohol-induced snoring and upper-airway obstructions that trigger arousals and motoric restlessness.

CHRONIC DAILY HEADACHES

The term chronic daily headache is ambiguous. It refers to very frequent primary headaches unrelated to defined lesions or systemic illness. In a series of 300 patients admitted for chronic refractory headaches, the majority had headaches attributed to overuse of medications. Headaches resulting from drug overuse and rebound represent a large subgroup of patients with chronic daily headache. Epidemiologic surveys have documented regular use of over-the-counter (OTC) analgesics by a substantial minority of the population, often to relieve chronic headaches. A controlled study has demonstrated that caffeine withdrawal tends to precipitate headaches. No placebo-controlled study has shown that analgesic withdrawal causes headaches but there are numerous reports based on uncontrolled investigations. When patients have become physically and emotionally dependent on medications, detoxification is warranted. Psychotherapeutic support and, in some cases, hospitalization may be helpful.

PSYCHOGENIC CONTRIBUTIONS

Headaches can be a manifestation of a functional problem. Just as when any psychogenic diagnosis is considered, it is essential to remember that a conversion-reaction–prone or somatizing personality does not protect against compounding organic disease. Every patient must be given the benefit of the doubt to the extent that the full range of relevant diagnostic alternatives is explored. Conversely, psychologic factors should be investigated and treated appropriately.

Pain can promote depression, and depressed individuals may feel pain most intensely. Psychologic factors should not be ignored, no matter what the underlying or organic cause of pain.

SINUSITIS

Sinus inflammation, infectious or allergic, can cause headaches. The location of the pain reflects the particular sinus or sinuses affected. For example, maxillary sinusitis often causes malar and frontal-sinusitis brow pain. Typically, there is a pressure type of pain associated with hyperesthesia. Often, sinus headaches are associated with nasal congestion and postnasal drip. If the pathogen is anaerobic, then nasal mucous may be malodorous. Sometimes, there is fever. Patients with symptoms and signs of sinusitis often undergo CT films of the sinuses and then are treated with decongestants and antibiotics. In my opinion, this approach can be excessive. When there is no fever, treatment can begin with warm, hypertonic-saline nasal lavage. Nasal lavage with 3.5% saline appears to increase mucociliary clearance and ciliary-beat frequency. The patient can do nasal lavage by instilling warm, hypertonic saline in one nostril and then the other, using a nasal douche tube or Neti pot. With the head bent forward and tilted to the side over a sink and the lower nostril occluded, the saline is gently sucked into the upper nostril to initiate flow through the nasopharynx and out the lower nostril. Then the procedure is repeated for the opposite nostril with the head tilted to the other side. When the sinus problem appears to be allergic, then the lavage can be followed once daily with use of a steroid nasal spray. If the patient will not try, cannot use, or fails to respond to hypertonic-saline nasal lavage, then treatment with appropriate antibiotics may be warranted. When there is fever, or the patient may be immunologically compromised, then CT of the sinuses should be expedited. Severe sinogenic-intracranial complications such as brain abscess, subdural empyema, meningitis, cavernous-sinus thrombosis, epidural abscess, and osteomyelitis may occur. Fatigue can be a symptom of chronic sinusitis. When the sinus inflammation is allergic, then minimization of environmental allergens can be very helpful, especially in the bedroom. Encasing mattresses, pillows, and comforters in mite-impermeable coverings may be worthwhile when nasal congestion intensifies when the patient is in bed.

OTHER CAUSES OF HEADACHE

Headaches have been attributed to other causes such as pyrexia, hypoxia, and endocrine disorders. In addition to sinusitis, diseases of eyes, ears, nose, and throat, such as the cranial neuralgias, also may cause headache. Temporomandibular joint dysfunction has been cited frequently as a cause of headache that may require specialized treatment, such as use of an intraoral splint.

GENERAL TREATMENT OF HEADACHE

While certain headaches have a singular, especially effective treatment (i.e., indomethacin for CPH), often a variety of strategies can be helpful. Relaxation training is especially useful for patients responding poorly to stress.

Biofeedback, hypnosis, meditation, acupuncture, and conditioning exercises also may be useful. These same measures may promote more restful sleep, and thereby reduce head pain resulting from excessive neck movement during sleep.

In general, opioid analgesics are not of long-term utility and should be avoided. A large variety of analgesics, including NSAIDs, aspirin, and acetaminophen are available. Tramadol is a relatively new nonnarcotic analgesic that is effective for some patients. Even in the absence of depression, amitriptyline, trazodone, and other antidepressants may reduce the intensity of pain. Anticonvulsants, particularly gabapentin, topiramate, and carbamazepine, can help in selective cases. Also, acupuncture, massage, and transcutaneous stimulation may help.

Overall, a good care-provider–patient relationship can be critical. It often is important to distinguish empathetically hurt from harm. Patients often benefit from understanding that the intensity of pain may bear no direct relationship to the severity of the cause. Upper-cervical root irritation may trigger excruciating pain or intracerebral tumor may not cause any pain at all.

The patient's level of activity should be considered. In some cases, certain movements, such as extreme neck movement in patients with headaches from cervical radiculopathy, need to be reduced or curtailed. In other instances, exercise, such as regular conditioning exercise to help alleviate stress, should be increased.

SELECTED READINGS

Ahlskogje, O'Neill BP. Pseudotumor cerebri. *Ann Intern Med* 1982;97:249–256.

Edlow JA, Caplan LR. Avoiding pitfalls in the diagnosis of subarachnoid hemorrhage. *NEJM* 2000;342:29–36.

Ekbom K. Lithium for cluster headache: review of the literature and preliminary results of long term treatment. *Headache* 1981;12:132–139.

Foley J. Benign forms of intracranial hypertension-"toxic" and "otitic" hydrocephalus. *Brain* 1955;78:1.

Gardner WJ. Traumatic subdural hematoma with particular reference to latent interval. *Arch Neurol Psychiatry* 1932;27:847.

Giammarco R, Edmeads J, Dodick D. *Headache Management.* Hamilton, Ontario: BC Decker, 1999.

Graham JR, Bana DS. Headache. In: Warfield C, ed. *Manual of Pain Management.* Philadelphia: J.B. Lippincott, 1991:65–97.

Graham JR, Wolff HG. Mechanism of migraine headache and action of ergotamine tartrate. *Arch Gen Neurol Psychiatry* 1938;39:737–763.

Hunter CR, Mayfield FH. Role of the upper cervical nerve roots in the production of pain in the head. *Am J Surg* 1949;78:743–749.

Joutel A, Bousser M, Biousse V, et al. A gene for familial hemiplegic migraine maps to chromosome 19. *Nat Genet* 1993;5:40–45.

Kittrelle JP, Grouse DS, Sybold ME. Cluster headache: local anesthetic abortive agents. *Arch Neurol* 1985;42:496–498.

Klein RG, Campbell RJ, Hunder GG, et al. Skip lesions in temporal arteritis. *Mayo Clin Proc* 1976;51:504–510.

Lance JW, Goadsby PJ. *Mechanism and Management of Headache.* Oxford: Butterworth Heinemann, 1999.

Moskowitz MA. The neurobiology of vascular head pain. *Ann Neurol* 1984;16:157–168.

O'Brien MD. Cerebral blood changes in migraine. *Headache* 1971;10:139–143.

Skinhoi E. Hemodynamic changes from the brain during migraine. *Arch Neurol* 1973;29:95–98.

Tourtellotte W, Henderson WA, Tucker RP, et al. A randomized double-blind clinical trial comparing the 22 versus 26 gauge needle in the production of the post-lumbar puncture syndrome in normal individuals. *Headache* 1972;12:73–78.

CHAPTER 8

Ear Pain

David M. Vernick

Ear pain (otalgia) is a common complaint in general practice. Up to 80% of pediatric visits involve some problem referable to the ear. Although children tend to have more frequent ear problems than adults, otalgia in an adult is not uncommon.

Ear pain is a symptom, not a disease. It can be caused by a local condition in the ear or be referred from pathology at adjacent sites (Figs. 8.1 and 8.2). Timely and appropriate treatment involves evaluation of all possible causes. Blanket treatment of otalgia with ear drops and antibiotics may lead to some very serious diagnostic oversights. Some have argued that no antibiotic coverage should be used for most bouts of acute otitis media unless there is an immunocompromised host, a major complication, or the patient fails to improve over the first few days. These recent efforts are motivated by a desire to reduce antibiotic prescriptions and try to avoid the increasing rate of resistant organisms. While most infections do clear without antibiotics, it is impossible to tell which ones will without frequent follow-up visits to check. The wisdom and savings of this approach has yet to be proven.

Causes of ear pain can be divided into two categories: those involving problems intrinsic to the ear and those secondary to an extrinsic problem.

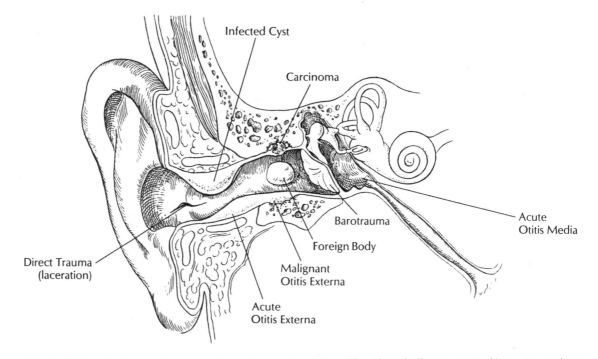

FIG. 8.1. Direct (intrinsic) causes of ear pain must be distinguished from indirect causes (those secondary to extrinsic problems) and treated accordingly. Direct causes of otalgia are acute otitis media, acute otitis externa (swimmer's ear), malignant otitis externa, barotrauma, infected cyst of the ear canal, foreign bodies, carcinomas, and direct trauma.

46

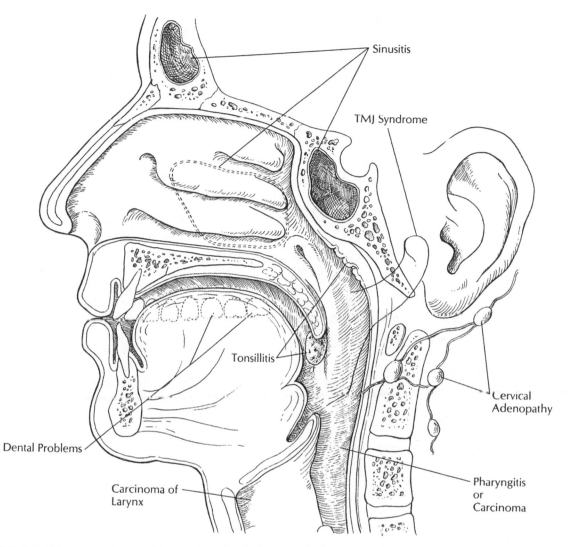

FIG. 8.2. When there is no evidence of local pathology, extrinsic causes of otalgia should be sought. These include temporomandibular joint syndrome, dental problems, pharyngitis and tonsillitis, sinusitis, cervical adenopathy, and carcinoma of the oropharynx or larynx.

INTRINSIC CAUSES

Acute Otitis Media

Acute otitis media is an infection in the middle ear, usually bacterial, although there is some evidence that viruses and Mycoplasma may be involved in some cases. It is more common in the wintertime, often with or following an upper-respiratory infection. Patients usually present with an acutely painful ear, fever, and diminished hearing. Examination shows a red, bulging drum, which may rupture and release bloody, purulent discharge. The ear canal itself is not tender. The severe pain generally lasts 24 to 48 hours, but may resolve sooner if the eardrum ruptures.

The causes of acute otitis media are, for the most part, age related. In neonates, coliform bacteria and *Staphylococcus aureus* are significant pathogens. In older children, *Streptococcus pneumoniae* and *Haemophilus*

influenzae are common. (Recent studies show that the incidence of *H. influenzae* does not decline until at least age 14.) In adults, *S. pneumoniae, Branhamella catarrhalis,* β-hemolytic streptococcus, and *H. influenzae* account for most infections.

Hospitalization and antibiotics usually are necessary for neonates because the infants are septic. For children and adults, a 10-day course of appropriate oral-antibiotic therapy usually is adequate to treat acute otitis media. Reevaluation after therapy may show that in many pediatric cases, the ears have not cleared. A second 10-day course of antibiotics should then be prescribed. If the ears have not shown significant improvement by then, an ear, nose, and throat (ENT) referral should be considered.

For children and adults, there are several choices for antibiotic therapy. Amoxicillin, cefaclor, and erythromycin are very effective. Combination drugs, such as trimethoprim-sulfamethoxazole and sulfisoxazole with erythromycin, also are effective. Newer, broad-spectrum antibiotics should be used only for treatment failures.

In most cases, if the drum does rupture, no further antibiotic therapy is needed beyond that recommended above. Ear drops can be used, however, if the canal is very irritated from the drainage. The patient must be very careful to keep water out of the ears until the eardrum has healed, which is usually about 1 week.

Pain medication should be prescribed as needed for 48 hours, until the antibiotics have had a chance to relieve the symptoms. If pain persists, the patient should be reexamined to determine the cause.

Acute Otitis Externa

Acute otitis externa (or swimmer's ear), an infection of the external ear canal, usually occurs in the summer but can occur in any season. It usually is caused by water trapped in the ear canal, with consequent maceration of the skin, or by direct trauma (e.g., from use of cotton swab sticks, which can cause a break in the skin in the ear canal). The ear canal becomes markedly tender and swollen. Pressure on the tragus exacerbates the pain. The eardrum is normal in appearance, and unless the ear canal is totally blocked, hearing is normal. With severe infections, periauricular swelling and cellulitis, along with cervical adenopathy, may be present.

Cultures of the ear canal usually grow *Pseudomonas, Proteus,* or *Staphylococcus.* Treatment involves cleaning out of the ear canal followed by the use of antibacterial ear drops (such as a combination of polymixin B sulfate, neomycin sulfate, and hydrocortisone) or drops that alter the pH of the canal (such as nonaqueous acetic acid). Addition of a steroid to the preparation seems to hasten the resolution of the canal edema. If the ear canal is almost totally occluded, use of an ear wick for about 48 hours will allow the medicine to diffuse into the canal. Oral antibiotics alone seldom are adequate therapy, but may be necessary in addition to ear drops in severe cases.

Adequate analgesics should be prescribed for 48 hours. In severe cases, it can take that long for the patient to begin to show improvement. Keeping the ear dry for several weeks is necessary to prevent recurrence of the pain and infection.

Malignant Otitis Externa

In patients who are diabetic or immunocompromised, an external ear infection may not be a simple swimmer's ear. If, in addition to otalgia, granulation tissue is present in the ear canal, or if the symptoms fail to respond to the usual treatment, a more serious infection must be suspected. Persistent pain usually means persistence of infection. Malignant otitis externa usually is caused by a *pseudomonas* infection of the skull base instead of just a superficial infection of the ear canal. When that condition

is suspected, ENT consultation should be sought, as treatment usually involves prolonged use of intravenous antibiotics and possible surgical debridement. Inadequate therapy can lead to a fatal outcome.

Barotrauma to the Ears

Changes in pressure outside the eardrum while flying or diving must be matched by changes in pressure in the middle ear. If this does not occur, the eardrum is stretched and pain ensues. Depending on the degree of pressure change involved, anything from mild discomfort and a "blocked" feeling to rupture of the eardrum and dislocation of the ossicles can occur. The best treatment is to equalize pressure through the eustachian tube either by swallowing or doing a Valsalva maneuver as the pressure changes. Use of nasal decongestants and antihistamines are intended to decrease any edema around the eustachian tube and allow for easier equalization of middle-ear pressures. After injury has occurred, only supportive therapy is of benefit. If the patient has an upper-respiratory infection, antibiotics may be beneficial to prevent an ear infection. If the patient is dizzy or has a sensorineural hearing loss after such injury, a perilymphatic fistula from rupture of the round or oval window membranes should be suspected. Surgical exploration of the ear and repair of the fistula should be undertaken.

Infected Cyst of the Ear Canal

Not all swelling and tenderness of the ear canal is otitis externa. The cartilaginous external ear canal has ceruminous glands and hair follicles that can become plugged-up and infected, causing severe otalgia with marked localized tenderness. These infections can be differentiated from routine otitis externa because only part of the ear canal is swollen and tender. Such cysts may totally occlude the ear canal if they become large enough, which makes prompt diagnosis difficult. Care must be taken not to overlook them, however, because they do not respond to local ear drops. They should be treated with oral antibiotics to cover for *Staphylococcus* and *Streptococcus*; often, the cyst will need to be incised and drained to promote healing.

Foreign Bodies

Foreign bodies in the ear can cause pain and discomfort. Almost everything that is small enough to fit into an ear canal has, at some point, been found there, including toys, beads, insects, paper, and food, to name a few. Removal of the foreign body is the only treatment. However, this may not be as simple as it sounds if it is a bead that fills the ear canal in a screaming two-year-old, or an insect clinging to the canal or drum. Care must be taken to do no harm to the ear canal and eardrum and other surrounding instruments while attempting to grasp the object. Occasionally, children may require a general anesthetic for extraction of the foreign body.

Carcinomas

Carcinomas, usually squamous-cell carcinoma or basal-cell carcinoma, can occur in the ear canal. When the tumors are superficial, they rarely cause pain. However, when they invade the bony ear canal and skull base, they can cause severe otalgia. They often present as an otitis externa that never seems to heal properly. Biopsy of the area can yield the diagnosis. Treatment depends on the extent and location of the cancer and may include surgery and radiation therapy.

Direct Trauma

Direct trauma can cause localized tenderness and swelling of the ear and ear canal and rupture of the eardrum. As with injuries in other areas, swelling usually progresses over 24 to 48 hours and then subsides. Eardrum rupture may be caused by a direct injury or by pressure changes (e.g., from a slap), with consequent otalgia and hearing loss. In severe injuries, ossicular disruption and a perilymphatic fistula can occur.

When there is only localized tissue bruising, ice and analgesics are adequate. When there is a break in the skin, local antibiotic coverage can be added to prevent infection. When there is a tear of the eardrum or ossicular disruption, treatment depends on the severity of the injury. Small, uncontaminated tears can be treated expectantly, with the ear kept dry to prevent possible infection. For small, contaminated ears, antibiotic ear drops should be added to the regimen. Most of those perforations will heal within a few weeks.

Patients with large drum tears or ossicular discontinuity after injury should be referred to an ENT physician. Early exploration, debridement, and surgical repair of severe injuries can avoid long-term problems. Patients who are dizzy after injury to the ear should be referred to an ENT physician immediately for suspected perilymphatic fistula. Early exploration and repair of the fistula may save the patient's hearing.

EXTRINSIC CAUSES

When examination of the ear reveals no pathology, a diagnosis of an early ear infection with no physical findings should not be made. A thorough search for other possible causes should be undertaken. Not all otalgia is otologic in origin.

Temporomandibular Joint Syndrome

Temporomandibular joint syndrome is one of the most common causes of referred ear pain. The temporo-mandibular joint makes up part of the external ear canal. Any stresses, strains, or inflammation of the joint can cause local pain and swelling. A history of increased pain on chewing or of recent dental work may give a clue to this diagnosis. Many patients also have radiation of pain up to the temple or down into the neck. Gentle pressure over the joint, either intraorally or externally, to reproduce the symptoms usually can confirm the diagnosis. Treatment is aimed at resting and relieving the stress on the joint. Heat to the area, aspirin or ibuprofen, and a soft diet are usually adequate for mild cases. When the problem persists, a specialist in this syndrome should be consulted.

Dental Problems

The first symptom of many dental problems is an earache. Children who are cutting teeth often pull at their ears, and many people with carious teeth or root abscesses complain that they have an earache. A good dental history and an examination often can turn up an occult cause for the otalgia. Appropriate treatment ranges from simple analgesics for tooth eruptions to dental referral for more significant pathology.

Pharyngitis and Tonsillitis

Pharyngitis and tonsillitis can cause an earache in addition to a sore throat. Ear pain is also a common complaint in patients who have undergone tonsillectomy. Clearly, acute otitis media can and frequently does accompany pharyngeal infections. However, a complaint of otalgia should not be interpreted as an imminent or early ear infection. Treatment of the pharyngitis is adequate therapy.

Sinusitis

Sinusitis can occasionally present with otalgia. A thorough exam of the perinasal sinuses is necessary for a patient with otalgia of no obvious cause. A thorough nasal exam, nasal endoscopy, and possibly sinus x-rays or computed tomography are important to make the diagnosis.

Cervical Adenopathy

Children are especially susceptible to cervical adenopathy. Often, the adenopathy is much more obvious and symptomatic than the underlying cause. Even minor injuries such as scrapes or cuts can cause notable adenopathy. Tender cervical nodes, especially high-anterior cervical nodes, can produce pain referred to the ears. When tender cervical nodes are found to explain the otalgia, the cause of the adenopathy must be sought and appropriate treatment instituted.

Carcinoma

Carcinoma of the oropharynx, nasopharynx, hypopharynx, or larynx may be signaled by unilateral otalgia in an adult, especially one who is a smoker or drinker. If no other source for the otalgia is found, a thorough ENT examination is mandatory. If nothing is found and the pain persists, radiologic and endoscopic evaluations of the upper airway may be necessary (with biopsies of such areas as the nasopharynx, tonsils, and base of the tongue, where occult malignancies can hide).

Other Extrinsic Causes

Glossopharyngeal neuralgia and some atypical facial neuralgias may present with pain radiating to the ear. Herpes zoster of the geniculate ganglion (Ramsey–Hunt syndrome) also often presents with otalgia associated with typical herpetiform lesions of the external canal. Treatment includes analgesics, antiviral medication, and steroids. Pain may persist long past the resolution of the external lesions.

SUMMARY

Otalgia is a symptom, not a diagnosis. Accurate diagnosis and appropriate therapy rest on careful history and physical examination. When the cause is unclear, continued observation and consultation should be the course of action.

SELECTED READINGS

Bass JW, Cashman TM, Frostad AL, et al. Antimicrobials in the treatment of acute otitis media. A second clinical trial. *Am J Dis Child* 1973;125: 397–402.

Buchanan BJ, Hoagland J, Fescher PR. Pseudoephedrine and air travel-associated ear pain in children. *Arch Pediatr Adolesc Med* 1999;153: 466–468.

Chandler JR. Malignant external otitis: further considerations. *Ann Otol Rhinol Laryngol* 1977;86:417–428.

Gacek RR, Goodman M. Management of malignancy of the temporal bone. *Laryngoscope* 1987;77:1622–1634.

Henderson FW, Collier AM, Sanyal M, et al. A longitudinal study of respiratory viruses and bacteria in the etiology of acute otitis media with effusion. *N Engl J Med* 1982;306:1377.

Ishiyama A. Why does air travel cause earaches? *West J Med* 1999;171: 106.

Kontiokari T, Koivunen P, Niemela M, et al. Symptoms of acute otitis media. *Pediatr Infect Dis J* 1998;17:676–679.

Laxdal OE, Merida J, Jones RH. Treatment of acute otitis media: a controlled study of 142 children. *Con Med Assoc J* 1970;102:263–268.

Lewis JS. Surgical management of tumors of the middle ear and mastoid. *J Laryngol Otol* 1983;97:299–311.

Licameli GR. Diagnosis and management of otalgia in the pediatric patient. *Pediatr Ann* 1999;28:364–368.

Loracy P, Houghten P. Treatment of acute suppurative otitis media. *J Laryngol Otol* 1977;91:331.

Parkin JL. Antimicrobial treatment of otitis media: penicillins, cephalosporins, sulfonamides. *Otolaryngol Head Neck Surg* 1981;89:376–380.

Peterkin GAG. Otitis externa. *J Laryngol Otol* 1974;88;15–21.

Rose DS. Acute suppurative otitis media. *Pediatrics* 1975;56:285.

Shumrick DA, Paparella MM, eds. Earaches. In: *Otolaryngology*, 2nd ed., vol. 2. Philadelphia: WB Saunders Co., 1980:1354–1357.

Saah AJ, Blackwelder WC, Kaslow RA. Treatment of acute otitis media. *JAMA* 1982;248:1071–1072.

Stickler GB, Rubenstein MM, McBean JB, et al. Treatment of acute otitis media in children. IV. A fourth clinical trial. *Am J Dis Child* 1967;114: 123–130.

Strohm M, ed. *Trauma of the Middle Ear*. New York: Karger, 1986.

Strome M, Kelly JH, Fried MP, eds. Ear. In: *Manual of Otolaryngology: Diagnosis and Therapy*. Boston: Little Brown Co., 1985:45–86.

Taylor JS. Otitis externa: treatment using a new expandable wick. *South Med J* 1975;68:698, 732.

Vernick DV. The painfully discharging ear. In: Branch WT, Jr., ed. *Office Practice in Medicine*. Philadelphia: WB Saunders Co., 1987.

Zaky DA, Bentley DW, Lowy K, et al. Malignant otitis externa, a severe form of otitis in diabetic patients. *Am J Med* 1976;61:298–302.

CHAPTER 9

Eye Pain

George K. Asdourian and Christine Peeters-Asdourian

Pain is not a common presentation of major blinding eye diseases, yet pain can be the first and presenting symptom of many diseases involving either the eye alone or its surrounding structures (Table 9.1). Pain in and around the eye is a common patient complaint that the physician cannot dismiss. Ocular pain requires prompt attention, as some conditions such as acute angle-closure glaucoma, if left untreated, may cause structural damage and blindness.

SENSORY INNERVATION OF THE EYE AND THE ORBIT

The optic nerve is an extension of the central nervous system arising from the retinal ganglion cells. It does not carry nociceptive information, though optic neuritis can be a painful condition. The ophthalmic V_1 and maxillary V_2 divisions of the trigeminal nerve provide the sensory innervation of the eye, the adnexa and the orbit. The sensory innervation of the globe is mediated through the ophthalmic division (V_1) of the trigeminal nerve (Fig. 9.1). The ciliary nerves, which are derived from the nasociliary branch of the ophthalmic nerve, provide a dense network of sensory endings to the cornea and the sclera. The conjunctiva has a lesser amount of innervation and thus is associated with minimal amount of pain. The iris and the choroid have a small network of sensory nerves while the ciliary muscle has no sensory nerve and the ciliary body, in contrast, has a rich sensory network, adjacent to the base of the iris. The ophthalmic nerve, before entering the superior orbital fissure, gives off several recurrent meningeal branches, which innervate the pain-sensitive dura, and segments of the blood vessels at the basis of the brain, the middle cerebral artery, and the circle of Willis. Pathology in those areas may refer pain to the eye. The lacrimal and the frontal nerves of V_1 provide sensory innervation of the orbit. The lacrimal nerve supplies the conjunctiva contiguous to the lacrimal gland. The frontal nerve supplies the forehead, scalp, and upper lid through the supraorbital and supratrochlear branches. Pain in the orbit can result from direct mechanical stimulation or from a combination of tissue distortion, vasodilation, and chemical inflammation. The maxillary division V_2 of the trigeminal nerve provides innervation to the lower eyelid via the infraorbital nerve.

TABLE 9.1. *Painful Conditions of the Eye and the Periocular Structures*

Eyelid
  Chalazion, tumor
Cornea
  Foreign body
  Keratitis
Sclera
  Scleritis
  Episcleritis
Uveal tissue
  Ciliary body spasm
  uveitis (anterior and posterior)
Intraocular pressure
  Acute angle-closure glaucoma
  chronic angle-closure glaucoma
Orbit
  Orbital cellulitis
  Orbital tumors
  Orbital pseudotumor
  Optic neuritis

OCULAR DISEASES CAUSING PAIN

For patients presenting with the symptom of pain in and around the eye, the physician first should rule out specific ocular diseases that may be responsible for the symptom. Often, pain is a nonspecific symptom and its description by the patient provides little insight as to the anatomical source of the pain. A careful history and thorough ophthalmic examination usually can pinpoint the cause of the pain and direct the physician to a definitive diagnosis and treatment of the condition. A systematic examination of the orbit, the

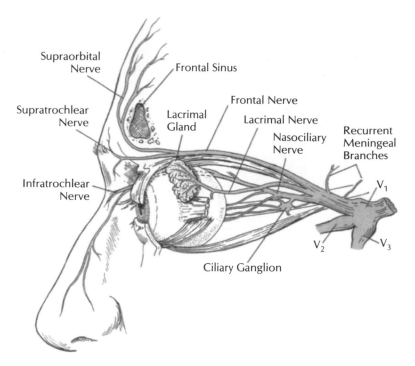

FIG. 9.1. The eye's extraordinary sensitivity to pain arises from the trigeminal nerve's ophthalmic (V_1) division. The nasociliary branch of the ophthalmic nerve supplies the whole eye and the side of the nose. The other branches supply the upper eyelid, the lacrimal system, the forehead, and the frontal sinus. Adapted from Tang RA, Pardo G. *Focal Points Volume XIV*. San Francisco: American Academy of Ophthalmology, 1996, with permission (illustration by Christine Gralapp).

eyelids, and the eye is essential. If no definite diagnosis is established, ancillary tests may be required as dictated by patient's history and clinical findings.

Eyelids

Acute infection and inflammation may involve any of the layers of the eyelid causing dermatitis, cellulitis, and blepharitis. Pain is a common symptom. A *hordeolum* (stye) is a localized staphylococcal infection of the meibomian gland (internal hordeolum) or the glands of Zeiss and Moll (external hordeolum). The eyelid swelling usually is obvious and the treatment involves hot compresses and (local/topical) antibiotics.

Lacrimal Gland and Lacrimal Drainage System

Acute infection of the lacrimal gland (dacryoadenitis) usually causes pain and swelling in the superotemporal aspect of the eye. It may be secondary to infection by different types of bacteria or viral in origin. Dacryocystitis (inflammation of the lacrimal sac) usually is associated with obstruction of the nasolacrimal duct. In acute dacryocystitis, which usually is caused by bacteria, there is an area of tender swelling below the lid margin, nasally.

For these conditions, the treatment is topical antibiotics and/or systemic antibiotics.

Conjunctiva

Conjunctivitis (inflammation of the conjunctiva) is a very common ocular condition and manifests itself with conjunctival injection, tearing, discharge, itching, and minimal pain. Bacterial conjunctivitis usually is accompanied by mucopurulent discharge while viral conjunctivitis produces copious tearing. The treatment of bacterial conjunctivitis is with the appropriate antibiotics, while most viral conjunctivitis have a self-limiting course and require no treatment.

Cornea

The cornea can be involved in a multitude of conditions that can cause extreme pain, as the cornea contains a dense plexus of nerves and is acutely sensitive to pain. Corneal pain usually is intense and may spread in the distribution of the trigeminal nerve to the forehead and periorbital region. The pain from a corneal pathology usually is accompanied by photophobia, lacrimation, and blepharospasm. Trauma to the cornea with foreign bodies is a common occurrence and usually is associated with corneal epithelial abrasion. The patient complains of considerable pain and foreign-body sensation beneath the upper lid as a result of eyelid movement over the foreign body. Inspection of the cornea with a penlight or the slit-lamp usually localizes the foreign body, which can be removed after instillation of a topical anesthetic. Topical antibiotics may be applied to prevent secondary infections.

Corneal abrasion from trauma without a foreign body also can cause severe pain and tearing. It may require patching of the eye for proper corneal epithelial healing. Recurrent corneal erosions sometimes follow because of deficiency of attachment of the regenerated epithelium to the corneal-basement membrane. Recurrent episodes of pain and tearing usually on awakening in the morning are typical symptoms. Ophthalmologic consultation is necessary for treatment of the condition. Corneal infections are not common, but when present and not recognized and properly treated can lead to corneal scarring, perforations, and intraocular infection with possible complete loss of vision and in rare cases, loss of the eye. Infectious keratitis and corneal ulcers can be secondary to infection by bacteria, viruses, and fungi. The majority of these infections follow trauma to the corneal epithelium. Referral for treatment is recommended.

Another very painful condition involving the cornea is ultraviolet keratitis or photophthalmia resulting from exposure to damaging ultraviolet rays from arc welders, sunlamps, or reflected sunlight on snow. Treatment for these conditions include patching and the use of cycloplegics.

Apart from trauma, keratitis also can be the result of toxic reaction to topical medications, chronic use of topical anesthetics, or allergic states causing bullous keratitis. In keratoconjunctivitis sicca or idiopathic dry-eye syndrome, the patient often complaints of a foreign-body sensation associated with itching, burning, redness, photophobia, and excessive tearing. This occurs most commonly in older women where the normal constituents of the tear film are progressively lost. Currently, there is no cure for keratoconjunctivitis sicca and therapy is directed for amelioration of symptoms. Treatment consists of eliminating most eye and facial cosmetics and using tear substitutes as needed for comfort during the day and ocular lubricants at bedtime.

Sclera and Episclera

Scleritis and episcleritis usually manifest themselves as localized areas of injection associated with an aching pain. The condition can occur in isolation or secondary to systemic disease such as rheumatoid arthritis. It usually responds to topical-steroid therapy.

Uveal Tract

Inflammation of the anterior uveal structures (iris and ciliary body) causes iritis, iridocyclitis, or cyclitis. Symptoms include blurry vision and periocular pain. The pain may be referred to the ear, teeth, or sinuses or may occur in the distribution of the ophthalmic division (V_1) of the trigeminal nerve. The pain, in part, is from ciliary muscle spasm. Examination reveals injection around the limbus, which has a purplish-red color (in contradistinction to the bright-red injection seen in conjunctivitis). Tearing, photophobia, and blepharospasm are common. The pupil is miotic and slit-lamp biomicroscopy reveals cells and flare in the anterior chamber as well as keratitic precipitate (KP) on the corneal endothelium.

In the majority of cases, no correlation with systemic disease is found, although one should always consider trauma, Reiter's syndrome, Behçet's disease, and ankylosing spondylitis in the differential diagnosis. Ocular treatment is usually with cycloplegics and steroids.

Glaucoma—Angle-Closure Glaucoma

In acute angle-closure glaucoma, which is a true ocular emergency, there is sudden elevation of the intraocular pressure (IOP). This occurs secondary to a mechanism termed "pupillary block." A middilated pupil causes a contact between the iris and the lens and obstructs the flow of aqueous from the posterior to the anterior chamber (Fig. 9.2). The increased pressure in the posterior chamber causes anterior bowing of the iris (iris bombé) and secondary obstruction of the anterior chamber angle. Exposure to dim light, emotional upset with associated sympathetic stimulation, and use of pharmacological agents with anticholinergic or sympathomimetic properties all result in pupillary dilation and potential angle closure in predisposed eye.

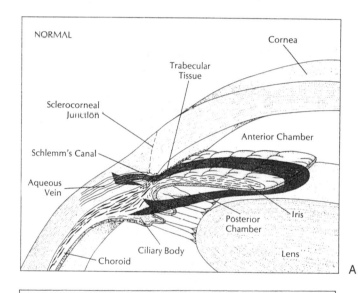

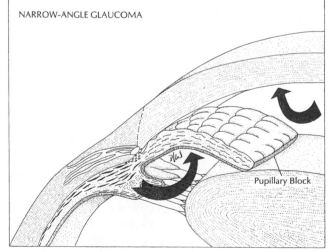

FIG. 9.2. A: Aqueous humor normally flows through pupil into anterior chamber, where it is reabsorbed by trabecular meshwork. B: In narrow-angle glaucoma, pupillary dilation occludes aqueous-flow channel between anterior lens and posterior iris, precipitating acute rise in intraocular pressure.

Patients with acute angle-closure glaucoma present with sudden onset of pain, decreased vision, eye injection, and seeing halos around lights. The pain may not be localized to the eye alone, but may spread to the forehead and temple and may mimic the pain of migraine and severe headache. The sudden increase of intraocular pressure may produce autonomic stimulation and associated nausea, vomiting, bradycardia, and diaphoresis. Examination reveals marked conjunctival injection, corneal edema, shallow anterior chamber, and a mid-dilated fixed pupil. The IOP is elevated, typically greater than 40 mmHg. The severe pain associated with the fixed pupil may lead emergency room physicians to an incorrect diagnosis of ruptured aneurysm with a lesion of cranial nerve III. Rarely, when vomiting and abdominal pain are severe and the patient cannot localize the eye as the source of pain, an abdominal crisis may be suspected. The medical management consists of medical therapy with antiglaucoma medications to break the acute attack.

Nausea and vomiting need to be controlled because they may contribute to further increase in IOP. Analgesic opioid and anti-emitting agents usually are required during the acute phase. The definitive treatment is an iridectomy to establish aqueous flow between the posterior and anterior chambers. The iridectomy usually is accomplished by laser therapy (argon or Nd:YAG)

Orbit And Optic Nerve

Pain is usually an uncommon feature of most orbital diseases. Pain is a prominent finding in orbital-inflammatory conditions or with lesions that cause bony destruction.

Orbital Cellulitis

This usually occurs secondary to orbital trauma especially when associated with penetration of the orbit with foreign bodies or secondary to spread of infection from the sinuses or other contiguous structures. Orbital cellulitis can be subdivided into different types, which include preseptal cellulitis, true orbital cellulitis with or without orbital involvement, subperiosteal abscess, and cavernous-sinus thrombosis. In preseptal cellulitis (the area anterior to the orbital septum), there is eyelid edema but normal ocular motility and globe integrity. Although preseptal cellulitis occurs in all age groups, it is more common in children under the age of 2 years and follows an upper-respiratory infection. In orbital cellulitis, the infection is localized posterior to the orbital septum. It is most commonly associated with sinusitis, although it can be posttraumatic or endogenous. It occurs in older children and young adults. The clinical manifestations include soft-tissue edema, limited eye movement, proptosis, and decreased vision associated with pain. Orbital cellulitis can be complicated by the formation of orbital and sub-

periosteal abscesses and this should be suspected when the patients do not clinically respond to parenteral antibiotic therapy, which is the standard of care for the treatment of orbital cellulitis. Cavernous-sinus thrombosis occurs either as a complication of orbital cellulitis or as the initial manifestation of spread of local infection (infection from the skin of the upper half of the face, the pharynx or ear) through the valveless veins tributary to the cavernous sinus. The clinical picture is one of pain in the distribution of V_1 and occasionally of V_2 accompanied by ophthalmoplegia from paresis of cranial nerves III, IV, or VI and a Horner's syndrome (miosis and ptosis). Vigorous systemic antibiotic therapy is required.

Orbital Pseudotumor

These include a heterogeneous group of nonspecific inflammatory processes that are generally acute or subacute. The classical clinical presentation is with signs of orbital inflammation—pain, proptosis, conjunctival injection, chemosis, and periorbital swelling. Orbital pseudotumor must be differentiated from orbital infections and from specific inflammations such as vasculitis, orbital amyloid, histiocytosis, and Graves' orbitopathy.

The clinical features vary. In *orbital myositis*, a disorder of young adults, there is pain, ophthalmoplegia, and enlargement of ocular muscles on computed tomography (CT). In *dacryoadenitis*, the inflammation may be localized to the superolateral orbit with downward placement of the globe. In the *Tolosa–Hunt* syndrome, a syndrome of painful ophthalmoplegia, there is inflammatory pseudotumor of the walls of the cavernous sinus.

All of these patients with signs of orbital pseudotumor require high-resolution CT or magnetic resonance imaging (MRI) to help localize and define the orbital process. Biopsy may be required for definitive diagnosis. Treatment with steroids may alleviate the signs and symptoms and support the diagnosis.

Orbital Tumors

Primary and secondary orbital tumors may cause pain by compression of vascular or nerve structure, destruction of bone, and invasion of orbital soft tissue. Most orbital tumors present with proptosis long before they cause pain. Symptomatic treatment with analgesics including nonsteroidal antiinflammatory drugs (NSAIDs) and opioids is appropriate.

Optic Neuritis

Optic neuritis refers to inflammation of the optic nerve and is referred to as anterior optic neuritis when there is swelling of the optic disc or retrobulbar neuritis when the disc appears normal. It is referred to as idiopathic optic neuritis in the absence of any systemic disease or symptoms of multiple sclerosis. Symptoms include loss of central vision and pain. The pain may be mild. However, some patients may complain of severe discomfort in the orbital and supraorbital area that is worsened by eye movement and pressure on the globe. Current recommendation for managing these patients includes obtaining an MRI of the brain for evaluation of prognosis regarding future development of multiple sclerosis.

The pain associated with optic neuritis responds well to intravenous corticosteroids when indicated. If corticosteroids are not used, pain may be managed by NSAIDs.

REFERRED OCULAR AND PERIOCULAR PAIN

Many syndromes associated with referred ocular or periocular pain (Table 9.2) are discussed elsewhere in this book. Migraine, as well as tension headache, can be accompanied by periocular pain and photophobia. The headache of giant-cell arteritis sometimes is associated with ischemic–optic neuropathy, and scintillating scotomata usually herald migraine.

Cluster headache and Raeder's paratrigeminal neuralgia are accompanied by oculosympathetic manifestations, lacrimation, and oculosympathetic palsy with ptosis, miosis, and anhydrosis (Horner's syndrome). Cluster headaches usually are benign in nature, while Raeder's neuralgia is associated with carotid and parasellar pathology such as pituitary tumor, meningioma, or internal carotid-artery aneurysm.

Herpes zoster involving the first division of the trigeminal nerve or herpes zoster ophthalmicus can present with vesicles over the eyelid. Treatment is the same as for herpes zoster in other areas of the body. Many tissues of the globe and orbit can be affected by highly varied types of lesions, including conjunctivitis, episcleritis, scleritis, keratitis, iritis, neuritis, and retinitis. Each of these condi-

TABLE 9.2. *Referred Ocular and Periocular Pain*

Aneurysms
Painful nerve third-palsy
Photo-oculodynia syndrome
Sinusitis
Trigeminal neuralgia
Raeder's paratrigeminal neuralgia (cluster headache)
Dental pain
Temporal arteritis
Herpes zoster/postherpetic neuralgia
Greater occipital neuralgia

tions require specific therapy. Postherpetic neuralgia is discussed in another chapter.

Trigeminal neuralgia rarely involves the ophthalmic division of the trigeminal nerve alone. The syndrome and treatment modalities are described elsewhere in this book.

Greater occipital neuralgia may present as eye pain that starts in the occipital region and extends over the temple. Palpation over the greater occipital nerve at the level of the occipital protuberance reproduces the pain, and local anesthetic infiltration of the nerve completely abolishes the pain. Treatment consists of heat, massage, NSAIDs, and local infiltrations with local anesthetic and steroid.

"Eye strain" often is blamed as a source of eye pain and headache especially in the presence of minor refractive anomalies. Correction of the refractive anomalies may improve the pain syndrome, but overcorrection or a refractive error may be a cause of eye strain.

SELECTED READINGS

Liu GT, Volpe NJ, Galetta SL. *Neuro-Ophthalmology—Diagnosis and Management.* Philadelphia: WB Saunders, 2001.

Rosen ES, Thompson SH, Cumming WJK, et al. *Neuro-Ophthalmology.* St. Louis: Mosby, 1998.

Tang RA, Pardo G. Ocular and periocular pain. In: *Focal Points Volume XIV.* San Francisco: American Academy of Ophthalmology, 1996:1–14.

CHAPTER 10

Orofacial Pain

Joel L. Dunsky and Cynthia H. Kahn

Citing a recent comprehensive investigation of the incidence of orofacial pain in 45,000 adult subjects, the results revealed 22% of those evaluated reported orofacial pain in the previous 6-month period. Thus, primary-care practitioners can reasonably expect to encounter patients with a chief complaint of orofacial pain.

When a patient presents for evaluation of acute or chronic facial pain, the cause can be difficult to determine and present a frustrating challenge for the practitioner. Orofacial pain can arise from a multitude of structures, e.g., teeth, jaws, periodontal tissues, salivary glands, paranasal sinuses, eyes, nose, ears, temporomandibular joints, muscles, and vascular structures. Origin of the pain may be of a neurologic nature and present as neuralgia or neuritis, or be referred to the orofacial area from intracranial pathology. Tumors of the gasserian ganglion, auditory neuromas, and multiple sclerosis are conditions known to have referred pain to the orofacial area.

For a clinician to properly evaluate pain complaints, he/she must be aware of the difference of the source and site of the pain. When the site of pain and the source of the pain are not the same, it can be quite confusing to both the patient and the clinician. Unfortunately, referred or heterotopic pain is extremely common in the orofacial area. It is important to note that therapy should be directed toward the source of the pain.

INNERVATION

The mouth and face are innervated by cranial nerves and nerves of the cervical plexus (Fig. 10.1). The cutaneous-sensory innervation to the face, head, and neck is supplied by the trigeminal nerve (V) and the cervical plexus (Fig. 10.2). The facial nerve (VII) supplies the muscles of facial expression and scalp as well as secretory and special taste senses. The facial nerve joins with the trigeminal nerve via the chorda tympani branch thus explaining why referred pain from dental structures may be perceived to be over a large area of the face and side of the head.

The first division of the trigeminal nerve (VI-ophthalmic branch) supplies the forehead and nose. The second division (V2-maxillary branch) supplies the upper jaw. The third division (V3-mandibular branch) supplies the lower jaw. The trigeminal ganglion (also called the gasserian, or the semilunar ganglion) contains pseudounipolar cell bodies, which send out processes that divide into central and peripheral fibers. The central fibers run in the sensory root of the trigeminal nerve to the brainstem, and the peripheral fibers conduct sensory impulses from the periphery to the ganglion cells. The ganglion rests in a dural invagination (Meckel's cavity), which is filled with cerebrospinal fluid. The structure is located in the middle cranial fossa, near the apex of the petrous part of the temporal bone and near the cavernous sinus.

The maxillary sinus is innervated by the maxillary branch of the trigeminal nerve (V2) and by the sphenopalatine ganglion. The ethmoidal sinus is supplied by the nasociliary nerve (a branch of V1) and the anterior and posterior ethmoidal branches. The frontal sinus is supplied by a branch of V1 called the frontal nerve. The tonsils are innervated by the lesser palatine nerve (V2), the lingual nerve (V3), and the glossopharyngeal nerve (IX), which are all closely situated in the pharyngeal plexus. The glossopharyngeal nerve exits the jugular foramen posterior and medial to the styloid process, and just anterior to the vagus (X) and accessory (XI) nerves. The glossopharyngeal nerve supplies the posterior third of the tongue, a major portion of the posterior pharynx, and the epiglottis. The vagus nerve supplies the larynx, the undersurfaces of the epiglottis, and the trachea.

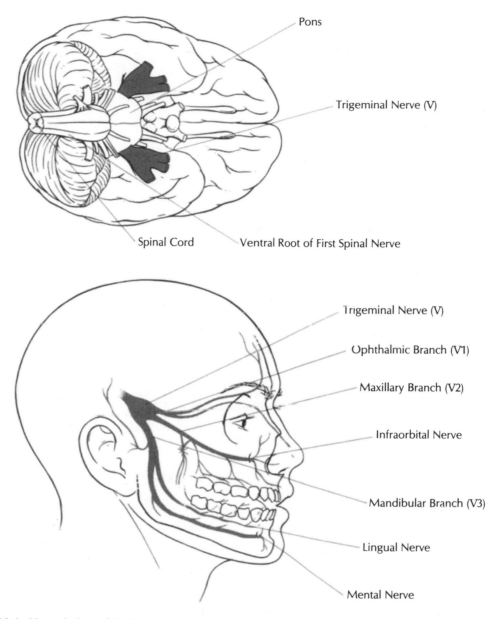

FIG. 10.1. Ventral view of the brain at top shows trigeminal nerve. The largest of all the cranial nerves, it has three major divisions—ophthalmic, maxillary, and mandibular—which are diagrammed with their branches at the bottom.

DENTAL DISEASE

The most common cause of facial pain is dental disease. Disease of the teeth and supporting structures can cause severe pain of both acute and chronic nature. If the pain can be localized to the teeth, the patient usually presents to the dentist for evaluation. However, a physician may be called on to perform an initial evaluation of facial pain in a patient who has not seen a dentist. After a complete history has been taken, a physical examination should be done. The examination requires good illumination and retraction in order to adequately evaluate the oral cavity. The visual examination should include the vestibule, cheeks, lips, tongue, palate, neck, and pharynx.

The orofacial complex is very vulnerable to traumatic-impact injuries. Automobile, motorcycle, and bicycle accidents, sports injuries, or blunt trauma from a variety of causes may result in damage to the teeth and surrounding structures. These occurrences may result in contusion, concussion, laceration, fracture, luxation, intrusion, and avul-

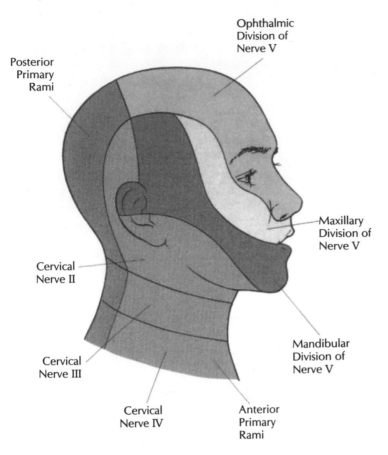

Posterior
Primary
Rami

Ophthalmic
Division of
Nerve V

Cervical
Nerve II

Cervical
Nerve III

Cervical
Nerve IV

Anterior
Primary
Rami

Maxillary
Division of
Nerve V

Mandibular
Division of
Nerve V

FIG. 10.2. Cutaneous-sensory information to the face, head, and neck is supplied by the trigeminal nerve and the cervical plexus in distribution shown.

sion. Sequelae following traumatic events can result in pulp necrosis, resorptions, calcifications, tooth mobility, and alveolar bone loss. The pain resulting from such injuries may arise from the dental pulp, periodontal tissues, or from the surrounding and supporting structures. Thus, careful and meticulous evaluation is required to determine the extent and severity of injury.

The examiner should look for soft-tissue lesions such as patches, discolorations, eruptions, and areas of induration. Fistulae, or sinus tracts, should be traced to their origin, as they often are caused by teeth with necrosis of the pulp. Discolored teeth should be noted as well as evidence of broken or fractured cusps. Extensive caries should be identified as this may be helpful in localizing a painful tooth. Lost or missing fillings as well as loose-fitting crowns or bridges require identification as well as partially or completely fractured teeth. Swellings both intraorally and extraorally should be noted for size, extent, and location. Periodontal disease including mobility, pocketing, and spacing of teeth may be implicated in painful occurrences.

PULPITIS

In the differential diagnosis of facial pain, inflammation of the pulp or pulpitis is the most common cause. It usually is characterized by intermittent bouts of acute pain, which may become continuous. The pain may be of a severe, constant throbbing, boring nature worsened by heat and sometimes relieved by cold. This is a nonreversible condition that requires either endodontic treatment or extraction of the tooth.

CRACKED TOOTH

A patient with a cracked tooth usually will have a transient sharp pain on biting. If the crack is superficial and does not involve the pulp, removal of the fractured segment and restoration of the tooth usually resolves the problem. However, if the crack extends into the pulp, then a pulpitis may ensue requiring either endodontic treatment or extraction if the tooth is not restorable.

An exposed root surface as a result of recent periodontal surgery or a recent deep restoration often will cause sharp, transient pain, aggravated by hot, cold, or sweet foods. Where the symptoms are merely slight sensitivity that do not linger when the stimulus is removed or do not come on spontaneously, it is an indication that the condition is reversible. Conditions such as caries or broken or missing fillings require dental intervention to resolve the pain. Many conditions may make a tooth tender to percussion and biting. The underlying cause of the problem must be determined to resolve the complaint.

PULP NECROSIS AND ALVEOLAR ABSCESS

Bacterial invasion of the pulp or severe traumatic impact injury can cause total necrosis and gangrene of the pulp. When the process extends from the tooth into the alveolar bone of either the mandible or maxilla, the condition may be described as an acute alveolar abscess. In this condition, there is a localized collection of purulence in the bone via the root canal of the tooth. The patient usually presents with severe, throbbing pain, a tooth or teeth that are exquisitely tender to the touch, and swelling of the soft tissues of the sulcus, lips, and cheek. In the case of the maxilla, the eye on the affected side may be partially closed because of the extension of the cellulitis. In the mandible, the swelling may be in the sublingual, submandibular, or submental areas and extend below the level of the mylohyoid ridge causing impingement on the trachea and airway. This latter condition, known as Ludwig's angina, usually requires hospital admission and treatment with intravenous (i.v.) antibiotics and/or incision and drainage. Where the condition is not as severe, dental treatment, including opening the tooth and draining the purulence, relieves the pain. This can be followed by endodontic treatment to salvage the tooth or extraction, if indicated.

GINGIVAL OR PERIODONTAL ABSCESS

The patient may present with a tooth that is painful to the touch and evidence of swelling around the tooth where the dental pulp is not involved. In this case, there may be an acute gingival or acute periodontal abscess present. Food impaction, foreign matter, filling materials, and bacteria may collect between the teeth or in gingival or periodontal pockets and cause a localized infection. In a severe case, this can mimic an acute alveolar infection but the treatment is different. Local measures such as cleaning out the material from the soft-tissue pockets and irrigation of the area with warm saline rinses are helpful. In the previously described conditions where soft-tissue swelling is present, incision and drainage along with appropriate antibiotics and analgesics may be indicated.

PERICORONITIS

Pericoronitis is the term used to describe a soft-tissue infection around the crown of an erupting tooth often present in wisdom teeth. Just as in other soft-tissue infections, there may be acute pain, swelling, fever, and trismus present. The infection may involve the jaw muscles on the affected side resulting in a very limited ability to open the mouth. Again, treatment consists of drainage, analgesics, antibiotics, and, after the acute symptoms have subsided, if there is insufficient space in the jaw for the tooth to erupt, extraction may be required.

OSTEOMYELITIS

Osteomyelitis can occur in both jaws but usually is found in the mandible. While the condition is rare, it can result in intense and difficult-to-manage pain. Evidence of the disease can be found on radiological and physical examination. Treatment consists of surgical debridement and long-term (months) i.v. antibiotics. It is important to treat these infections aggressively in the early stages as they may extend into the lateral pharyngeal space or cause a cavernous sinus thrombosis.

DRY SOCKET

Dry socket is a term used to describe pain radiating to the chin or cheek that can occur following the extraction of a tooth, often a mandibular molar. It is a form of localized osteitis thought to occur when an intraalveolar blood clot becomes infected and degenerates, leaving exposed bone in the empty socket. The pain, often described as severe and constant, usually starts 2 to 3 days after extraction and lasts 10 to 14 days. Resolution of this painful condition can be hastened by regular irrigation and dressing of the socket, allowing granulation tissue to form over the affected area. Analgesics may be required. Phantom tooth pain has been known to occur in these areas long after the socket has healed. Such pain in the supporting structures often is quite refractory to various forms of therapy.

ACUTE NECROTIZING ULCERATIVE GINGIVITIS

Acute necrotizing ulcerative gingivitis (ANUG), previously known as "trench mouth," is characterized by painful, swollen gingiva and punched-out interdental papilla. A gray, necrotic pseudomembrane covers the tissue, which bleeds quite easily. The patient often has difficulty in eating and usually presents with general malaise, headache, and fever. Poor oral hygiene, fatigue, smoking, poor diet, or improper sanitary conditions are some of the predisposing factors. A foul, fetid breath odor is present. Treatment consists of dental prophylaxis and scaling utilizing local anesthesia, chlorhexidine mouth rinses, antibiotics (e.g., tetracycline or metronidazole), rest, and nutritional support.

HETEROTOPIC OR REFERRED PAIN

Referred pain is a phenomenon that frequently is encountered and is most baffling. It is quite common to have patients with pulpal involvement of lower molar teeth, often wisdom teeth, complain they have pain in the ear, angle of the mandible, and occasionally to the superior laryngeal area (Fig. 10.3). Maxillary incisor teeth may refer pain to the frontal area of the head, while max-

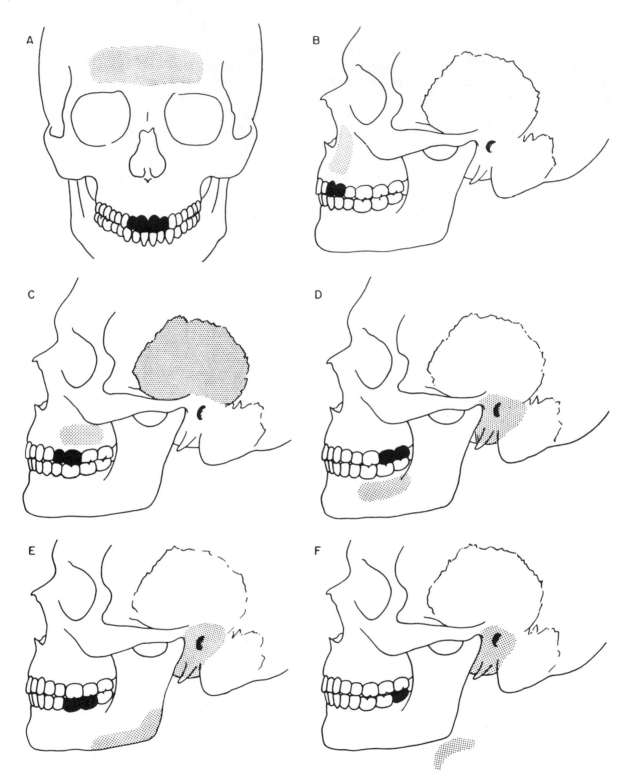

FIG. 10.3. Pain referred from pulpalgia to structures remote to involved tooth. *Black* indicates teeth involved in pulpalgia; *stippled areas*, remote areas of referred pain. **A:** Maxillary incisors may refer pain to frontal areas. **B:** Maxillary canine and first premolar may refer pain into nasolabial area and into orbit. **C:** Maxillary second premolar and first molar may refer pain to maxilla and back to temporal region. **D:** Maxillary second and third molars may refer pain to mandibular molar area and occasionally into ear. **E:** Mandibular first and second molars may commonly refer pain to ear and to angle or mandible. **F:** Mandibular third molar may refer pain to ear and occasionally to superior laryngeal area. (Adapted from Glick DH. Locating referred pulpal pains. *Oral Surg* 1962;15:613, with permission.)

illary canine and first premolars may refer pain into the nasolabial area and into the orbit. Maxillary second and third molars may refer pain to the mandibular area on the same side.

A complete dental examination is required in these cases to localize the offending tooth or source of the pain. Radiographs, pulp-vitality tests, thermal tests, percussion, palpation, and not infrequently the use of diagnostic local anesthesia, may be required to isolate the source of pain. Where the use of local anesthesia blocks the source of the pain, the pain decreases at both the source and site of pain. Conversely, where the use of local anesthesia blocks the site of pain and not the source, the pain is not decreased. Partially fractured teeth where the pulp is involved often are implicated in this pain phenomenon.

DISEASES OF THE SINUSES

Much less common is pain that is referred to the face from the nose and paranasal sinuses. Acute infection of the maxillary sinuses can cause severe pain over the sinus and maxillary posterior teeth. In that the roots of the maxillary premolar and molar teeth may be in the wall or adjacent to the maxillary sinus, it is necessary to rule out acute alveolar abscess of the teeth extending into the sinus as the causative factor. Pain on positional change of head, a metallic taste, and teeth sensitive to biting often are reported in sinus infection. The use of transillumination of the sinuses, sinus x-rays, and pulp-vitality tests are very helpful. There may be nasal congestion and discharge because of the fact that the maxillary sinus communicates with the middle meatus of the nasal cavity. Often, there are symptoms of fever and general malaise present. The sinus often is tender to palpation. Chronic sinusitis rarely causes facial pain, except during an acute exacerbation. Treatment consists of antibiotics and vasoconstrictors, and possible antrostomy and drainage.

Tumors can occur in the sinuses and have been known to cause a variety of symptoms including pain, swelling, and loss of sensation. Appropriate treatment is contingent on the type and extent of tumor involvement. Trotter syndrome, referred pain in the lower jaw, tongue, and side of the head caused by a tumor of the nasopharynx, occurs very rarely.

HERPES ZOSTER

Herpes zoster infection of the face and head may be extremely painful and protracted. As in zoster infection elsewhere in the body, an acute, ticlike pain precedes the appearance of vesicles. The eruptions tend to follow the course of the affected nerve in a linear pattern and tend to be unilateral. If the vesicles rupture, ulcerative-type lesions remain. These lesions may occur on the lips, cheek, labial, palatal, or buccal mucosa. Sequelae of this infection may be protracted periods of paraesthesia, neu-ralgia, and corneal involvement. The infection usually is self-limiting.

SALIVARY GLANDS

The salivary glands can be painful if they become obstructed or infected. The submandibular gland is the most common site. Submandibular sialolithiasis can occur when Wharton's duct of the submandibular salivary gland becomes blocked by a stone or by sludge consisting of inspissated mucus or cellular debris. Some predisposing factors are gout or diuretic therapy. Pain increases at the sight, smell, or thought of food, as well as in the course of eating, and decreases after a meal, only to reappear at the next mealtime. Surgical removal of the stone, or the entire gland if it has become infected, often is curative. Infection of the parotid gland occurs rarely and is most common in elderly patients. Sialolithiasis also can occur in Stensen's duct of the parotid gland. Treatment includes hot-saline mouthwashes and ingestion of fruit drinks (which stimulate acid taste) to increase the salivary secretions, removal of calculi or sludge, and establishment of drainage if infection is present; antibiotics are indicated if the patient manifests signs of systemic infection.

ORAL MUCOSA

Disorders of the oral mucosa can be severe enough to cause oral and facial pain. Especially painful are those that have an ulcerative component. The most common painful oral-mucosal disorders are those resulting from trauma (e.g., cheek biting or abrasion by dental appliances), herpes simplex infection, *Candida* infection, acute ulcerative stomatitis, lichen planus, and aphthous stomatitis. Less commonly, neoplastic disease, systemic HIV, immunologic disorders, and psychiatric disturbances may result in painful oral mucosa.

Extremely painful mucositis may occur following radiotherapy and/or chemotherapy. Usually, desquamation and ulcerations occur resulting in painful mucosa, thus eating is almost impossible. Treatment consists of palliation and attempts to reduce secondary infection, which, in most cases, begins with candidiasis. In the case of chemotherapy, pain begins about 1 week after administration of the drug. In the oral cavity, there is decreased cell renewal, which results in epithelial thinning thus producing the mucositis followed by ulceration, invasion of oral bacteria, and occurrence of secondary infection and sepsis. The affect on bone marrow results in reduced myeloproliferation, neutropenia, and thrombocytopenia, and thus the sepsis in the susceptible oral tissues is enhanced.

Treatment for oral mucositis may consist of mouth rinses containing topical anesthetics such as viscous lidocaine, dyclonine hydrochloride, and benzocaine products.

Also, a mixture of Benadryl (Parke–Davis, Morris Plains, NJ, U.S.A.) and Kaopectate (Pharmacia & Upjohn Company, Bridgewater, NJ, U.S.A.) in equal amounts has been used to provide relief. In addition, analgesics may be used as required.

BONE DISEASE

Bone tumors and metastases from other primary cancer sites can cause facial pain. Necrosis of the bone can occur after radiation therapy that involves the facial bones or jawbones. This can result in severe pain, which is definitively treated only by surgical excision of necrotic bone.

Jaw and facial fractures are very painful; they often require open reduction and internal fixation under anesthesia. In the course of healing, analgesia can be achieved with a variety of nonsteroidal antiinflammatory drugs (NSAIDs) or low-dose narcotics until the acute pain subsides.

JOINT AND MUSCLE DISORDERS

Temporomandibular joint dysfunction is another common cause of facial pain. However, it is important to rule out degenerative joint disease, congenital abnormalities, tumors, and history of trauma. Pain in the ears, eyes, and muscles of the face and neck are common symptoms of temporomandibular joint syndrome (also known as myofascial pain dysfunction). Patients also may complain of ringing in the ears, blurred vision, and facial dysesthesias.

On examination, there may be a significant deviation of the mandible as a patient opens and closes his mouth. Mouth opening may be very limited. With movement of the jaw, it may be possible to palpate joint crepitus. In most cases, no radiographic abnormalities are detected. Treatments include rest, reassurance, heat application to the tender areas, ultrasound, short-wave diathermy, NSAIDs (low doses for 2 weeks), anxiolytics (diazepam two to four times daily for 2 weeks), antidepressants (amitriptyline or doxepin at bedtime tapered to a low-maintenance dosage over 2 to 4 months), interocclusal appliances, and behavior modification (relaxation, biofeedback). Each of these therapies, alone or in various combinations, has resulted in some relief of the painful symptoms of temporomandibular joint syndrome.

Myofascial pains of the muscles of mastication occur mostly in the lateral face. The pain is described as cramping, aching, or burning and as increasing with use of the jaw or its muscles, as when talking or chewing. The muscles may be tender to palpation. Trigger points may be present. The pain also may radiate to the scalp and neck. Treatment is similar to that for temporomandibular joint syndrome.

Muscle pain such as that from a muscle-contraction headache, posttrauma headache, trismus, myositis, or benign masseteric dystrophy also may cause facial pain.

Therapy consists of treatment of the primary cause and symptomatic relief with analgesics, antidepressants, phenothiazines, biofeedback, and psychotherapy, as appropriate.

CRANIAL NEURALGIAS

The cranial-nerve neuralgias are among the most excruciating entities known. The trigeminal nerve is affected most often.

Trigeminal neuralgia has been called *tic douloureux* ("painful tic") because squinting or twitching often occurs on the affected side during an attack. The pain associated with this syndrome has been likened to that of electric shock or stabbing. It is restricted to the distribution of the trigeminal nerve (involving one or more branches). Three percent of patients have bilateral tic pain, but only one side is affected during any episode. Onset and termination of attacks are equally abrupt, and patients usually are pain free between episodes. Some patients may have an aching or burning sensation between paroxysms or may have disturbances in sensation in the affected areas. Attacks last only a few seconds, but it is not uncommon for a series of attacks to occur in rapid succession over several hours. Nonnoxious stimulation triggers the pain, which does not always affect the same area of the face. The trigger zone often is in the nasolabial fold or the upper or lower lip and can be touched off by washing, shaving, talking, or any slight movement. The trigger almost always is ipsilateral to the pain but may be in the same or a different division of the trigeminal nerve.

Most commonly, tic pain occurs in the combined distribution of the second and third divisions. The rarest combination is a tic involving the first and third divisions. More than 44% of patients with trigeminal neuralgia have pain in the second division, 35% have pain in the third division, and 19% have pain in the first division. There is minimal or no sensory loss in the region of pain. (If the patient has sensory loss in the painful area, tumor or infection must be ruled out.) The pain often is severe enough to interrupt all purposeful activities. The patient may present in an unkempt state, drooling, and unwilling to move or touch the trigger area. Emotional and physical stress intensify the pain

Although the etiology of trigeminal neuralgia most often is idiopathic, many patients with classical tic have mechanical compression of the trigeminal nerve as it leaves the pons and traverses the subarachnoid space toward Meckel's cavity. On surgical decompression, it is most often found that the nerve has been compressed by one of the major cerebellar arteries. The region of impingement of the blood vessel on the nerve frequently corresponds to the region of facial pain. Rarely, arteriovenous malformations, aneurysms, or tumors in the cerebellopontine angle have been found to compress the trigeminal nerve. Trigeminal neuralgia also can occur after an episode of acute herpes zoster, after trauma to the face, or after facial or dental surgery. There is an increased incidence of trigeminal neuralgia in patients with multiple sclerosis. The peak incidence of trigeminal neuralgia is in patients between the ages of 50 and 70; 60% are female.

There is no test that can confirm the diagnosis of trigeminal neuralgia. If injection of local anesthetic into the trigger area abolished the trigger effect for the duration of anesthesia, however, the diagnosis is presumptive. In rare cases, the block may induce a spontaneous remission, which can last for months or years.

Most patients will require medical or surgical intervention in order to obtain relief from their pain. Two thirds of patients who are given carbamazepine will have improvement in their symptoms. Response varies, but many patients obtain complete relief. Treatment may have to continue for years. Total daily doses as high as 800 to 1,800 mg may be required. Twenty-five percent of patients obtain good relief from phenytoin. Serum levels of phenytoin must be at least 15 μg/mL for the drug to be effective in trigeminal neuralgia. Some patients respond to baclofen. Antidepressants have been tried with some success, as have analgesics, hypnosis, acupuncture, transcutaneous-nerve stimulation, phenothiazines, and psychotherapy.

Some practitioners perform regular nerve blocks to provide pain relief until drugs reach adequate analgesic levels or until surgery is done. (Patients undergoing nerve block will experience the effects of neurectomy or total rhizotomy.) Alcohol blocks are not commonly performed, because the pain relief rarely lasts longer than 1 year and the success rate is low. Moreover, morbidity is high because the amount of hypalgesia and anesthesia is difficult to control.

Surgery is warranted only if drug therapy has failed. Several surgical techniques have been developed for treatment of trigeminal neuralgia (see also Chapter 59). Gangliolysis is a procedure in which a needle is inserted through the cheek into the foramen ovale and into the rootlets behind the trigeminal ganglion. Radiofrequency heat then is applied to portions of the posterior rootlets or glycerol is injected into the cistern of the trigeminal ganglion. Radiofrequency heat destruction can be associated with significant loss of facial sensation, whereas the glycerol infection provides excellent analgesia without anesthesia. Eighty percent of patients have at least 1 year of pain relief; 60% have 5 years or more of relief. The complication rate is less than 0.5%.

Some neurosurgeons prefer the technique of microvascular decompression. This is performed under general anesthesia via a suboccipital craniotomy; a microscope is used to visualize the trigeminal nerve as it leaves the pons. The vessels found to be compressing the nerve are either repositioned or coagulated. There is an 85% long-term success rate, and there is no sensory loss. The complication rate is 3%, with a mortality rate of less than 1%.

If gangliolysis fails and the patient cannot safely undergo craniotomy, peripheral neurectomy is done. This procedure produces a dense numbness, with relief lasting about 1 year. Repeat avulsions of the peripheral branches of the trigeminal nerve have a low success rate. A retro-gasserian neurotomy is performed if no microvascular compression is found on suboccipital craniotomy or if pain returns after decompression surgery. The trigeminal root is sectioned between the trigeminal ganglion and the pons. A partial rhizotomy also is performed to decrease the likelihood of anesthesia dolorosa or of a totally numb face.

If all other measures have failed, a trigeminal tractotomy can be performed via a suboccipital craniotomy and laminectomy at C1 and C2. The descending trigeminal tract is sectioned in the medulla to produce loss of pain and temperature sensation in the ipsilateral face and pharynx. This procedure can be performed in patients with other cranial neuralgias — such as glossopharyngeal, vagal, or nervus intermedius (VII) neuralgias — because their pain and temperature fibers all travel in the medial aspect of the descending trigeminal tract (Fig. 10.4).

Glossopharyngeal Neuralgia

Glossopharyngeal neuralgia is at least 100 times less common than trigeminal neuralgia. It is characterized by shocklike pain in the tonsillar fossa, lateral pharyngeal wall, or base of the tongue, which may radiate to the ear, angle of the jaw, or upper neck. Triggering stimuli may include swallowing, yawning, clearing the throat, or talking. Some patients have loss of consciousness, arrhythmias, or even asystole with an attack of pain. Treatment includes carbamazepine or phenytoin. If medical therapy fails, a trigeminal tractotomy can be performed.

Geniculate Neuralgia

Geniculate neuralgia, or nervus intermedius tic douloureux, is so rare that no incidence data have been reported. Herpes zoster is the most common cause. Symptoms include otalgia and pain located deep in the face behind the orbits, or in the posterior nasal cavity. Pain often is perceived in the inner ear or in the anterior external canal and may be triggered by touching the ear canal or by swallowing or talking. Bitter taste, salivation, vertigo, and tinnitus are associated with painful attacks in some patients. Frequently, there are sensory and motor disturbances in the distribution of the facial nerve. Cases of facial paralysis have been associated with geniculate neuralgia. A trial of medical and nonmedical therapies, as described for trigeminal neuralgia, is indicated. A trigeminal tractotomy can be performed if medical therapy fails to relieve the symptoms.

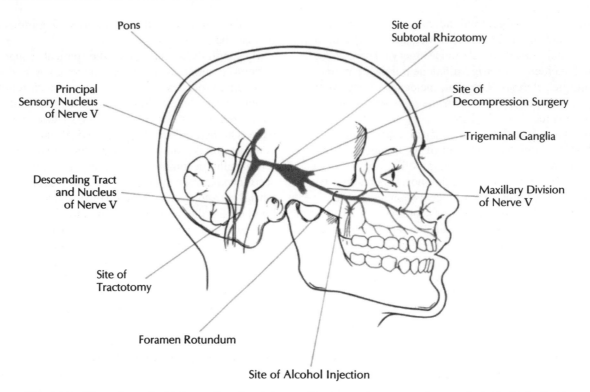

FIG. 10.4. Sites of surgical intervention (tractotomy, rhizotomy, decompression, and alcohol injection) are indicated along various trigeminal structures—nuclei and tracts, root, ganglion, and maxillary division.

Idiopathic Cranial Polyneuropathy and Tolosa–Hunt Syndrome

Idiopathic cranial polyneuropathy and Tolosa–Hunt syndrome (a variant) involve the motor components of the cranial nerves. Patients complain of deep and constant unilateral aching, which can be punctuated with sharp bursts of pain. The pain is located in the temporal, frontal, or vertex regions and radiates to the orbit as well as to the cheek, earlobe, lateral neck, nose, or scalp. There may be a transient diminution in visual acuity, hearing, and taste; anisocoria, ptosis, mild proptosis, conjunctivitis, sustained nystagmus, eyelid edema, and tinnitus also may be noted.

Cranial nerves II to XII (in a variety of combinations) have been found to be involved in these syndromes. Abnormalities occasionally can be found in the cerebrospinal fluid (pleocytosis and a mild increase in protein), but laboratory tests usually are within normal limits, as are carotid angiograms and computed tomographies (CTs). Cranial polyneuropathy has been associated with mycoplasmal infection, Guillain–Barré syndrome, herpes zoster, herpes simplex, Wegener's granulomatosis, giant-cell tumors, lymphomas, chordomas, and epidermoid tumors. It also has been described in a patient who had a severe upper-respiratory infection and a transient rise in intracranial pressure.

Corticosteroids provide relief of pain and associated ophthalmoplegia within 12 hours to a few days after initiation of therapy. Untreated, the syndrome may last 3 days to 20 weeks before resolving spontaneously.

Other diseases associated with facial pain caused by lesions in the central nervous system are Paget's disease, disseminated sclerosis, tertiary syphilis, and syringobulbia. Referred pain from the ears and eyes may affect the face. In patients with myocardial ischemia, cardiac pain can radiate to the arms, throat, and jaws. Cervical spondylosis, cervical muscle spasm, or neoplasms affecting the upper-cervical vertebrae can cause pain that radiates to the head and face. Treatment of the primary cause is indicated in such cases, with appropriate use of analgesics.

VASCULAR PATHOLOGY

Vascular headaches often cause pain that involves facial structures (see also Chapter 7). Migraine headaches, cluster headaches, temporal or giant-cell arteritis, and less-common vascular abnormalities (such as internal carotid-artery aneurysms and compression of the cavernous sinus by an aneurysm or granuloma associated with Wegener's granulomatosis) all can cause facial pain. Traumatic or spontaneous dissection of an internal carotid artery can cause symptoms of Horner's syndrome and a dull ache over the face on the affected side. Raeder's syndrome is caused by chronic dilation of the internal carotid artery as it enters the middle-cranial fossa. It can be idiopathic or secondary to a carotid body tumor. Patients with Raeder's syndrome present with a partial or complete Horner's syndrome and a throbbing pain in the first division (ophthalmic) of the trigeminal nerve. Rapid relief often is obtained with the administration of steroids.

Patients with migraine may describe auras before the onset of pain and may complain of photophobia, nausea, and vomiting. The pain usually is throbbing or burning. Onset of the headache may be associated with stress or the ingestion of particular foods. Relief can be obtained by use of antidepressants, β blockers, analgesics, ergot compounds, methysergide, and cyproheptadine, alone or in combination. Migraine headaches are more common in women, whereas cluster headaches occur more often in men.

Patients with cluster headache may present with unilateral ocular, frontal, or temporal pain. Less commonly, the pain may be in the infraorbital region and maxilla. Men between the ages of 18 and 40 most often are affected. The attacks occur in bouts over a period of weeks to months, followed by pain-free intervals of several months' duration. Bouts often last 4 to 8 weeks, with one to three attacks during a 24-hour period. Some patients have described up to eight attacks a day. The pain is excruciating, constant, stabbing, burning, and throbbing. Ipsilateral ptosis, miosis, tearing, rhinorrhea, facial sweating, flushing, and nasal congestion may be concurrent manifestations. Ergotamine tartrate, methysergide, prednisolone, and lithium have been helpful in decreasing the number and intensity of the attacks. Interestingly, inhalation of oxygen (7 L/minute) for 15 minutes may abort an attack.

Temporal and giant-cell arteries have been associated with temporal pain and headache. The patient, who is commonly over 60, may describe a dull, persistent pain in the temples that is exacerbated by chewing. A Horner's syndrome may be noted on examination. The temporal artery often is nonpulsatile, tortuous, and tender. Diagnosis is confirmed by a temporal-artery biopsy. The patient should be referred to an ophthalmologist to rule out ophthalmic-artery involvement. Prompt treatment with corticosteroids may prevent permanent blindness.

Chronic paroxysmal hemicrania occurs most often in women. Attacks occur daily and last 15 to 30 minutes. Patients most commonly complain of ocular, frontal, and temporal pain. Less often, pain occurs in the ipsilateral occipital, infraorbital, aural, mastoid, and nuchal areas. The pain is described as excruciating and fluctuating in frequency and severity. It can be associated with ipsilateral conjunctival injection, lacrimation, and nasal congestion. Indomethacin provides immediate relief of symptoms.

ATYPICAL FACIAL PAIN

Bilateral, atypical, facial pain has no known etiology. It occurs most commonly in women, with no age predominance. The pain is constant and burning and has no trigger points. On examination, a slight hypoesthesia, paraesthesia, or dysesthesia may be noted. Some patients may have undergone ablative surgery or nerve blocks, which only exacerbate their complaints. Significant emotional stressors or psychopathology often is present. Patients may benefit from a combination of tricyclic antidepressants and phenothiazines.

Unilateral, atypical, facial neuralgia is most commonly seen in young and middle-aged women. The pain is not as severe as trigeminal neuralgia and is characterized as burning, aching, stabbing, or throbbing. Patients describe their pain as being located in the hard tissues of the affected area, often in the distribution of the trigeminal nerve, with radiation to the upper neck or posterior scalp. Unlike tic pain, however, the pain of atypical facial neuralgia crosses divisions of the trigeminal nerve and radiates across the midline. Stress may exacerbate pain, so can the stimulation of the affected area. There are no trigger points. The pain usually is constant, with intermittent increases in intensity. There are rarely any pain-free intervals. Autonomic reactions in the area of facial pain are rarely seen in patients with atypical facial neuralgia.

The condition has been described in patients with the following pathologies: infection of the paranasal sinuses, jaws, or base of the skull; malignant neoplasms invading the base of the skull and traumatizing the branches of the trigeminal nerve or the meninges; vascular compression of the trigeminal nerve; and trauma to peripheral branches of the trigeminal nerve from facial lacerations and contusions. However, the vast majority of cases of atypical facial neuralgia are without any known cause.

Because of the multiple possible etiologies, an extensive diagnostic evaluation must be made to rule out treatable lesions. It often is necessary to obtain skull films; a CT (with particular attention to the base of the skull); a complete dental and ear, nose, and throat evaluation; and a complete neurologic examination. If a treatable lesion is excluded, tricyclic antidepressants and phenothiazines can be given for symptomatic relief. Surgical therapy for atypical facial neuralgia has not been successful.

MISCELLANEOUS CAUSES OF OROFACIAL PAIN

Glossodynia

Some patients complain of a painful burning sensation of the mouth and tongue associated with abnormal taste sensations. There is subjective xerostomia and a sensation of lumpy, gritty saliva. Patients may report areas of circumoral numbness. To evaluate this disorder, a complete physical examination must be performed. Radiographic evaluation of the face and skull also may be helpful, as well as a full battery of laboratory tests.

These measures are necessary to rule out vitamin B_{12}, iron, and folate deficiencies, as well as oral candidiasis, diabetes, peripheral neuropathy, amyloidosis, multiple myeloma, malignant lesions with metastases to the tongue, neuropathy of the lingual nerve, glossopharyngeal neuralgia, temporomandibular joint syndrome, xerostomia, geographic tongue, median rhomboid glossitis, trauma, and psychogenic factors. Hysteria, schizophrenia, and hypochondriasis may be primary or contributing causes of the pain. Patients have had good responses to a combination of medications appropriate to their conditions. Antidepressants, monoamine oxidase inhibitors, lithium, minor tranquilizers such as chlordiazepoxide and diazepam, meditation, hypnotherapy, behavior therapy, and biofeedback have been helpful.

Occipital Neuralgia

Occipital neuralgia may occur spontaneously or be secondary to trauma or cervical radiculopathy. The pain radiates along the entire distribution of the occipital nerve. It often is possible to elicit pain by pressure on the trigger point located along the nuchal ridge. A series of nerve blocks with a combination of local anesthetic and steroids often is necessary to relieve the pain.

Eagle Syndrome

Eagle syndrome, also known as styloid-process syndrome, is caused by an elongated styloid process, which occurs in 4% of the population. It rarely produces discomfort, but it can impinge on the soft tissue of the throat and on the external carotid artery during movement of the neck. This results in headache, carotid artery and ear tenderness, dizziness, and occasional loss of consciousness. Eagle syndrome also has occurred after tonsillectomy, with pain that is referred to the ear. Radiographic confirmation of the diagnosis indicates surgical excision of the styloid process, which is the definitive treatment for this syndrome.

Ictal Facial Pain

This is an unusual manifestation of sensory epilepsy, which is thought to be caused by paroxysmal discharges within the reticular formation. Patients describe the pain as being deep in the facial numbness, tightness, and tingling that later develops a burning quality. These symptoms last for 15 to 20 minutes before gradually subsiding. Afterward, the affected areas feel numb and cold for several hours. Onset usually is in adulthood; patients often have an extensive family history of seizure disorders. Treatment consists of anticonvulsant therapy.

Once dental disease has been excluded as the etiology of facial pain, the clinician will be left with a challenging range of possible diagnoses (Table 10.1). A thorough physical and psychological examination, as well as laboratory tests and radiographs often will be informative.

TABLE 10.1. *Characteristics of Facial-Pain Syndromes*

	Cranial neuralgias	Atypical facial pain	Vascular pathology	Temporomandibular joint syndrome	Local pathology
Pattern of occurrence	Intermittent, with pain-free intervals	Constant	Intermittent or clustered	Constant or fluctuating	Constant
Type of pain	Stabbing, electric shocklike, sharp	Burning, aching, jabbing	Throbbing, burning	Aching, radiating, associated with jaw use	Aching, throbbing, burning
Side affected	Unilateral	Unilateral or bilateral	Unilateral	Unilateral	Usually unilateral
Area involved	Areas innervated by V, VII, IX, X	Areas innervated by V or upper cervical plexus	Mid or upper face	Lateral face	Corresponds to pathology
Sensory changes	Minimal or none	Frequent	None	None	Frequent
Trigger points	Respond to nonpainful stimuli; always ipsilateral, usually anterior face	In the area of pain when present	None	None	None
Facial flush	Absent	Absent	Present	Absent	Absent
Lacrimation and rhinitis	Absent	Absent	Present	Absent	Absent
Local tenderness	None	Possible dysesthesias	Rare, usually mild	Over temporomandibular joint or muscles of mastication	Often in area of pathology

SELECTED READINGS

Alpert JN, Armbrust CA, Akhavi M, et al. Glossopharyngeal neuralgia, asystole, and seizures. *Arch Neurol* 1977;34:233–235.

Bullitt E, Tew JM, Boyd J. Intracranial tumors in patients with facial pain. *J Neurosurg* 1986;64:865–871.

Drinnan AJ. Differential diagnosis of orofacial pain. *Dent Clin North Am* 1987;31:627–643.

Dubuisson D. Root surgery In: Wall PD, Melzack R, eds. *Textbook of Pain*. New York: Churchill Livingstone, 1984:590–600.

Feinmann C, Harris M, Cawley R. Psychogenic facial pain: presentation and treatment. *Br Med J [Clin Res]* 1984;288:436–438.

Hakanson S. Trigeminal neuralgia treated by injection of glycerol into the trigeminal cistern. *Neurosurgery* 1981;9:638–646.

Heir GM. Facial pain of dental origin — a review for physicians. *Headache* 1987;27:540–547.

Ingle JI, Backland LK. *Endodontics*, 4th ed. Philadelphia: Williams & Wilkins, 1994.

Juncos JL, Beal MF. Idiopathic cranial polyneuropathy. A fifteen-year experience. *Brain* 1987;110:197–211.

Kashihara K, Ito H, Yamamoto S, et al. Raeder's syndrome associated with intracranial internal carotid artery aneurysm. *Neurosurgery* 1987;20:49–51.

Loeser JD. Tic douloureux and atypical face pain. In: Wall PD, Melzack R, eds. *Textbook of Pain*. New York: Churchill Livingstone, 1984:426–433.

Moffat DA, Ramsden RT, Shaw HJ. The styloid process syndrome: aetiological factors and surgical management. *J Laryngol Otol* 1977;91:279–294.

Okeson JR. *Bell's Orofacial Pain*, 5th ed. Chicago: Quintessence Publ Inc., 1995.

Poswillo DE. Prevention and early recognition of major orofacial disorders. *Br Dent J* 1980;149:326–333.

Sachs E Jr. The role of the nervus intermedius in facial neuralgia. Report of four cases with observations on the pathways for taste, lacrimation, and pain in the face. *J Neurosurg* 1968;28:54–60.

Sweet WH. The treatment of trigeminal neuralgia (tic douloureux). *N Engl J Med* 1986;315:174–177.

Watts PG. Intractable trigeminal neuralgia. *J R Soc Med* 1987;80:561–562.

CHAPTER 11

Neck Pain

Richard L. Gilbert and Hilary J. Fausett

Neck pain is almost as common a complaint as low-back pain. The neck contains many pain-sensitive tissues, which are vulnerable to a variety of painful conditions. The cervical spine is quite mobile; situated between an immobile thorax and a relatively weighty head, and thus it is subject to varying degrees of trauma.

In the evaluation of a patient with neck pain, it is necessary to be aware of serious pathology that will require referral to an orthopedist or neurosurgeon. A patient with minor, self-limited neck pain may never consult a physician. Those who present to a primary-care physician often can be helped by conservative management. Patients with severe and chronic neck pain usually can be helped by the therapeutic modalities offered by an anesthesiologist and a pain-management center.

The causes of neck pain are multiple and varied (Table 11.1). Many result in pain that may be self-limited, requiring little intervention and conservative management. Some causes of neck pain, however, may be from conditions that may cause significant morbidity and require immediate intervention. Knowledge of the causes of neck pain and the anatomy of the neck and a thorough history, physical exam, and appropriate tests are invaluable to the clinician called upon to diagnose and treat painful cervical conditions. Acute trauma requires careful neurologic examination as well as radiologic investigation. A history of significant or progressive arm weakness or long-tract signs necessitates neurosurgical or orthopedic referral. The presence of meningeal signs in the appropriate setting mandates hospitalization, and often the empiric dosing of antibiotics.

It is important to ascertain from the patient any history of precipitating events and associated conditions (e.g., trauma, infection, other illnesses, emotional stress, or use of medications). The duration of symptoms (i.e., acute, subacute, or chronic); aggravating and alleviating factors; area of maximum pain; points of origin and radiation; and character of pain (i.e., sharp, dull, burning, or throbbing) may aid in diagnosis. The presence of neurologic symptoms (e.g., weakness, numbness, clumsiness, long-tract signs, or evidence of bladder and bowel dysfunction) requires expeditious investigation. The presence of medical symptoms (e.g., constitutional symptoms, dyspnea, fever, or chest tightness) other bony or muscular pain, may lead to a diagnosis of systemic disease or malignancy. It also is important to inquire about the past medical history, including other medical problems and any prior surgeries. To formulate a treatment plan, previous therapeutic modalities should be discussed, and the response to previously tried medications and any side effects also need to be discussed.

A complete physical examination is essential for evaluation of the patient with neck pain. The neck region should be inspected for normal characteristics as well as pathology, including masses, muscular asymmetries, scars, discolorations, and cutaneous lesions. Palpation of the neck is best performed on the supine patient. The anterior bony structures of the neck (the humid bone, thyroid cartilage, cricoid cartilage, and the first-cricoid ring) are assessed for normal contour and motion. The thyroid gland is assessed for enlargement, tenderness, nodules, and bruits. The carotid arteries are assessed for bruits, tenderness, carotodynia, and carotid body tumors. Lymphadenopathy may indicate infection or malignancy. Parotitis should be ruled out. The sternocleidomastoid is palpated for trigger points (as in myofascial pain syndrome), hypertrophy (torticollis), tenderness, and swelling (viral myalgia, hematoma). The supraclavicular fossa is assessed for masses (tumor, subclavian-artery aneurysm, pathologic lymphadenopathy) and plethora (superior vena cava syndrome). Muscles that may refer pain of myofascial origin to the throat and front of the neck include the sternocleidomastoid, the medial pterygoid, and the digastric; they should be carefully palpated for trigger points.

With the patient still supine, the examiner palpates the posterior neck. Palpation of the occiput may elicit the

TABLE 11.1. *Sources of Neck Pain*

Soft tissue
Pharynx: pharyngitis, Ludwig's angina, inflamed pharyngeal cyst (branchial cleft remnants)
Tonsils: tonsillitis, neoplasm
Tongue: ulcers, neoplasm
Esophagus: inflamed diverticulum, peptic esophagitis, radiation esophagitis
Skin and subcutaneous tissues: furuncle, carbuncle, erysipelas, soft-tissue calcemia of the first and second cervical vertebrae

Glands
Thyroid gland: acute, suppurative thyroiditis, subacute thyroiditis with pain radiating to the ear, hemorrhage
Salivary gland: mumps, suppurative parotitis, calculus in duct
Lymph node: acute adenitis, chronic conditions (Hodgkin's disease, scrofula, gummas, actinomycosis, carcinomatous metastases)

Blood vessels
Carotodynia: carotid body tumor, subclavian artery aneurysm

Bones and ligaments
Mandible: fracture, osteomyelitis, periodonitis
Cervical vertebrae: whiplash, subluxation, acute or subacute fracture, spondylosis, primary metastatic neoplasm, osteomyelitis, tuberculosis
Ligamentous: rupture, cervical spine strain

Joints
Temporomandibular joint: associated with myofascial pain syndrome in neck
Facet joint: facet joint syndrome and dislocation
Infectious arthritis
Occipital neuralgia: with C1, C2 arthrosis syndrome

Discs
Herniated intervertebral disc

Muscles
General: myofascial pain syndrome, viral myalgia, fibrositis (transient stiff neck), hematoma, intramuscular gummas, calcific tendonitis of the musculus longus colli, reflex spasm (meningitis, adenitis, acute pharyngitis)
Sternocleidomastoid: torticollis (acquired, congenital)

Compression syndromes
Anterior scalenus syndrome, costoclavicular syndrome, pectoralis minor (hyperabduction) syndrome

Nerves
Cervical herpes zoster, spinal-cord tumor, epidural abscess or hematoma, poliomyelitis, occipital neuralgia, suprascapular neuralgia, reflex sympathetic dystrophy

Referred pain
Bronchial tumor, Pancoast's tumor, angina from the sixth cervical dermatomal band, spontaneous pneumomediastinum

pain characteristic of occipital neuralgia. The mastoid process and the superior nuchal lines are examined. To examine the cervical spine, each vertebral spinous process is palpated, beginning with C2; tenderness, irregularity, malalignment, and "step-offs" (i.e., when one spinous process protrudes more than the adjacent one) are noted. One can assess the facet joints for tenderness (facet-joint syndrome) by moving each hand laterally about 1 inch from the spinous process. Pain localized to the facet joint on rotation and extension of the neck supports the diagnosis of facet-joint syndrome.

Soft tissues of the posterior neck are examined next: the trapezius and posterior cervical muscles are palpated for spasm, trigger points, and tenderness. Muscles that may refer pain of myofascial origin to the back of the neck are the trapezius, multifidi, levator scapulae, splenius cervices, and infraspinatus. These muscles should be palpated carefully for trigger points to elicit local pain as well as the patient's characteristic pain, which may radiate from the trigger points.

If there is no evidence of an unstable cervical spine, full range of motion as well as cervical-muscle strength should be tested. The presence of atrophy or hypertrophy as well as reproduction of the pain symptomatology is assessed. The arms and hands are observed for signs of atrophy, cyanosis, and differences in skin temperature. A history of hyperesthesia is sought. Positive findings suggest complex regional pain syndrome, especially in the patient with a history of trauma or surgery.

The arms are maneuvered to elicit the characteristic pain and diminished radial pulse of the compression syndromes (anterior scalenus, costoclavicular, and pectoralis minor syndromes), as illustrated in Figure 11.1. The anterior scalenus test tenses the scaleni and elevates the first rib, thus trapping the subclavian artery, brachial plexus, and sometimes the subclavian vein. The examiner abducts and extends the involved arm while monitoring the radial pulse. The patient faces the involved side, extends the neck, and takes a deep breath. Reproduction of symptoms as well as obliteration of the radial pulse constitutes a positive test.

Compression of the neurovascular bundle between the first rib and clavicle (the costoclavicular syndrome) is assessed by having the patient stand at attention (with chest elevation and shoulder retraction). Obliteration of the radial pulse and reproduction of symptoms constitute a positive test.

To stretch the pectoralis minor, the patient's arms are raised overhead and rotated externally and backward. Compression of the neurovascular bundle between the pectoralis minor and the thorax elicits the characteristic symptoms and obliteration of the radial pulse seen in patients with pectoralis minor (hyperabduction) syndrome.

Neurologic examination is critical in evaluating the patient with neck pain, as radicular symptoms and neurologic deficits localize the area of pathology. The brachial plexus is formed by the anterior primary rami of C5 through T1 and serves to provide motor and sensory innervation to the arms. The pattern of radicular symp-

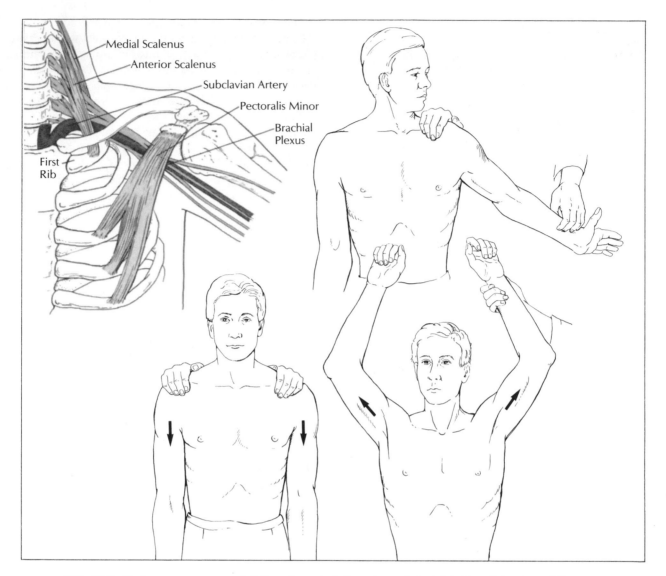

FIG. 11.1. Various maneuvers elicit the characteristic pain and diminished radial pulse of the compression syndromes. A test is positive if symptoms are reproduced and pulse is obliterated. To test for anterior-scalenus syndrome (upper right), patient faces the involved side, extends neck, and takes a deep breath. The examiner abducts and extends involved arm while monitoring radial pulse. For the costoclavicular syndrome (lower left), examiner exerts downward pressure and radial pulse is monitored while patient stands at attention. For the pectoralis-minor (hyperabduction) syndrome (lower right), examiner monitors radial pulse while patient's arms are elevated, extended, and hyperabducted

toms and the motor, sensory, and reflex deficits localize the nerve root involved. Acute neurologic deficits in a patient with neck trauma mandate immediate referral to a neurosurgeon or orthopedist.

The history and physical exam may indicate a need for x-rays and further laboratory tests. Anteroposterior and lateral views of the cervical spine are the basic x-ray film studies. All seven cervical vertebrae must be visualized. Some suggest including an anteroposterior film of the atlanto-axial articulation (open-mouth view) as well as oblique views. A lateral flexion and extension view could be ordered for flexion–extension injuries (e.g., whiplash) once an unstable cervical spine has been ruled out. X-

rays should be assessed not only for bone damage but for soft-tissue injury as well.

Neurologic or chronic symptoms may warrant further investigation, possibly including a computed tomography (CT), magnetic resonance imaging, or myelography. It may take 3 weeks for an electromyography to become positive after nerve injury, and so taking a careful history prior to ordering any tests is necessary. A history and physical exam consistent with an inflammatory process (e.g., osteomyelitis or metastatic disease) may warrant a bone scan, erythrocyte sedimentation rate, white blood cell count, or other laboratory tests. More common diagnoses are minor cervical trauma (the whiplash syndrome), neck pain of myofascial origin, cervical spondylosis, and torticollis.

WHIPLASH

The anatomic characteristics of the cervical spine predispose it to injury by direct as well as indirect forces. According to published reports, as many as 85% of neck disorders result from acute or repetitive injuries (often sustained in automobile accidents) or chronic stress and strain. The term "whiplash" describes the injury caused by an abrupt hyperextension of the neck from an indirect force, as in a rear-end motor vehicle collision. The body is propelled forward in a linear and horizontal manner. The head is then thrown backward, which causes acute hyperextension of the cervical spine. Recoil of the head with marked cervical neck flexion occurs, and then, the head and neck return to the neutral position. Head-on motor vehicle collisions initiate an opposite sequence of events. Whiplash injury is severe because backward hyperextension of the head stops when the occiput hits the posterior upper thorax, which is a position that is not within the normal physiologic range of motion. In contradistinction, forward flexion of the head stops when the chin hits the chest; lateral flexion stops when the ear hits the shoulder. Those movements are physiologic and place no strain on the intervertebral joints.

After a whiplash injury, the cervical flexor muscles, the sternocleidomastoid, the scalenus, and the longus colli, undergo an acute stretch reflex. Fibers are traumatized and torn, often with consequent muscular edema and hemorrhage. Patients usually do not exhibit symptoms for the first 12 to 24 hours. Most commonly, they complain of neckache and stiffness, as well as headache, shoulder pain, and intrascapular pain. Less commonly, patients with whiplash injuries complain of pain or numbness in the arm or hand (usually unilateral, but it may be bilateral), and some report loss of consciousness. Neurologic deficit is rare in soft-tissue injuries associated with whiplash. Stretching of the esophagus with resulting edema, dysphagia, and retropharyngeal hemorrhage may occur. Vocal-cord damage with hoarseness has been reported. Trauma to the cervical sympathetic chain may occur with symptoms of nausea, vomiting, dizziness, Horner's syndrome, and even complex regional pain syndrome, type I. Persistent radicular pain after cervical trauma requires further investigation to rule out nerve root involvement.

Psychosomatic reactions to soft-tissue injuries of the neck may be related to a variety of factors. Chronicity of symptoms may be associated with emotional reaction to the accident or with secondary gain. Studies show that if litigation claims were settled within the first 6 months of injury, more than 80% of patients were symptom free at 5-year follow-up. If settlement of litigation was delayed to 18 months after the accident, 5-year follow-up showed that only 40% of patients were symptom free. Even without pending litigation, however, some patients become significantly impaired by soft-tissue injuries.

Minor cervical trauma resulting in acute cervical pain often is secondary to musculoskeletal injury and usually is self-limited with conservative treatment. In patients who have no evidence of neurologic deficit and have unremarkable radiologic studies, initial treatment is conservative. Most authors recommend a soft cervical collar, analgesics, bed rest, and gradually increased activity for the first 1 to 2 weeks. In addition, physiotherapy, isometric exercises, heat, traction if symptoms improve, and transcutaneous–electrical nerve stimulation have been useful for the acute cervical strain associated with whiplash injuries.

Patients with chronic pain often are referred to a pain management center. A detailed history, physical examination, and review of radiologic information will identify those who require neurosurgical or orthopedic referral. Patients with chronic neck pain after soft-tissue injury of the neck often can be helped by a nerve block with local anesthetic and sometimes with steroids. These include patients with complex regional pain syndrome (amenable to stellate ganglion block), occipital neuralgia (amenable to occipital nerve block), traumatic torticollis (amenable to accessory nerve block or injection into the muscle belly), traumatic myofascial pain syndrome (amenable to trigger point injections as well as stretch and spray techniques), and suprascapular pain (amenable to injection of the suprascapular nerve). Additionally, patients with radicular neck pain can benefit from cervical–epidural steroids, which may be administered by the anesthesiologist in a pain-management center. Patients also should be examined for evidence of facet syndrome, which may respond to facet-joint injections.

MYOFASCIAL PAIN SYNDROME

The myofascial pain syndrome is one of the most common and often overlooked causes of neck pain. Myofascial pain is characterized by pain referred from active trigger points. A myofascial trigger point is a hyperirritable locus, which may be palpable as an exquisitely tender, taut band within skeletal muscle. The examiner carefully palpates head, neck, and shoulder muscles, attempting to detect trigger points. Compression at those points elicits a characteristic and reproducible pattern of referred pain remote from the location of the tender trigger point (Fig. 11.2). Often, the pain is described as steady, deep, and aching in quality, although it is not uncommon for patients to use words like burning or crushing. The pain pattern is not limited to a specific dermatome or peripheral-nerve segment. Neck pain of myofascial origin is essentially a diagnosis of exclusion, as the character of the pain may mimic other cervical pathology. Myofascial pain may be abrupt in onset (perhaps after an injury) or

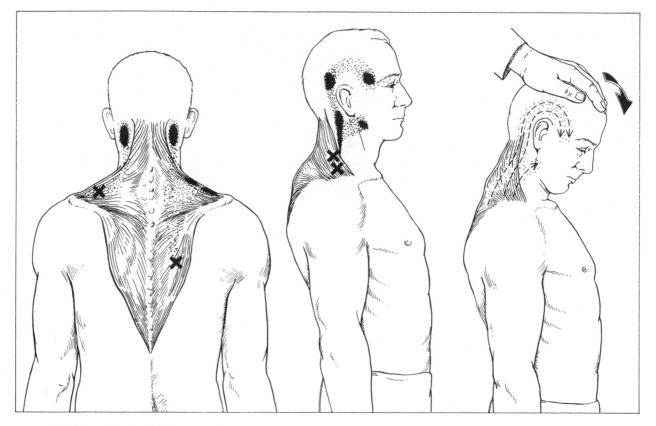

FIG. 11.2. Myofascial trigger points can be a source of referred pain. The "*X*" marks the hyperirritable locus that can be palpated as a tender, taut band of muscle or a "knot." The *stippled area* outlines the patient's area of pain. Pressure on the trigger point may reproduce the patient's symptoms.

of more gradual onset (from chronic overutilization of muscles). Psychogenic stress, viral illness, visceral disease, exposure to cold or damp weather, strenuous exercise, or prolonged tension of the involved muscle may precipitate or exacerbate a myofascial pain syndrome.

Trigger points commonly responsible for pain referred to the cervical area are located within several muscle groups (Table 11.2). Pain referred from identified trigger points may be alleviated by spraying the involved muscles with vapo-coolant, coupled with passive stretching of the muscle. Alternatively, needling of the trigger point and injection with local anesthetic and sometimes steroid,

followed by passive stretching, may be performed. Hot packs are applied after either modality.

Additionally, physical therapy (involving muscle strengthening and stretching) and application of moist heat, ultrasound, electrical stimulation, or iontophoresis have been useful. Effective medical therapies include nonsteroidal antiinflammatory drugs, muscle relaxants, and a bedtime tricyclic antidepressant. Stress-reduction therapy (including biofeedback, hypnosis, and behavior modification) also may be helpful. Many patients will seek out alternative therapies, such as Gua-shua, Reikii, or acupuncture in their search for relief.

TABLE 11.2. *Cervical Myofascial Trigger Points*

Muscle	Area of referred pain
Trapezius	Neck, shoulder, and temporal region
Splenius capitis and cervicis	Head, occiput, shoulder and neck; vision may be blurred
Posterior neck muscles, semispinalis capitis and cervicis, and multitifidi	Suboccipital area, neck, and shoulders
Levator scapulae	Angle of the neck and along the vertebral body of the border of the scapula
Scalene	Chest, upper-central border of the scapula, and along the arm
Supraspinatus	Posterior neck and suboccipital area of the deltoid, deep in the shoulder joint, and the front and lateral aspects of the arm and forearm

CERVICAL SPONDYLOSIS

Disc degeneration and cervical spondylosis are common causes of neck pain. An estimated 50% of people over the age of 50 and 75% of those over 65 have radiologic evidence of cervical spondylosis, most of them without symptoms. Cervical spondylosis comprises the process in which wear and tear of the cervical spine results in disc degeneration, calcification, new bone formation, and osteophyte formation. The bone formation may lead to intervertebral foramen narrowing, with nerve-root irritation or spinal-canal narrowing with cord compression.

The process starts with disc degeneration, which occurs with aging as the vascular supply and nutritional supply to the disk are compromised. Nerve roots most often involved with nerve-root compression are C5 and C6, which represent the locale of maximum mobility, angulation, and degeneration of the cervical spine. The manifestations of cervical disc degeneration and cervical spondylosis encompass a wide spectrum: brachial radiculopathy, suboccipital neuralgia, localized neck pain, cord compression, vertigo, and vertebral basilar-ischemic symptoms. Symptoms may be acute and associated with minor trauma or of a more chronic and progressive nature.

The patient who presents with neck pain or cervical–radicular symptoms but with normal neurologic and radiographic findings may be treated conservatively. Therapeutic modalities include a soft cervical collar, analgesics, antiinflammatories, local heat, possibly traction (although some individuals find this to be an irritant), and isometric exercises. Secondary myofascial trigger points or occipital neuralgia may be treated with injection of local anesthetics, possibly mixed with steroids. Surgery usually is recommended for progressive neurologic deficits or signs of cord compression; however, surgery for pain alone is controversial. The use of cervical–epidural steroids or selective nerve root block for chronic neck pain and cervical radiculitis has been reported to be effective in a number of studies.

CERVICAL HERPES ZOSTER AND POSTHERPETIC NEURALGIA

The patient with cervical herpes zoster or cervical postherpetic neuralgia may present to the primary-care clinician with severe pain. In the patient with herpes zoster, early institution of antiviral therapy and tricyclic antidepressant can reduce the incidence of postherpetic neuralgia. Patients with severe pain with zoster need to be treated aggressively with anticonvulsants, opiates, and possibly injections such as stellate ganglion block or intralesional injection with local anesthetic and steroid. Similarly, stellate ganglion block or intralesional injection with local anesthetic and steroid have been used in patients presenting with cervical postherpetic neuralgia. Application of transcutaneous electrical nerve stimulation in the adjacent half of the involved dermatomes (those without lesions) has successfully relieved pain in some patients, whereas others report an increase in pain.

The neuropathic pain of postherpetic neuralgia is rarely responsive to spinal-cord stimulation, but this has been tried for patients suffering from intractable pain.

SELECTED READINGS

Borenstein DG, Wiesel SW, Boden SD. *Neck Pain : Medical Diagnosis and Comprehensive Management*. London: W B Saunders Co, 1996.

Cote P, Hogg-Johnson S, Cassidy JD, et al. The association between neck pain intensity, physical functioning, depressive symptomatology and time-to-claim-closure after whiplash. *J Clin Epidemiol* 2001;54: 275–286.

Giles L, Singer KP. *Clinical Anatomy and Management of Cervical Spine Pain*. Woburn, Massachusetts: Butterworth-Heinemann Medical, 1998.

Hanten WP, Olson SL, Butts NL, et al. Effectiveness of a home program of ischemic pressure followed by sustained stretch for treatment of myofascial trigger points. *Phys Ther* 2000;80:997–1003.

Leak AM, Cooper J, Dyer S, et al. The Northwick Park Neck Pain Questionnaire, devised to measure neck pain and disability. *Br J Rheumatol* 1994;33:469–474.

Lucente FE, Cooper BC. *Management of Facial, Head and Neck Pain*. London: W B Saunders Co, 1989.

M Peeters GG, Verhagen AP, de Bie RA, et al. The efficacy of conservative treatment in patients with whiplash injury: a systematic review of clinical trials. *Spine* 2001;26:E64–E73.

Sist T, Wong C. Difficult problems and their solutions in patients with cancer pain of the head and neck areas. *Curr Rev Pain* 2000;4:206–214.

Slipman CW, Lipetz JS, Plastaras CT, et al. Therapeutic zygapophyseal joint injections for headaches emanating from the C2-3 joint. *Am J Phys Med Rehabil* 2001;80:182–188.

Slipman CW, Lipetz JS, Jackson HB, et al. Therapeutic selective nerve root block in the nonsurgical treatment of atraumatic cervical spondylotic radicular pain: a retrospective analysis with independent clinical review. *Arch Phys Med Rehabil* 2000;81:741–746.

CHAPTER 12

Shoulder Pain

Tobin N. Gerhart and Lena E. Dohlman

The patient with a chief complaint of pain in the region of the shoulder is a common clinical challenge to the practicing physician. Causes can include disorders of the glenohumeral joint, surrounding soft tissues, neurologic structures extrinsic to the shoulder, and even intrathoracic and abdominal organs. Correct diagnosis can be difficult but is crucial for proper therapy. It is important to differentiate shoulder pain caused by some serious underlying medical condition from tendinitis or bursitis.

An organized and systematic approach is the best way to avoid missing the diagnosis (Table 12.1). The pathologic causes of shoulder pain can be divided into two categories: intrinsic and extrinsic disorders. Intrinsic disorders involve the shoulder itself and characteristically involve three findings: (a) pain is aggravated by using the shoulder (e.g., raising the arm); (b) tenderness, either localized or diffuse, is present on physical examination; (c) pain can be elicited by active or passive motion of the arm. Extrinsic disorders (originating outside the shoulder) do not fulfill those three criteria. Usually, the distinction is easy to make, but sometimes the boundaries can be blurred, particularly with neurologic causes.

Neurologic disorders are the most common extrinsic cause of shoulder pain (Fig. 12.1). The patient typically complains of a pain that either radiates down into the shoulder from the neck or starts in the shoulder and radiates down the arm. Sensory or motor deficits are often present, which mandates a careful neurologic exam in all patients with this complaint. An attempt should be made to correlate any findings of sensory or motor deficit with either a specific dermatome or peripheral-nerve distribution. Shoulder pain may originate with neurologic pathology in the cervical roots, the brachial plexus, and the axillary or other peripheral nerves. Electromyographic and nerve-conduction studies can help to determine the location of the lesion.

Cervical radiculopathy with impingement affecting the C5 to T1 roots is a common neurologic cause of shoulder pain. The most frequent cause of cervical radiculopathy, particularly in middle-aged or older patients, is cervical spondylosis. Spondylosis is a degenerative condition of the cervical intervertebral region, causing disc-space collapse, subsequent annular protrusion, and an osteophytic reaction. Spondylitic changes can occur at one or several intervertebral levels and may be considered a normal process of aging. Patients become symptomatic when the condition is sufficiently severe to cause impingement on the nerve root as it exits from the spinal canal.

Disc-space narrowing is seen on lateral-view x-rays. On physical exam, the patient typically has some tender-

---

TABLE 12.1. *Clinical Diagnosis of Shoulder Pain*

Extrinsic causes
Neurologic
   Cervical radiculopathy (spondylosis, herniated disc)
   Thoracic outlet (cervical rib, scalenus anticus)
   Brachial plexus (neuritis)
   Peripheral nerve (suprascapular, spinal accessory,
     long thoracic, dorsal scapular)
Referred
   Somatic (free air under diaphragm)
   Visceral (gallbladder)
Intrinsic causes
   Acromioclavicular separation (acute with instability;
     chronic with degenerative joint disease)
   Adhesive capsulitis (idiopathic, secondary)
   Glenohumeral arthritis (osteoarthritis, rheumatoid
     arthritis, gout, septic arthritis)
Periarticular
   Bursitis, tendinitis (supraspinatus, coracoid, bicipital,
     deltoid)
   Impingement (subacromial)
   Rotator-cuff tear
Other
   Fracture (proximal humerus)
   Myofascitis
   Tumor (metastatic, primary)

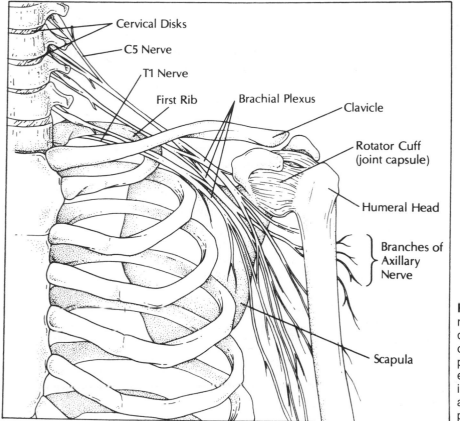

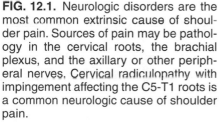

FIG. 12.1. Neurologic disorders are the most common extrinsic cause of shoulder pain. Sources of pain may be pathology in the cervical roots, the brachial plexus, and the axillary or other peripheral nerves. Cervical radiculopathy with impingement affecting the C5-T1 roots is a common neurologic cause of shoulder pain.

ness in the back of the neck and increased pain in the neck and shoulder with hyperextension of the neck.

Younger patients may have cervical radiculopathy secondary to a herniated disc and consequently a more acute presentation. Material from the nucleus pulposus extrudes through a defect in the disc's annular wall and can cause dramatic pain, weakness, and numbness in the shoulder and arm. To relieve some tension on the nerve root, the patient may elevate his arm and present holding his hand on his head. Magnetic resonance imaging (MRI) will show disc herniation and dural-sac or nerve-root impingement.

Most patients with cervical radiculopathy respond to conservative therapy, which may consist of antiinflammatory drugs, local heat, and limitation of the neck motion with a cervical collar. Those who do not respond to conservative therapy may benefit from cervical-epidural steroids, which should be administered by an experienced clinician on an outpatient basis. Rarely, surgery is required for severe and persistent symptoms.

Thoracic-outlet syndrome is a common neurologic cause of intermittent pain in the shoulder. Patients characteristically have symptoms associated with specific activities, such as work involving use of the arm in an elevated position. The pathophysiology usually involves compression of neural elements between the first rib and some other anatomic structure, such as the clavicle, cervical rib, or scalenus-anticus muscle. The examining physician can elicit symptoms by specific maneuvers, such as placing the arm in an abducted and elevated position and having the patient face toward the affected shoulder and take a deep breath. In addition to reproducing the patient's pain, that maneuver commonly extinguishes the radial pulse. Thoracic-outlet syndrome usually responds to a physical-therapy program, but severe cases may require surgery (usually resection of the first rib) for relief.

Brachial-plexus neuropathy is a somewhat enigmatic disorder for which no etiologic factor has been convincingly identified. Tenderness and pain in the shoulder may radiate into the scapula or arm. Sensory and motor deficits are common. Extension of the arm may aggravate symptoms that are caused by irritation of the plexus. Electrodiagnostic studies are useful, as patients often have abnormal fibrillation potentials in the muscles of the shoulder and upper arm. Brachial-plexus neuropathy may involve a prolonged course, taking more than 1 year to resolve in some cases, but the prognosis for a complete recovery is excellent. Only symptomatic treatment is indicated.

Persistent pain and weakness localized to a specific shoulder muscle can be caused by injury or entrapment of a peripheral nerve. Etiologic factors include blunt impact or traction (e.g., contact sports), overuse syndromes (e.g., competitive swimming), impingement by a ganglion cyst, or entrapment by a fibrous band. Suprascapular nerve involvement produces supraspinatus muscle pain and weakness. The clinical signs and symptoms mimic those of a rotator-cuff tear. Scapular winging, or abnormal tilting of the scapula secondary to muscle imbalance, results from weakness of the parascapular muscles. Spinal-accessory nerve palsy causes trapezius-muscle atrophy with depression and counter-clockwise rotation of the scapula. Long thoracic-nerve palsy causes serratus anterior-muscle atrophy with elevation and clockwise rotation of the scapula. Dorsal scapular nerve palsy, rarer than the previous conditions, causes rhomboid-muscle atrophy. Suspected peripheral nerve palsies can be confirmed by electromyography (EMG) studies. Most patients eventually respond well to physical therapy for muscle strengthening and range-of-motion exercises. Some patients, particularly those with ganglions or fibrous-band entrapment, may require surgery.

Thoracic or intraabdominal pathology occasionally may present as shoulder pain. Cholecystitis, a ruptured abdominal viscus, and cardiac or pulmonary disease, can all cause pain to be referred to the shoulder. Free air under the diaphragm characteristically causes a dull ache in the scapular area. Referred pain should be suspected when symptoms seem unrelated to activity involving the shoulder and when other symptoms or signs of systemic illness are present.

Intrinsic shoulder pain may result from pathology of the joint proper, periarticular soft tissues, or surrounding musculoskeletal structures. Orthopaedic examination of the shoulder should involve careful measurement of its range of motion. Findings on physical examination are compared with those of the contralateral shoulder as well as with accepted normal values. To assess internal rotation, the examiner should note how high the patient can place the hand behind the back with the elbow bent. External rotation, measured with the patient holding the elbow at the side and rotating the arm outward, will range between 45 and 90 degrees from the sagittal plane, depending on the joint's flexibility. Forward elevation of the arm in front of the body to an overhead position should be assessed while the patient is sitting and while supine, with both active and passive motion. Decreased range of motion and pain at the extremes of motion are important signs of intrinsic shoulder pathology.

The glenohumeral joint is susceptible to all forms of arthritis, including osteoarthritis, rheumatoid arthritis, gout, pseudogout, and septic arthritis. Osteoarthritis restricted to the shoulder usually is associated with a history of trauma, whereas systemic forms of arthritis usually have manifestations in other joints. Osteoarthritic changes on x-ray include narrowing of the joint space, cyst formation, spurs, and sclerosis. The acromioclavicular joint also is susceptible to osteoarthritis, often as a sequelae to a traumatic shoulder separation.

Stability of the glenohumeral joint depends mostly on muscular forces and capsular attachment, because the glenoid articulation is very shallow and provides little bony constraint. As a result, the shoulder has a very wide range of motion but is vulnerable to instability when the capsule and ligaments are torn by trauma. Complete disruption of the joint is called a dislocation and may occur with humeral head being driven either anteriorly or posteriorly. Anterior dislocations are much more common and usually are unmistakable, as the patient is unable to move the arm. X-ray, preferably both anteroposterior and axillary lateral views, will confirm dislocation of the humeral head. Elderly patients often present with chronic dislocations that have gone unrecognized. The patient may be fairly asymptomatic, except for a very limited range of active motion. X-ray examination confirms the diagnosis. Patient should be referred to an orthopaedist, as chronic dislocations may require surgical intervention.

The less common, posterior, glenohumeral dislocations often present in an atypical fashion and are therefore more frequently missed. The history need not involve acute trauma, as posterior dislocations are common sequelae of convulsions. Because the anteroposterior x-ray often gives the false impression of a normal glenohumeral relationship, owing to superposition, a lateral view is mandatory.

When the glenohumeral disruption is only partial and transitory, it is termed subluxation. It occurs in younger patients and usually is associated with physical activity, such as throwing a ball. The patient feels that the arm goes "dead," and shoulder hurts afterward. The physician can elicit the symptoms by abducting the arm 90 degrees and then pressing from behind directly on the humeral head. If instability is present, the patient will have discomfort and a feeling that the arm will dislocate — a positive "apprehension test."

Adhesive capsulitis is a serious problem that can result after seemingly minor trauma or is secondary to a primary condition that immobilizes the shoulder. The patient notes poorly localized pain and tenderness in the shoulder and a limitation of range of motion, especially external rotation and elevation. The pathophysiology is adhesion and contraction of the inflamed capsular surfaces. The primary aim of treatment should be prevention. Thus, in all patients with a shoulder disorder, daily range-of-motion exercises should be instituted as soon as possible. They include pendulum exercises in which the patient bends forward and lets the hanging arm swing in widening arcs. As motion improves, the patient should lie supine and slowly raise the involved arm fully overhead, using the contralateral hand. Physical-therapy referral for modalities and range-of-motion exercises is appropriate. Once full-blown adhesive capsulitis occurs, treatment can be very difficult and prolonged. In moderate cases, intraarticular injections of lidocaine and corticosteroids can provide temporary relief of symptoms, and thus facilitate progress with range-of-motion exercises. In recalcitrant cases, patients may benefit from a suprascapular nerve block just before their physical-therapy session. The suprascapular nerve contains sensory fibers to the shoulder joint and surrounding structures. It is a fairly superficial nerve and can be blocked without great difficulty.

CASE REPORT

A 66-year-old man presented with pain in his left arm and shoulder and a frozen left shoulder resulting from a cerebrovascular accident. He had been treated by a physical therapist for several months with little improvement in range of motion or symptoms. He was seen several times in the pain clinic at 2-week intervals and received a left suprascapular nerve block at each visit, after which he was seen by the physical therapist. Each block resulted in complete relief of shoulder pain for about 2 hours. He continued range-of-motion exercises at home between clinic visits. After several months, the range of motion of his left arm was markedly increased, and his shoulder and arm pain significantly decreased.

Intrinsic periarticular shoulder problems are characterized by localized tenderness on physical examination. Pain occurs with active motion, but usually the arm can be passively moved, at least through a limited range of motion, with minimal discomfort.

The most common causes of shoulder pain seen by the practicing physician are bursitis and tendinitis. Both of those conditions represent an inflammatory response to injury resulting from overuse of the shoulder. The history typically includes participation in some activity that involves vigorous use of the arm, such as painting a wall or playing tennis. The patient usually does not experience maximal discomfort until 12 to 24 hours afterward. Often, the condition is chronic, characterized by asymptomatic periods between acute exacerbations.

Numerous structures are at risk, most commonly the supraspinatus tendon and bursa, the long head of the biceps tendon, the deltoid insertion, and the coracoid process. Patients have pain referred to the specific location when they are actively moving the involved muscle against resistance. With supraspinatus bursitis, for instance, the first 30 degrees of elevation or abduction of the arm can be the most painful. On x-ray, the presence of calcifications corresponding to the area of the tenderness indicates that a long-standing process exists. Treatment consists of antiinflammatory medication and sling immobilization, followed by gentle, daily range-of-motion exercises to prevent stiffness. Corticosteroid injections are indicated in selected cases.

Impingement syndrome involves rubbing of the rotator cuff underneath the coraco-acromial ligament and anterior acromion. Patients often complain of painful snapping and have a painful arc-of-arm motion from 70 to 100 degrees of elevation. The diagnosis is supported by good pain relief from a subacromial injection of Xylocaine.

Most patients respond to antiinflammatory medication, modification of activities, and physical-therapy exercises, but some may require arthroscopic surgery.

Rotator-cuff tears need to be differentiated from acute-inflammatory conditions, as they may not heal without operative treatment. The etiology is acute or chronic trauma to the rotator cuff, the aponeuroses of the muscles responsible for internal and external rotation of the shoulder. On physical examination, patients have tenderness directly over the proximal humerus and weakness of external or internal rotation as determined by testing muscle strength. The diagnosis can be confirmed by MRI. Small tears can heal with antiinflammatory medications and immobilization. Large tears in the cuff may require surgical repair.

Miscellaneous conditions causing pain about the shoulder include fractures, tumors, and myofascitis. A fall on the outstretched arm is a very common cause of proximal-humeral fracture, particularly in postmenopausal women and elderly men. The fracture line usually occurs between the tubcrosities, an area referred to as the surgical neck. If there is a minimal displacement, most fractures are fairly stable and require only immobilization and a sling for comfort. It is important to begin some range-of-motion exercises as early as possible to prevent stiffness. Elderly patients generally should start arm movement within 1 to 2 weeks.

If shoulder pain is unrelated to activity, seems to be worse at night, and is relieved only by narcotics, malignancy should be suspected. Metastatic lesions are much more common than primary lesions. The bone scan is the most sensitive test for skeletal involvement. Malignant lesions are distinguished from benign process by their relatively large size, destruction of cortical bone, and presence of a soft-tissue mass. An apical (Pancoast) lung tumor can invade the cervical-thoracic sympathetic nerves and cause Horner's syndrome.

Myofascitis is one name for a common and perplexing shoulder syndrome usually involving the medial and superior borders of the scapula. There often is a discrete area of tenderness and a trigger point from which the pain radiates. Occasionally, autonomic phenomena can result from palpation of the trigger point. Activities involving lifting or pulling motion usually are painful. The diagnosis is clinical, as x-rays and scans are normal. The pathophysiology of myofascial trigger points is controversial. Most evidence suggests that the syndrome begins with muscular strain that affects the site of hypersensitive nerves, increases metabolism, and decreases circulation. Treatment can begin with antiinflammatory medication, heat, and rest, but symptoms often are unresponsive to those measures. Early treatment with a transcutaneous-electrical nerve stimulation (TENS) unit or trigger-point injections (see also Chapter 47) of a local anesthetic can be helpful and sometimes can prevent progression to the dystrophic phase.

In summary, shoulder pain can have a myriad of etiologies. An organized and systematic approach to diagnosis will help avoid errors in treatment. A useful starting point is differentiation of pain of intrinsic origin from that of extrinsic origin. A careful history and physical exam usually will reveal the diagnosis.

SELECTED READINGS

Biglioni L, Levine WN. Subacromial impingement syndrome. *J Bone Joint Surg Am*1997;79:1854–1868

Kuhn JE, Plancher KD, Hawkins RJ. Scapula winging. *J Am Acad Orthop Surg* 1995;3:319.

Warner JJ. Frozen shoulder: diagnosis and management. *J Am Acad Orthop* 1997;5:130–140.

CHAPTER 13

Elbow Pain

Jeffrey L. Zilberfarb

Elbow pain is a frequent patient complaint seen by both the primary-care physician and in general orthopedic practice. The common etiologies of elbow pain are listed in Table 13.1. Pain from overuse activities at work or from recreation is most commonly seen.

The vast majority of elbow problems can be diagnosed based on history and physical examination. Radiographs are useful in ruling out loose bodies, arthritis, or serious, rare disorders such as tumors or chronic osteomyelitis. Magnetic resonance imaging (MRI) is infrequently required to secure the diagnosis.

INFLAMMATORY DISORDERS

Lateral Epicondylitis/Medial Epicondylitis

Lateral epicondylitis is commonly referred to as "tennis elbow," although it is frequently seen in other activities such as prolonged use of a computer keyboard, lifting a heavy briefcase or suitcase, or any activity that puts strain on the elbow. It also may be seen in the left arm of right-handed golfers, although golfers also may have a distinct syndrome known as "golfer's elbow" (*medial epicondylitis*). This is thought to occur because of improper swing mechanics.

TABLE 13.1. *Common Etiologies of Elbow Pain*

Lateral epicondylitis
Medial epicondylitis
Bursitis
Septic arthritis
Osteomyelitis
Fractures
Ligament injuries
Bicep-tendon injuries
Osteochondritis dessicans
Cubital tunnel syndrome
Arthritis

With lateral epicondylitis, patients complain of pain at the lateral aspect of the elbow; with medial epicondylitis they complain of medial-elbow pain.

Physical examination in lateral epicondylitis reveals tenderness to palpation overlying the lateral epicondyle, which is the origin of the wrist and finger extensor musculature. Occasionally, there is soft-tissue swelling in this area. With medial epicondylitis, tenderness occurs overlying the medial epicondyle.

Initial treatment should include rest, icing, and the use of nonsteroidal antiinflammatory drugs (NSAIDs,) along with a gentle wrist-stretching program. Physical therapy with ionto- or phonophoresis may help reduce inflammation. These modalities use corticosteroid topical preparations and either electrical current (iontophoresis) or ultrasound (phonophoresis) to provide transcutaneous dispersion. For recalcitrant cases, the physician may perform one or two direct corticosteroid injections overlying the inflamed tendinous origin. Direct tendon injection should be avoided as this may lead to tendon rupture. Once the inflammation and pain have resolved, a gentle wrist-extensor strengthening program is indicated.

The vast majority of these patients will respond to nonoperative treatment. If this is not successful, surgery to excise the inflamed tissue and a limited epicondylectomy are indicated.

It is important to determine the etiology of this overuse syndrome so that the behavior can be modified. Tennis players and golfers should have a professional evaluate their swing; computer workers may benefit from an ergonomics evaluation of their workstation.

Noninfectious Bursitis

Noninfectious bursitis is caused by inflammation of the olecranon bursa, which overlies the posterior aspect of the elbow. It may be seen in computer workers who rest their elbows on hard surfaces for prolonged time periods (e.g., hard arm rests on chairs) or in those whose occupations require repetitive elbow flexion or crawling (such as coal miners or construction workers). Alcoholics may develop this from spending many hours at the bar leaning on their elbows.

Physical examination reveals a swollen, slightly tender olecranon bursa without erythema and with minimal warmth. Patients are afebrile. These findings are very different in patients with septic bursitis, which is characterized by fever, erythema, and severe tenderness to palpation overlying the bursa. Radiographs may infrequently reveal an olecranon osteophyte.

Inflammatory bursitis typically responds slowly to rest, icing, NSAIDs, compression wrapping of the elbow, and avoidance of the instigating behavior. A direct bursal corticosteroid injection may be useful for patients who do not get the relief they seek. Chronic cases may require a surgical approach with bursal excision and osteophyte removal, if present.

INFECTIOUS DISORDERS

Septic Bursitis

Septic bursitis may occur after a skin abrasion or puncture wound. Physical-examination findings are as described above: fever, erythema, and severe tenderness to palpation overlying the bursa. Aspiration of the olecranon bursa may reveal a cloudy aspirate, and subsequent examination with gram stain and culture will confirm the diagnosis.

Treatment is with oral antibiotics and repeated needle aspiration in mild cases. For patients with more severe symptoms, intravenous antibiotics, possibly in conjunction with surgical drainage, is indicated.

Septic Arthritis

Patients with septic-elbow arthritis have severe pain with active and passive range of motion of the elbow. They may be febrile, and may have an effusion. Diagnosis is confirmed by elbow-joint aspiration, gram stain, and culture. Radiographs are expected to be normal, although they may reveal osteomyelitis in advanced, chronic cases. Treatment consists of intravenous (i.v.) antibiotics and surgical drainage.

Osteomyelitis

Osteomyelitis may develop secondary to direct local causes (e.g., open fracture) or by systemic infection. Patients may complain of localized or diffuse pain, may or may not be febrile, and may or may not have abnormal motion.

Radiographs may reveal lytic bone abnormalities in chronic cases, but often are unremarkable early. Nuclear imaging using bone scans or white blood cell-labeled scans may be required to make the diagnosis. MRI also may be helpful.

Bone biopsy for gram stain, culture, and pathology often is needed to confirm the diagnosis and choose appropriate antibiotic therapy. Treatment consists of several weeks of i.v. antibiotics and usually requires surgical debridement.

TRAUMATIC INJURIES

Fractures

Elbow fractures are often easily diagnosed, as there usually is a history of a fall. The physical examination and radiographs confirm the diagnosis. The majority of elbow fractures can be treated without surgery. Most simple fractures heal without consequence. Complications such as malunions and nonunions may lead to joint stiffness and pain. Surgery usually is required for displaced fractures.

Ligament Injuries

The elbow has two primary ligamentous constraints: the medial collateral and lateral collateral ligaments. The medial collateral ligament is the primary elbow stabilizer. These ligaments may be injured from a fall or repetitive stress injury (e.g., a baseball pitcher).

Physical examination reveals tenderness directly overlying the ligament, possibly with soft-tissue swelling. If the ligament is stretched or torn, there may be laxity with stress testing (Fig. 13.1).

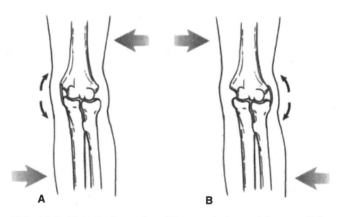

FIG. 13.1. Test the integrity of ligaments by exerting medially and laterally directed pressure as shown. If the ligaments are ruptured, abnormal opening of the joint space will occur. **A:** Medial–collateral ligament stress test. **B:** Lateral–collateral ligament stress test. (Reprinted from Gates SJ, Mooar PA, eds. *Musculoskeletal Primary Care*. Philadelphia: Lippincott Williams & Wilkins, 1999, with permission.)

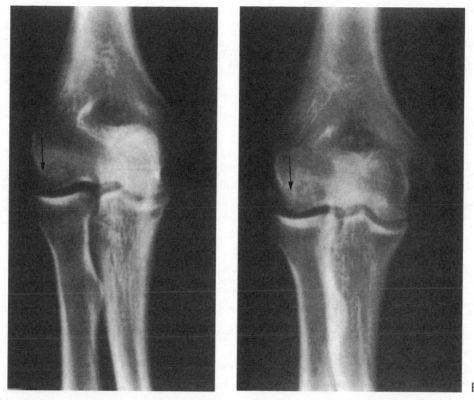

FIG. 13.2. A: Anteroposterior (AP) view, type I lesion in a 14-year-old boy with osteochondritis dissecans. **B:** AP view 1 1/2 years later. The zone of rarefaction surrounding the lesion is becoming less distinct, and the patient is asymptomatic. (Reprinted from Gates SJ, Mooar PA, eds. *Musculoskeletal Primary Care.* Philadelphia: Lippincott Williams & Wilkins, 1999, with permission.)

Treatment for simple sprains consists of rest, bracing, icing, NSAIDs, and physical therapy. Completely torn ligaments may require surgical reconstruction.

Biceps-Tendon Injuries

The insertion of the biceps tendon on the proximal radius may be injured by lifting very heavy objects (e.g., a large television set). Physical examination reveals tenderness to palpation with simple strains, and the absence of a palpable tendon in complete tears. Radiographs are normal. MRI is infrequently required to confirm the diagnosis. Treatment of strains is conservative; complete tears often require surgical repair for optimum function.

Osteochondritis Dissecans

This condition often is seen in athletes who throw (i.e., pitcher, quarterback, shot-putter) and is characterized by dull, achy elbow pain. Physical examination may reveal limited range of motion but often is benign. Radiographs depict a bony lesion most commonly affecting the capitellum (Figure 13.2). Computed tomography provides better detail and may be needed for diagnosis.

Those patients who do not respond to conservative modalities may benefit from arthroscopic debridement.

NEUROLOGIC DISORDERS

Cubital Tunnel Syndrome

The ulnar nerve is relatively superficial at the posteromedial elbow, and thus is subject to direct traumatic injury. The ulnar nerve also is vulnerable to repetitive stress from repeated elbow flexion, and it may become compressed in the cubital canal. Some patients with a lax medial collateral ligament may become symptomatic from stretch on the ulnar nerve. Others may have a history of lateral elbow fracture (tardy ulnar nerve palsy) from a similar mechanism.

Patients may complain of medial elbow pain, and usually of paresthesias and numbness along the medial forearm and the ring and little fingers. In more severe cases, patients may have intrinsic hand-muscle weakness.

Physical examination may reveal a positive Tinel's sign overlying the ulnar nerve at the cubital tunnel, decreased sensation in the ulnar nerve distribution, and intrinsic muscle weakness/atrophy. Electrodiagnostic studies confirm the diagnosis and eliminate other abnormalities (e.g., cervical radiculopathy). In mild cases, extension nighttime elbow bracing is helpful, but in more severe cases, ulnar-nerve decompression and transposition is indicated.

ARTHRITIS

Osteoarthritis

Degenerative arthritis of the elbow is less common than in the lower extremities and may be secondary to trauma but more often idiopathic. Patients complain of pain with motion, stiffness, and occasionally swelling.

Treatment consisting of NSAIDs and icing usually is helpful. An occasional cortisone intraarticular injection with flare-ups may be indicated. Arthroscopic or open debridement can provide pain relief in mild to moderate cases unrelieved by conservative treatment; total elbow replacement generally is reserved for severe cases in patients over 60 years old.

Rheumatoid Arthritis

This form of erosive inflammatory arthritis can be quite debilitating. Patients often respond to those med-ications used typically with rheumatoid arthritis (NSAIDs, methotrexate, etc.). In addition, arthroscopic synovectomy can provide significant pain relief. As with osteoarthritis, total elbow arthroplasty is indicated in severe cases.

SELECTED READINGS

Andrews JR, Whiteside JA. Common elbow problems in the athlete. *J Orthop Sports Phys Ther* 1993;17:289–295.

Conway JE, Jobe FW, Glousman RE, et al. Medial instability of the elbow in throwing athletes. *J Bone Joint Surg Am* 1992;74A:67–73.

D'Alessandro DF, Shields CL Jr., Tribone JE, et al. Repair of distal biceps tendon ruptures in athletes. *Am J Sports Med* 1993;21:114–119.

Ellenbecker TS. Rehabilitation of shoulder and elbow injuries in tennis players. *Clin Sports Med* 1995;14:87–110.

Gates SJ and Mooar PA, eds. *Musculoskeletal Primary Care.* Philadelphia: Lippincott Williams & Wilkins, 1999.

Morrey BF. Complex instability of the elbow. *J Bone Joint Surg Am* 1997; 79:460–469.

Morrey BF. *The Elbow and its Disorders.* Philadelphia: WB Saunders, 1993.

Safran MR. Elbow injuries in athletes: a review. *Clin Orthop* 1995;1: 257–277.

Wilk KE, Arrigo C, Andrews JE. Rehabilitation of the elbow in the throwing athlete. *J Orthop Sports Phys Ther* 1993;17:305–317.

CHAPTER 14

Chest Pain

Joseph P. Kannam

Chest pain is an extremely common complaint that causes individuals to seek medical attention. The etiology of the patient's complaint can be from something as benign as a pulled muscle or mild osteoarthritis, or as serious as a myocardial infarction or an aortic dissection.

To identify the cause of the chest pain, an accurate history, a brief physical exam, and selected laboratory tests and imaging tests are needed. An easy way to think about chest pain is to think of the organs and structures that reside in the thorax: ribs/chest wall, the heart and great vessels, the lungs, the esophagus, and the nerves that innervate the thorax. Occasionally, gastrointestinal pain other than esophageal pain will radiate to the thorax but there usually is associated abdominal pain. For the most part, chest pain originates from structures that reside in the thorax.

When encountering a patient with chest pain, it is important to identify quickly whether it could be a life-threatening and emergent condition or if it is a benign condition. Of all the things that can cause chest pain, only a few truly are life threatening. In the cardiovascular category, ischemia or myocardial infarction or an aortic dissection are life-threatening emergencies. In the pulmonary category, pulmonary embolus and pneumothorax are two very important diagnoses to make promptly. These four conditions, if truly life threatening, usually can be identified rapidly with a pointed history and physical examination, measuring oxygen saturation, and reviewing the electrocardiogram (ECG) and chest x-ray. Although at times a pulmonary embolus or intermittent myocardial ischemia may be difficult to diagnose, if it is truly life threatening, it usually is obvious from the vital signs, oxygen saturation, and ECG.

An accurate history is essential in making the correct diagnosis. What is the quality of the pain? What is the location of the pain? Does the pain radiate? What provokes the pain? What relieves the pain? How long does the pain last?

The physical exam can be limited to vital signs (including heart rate, blood pressure in both arms, and oxygen saturation measured by pulse oximetry), cardiovascular exam (including pulses), lung exam, and abdominal exam. It is important for the clinician to evaluate the patient critically. Are the vital signs stable? Is the blood pressure equal in both arms? Are there any murmurs or rubs? Are the breath sounds equal bilaterally? Is there pain to palpation of the chest wall? Is the abdomen tender?

The ECG can determine if there is evidence of significant myocardial ischemia (i.e., is there significant ST segment depression or elevation)? A prompt chest x-ray can determine if there is significant pulmonary pathology or a widened mediastinum. Within 15 minutes, you will be able to determine if this is a life-threatening condition or not. If not, a more leisurely approach may be taken including observation and the patient's response to medications such as antacids, nitroglycerin, or nonsteroidal antiinflammatory drugs (NSAIDs). Additional testing should be ordered, such as stress testing, chest scans, or lungs scans, as indicated by the initial evaluation.

CARDIOVASCULAR CAUSES

Myocardial Ischemia/Infarction

Angina occurs when myocardial oxygen demand exceeds oxygen supply. This usually occurs in the setting of coronary-artery disease but can occur with coronary vasospasm. In stable angina pectoris resulting from a fixed coronary stenosis, the pain usually is retrosternal and may feel like a burning, squeezing, or suffocating feeling. It often radiates to the left arm, neck, or jaw. It usually is provoked with exertion or emotional distress and is relieved with rest or nitroglycerin. The pain may be associated with shortness of breath. The pain may not occur in the chest but may isolated to the neck, jaw, or arm. A patient at high risk for coronary disease include those with coronary risk factors such as diabetes mellitus, smoking, hypertension, family history of premature coronary disease, or hypercholesterolemia.

The physical examination may be benign but may include hypertension or an S4 on a cardiac exam. The ECG may not show evidence of acute ischemia (i.e., ST segment changes) but may show evidence of a prior myocardial infarction such as Q waves. The diagnosis is confirmed in most cases with an exercise test with or without imaging such as thallium or echocardiography. In some cases, a definitive diagnosis is obtained with the use of cardiac catheterization.

Treatment consists of aspirin, antianginal medication, and possibly revascularization with either angioplasty or bypass surgery. Acute myocardial ischemia with either unstable angina or acute myocardial infarction requires prompt diagnosis and treatment.

Acute coronary syndromes are the result of cholesterol plaque rupture and coronary thrombosis that either transiently or permanently occludes the coronary vessel. The pain is similar in quality to that of stable angina but it tends to be more severe and unremitting. It typically lasts more than 30 minutes (in the case of an infarction), can occur at rest, can awake the individual from sleep, and may be associated with nausea, vomiting , diaphoresis, or an impending sense of doom. The pain often is unrelieved with sublingual nitroglycerin.

On examination, the patient may be in distress, clammy, and with hypertension or hypotension and tachycardia. The ECG will show evidence of acute ischemia, such as ST-segment depression or elevation, or hyperacute T waves. Prompt treatment with aspirin, intravenous heparin, oxygen, and intravenous nitroglycerin is warranted. If the patient has ST elevation on the ECG from an acute infarction, reperfusion therapy with either thrombolytic therapy or angioplasty is warranted.

Aortic Dissection

An acute aortic dissection is another diagnosis that must be made promptly. Dissection of the aorta causes severe anterior chest pain with abrupt onset that can last for hours. It often radiates straight through to the back or between the shoulder blades. It often has a tearing, knife-like quality and the patients just can't get comfortable. Risk factors for dissection include hypertension, Marfan's syndrome, cystic medial necrosis, or blunt trauma to the chest. If the dissection involves the great vessels, there may be associated neurological sequelae or numbness/tingling in the arms. If the dissection involves the aortic valve, there may be acute aortic regurgitation and symptoms of congestive heart failure. If it involves one or more of the coronary arteries, there may be acute myocardial ischemia. The dissected aorta may rupture into the pericardium leading to signs and symptoms of pericardial tamponade.

On physical examination, unequal blood pressures or pulses may be seen, necessitating measurement in both arms. There may be a diastolic murmur of aortic regurgitation. There may be a palpable aneurysm in the abdomen. The ECG usually is nondiagnostic unless there is associated myocardial ischemia. The chest x-ray may reveal a widened mediastinum. A definitive diagnosis is made with either transesophageal echocardiogram (TEE), chest computed tomography (CT) angiogram, or a chest magnetic resonance imaging (MRI). The hemodynamic stability of the patient determines whether a TEE, CT, MRI is indicated. In general, visualization of the aortic arch is better with a CT or MRI, therefore these modalities are preferred if the patient is stable. The advantage of the TEE is that it can be done portably in the emergency room or intensive-care unit if necessary. Once the diagnosis is confirmed, if the dissection involves the ascending aorta, emergency surgery is indicated.

Pericarditis

The pain of acute pericarditis is not related to exertion. It usually is sharp and may radiate to the shoulder or neck. The pain usually is worse with inspiration and may be relieved with sitting forward. The pain may last for hours to days and may wax and wane. There may be an associated viral upper-respiratory infection but this is not always the case. A pericardial rub may be heard on physical examination. The electrocardiographic findings of acute pericarditis include diffuse ST-segment elevation (never more than 5 mm), diffuse PR-segment depression (except for AVR where there is PR-segment elevation), and T wave inversions. An echocardiogram can help determine if there is an associated pericardial effusion but the absence of an effusion does not rule out pericarditis. The most common etiology of pericarditis is a viral infection but it may be from a recent myocardial infarction, uremia, radiation, drugs, or an autoimmune disorder. Treatment consists of NSAIDs and eliminating any potential underlying causes.

Aortic Stenosis

Aortic stenosis can cause exertional angina as a result of subendocardial ischemia from increased left ventricular wall stress. It is never associated with rest chest pain. Aortic stenosis may be associated with the other cardinal symptoms such as exertional dyspnea or lightheadedness/syncope. Physical examination reveals a crescendo/decrescendo murmur at the left sternal border. Carotid pulses may be diminished or delayed. There may be evidence of congestive heart failure on examination. The ECG commonly reveals left-ventricular hypertrophy with a strain pattern. The diagnosis is confirmed with an echocardiogram.

PULMONARY CAUSES

Pulmonary causes of chest pain typically are pleural in nature, which is typically sharp or stabbing pain related to breathing or coughing.

Pleurisy

Inflammation of the pleura is the most common cause of pulmonary-related chest pain. The pain usually is unilateral and worse with deep breathing and sometimes with movement. Etiologies include a respiratory-tract infection either viral or bacterial, pulmonary embolus, pulmonary infarction, cancer, or a connective disease disorder such as systemic lupus erythematosus. Physical examination may reveal a pleural rub, and chest x-ray may reveal a pleural effusion. Treatment consists of NSAIDs and eliminating any potential underlying causes.

Pulmonary Embolus

A pulmonary embolus may be associated with pleuritic chest pain and, if large enough, severe substernal chest pain. The diagnosis may be elusive and potentially life threatening, therefore one must think of it in the differential diagnosis of chest pain. More than 95% of pulmonary emboli arise from deep-venous thrombosis (DVT). Risk factors for DVT include prolonged bed rest, fracture of lower extremity, postpartum status, carcinoma, and congestive heart failure. In addition to pleuritic chest pain, there may be associated acute onset of dyspnea, hyperventilation, hemoptysis, and palpitations. The physical examination may be deceptively normal. There may be tachycardia, decreased oxygen saturation, or a pleural rub. The ECG may reveal right-axis deviation and evidence of right-heart strain. The chest x-ray may be normal but may show a pleural effusion or infarction. An arterial blood gas may reveal arterial hypoxemia and/or hypocapnia. The diagnosis is supported by a suggestive ventilation/perfusion scan (V Q scan) or a pulmonary CT angiogram, although sometimes it is necessary to do a contrast pulmonary angiogram to confirm the diagnosis. An echocardiogram may be helpful in determining if there is significant right-heart dilatation or dysfunction. Therapy consists of intravenous heparin. In cases of massive pulmonary emboli, intravenous thrombolytics or an embolectomy may be necessary.

Pneumothorax

A pneumothorax is another urgent diagnosis. Spontaneous pneumothorax can occur in tall, lean individuals, but most commonly, it occurs with associated chest trauma. The pain is acute in onset and usually is severe and disabling, although a very small pneumothorax may be asymptomatic. There often is a pleuritic component of pain and the patient will exhibit splinting. Physical examination will reveal decreased breath sounds and a chest x-ray will confirm the diagnosis. A tension pneumothorax can lead to hemodynamic compromise and requires immediate therapy with expansion of the affected lung, usually with a chest tube.

Chest Tumors

Mediastinal or lung tumors can cause a poorly localized, dull chest pain. They may be associated with other constitutional symptoms and usually are diagnosed with a chest x-ray or chest CT.

GASTROINTESTINAL CAUSES

Esophageal

Esophageal spasm can mimic angina and it often can be hard to distinguish the two, especially because both conditions are fairly common. Esophageal spasm may present as a substernal chest pain that radiates to the neck, arms, and back and may be relieved with nitroglycerin. It is not associated with exertional pain or dyspnea and may be precipitated by acid reflux. Esophageal reflux pain may be a substernal epigastric burning pain worsened by eating or recumbent position and may be relieved with antacids. Diagnostic studies such as exercise testing and esophageal manometry may be needed to distinguish between cardiogenic and esophageal pain. Endoscopy may reveal esophagitis and a barium swallow may reveal a hiatal hernia. Treatment consists of antacids and H2 blockers.

Peptic Ulcer Disease

The pain of a gastric or duodenal ulcer or of gastritis typically is a gnawing, epigastric pain that often radiates to the substernal area. It rarely radiates to the neck and shoulders and is never associated with dyspnea. It typically begins 60 to 90 minutes after meals and is relieved with antacids but not with nitroglycerin. Endoscopy is useful in confirming the diagnosis.

Biliary/Gall Bladder Colic

The pain of biliary colic usually originates in the right upper quadrant, but epigastric chest and back pain are not uncommon. The pain usually is colicky in nature typically occurring after meals. There may be associated right upper-quadrant tenderness, fever, elevated white blood cell count, and abnormal liver-function tests. Abdominal ultrasound can examine the gall bladder for stones, evidence of inflammation, or biliary obstruction.

MUSCULOSKELETAL CAUSES

Pain of the various musculoskeletal disorders is precipitated by particular movements, change in position, or palpation of the ribs, spine, or costochondral junction.

Costochondritis

Costochondritis consists of pain and tenderness of the costochondral junction. Pain usually is dull and can be elicited with palpation. Treatment consists of NSAIDs and occasionally infiltration with local anesthetics or corticosteroids may be indicated.

Cervical Osteoarthritis

Pain arises from nerve-root compression and is referred to the dermatomes affected by the nerves. The pain may be in the upper extremities, shoulder, or neck. Activities involving the upper body and arms can exacerbate the pain. X-rays of the cervical spine may show the typical findings of osteoarthritis. Treatment consists of physical therapy and NSAIDs. If conservative treatment fails, laminectomy may be required.

Muscular Strain

Strain of the accessory thoracic muscles can result in chest pain. It is worse with movement of the torso and is relieved with stretching and NSAIDs.

NEUROLOGICAL CAUSES

Herpes Zoster and Postherpetic Neuralgia

Herpes zoster occurs when dormant varicella viruses become reactivated. Pain can spread along one or more thoracic dermatomes, which can appear days before the characteristic rash appears. Postherpetic neuralgia can develop long after the rash disappears. Management includes antivirals and pain medication. Postherpetic neuralgia is extremely difficult to treat. Tricyclic antidepressants, steroids, transcutaneous electrical nerve stimulation, and local nerve blocks all have been tried with inconsistent results.

SELECTED READINGS

Goldman L. Approach to the patient with chest pain. In: Goldman L, Braunwald E, eds. *Primary Cardiology*. Philadelphia: WB Saunders Co., 1998:84—97.

Goldman L. Chest discomfort and palpitation. In: Fauci AS, Braunwald E, Isselbacher KJ, et al., eds. *Harrison's Principles of Internal Medicine*, 14th ed. New York: McGraw–Hill, 1998:58–65.

Vanden Belt RJ. The history. In: Chizner MA, ed. *Classic Teachings in Clinical Cardiology; A Tribute to W. Proctor Harvey*. New Jersey: Laennec Publishing Co., 1996:42–46.

CHAPTER 15

Low-Back Pain

Paul A. Glazer and Liane Clamen Glazer

THE EPIDEMIOLOGY OF LOW-BACK PAIN

Back pain is a very common affliction that has a tremendous impact on society through lost productivity and increased healthcare costs. The second leading cause of work absenteeism in this country, back pain, leads to more productivity loss than any other medical condition. According to population surveys, the number of people in the United States who sought professional healthcare for back pain in 1990 was 24 million (9.4% of the population). Every year in this country, more than $33 billion is spent on healthcare for back pain. When additional costs such as disability and lost productivity are included, total costs for back pain in this country add up to more than $100 billion per year.

In the United States, approximately 80% of adults will at some point during their lives experience low-back pain that will affect their daily activities; 1% to 2% of these will require surgery. The first episode of low-back pain typically occurs in the third decade of life. The incidence of low-back pain peaks between ages 55 and 64, and then decreases. The severity of pain at onset increases with increasing age of presentation. About 10% to 12% of patients with low-back pain have concomitant sciatica.

One way to improve upon current healthcare treatment of back pain is to increase the accuracy with which the various causes of back pain are properly diagnosed. We hope this chapter will prove useful to healthcare providers as they attempt to differentiate and treat different types of back pain.

RISK FACTORS FOR LOW-BACK PAIN

There are two categories of risk factors associated with back pain: extrinsic and intrinsic. Extrinsic risks include heavy physical labor, frequent bending and twisting, lifting and forceful movements, repetitive work, vibration, sedentary office work, and smoking. For example, truck drivers, athletes, and nurses are more likely than others to suffer from back pain. Intrinsic risk factors for disc degeneration include anthropometrics, spinal abnormalities, and genetic predispositions.

Job-Related Risk Factors

Heavy physical labor often is associated with low back pain. A 5-year prospective study recently concluded that people with jobs requiring heavy physical labor were almost twice as likely to report low-back pain as those who worked in jobs that involved no heavy physical activity. Unfortunately, colleagues who are too sedentary may suffer as well. Some investigators have noted a positive relationship between sedentary occupations and low-back pain. Sedentary labor may contribute to low-back pain by way of increased intradiscal pressures that occur with sitting versus those while standing, fluid exudation from the disc nucleus leading to harmful load transfer to the anulus, and a decrease in normal nutrient delivery as a result of intermittent disc compression.

There is a strong correlation between disc prolapse and long-distance driving. The risk ratio of disc herniation for truck drivers is as high as 3:1 in the United States. This increased risk of back disorders in drivers has been attributed both to posture and vibration. Whole-body vibration reportedly causes damage to the back by way of a reduction of strength and stiffness of ligaments, disc fluid loss, and disc hardening.

Nonoccupational Risk Factors

Studies have shown a positive association between low-back pain and participation in sports such as golf, gymnastics, rowing, and bowling. In a survey of 142 athletes involved in activities such as soccer, tennis, wrestling, and gymnastics, 50% to 85% reported low-back pain and 36% to 55% had radiologic spinal abnor-

87

malities. Of course, insufficient exercise also has been linked with an increased risk of disc herniation. In general, good muscle strength and good overall fitness is suggested for reducing the risk of low-back pain and disc herniation.

Many retrospective and prospective studies have implicated smoking as a risk factor for back pain. A biomechanical hypothesis is that repetitive increases in intradiscal pressure, as occurs with frequent coughing, could be a cause of discogenic back pain. This theory is supported by the observation that coughing and chronic bronchitis among nonsmokers have independently been associated with back pain.

A second hypothesis is that smoking reduces blood flow to the vertebral body and inhibits diffusion to the intervertebral disc, thereby interfering with systemic nutrient delivery and facilitating disc degeneration. A magnetic resonance imaging (MRI) study of smoking and nonsmoking identical twins found that those who smoked had an increased frequency of disc degeneration throughout the entire lumbar spine.

Risk Factors Associated with Body Habitus

Both increased height and increased body mass are associated with an increased risk of disc prolapse. Obesity independent of height has been correlated with both disc degeneration, as diagnosed by radiographic abnormalities, and with the presence of low-back pain. Likewise, height independent of weight has been associated with disc prolapse: one study found that men taller than 180 cm had a relative risk of disc herniation of 2.3, while women taller than 170 cm had a relative risk of 3.7.

Taller and larger people probably place greater loads on their intervertebral discs, but they also typically have correspondingly larger discs. Therefore, people of different statures should not experience significant differences in disc stress related to a given task. Rather, the increased disc pathology in individuals of large stature may be explained by factors such as problems with nutrient diffusion or the fact that large individuals are more likely to work in awkward postures.

Genetic Predisposition to Low-Back Pain

Postacchini and colleagues suggested that there may be a genetic predisposition for disc herniation. In a review of 63 patients under the age of 21 who had lumbar disc herniations, 32% had a positive family history for that same lesion; in the control group, only 7% had a positive family history. Although no genetic markers have been proposed, certain congenital spinal abnormalities such as asymmetric facet orientation and a small vertebral canal hypothetically predispose certain individuals to symptomatic disc herniations.

EVALUATION OF LOW-BACK PAIN

History

A careful history aids the healthcare provider in formulating a differential diagnosis for each patient. A history should include the patient's own clear description of the back pain, and whether or not there is associated leg pain. Determine if there were any precipitating events or if the onset of the pain was more insidious in nature. Find out if the patient's low back pain is a recurrent or a progressive problem. Ask when the pain occurs, and if the pain is exacerbated or alleviated when the patient lies down. Mechanical low-back pain is aching in nature; it is typically worse toward the end of the day and better with rest. Discogenic pain often is burning and aching in nature, and may be constant. Radicular pain radiates below the knee, may be coupled with numbness and/or paresthesias, and often improves with rest. Spinal tumors are frequently associated with pain that is boring in nature, worse at night, and unrelieved by bed rest. Flexion of the spine often causes an increase in pain related to discogenic disease, whereas extension worsens facet pain.

Is there any history of systemic disease that may be affecting the spine? Find out if there is a family history of back problems, or if there is any history of psychiatric illness. It is important to know the medications and alternative treatments (e.g., spinal manipulations) currently used by the patient and for what period of time they have been used. Also, ask the patient what medications and treatments they have tried in the past, and why those modalities were abandoned. Note the present occupational and social history of the patient, and whether or not there is any litigation involved with the current illness.

A careful neurologic history is essential. In the elderly, one often has to distinguish between neurogenic claudication and vascular claudication. For example, neurogenic claudication often is alleviated by walking uphill or by leaning forward in a chair, and exacerbated by walking downhill. Vascular claudication, however, is exacerbated by any exercise, and alleviated with rest.

Question the patient for a history of paresthesias or weakness. If paresthesias are present, determine their exact location. Pain drawings often are helpful in demonstrating the dermatomal distribution of the patient's radicular pain. These pain drawings in conjunction with Waddell signs (see The Neurologic Examination, below) help in distinguishing nonorganic pain patterns. Patients presenting with weakness of the lower extremities, incontinence, or constipation of either bowel or bladder, require an acute neurologic evaluation.

Physical Examination

The physical examination of a patient presenting with low-back pain should begin with an observation of gait, mobility, and posture. For example, the patient with acute pain and spasm avoids bending and twisting motions.

To perform a thorough physical examination, it is essential to have the patient completely disrobe. Inspect the skin over the lower back; hairy patches, lipomas, or neurofibromas may indicate the presence of spinal dysraphism. Check for asymmetry or scoliosis. Determine if there is a normal lumbar lordosis. The loss of lordosis may be secondary to a loss of disc height or anterior compression fractures. Conversely, an exaggerated lumbar lordosis is characteristic of obese patients and those with a high-grade spondylolisthesis.

Palpate all tender areas. Sciatic-notch tenderness may indicate a radicular disorder. Low-back spasm can be appreciated by manual palpation and may be associated with a scoliosis or loss of lordosis.

An accurate measurement of range of motion of the spine is difficult. Furthermore, there is a wide variance in normal range of motion in the general population. However, one can easily test flexion motion quantitatively by assessing how far the patient can bend forward as if to touch the toes with the knees straight. If the patient cannot touch the floor, measure the distance from the fingertips to the floor with a tape. Similarly, one can determine whether the range in lateral bending and hyperextension is decreased or whether it causes an increase in pain. Spondylolisthesis, spondylolysis, and spinal stenosis cause increased back pain with extension.

The Neurologic Examination

The neurologic examination of the lower extremities, as it relates to the lumbar spine, consists of a careful evaluation of motor strength, sensation, vibratory sense, reflexes, and evidence of nerve-tension signs. True muscle weakness is the most reliable indicator of persistent nerve compression. Muscle strength should be assessed on a zero- to five-point scale. One should carefully document the strength of hip flexion, extension, abduction and adduction; knee flexion and extension; ankle dorsi-flexion and plantar-flexion; extensor and flexor hallucis and digitorum communis; and peroneal and posterior tibialis muscles. Fatigue testing, as with repetitive, isolated calf raises, often is beneficial. Sensory changes are important but are subjective findings.

Much can be learned by testing knee and ankle reflexes. Hyperreflexia may indicate an upper motor-neuron lesion. Upper motor-neuron dysfunction also may be indicated by the absence of the following reflexes: the superficial abdominal reflex, the superficial cremasteric reflex, and the superficial anal reflex. A positive Babinski sign may be elicited in the presence of an upper motor-neuron lesion.

Vibratory sensation is lost in peripheral neuropathy, spinal stenosis, and in the elderly. One should accurately record the proximal level of intact vibration sense. Proprioceptive function, indicative of posterior-column disease, also should be assessed. Lower motor-neuron problems, as seen in degenerative lumbar spinal stenosis, can cause pain, dysesthesias, motor weakness, and diminished reflexes.

With the straight-leg-raise test, one can assess the extent of nerve-root tension by noting the angle made between the table and the extended leg when pain is produced. This test for sciatica is only considered positive if the pain extends below the knee. The straight-leg-raise test should be performed on both the affected and the unaffected leg. Radicular pain in the affected leg during straight leg raising of the unaffected leg is a positive contralateral test.

As one performs the physical exam, it is important to remember extraspinal sources of low-back pain. For example, abdominal aortic aneurysms and renal disease secondary to nephrolithiasis also can cause low-back pain. Rectal and pelvic exams should be performed to evaluate for prostatic or rectal cancer, as they may present as low-back pain.

To evaluate whether or not a patient has nonorganic pathology such as malingering, Waddell developed a series of five tests. If three of the five Waddell signs are positive, this implies a high probability of nonorganic pathology. The first sign is positive if there is tenderness in a nonanatomic distribution. The second involves the use of axial pressure on the skull, or rotation of the pelvis and shoulders in the same plane to reproduce low-back pain. The third sign is positive if the patient's symptoms disappear when they are distracted. The fourth sign is a giving way or voluntary release during testing of muscle strength, or the presence of a nondermatomal distribution of sensation loss. The fifth sign is a patient's overreaction to stimuli.

Diagnostic Studies

Plain radiographs in the anteroposterior and lateral planes are an essential component of the evaluation of patients with persistent low-back pain. These should be taken in the standing position to assess the effect of gravity on any deformity present. The diagnosis of a spondylolisthesis may be missed if plain films are taken with the patient supine, as 30% of spondylolistheses may reduce in this position. One should carefully document any decompensation in the frontal and lateral planes in patients with severe kyphosis or scoliosis.

MRI is currently the gold standard for evaluating patients who may have disc problems, infections, or stenosis. Computed tomography (CT) is the study of choice in trauma because of its ability to assess the spine's bony architecture. Myelography in conjunction with CT is the imaging modality of choice in patients with deformity. Radionuclide imaging or bone scans allow evaluation of any process that disturbs the normal balance of bone production and resorption. Discography, which involves the injection of saline into the disc to determine a concordant pain response, remains a controversial technique.

Laboratory Tests

In patients who have suspected malignancies, infections, or metabolic abnormalities, a complete blood count with differential is helpful. The erythrocyte sedimentation rate (ESR) is nonspecific, but often is a useful indicator of disease severity. Calcium and alkaline phosphatase activity may demonstrate an increased osteoblast activity secondary to malignancy or to metabolic diseases such as Paget's disease of bone. Protein electrophoresis of urine and serum are helpful in demonstrating the presence of multiple myeloma. HLA-B27 antigen testing provides evidence for ankylosing spondylitis and Reiter's syndrome.

GENERAL MANAGEMENT STRATEGIES

Treatment of low-back pain should be directed to the patient's specific diagnosis (Table 15.1). One must remember that the differential diagnosis includes extraspinal diseases such as the following, which may produce symptoms similar to those caused by degenerative spinal disorders: hip osteoarthritis, diffuse idiopathic-skeletal hyperostosis, cervical-spinal stenosis, central-neurological syndromes, psychological disorders, tumors, renal disease, abdominal-aortic aneurysms, and peripheral vascular disease.

There are no specific exercise or physical-therapy regimens that have been demonstrated to be better than any other in the prevention of back pain. However, patients may benefit from physical-therapy regimens as these modalities encourage them to take a more active role in their recovery process. Braces offer little biomechanical support but can provide a proprioceptive function and may subjectively reduce back pain.

Epidural steroid injections are commonly used to treat low-back pain. They also have been shown to provide temporary relief in patients with sciatica. However, epidural steroid injections have inherent risks as well. These include the systemic effects of the steroids, persistent cerebrospinal fluid leak, and meningitis. Furthermore, they have been found to have a decreased efficacy in patients with previous surgery, those with symptoms greater than 1 year in duration, and in smokers. We currently advocate steroid injections only for those patients who have either spinal stenosis or disc herniations with sciatica, and who are nonoperative candidates for temporary relief of symptoms.

In the United States, approximately 40% of patients with back pain prefer to seek chiropractic care. Many studies have attempted to demonstrate the benefit of spinal manipulation for patients with low-back pain. However, recent reviews have indicated that the efficacy of spinal manipulation has not been demonstrated by sound, randomized clinical trials.

DIFFERENTIAL DIAGNOSIS AND SPECIFIC MANAGEMENT STRATEGIES

MUSCLE STRAIN

Acute muscle strain is a common cause of low-back pain. When a patient presents with a history of pain after exertion, and without evidence of neurologic deficits or structural abnormalities, the most likely diagnosis is acute muscle strain. The majority of muscle strains improve with rest and soft-tissue modalities such as ultrasound, ice, heat, and massage. Prolonged bed rest should be avoided as muscle atrophy and stiffness may result. In addition, bed rest longer than 2 to 3 days may induce a dependency role. The use of nonsteroidal antiinflammatory drugs (NSAIDs) as well as flexibility and strengthening exercises often are beneficial. Patients whose symptoms persist greater than 3 weeks after initiation of treatments should be further evaluated for other structural or systemic abnormalities. Disorders such as fibromyalgia must be considered in the differential diagnosis when patients present with prolonged pain in multiple muscle groups.

TABLE 15.1. *Differential Diagnosis of Low Back Pain*

Musculoskeletal
Spinal degenerative diseases
   Disc degeneration
   Disc herniation
   Spinal stenosis/osteoarthritis/facet degeneration
   Degenerative spondylolisthesis/osteoarthritis
   Facet degeneration
   Spinal instability (normal loads produce abnormal motion)
Spinal deformities
   Scoliosis
   Spondylolisthesis
   Kyphosis
   Hyperlordosis
   Spina bifida
Trauma
   Spondylolysis
   Spondylolisthesis
Systemic problems
   Metabolic: Paget's, osteoporosis
   Infections: Discitis, osteomyelitis
   Neoplasia
   Inflammatory: Rheumatoid, Reiter's syndrome, ankylosing spondylitis
   Back pain during pregnancy
Iatrogenic
   Flat back
   Instability

Spinal Degenerative Diseases

Disc Degeneration and Herniation

Intervertebral disc pathology is a common cause of low-back pain. Disc disorders encompass many conditions, from subtle disc degeneration to dramatic disc herniation. Annually, an estimated 4.1 million people in the United States report a prolapsed disc. From 1985 to 1988, intervertebral disc disorders were the cause of an average of 334,000 hospitalizations annually, or 2.3 million annual hospital days.

As common and troubling as intervertebral disc disorders are, there is little agreement regarding their etiology. Most researchers believe that disc disruption generally results from a chronic or degenerative process. Researchers agree, however, with the observation that disc degeneration tends to occur in people who either exercise too much or too little.

Epidemiology of Degenerative Disc Disease

While many patients with low-back pain have disc degeneration, a significant number of patients with degeneration are completely asymptomatic. Consequently, disc degeneration is not a precise indicator of back pain. As a corollary, in a patient with both back pain and disc degeneration, the degeneration does not always account for the pain.

Approximately 95% of herniated intervertebral discs occur at the L4 and L5 levels in people between the ages of 25 and 55 years. The high prevalence of pathology at L4 and L5 can be explained by several factors unique to the lower lumbar spine. First, the posterior longitudinal ligament is narrow, and thus provides less support to the posterior anulus. Secondly, this site experiences a great deal of flexion, bending, and torsion, placing greater structural demands on the connective tissue. Finally, lumbar lordosis causes the vertebrae at L4 and L5 to bear more force in shear. Although the disc between L5 and S1 usually is the smallest of the lower three lumbar discs, it bears the heaviest loads. Thus, L5-S1 disc stresses are much greater than those found in the other lumbar discs. While disc degeneration typically begins in the lower lumbar spine, it progresses to successively higher levels as the affected discs become stiffer and an increased demand is placed on the superiorly adjacent discs.

Treatment for Disc Herniation

Surgical intervention is indicated for patients who have pain refractory to 6 to 8 weeks of nonoperative therapy. Any patient with a neurologic deficit secondary to disc herniation should be considered an operative candidate, initially. Current surgical interventions for isolated herniated discs include microdiscectomy, routine laminotomy, and modern endoscopic approaches. Because these procedures are minimally invasive, length of hospital stay and overall cost for these procedures have been dramatically reduced.

Spinal Stenosis/Osteoarthritis/Facet Degeneration

Degenerative lumbar-spinal stenosis results from chronic disc degeneration, facet arthropathy secondary to osteoarthritis, spinal instability, and the body's attempt to compensate for these changes. A disease spectrum exists from minimal symptoms of mechanical low-back pain caused by early facet degeneration to severe spinal stenosis. Stenosis can lead to compression of the cauda equina or exiting nerve roots, and lead to significant pain and functional disability. Symptoms may include isolated nerve-root irritation, back pain, and frank neurogenic claudication.

Primarily a diagnosis of the elderly, lumbar-spinal stenosis is the most common diagnosis among Medicare patients undergoing lumbar spine surgery. Each year, more than 30,000 surgeries are performed for degenerative spinal stenosis.

Treatment for Spinal Stenosis/Osteoarthritis/Facet Degeneration

Spinal stenosis is caused by a combination of hypertrophy of the facet joints and degeneration of the ligamentum flavum. Therefore, surgical intervention for spinal stenosis consists of a decompression of the neural elements. This is accomplished by performing laminectomies, partial facetectomies, bilateral foraminotomies, and removal of the hypertrophic soft tissue. Decompression should provide adequate space for the passage of the nerve roots through the foramen.

Preoperative assessment of the structural integrity of the spine should be performed to assess whether a fusion also should be performed. The indications for performing a fusion include a degenerative spondylolisthesis, scoliosis and/or kyphosis, or recurrent spinal stenosis. Intraoperative structural alterations that require a fusion include excessive facet joint removal (greater than 50% bilaterally) and radical disc excision. In patients who are nonoperative candidates, temporary relief of symptoms may be achieved through the use of epidural steroid injections.

Degenerative Spondylolisthesis

Degenerative spondylolisthesis is a form of spinal stenosis that is caused by chronic disc degeneration and subsequent motion segment instability. Patients with a sagittal orientation of their facet joints are predisposed to acquiring this form of spinal stenosis. Conservative treatment is similar to that for spinal stenosis.

Treatment for Degenerative Spondylolisthesis

Surgery for degenerative spondylolisthesis is indicated when symptoms become functionally incapacitating despite 2 to 3 months of nonoperative treatment. Ten percent to 15% of patients have surgery as a result of failure of conservative treatment. Operative treatment involves decompression with the addition of stabilization-fusion procedures. The use of pedicle-screw instrumentation has been found efficacious in the treatment of multisegmental instability of the lumbar spine, such as degenerative spondylolisthesis. Pedicle screw instrumentation allows fixation of the strongest portion of osteopenic vertebra, maintains lordosis, and achieves torsional stability.

Spinal Deformities

Scoliosis

Scoliosis is a structural abnormality that should not be confused with poor posture. Patients with thoracic and lumbar scoliosis often present with one shoulder higher, and one scapula more prominent. With the arms at the side, more space is seen between the arm and body on one side, and one hip appears higher. Often, the head is not centered over the pelvis.

The majority of scoliosis (85%) is idiopathic, having no known cause. It commonly affects adolescents during the growth spurt. It has been found to run in families, showing some genetic or hereditary influences. Congenital scoliosis is from defects of the spinal vertebrae present at birth. Neuromuscular scoliosis is from chromosomal abnormalities or disorders of the central nervous system, muscle, and connective tissue. Representative examples of neuromuscular scoliosis include cerebral palsy, arthrogryposis, Marfan's syndrome, and Down's syndrome.

There are currently over 500,000 adults with scoliosis greater than 30 degrees in the United States. It now is recognized that scoliosis greater than 50 degrees may progress after skeletal maturation. Furthermore, untreated spinal deformity of childhood can lead to severe back pain, cardiopulmonary dysfunction, and neurologic compromise.

Often, adults present with scoliosis, but documentation of the progression of the scoliosis is missing. Patients notice an increasing deformity, with loss of overall height. There is a high incidence of pain in adult patients with thoracolumbar or lumbar curves greater than 45 degrees. Standing anteroposterior and lateral plain radiographs of the lumbar spine demonstrate an apical vertebral rotation and coronal imbalance. Neurologic dysfunction is uncommon. Rather, patients present with radiculopathy as well as signs and symptoms of spinal stenosis. Paraplegia secondary to scoliosis has not been reported.

Radiographic studies should include standing anteroposterior, lateral, and bending x-rays. Pulmonary function testing should be considered in those with significant thoracic scoliosis and pulmonary compromise. MRI and CT myelograms should be used to evaluate the neural axis. In the older adult population with scoliosis, it often is beneficial to perform a thorough medical evaluation. These patients may have cardiorespiratory problems, nutritional deficiency, poor body conditioning, and osteopenia.

Treatment for Scoliosis

Nonoperative treatment for scoliosis includes soft-tissue modalities, analgesics, and NSAIDs. Exercises demonstrated by a competent therapist with a "sports-medicine approach" can restore many patients to a higher degree of overall function. Bracing in the adult population will not permanently change the curvature. However, braces may provide beneficial pain relief for older patients.

The indications for surgical intervention include progression of deformity, pain, deterioration of pulmonary function, and cosmesis. The surgical goals are to improve deformity and prevent increasing deformity. Surgery involves the fusion of the spine at the optimum degree of safe correction of the deformity. Correction in adults in general does not equal that of adolescents who have more flexible curves. The surgical complications include pseudarthrosis (0% to 25%), residual pain (5% to 15%), neurologic problems (1% to 5%), and infection (0.5% to 5%).

Spinal fusion instrumentation includes metallic rods, hooks, and screws that hold the spine in the corrected position while the fusion heals. Instrumentation is rarely removed. Modern scoliosis surgical techniques provide maximum stability with early mobilization of patients postoperatively. Combined anterior and posterior procedures allow greater correction of the curves and obtain higher fusion rates. Comprehensive preoperative conferences involve discussion of the risks versus benefits of surgical intervention.

Kyphosis, Hyperlordosis, Spina Bifida

The lumbar spine has a natural swayback, or lordosis. The thoracic spine has a normal kyphosis. Patients who have an excessive thoracic curvature (kyphosis) often compensate to maintain sagittal plane balance by increasing their lumbar lordosis. This commonly causes pain in the lumbar region secondary to the hyperextension stress on the facet joints. Treatment should be directed to correct the thoracic deformity.

Hyperlordosis can be a congenital deformity, but most commonly is secondary to obesity with weakness of the anterior wall musculature. Treatment should include an appropriate nutritional regimen and exercise program.

Spina bifida refers to a congenital absence of a portion of the bony elements of the posterior spine. There is a wide spectrum of the defect. The majority of the population are not aware that they have this abnormality (thus the term, spina bifida occulta). No treatment typically is necessary for these patients who have no neurologic deficit. However, there is an increased incidence of spina bifida in patients with lumbar spondylolysis or defects in the pars interarticularis.

Trauma

Adolescents

Low-back injuries from trauma often occur in the adolescent population. Adolescents have an increased susceptibility to back injury because of the young spine's immature bony and ligamentous structures. Sports such as football and gymnastics can cause low-back pain secondary to the hyperlordotic postures required by these sports. Conservative treatment for this type of low-back pain caused by muscle strain consists of rest, abstinence from sports, and flexibility exercises for the hamstrings as well as strengthening exercises for the abdominal muscles.

If the back pain persists despite conservative treatment, then further evaluation should be performed to determine whether the patient has a spondylolysis, a fracture in the pars interarticularis. This type of fracture may lead to a spondylolisthesis, or slippage, of one vertebrae on another. On physical examination, these patients often have pain exacerbated when they assume a hyperlordotic stance. This diagnosis can be confirmed with the use of plain films and CT. If no pathology is seen with these studies, it is often useful to use bone scans and single-photon emission computed tomography (SPECT). Nonoperative treatment includes the use of a brace and NSAIDs. If the pain persists despite these interventions, operative treatment involves either a direct repair of the pars interarticularis fracture or an *in situ* fusion.

Adults

Evaluation of a patient after a serious traumatic insult requires a thorough history and physical evaluation including a neurologic examination. Plain radiographs including flexion-extension views provide information regarding lumbar-spine stability. The use of CT and MRI also are beneficial in assessing bony and soft-tissue injuries. The principles of treatment of fractures in the spine are similar to those for the management of long bone fractures. It is essential to obtain immediate stability so that early mobilization of the patient can occur. One performs a fusion of the involved spinal segments only, attempting to maximize the remaining number of levels for motion.

Systemic Problems

Metabolic Diseases

Paget's Disease of Bone

Paget's disease of bone is a common disorder in adults over 40 and affects up to 10% of the general population of octogenarians. It is an idiopathic disorder of skeletal remodeling. The primary dysfunction involves an increase in osteoclastic resorption of bone with the production of structurally weak and immature woven bone that leads to deformities and fractures. Paget's disease of bone usually is asymptomatic. However, aching bone pain may be present in severe cases. The progressive enlargement of vertebral bodies involved with Paget's disease of bone may cause a secondary spinal stenosis. In patients with extensive disease, high-output congestive heart failure may occur. One must be aware of the possibility of the development of a secondary sarcoma in pagetoid bone.

Pain may be associated with an increase in metabolic activity. The major therapeutic agents used to relieve clinical symptoms are bisphosphonates and calcitonin. Surgical interventions are indicated for nerve compression, fractures, and end-stage arthritis.

Osteoporosis

Osteoporosis currently affects more than 20 million individuals in the United States. Osteoporosis is characterized by decreased bone mass and increased susceptibility to fracture. Given the increasing longevity of the general population, the number of people who will sustain osteoporotic compression fractures grows each year. Although osteoporosis is the most common cause of vertebral compression fractures in the elderly, such fractures also might be secondary to other metabolic bone diseases that affect the spine, such as osteomalacia. Therefore, any elderly patient who presents with a compression fracture requires a thorough medical work-up to assess the true cause of the patient's osteopenia. Osteoporosis is now a subject of major interdisciplinary research efforts, and treatment should be focused on prevention.

Infections

The goal of treatment of spinal infections includes early diagnosis with eradication of infection and prevention of neurologic deficit. This involves an aggressive approach to prevent the development of osteomyelitis and secondary deformities. The incidence of postoperative infections has been greatly reduced with the use of current antibiotic regimens. However, there has been a resurgence of diseases such as tuberculosis of the spine in patients with compromised immune systems. In this population of immunocompromised patients, any suspicion of spinal infections should be investigated promptly.

Most epidural abscesses are associated with vertebral osteomyelitis, discitis, or postoperative infections. These abscesses occur commonly in the lumbar region. The imaging modality of choice for the diagnosis of epidural abscesses is the MRI. Treatment with surgical decompression and antibiotics must be performed emergently because the prognosis is directly related to the timing of the intervention.

Tumors

Although primary malignancies of the spine are rare, many types of cancers can metastasize to the spine. The most common tumors that metastasize to the vertebral column include breast, prostate, lung, kidney, and thyroid.

Tumors may present with progressive low-back pain which is not relieved with rest. Often, patients relate a history of severe night pain. Suspicion of metastatic involvement can be evaluated with the use of plain radiography and bone scans. Treatment goals should include the maintenance of spinal stability as well as oncologic treatment of the primary cancer.

Inflammatory

Low-back pain may occur secondary to inflammatory diseases such as rheumatoid arthritis, ankylosing spondylitis, and Reiter's syndrome. Severe spinal deformities and pain may occur in patients with these diseases. Surgical intervention should be considered in coordination with rheumatologic consultation. In certain conditions, such as ankylosing spondylitis, the surgical correction of spinal deformities may provide patients with a dramatic improvement in overall outlook and quality of life.

Back Pain During Pregnancy

In a recent prospective study of 200 pregnant women, 76% of the women reported back pain at some time during pregnancy, with 61% experiencing new onset of their back pain during the present pregnancy. The prevalence of pain in the latter group declined to 9.4% after delivery. Thirty percent of the pregnant women with back pain reported significant difficulty with activities of daily living and significant time lost from work.

Iatrogenic Spinal Deformities

One of the most common and preventable forms of iatrogenic lumbar-spine deformities is the flat-back syndrome. This syndrome consists of a loss of lordosis in the lumbar spine. It is most commonly created by the use of distraction instrumentation. Historically, use of Harrington instrumentation was the primary reason for this severe iatrogenic deformity. Patients present with a loss of sagittal-plane imbalance and a flexed hip and knee posture. Surgical correction of this deformity involves anterior and posterior spinal reconstruction with osteotomy of the spine.

CONCLUSION

Low-back pain may result from a variety of different medical conditions. To provide appropriate care and minimize disability, it is essential to obtain the appropriate diagnosis and institute the proper treatment.

SELECTED READINGS

Deyo RA, Ciol MA, Cherkin DC, et al. Lumbar spinal fusion: a cohort study of complications, reoperations, and resource use in the Medicare population. *Spine* 1993;18:1463–1470.

Kelsey JL, White AA. Epidemiology of low back pain. *Spine* 1980;6: 133–142.

Koes BW, Assendelft WJJ, Van der Heijden GJMG, et al. Spinal manipulation for low back pain. An updated systematic review of randomized clinical trials. *Spine* 1996;21:2860–2873.

Leboeuf-Yde C, Lauritsen JM, Lauritzen T. Why has the search for causes of low back pain largely been nonconclusive? *Spine* 1997;22:877–881.

Mardjetko SM, Connolly PJ, Schott S. Degenerative lumbar spondylolisthesis. A meta-analysis of literature, 1970–1993. *Spine* 1994;19: 2256S–2265S.

Taylor VM, Deyo RA, Cherkin DC, et al. Low back pain hospitalization: recent United States trends and regional variations. *Spine* 1994;19: 1207–1213.

Twomey L, Taylor J. Exercise and spinal manipulation in the treatment of low back pain. *Spine* 1995;20:615–619.

Waddell G. Low back pain: a twentieth century health care enigma. *Spine* 1996;21:2820–2825.

Wheeler AH, Hanley EN Jr. Nonoperative treatment for low back pain. Rest to restoration. *Spine* 1995;20:375–378.

CHAPTER 16

Sacroiliitis

Barry R. Chi

Low-back pain located around the parasacral area is a common presenting complaint of many patients. The differential diagnosis for the etiology and the source of this pain is varied. One of the causes of low-back pain that often is overlooked by clinicians is sacroiliac-joint dysfunction. A lack of awareness of this potential etiology for low-back pain results in inappropriate and inadequate treatment.

The sacroiliac joint is formed from the junction between the sacrum and the iliac portion of the pelvis (Fig. 16.1). It is a true synovial joint anteriorly and a syndesmotic joint posteriorly. The primary function of the sacroiliac joint is to provide weight transfer from the spinal column to the lower extremities in equal weight distribution when a person is standing in a neutral erect position. Pain to the sacroiliac joint is caused by a variety of pathologies including ligamentum laxity or injury, pelvic obliquity, trauma, or collagen-vascular diseases, all which culminate in an increased stress to the sacroiliac joint. This can occur either unilaterally or bilaterally, which then becomes focally hypermobile, inflamed, and painful, resulting in sacroiliitis.

Sacroiliac-joint dysfunction is seen from the teenage years to the elderly. However, the most common age group to suffer from sacroiliitis are young adult and those from the third through the sixth decades. This is thought to be because of the ability of the sacroiliac joints to remain relatively mobile during this age group. With

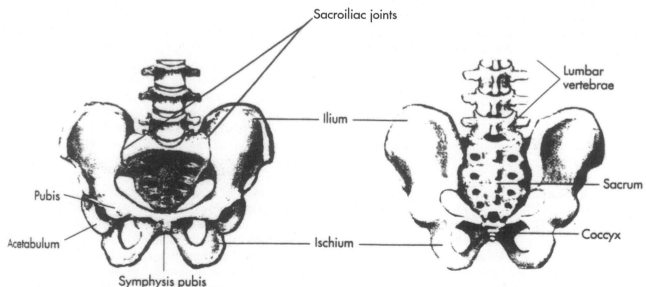

A   B

FIG. 16.1. A: Anterior view of the trunk showing both sacroiliac joints. **B:** Posterior view of the trunk showing the sacrum and both bones of the ilium with the posterior view of the sacroiliac joints. (Modified from Seidel HM. *Mosby's Guide to Physical Examination*, 4th ed. St. Louis: Mosby, 1999.)

advancing age, the sacroiliac joints become less mobile, more stable through the normal aging processes, which includes sclerosis, and osteophytosis formation of the joint spaces. Partial autoankylosis of the sacroiliac joints in otherwise healthy, elderly patients is commonly seen radiographically but are asymptomatic. It is with these stabilization processes that may, in fact, contribute the decline in the incidence of sacroiliitis in the elderly.

Patients with sacroiliitis, as with other causes of low-back pain, present with a variety of symptoms. The onset may be immediate or progressive from a few hours to days. Patient may or may not be able to recall the specific inciting event, and the pain may be either unilateral or bilateral in presentation.

Some of the common causes of sacroiliitis include trauma to the sacroiliac joint stemming from slipping, falling, landing on the lower back, or buttocks area, or seatbelt traction injury as a result of a high-speed decelerating automobile accident. Obesity, poor posture, and body mechanics are additional causes of sacroiliitis. Altered gait mechanics as a result of lower-extremity pain stemming from soft-tissue injuries such as sprain, strains, and tendonitis, as well as arthritis and other collagen-vascular diseases, also cause this condition. Lastly, running or walking on uneven or significantly cambered surfaces also can cause sacroiliitis.

Congenital and acquired leg-length discrepancies also may lead to development of sacroiliitis. These syndromes include scoliosis and other congenital birth defects, leg fractures with uneven bone-length healing, and poorly performed hip and knee joint replacement surgeries without correcting for the resultant leg-length differences. Endocrinological causes of sacroiliitis include a hormone known as relaxin. Relaxin is present in high concentration in antepartum women as it promotes ligamentum laxity especially around the pelvic girdle region, which aides in the process of labor and delivery. Relaxin is also the major factor that contributes to the development of the classic "waddling gait" seen in antepartum women because of the laxity effect. And through these effects, sacroiliitis frequently is seen in peripartum women. Patients frequently noticed the onset of their pain beginning in the last trimester of their pregnancy and persisting well beyond their usual postpartum period where soft-tissue injuries related to the delivery process have long since healed. This low-back pain may be either unilateral or bilateral in location but it will have signs and symptoms that typify sacroiliitis.

The diagnosis of sacroiliitis is based almost entirely on history and physical examination. Presently, there are no reliable radiographic or laboratory tests that can aide in the diagnosis of symptomatic sacroiliitis. Plain films and CT of the pelvis may indicate sacroiliac-joint sclerosis such is seen in ankylosing spondylitis or in other collagen-vascular diseases, as well as in many asymptomatic elderly patients. Their presence does not necessarily indicate symptomatic sacroiliitis. Clinicians, therefore, must be weary of these radiologic findings and correlate it to the patient's history and physical findings.

The location of sacroiliac joint pain is highly variable. Some patients experience focal-point tenderness located at and around the posterior–superior iliac spine region, while others complain of diffuse, poorly localized low-back and parasacral pain that may radiate to the contralateral side or, more frequently, down the ipsilateral–posterior buttock and proximal thigh regions (Fig. 16.2). Rarely would sacroiliac pain radiate beyond the popliteal area, and pain which does, suggests another etiology may be involved.

Patients commonly characterize sacroiliitis pain as a dull, burning, pressurelike baseline pain that may give way to become a sharp, jabbing pain lasting seconds to minutes with each exacerbation event. Additional symptoms described by patients include achy and throbbing pain. Numbness and tingling are not typical symptoms of sacroiliitis and their presence suggests other pathologies. Exacerbating factors of sacroiliitis pain include sitting, bending, and twisting of low back, supine lying, bed mobility, transferring from supine to sitting, and sitting to standing and vice versa. In essence, all activities involving the movement of the low back and pelvis may worsen a patient's sacroiliac pain because of increases in the stress-force imparted upon the sacroiliac joints by the activities involved.

There are numerous physical-examination tests that are employed to test for the presence of symptomatic sacroiliitis. Clinicians should become familiar with a few of the tests and apply them in combination to confirm and enhance the accuracy of the diagnosis. Some of the tests include Gillet test, side-lying iliac-compression test, standing and sitting forward-flexion test, supine iliac-gapping test, and Patrick's test with pain localized to sacroiliac joint area. Patrick's test is sometimes called the FABER test (flexion, abduction, and external rotation of the hip).

There are more than ten distinct manners in which there may be sacroiliac-joint dysfunction, but the most common type of dysfunction seen in athletes and nonathletes alike is the right-innominate anterior rotation. This involves muscle imbalances in the pelvis and proximal lower extremities that frequently result in an apparent leg-length discrepancy.

Treatment of sacroiliitis depends on the severity of the symptoms. A provider may initially treat conservatively with a course of nonsteroidal antiinflammatory drugs when there is no contraindication to do so. Other medications used to treat symptomatic sacroiliitis include a brief course of oral steroids, opiate pain medications for patients with severe pain, and muscle relaxants for muscle spasms. Clinicians should consider referring patients who do not respond to conservative therapy to undergo fluoroscopically guided, intraarticular sacroiliac-joint

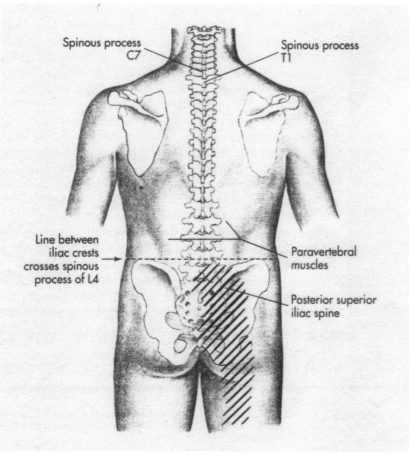

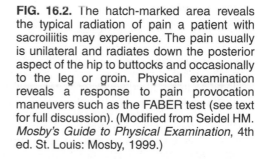

FIG. 16.2. The hatch-marked area reveals the typical radiation of pain a patient with sacroiliitis may experience. The pain usually is unilateral and radiates down the posterior aspect of the hip to buttocks and occasionally to the leg or groin. Physical examination reveals a response to pain provocation maneuvers such as the FABER test (see text for full discussion). (Modified from Seidel HM. *Mosby's Guide to Physical Examination*, 4th ed. St. Louis: Mosby, 1999.)

injection with injectable steroids such as betamethasone, triamcinolone, or Depo–Medrol (Pharmacia & Upjohn Company, Bridgewater, NJ, U.S.A.) mixed with injectable anesthetics agents such as lidocaine and/or bupivacaine (Fig. 16.3). Intraparticular sacroiliac-joint injection is considered by many to be the most rapid and effective treatment for painful sacroiliitis. Another key benefit of fluoroscopically guided sacroiliac-joint injection, aside from its well-known therapeutic effect, is the resultant pain pattern felt by the patient after the injection may aid in the differential diagnosis of patient's parasacral low-back pain.

In an intraarticular sacroiliac-joint injection (Fig. 16.4), it is routine to inject some form of anesthetic agent into the putative joint space along with a steroid. The anesthetic's effect produces the immediate onset of pain relief in patients with symptomatic sacroiliitis indicating that the sacroiliac joint is the cause of the patient's chief complaint. Therefore, if no significant immediate pain relief is noticed after the procedure, this usually indicates that other pathologies may be the source of the patient's pain, and not sacroiliitis.

Patients who do have good relief of their symptoms with local anesthetic blockade may be candidates for radiofrequency denervation of the sacroiliac joint. There are a number of techniques described for denervating the sacroiliac joint with radiofrequency lesioning. Using

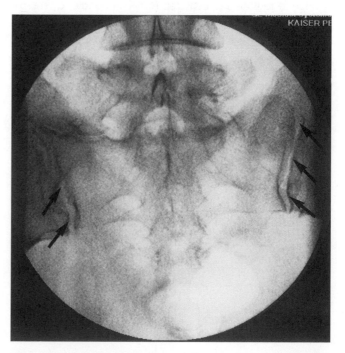

FIG. 16.3. Fluoroscopic view of the sacrum and bilateral sacroiliac joints. The patient is in the prone position and the fluoroscope is angled to give a full anterior-posterior view. The overlying ilium can be seen as a shadow over the underlying sacrum. *Arrows* indicate the sacroiliac joint.

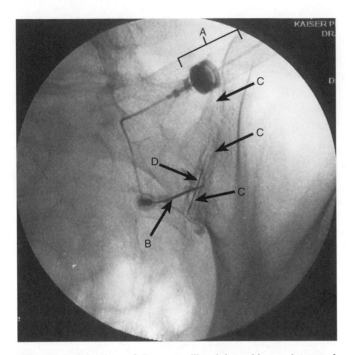

FIG. 16.4. Injection of the sacroiliac joint with a mixture of local anesthetic and steroid may provide both short-term and long-term relief of pain for patients with sacroiliitis. The joint is identified under fluoroscopic guidance. A long, thin needle is advanced into the joint and radioopaque contrast media is injected into the joint to confirm placement. Once proper position of the needle is assured, the medication mixture is injected. The fluoroscopic image above shows successful needle placement in the inferior portion of the sacroiliac joint and outline of the joint capsule with contrast media. *A*, syringe in radiopaque contrast; *B*, spinal needle; *C*, sacroiliac joint; *D*, conrast in sacroiliac joint.

radiofrequency probes that have been modified to create a bipolar system, the joint itself can be sequentially denervated, one centimeter at a time. Other experts prefer to view the sacroiliac joint as a "facet" joint and attempt to lesion the nerves that supply the joint as they leave the neural foramen of the sacrum. Radiofrequency lesioning may provide as much as 1 year's worth of pain relief, according to some studies. There is disagreement in both the literature and among pain-management specialists as to whether subsequent lesioning can provide relief. This area is controversial, and as of yet, radiofrequency lesioning of the sacroiliac joint is not a commonly performed procedure.

The objective of treating painful sacroiliitis with medications and/or injection is to reduce the pain and symptoms of the problem. The most important intervention that clinicians should offer to patients to prevent the recurrence of sacroiliitis, however, is to first diagnose and correct the underlying pathology that led to the development of sacroiliitis. Referring patients to physical therapy after the acute, painful symptoms have abated is the second-most important treatment. Therapists are asked to teach patients home-exercise programs with emphasis on sacroiliac-joint stabilization, self correction, and ligamentum-strengthening exercises, as well as posture and gait retraining, if indicated. Periodic reexacerbation of sacroiliitis is not uncommon. It is with the correction of the underlying cause in combination with routine participation in a home-exercise program that stabilizes the sacroiliac joint and its surrounding ligaments that results in patients having the best outcomes.

SELECTED READINGS

Cibulka MT. Classifying sacroiliac dysfunction. *J Orthop Sports Phys Ther* 1999;29:556–557.

Cibulka MT, Koldehoff R. Clinical usefulness of a cluster of sacroiliac joint tests in patients with and without low back pain. *J Orthop Sports Phys Ther* 1999;29:83–89, 90–92.

Ferrante FM, King LF, Roche EA, et al. Radiofrequency sacroiliac joint denervation for sacroiliac syndrome. *Reg Anesth Pain Med* 2001;26: 137–142.

Kibler W, Herrin S, Press J, et al. Rehabilitation of the hip, pelvis, and thigh. In: Kibler WB, Herring SA, Press JM, eds. *Functional Rehabilitation of Sports and Musculoskeletal Injuries.* Gaithersburg, Maryland: Aspen Publications, 1998.

Magee DJL. *Orthopedic Physical Assessment*: Philadelphia: WB Saunders, 1987.

Reid D. Problems of the hip, pelvis, and sacroiliac joint. In: Reid DC, ed. *Sports Injury Assessment and Rehabilitation.* New York: Churchill Livingstone, 1992:661–664.

Rothstein J, Roy S, Wolf S. Commonly used orthopaedic tests. In: Rothstein J, Roy S, Wolf S, eds. *The Rehabilitation Specialist's Handbook.* Philadelphia: FA Davis Company, 1991:128–131.

Vleeming A, Stoeckart R, Volkers ACW. Relationship between form and function in the sacroiliac joint I: clinical anatomical aspects. *Spine* 1990; 15:130–132.

Vleeming A, Stoeckart R, Volkers ACW. Relationship between form and function in the sacroiliac joint II: biomechanical aspects. *Spine* 1990;15: 130–132.

CHAPTER 17

Knee Pain

Donald T. Reilly, David B. Golden, and Ralph J. Di Libero

Knee pain is a very common complaint. According to the American Academy of Orthopaedic Surgeons, more than 11.2 million Americans visit physician offices each year because of knee problems, and the knee is the most often treated area of the body by orthopaedic surgeons. Knee pain is a subjective complaint that is confirmed by objective factors in the physical examination.

EVALUATION OF THE PATIENT WITH KNEE PAIN

Knee pain first should be evaluated from a holistic point of view. The etiology of pain in the knee can be extremely variable. Impairment problems resulting from knee pain must be viewed in reverse order by also considering pain problems caused by knee impairment. Overuse of the knee joint or underuse because of impairment elsewhere in the body also must be considered. There may be radicular pain that manifests as knee pain and yet results from nerve-root pathology. Abnormal gait mechanics resulting from a subtle, asymptomatic foot impairment may present with knee pain. There may be referred pain from hip pathology such as a slipped capitol–femoral epiphysis. A common obturator nerve serves the hip and the medial side of the knee. Phlebitis versus popliteal-capsule rupture can be a diagnostic dilemma. The possibility of gastrocsoleus mechanism tear at either tendon end or muscular origin can add more confusion to the conundrum. Therefore, one first must determine whether the knee pain is intrinsic or extrinsic.

The knee is subjected to stresses as great as five times body weight. Such stresses cause knee pain when combined with minor mechanical injuries or degenerative changes. Intrinsic causes of knee pain arise from a variety of disorders (Table 17.1). Understanding the complex anatomy of the knee is necessary for the appropriate diagnosis and treatment of knee pain. A helpful method to discern an exact diagnosis would be to determine whether the pain was limited to a specific area or quadrant, or whether there was generalized knee pain. Quadrant pain can be listed as anterior, posterior, medial, or lateral, and then is further defined in relation to the joint, intracapsular or extracapsular. There often is great overlap in quadrant pathology as well as in traumatic and nontraumatic etiologies, which must be accurately defined before proper treatment can be initiated.

Intrinsic knee pain may be elicited by stretching of the joint capsule. Capsular knee pain may be from effusion alone, increased capsular stretching from range of

TABLE 17.1. *Causes of Knee Pain*

Traumatic
Sprain
Strain
Meniscal injury
Ligament injury
Fracture
Bursitis/tendonitis
Contusion
Dislocation
Subluxation
Atraumatic
Arthritis
Rheumatoid
Degenerative
Seronegative and seropositive arthropathies
Infection
Neoplasm
Metabolic disorders
Gout
Pseudogout
Endocrine disorders
Tibial tubercle apophysitis (Osgood–Schlatter)
Neuropathy (i.e., diabetes mellitus)
Patellofemoral syndrome (chondromalacia patellae)
Regional-pain syndrome (reflex sympathetic dystrophy)
Popliteal cyst (Baker's cyst)
Referred pain (from the hip)
Postsurgical neuroma

motion, or capsular trauma or inflammation with or without effusion. Capsular knee pain tends to be generalized. Patients with rheumatoid arthritis experience pain because of both joint deterioration and increased capsular pressure from effusion. Excessive, abnormal, and mechanically obstructive knee range-of-motion patterns also produce knee pain in accordance with normal, protective proprioceptive functioning to mediate and maintain knee-joint stability. Among the many conditions that fall into this category are meniscal tears and "joint mice," or free-floating cartilage. The knee synovium, ligaments, infrapatella fat pad, meniscal attachment areas, bone, and periosteum are manifestation sites for localized pain.

A thorough physical examination and history is of paramount importance in diagnosing the cause of knee pain. In the course of an initial patient encounter with a chief complaint of knee pain, there are certain red flags that alert a physician to serious injury that needs immediate referral. A patient reveals most diagnoses during the history of the present illness portion of the visit. A buckling, locking, suddenly stiff, popping, suddenly swelling, or immediately handicapping injury is most likely a severe injury.

Findings during the physical examination that indicate severe injury are severe pain precluding an adequate examination, a tense effusion, a locked or unstable knee, neurocirculatory abnormalities, muscle atrophy, palpation of a mass, discoloration, and a deformity or abnormal extremity alignment.

Palpation or stretch of the structures about the knee may elicit extrinsic knee pain from muscles, tendons, bursae, apophyses, epiphyses, periosteum, and bone. A warm, red joint and evidence of painful knee inflammation may be from trauma, infection, metabolic alterations, neurologic dysfunction, or even tumor processes. Traumatic injuries that cause pain may be acute, chronic, repetitive, or mixed.

Because trauma is the most common cause of knee pain, obtaining appropriate imaging is important to compliment the evaluation. Initial evaluation should include radiographs with anteroposterior (AP) and lateral films, and sunrise view of the patella. Oblique AP views at 90 degrees to each other, AP 30 degrees flexed or tunnel view, and AP 15 degrees caudad or tangential view sometimes are indicated, especially when tibial plateau fracture is suspected.

X-rays can determine if a fracture is present and other imaging modalities, including magnetic resonance imaging (MRI) and computed tomography (CT) can help determine the nature of the injury or cause of the knee pain. If a fracture is present but not well visualized on x-rays, CT can aid in evaluating the bony anatomy and fracture pattern. MRI, when indicated, can help delineate injury patterns and difficult-to-visualize, soft-tissue injuries.

Aspiration of the knee joint is indicated for obtaining a diagnosis and temporary relief of pain. Blood in the aspi-

rant indicates internal derangement and possible ligament tearing. Fat in the blood indicates fracture. Cloudy fluid indicates inflammation or infection. Questionable synovial fluid should be tested for viscosity, clarity, sugar, differential cell count, gram stain, crystals, and various cultures and sensitivities.

General Treatment Management

With the exception of a true knee dislocation, very few knee injuries require specialized treatment in the acute setting. Knee dislocations occur with severe trauma, often seen in motor-vehicle crashes or falls from great heights. Evaluation of a dislocation requires the help of specialists, including the orthopaedic and vascular surgeon as well as the diagnostic equipment and specialists trained in angiography to rule out arterial injury.

Most fractures should be evaluated in the emergency department by an orthopaedist to plan for definitive treatment. Without evidence of fracture, treatment with protected weight bearing, rest, ice, compression, and elevation (eponym: "RICE") usually is sufficient until a referral can be made. The addition of nonsteroidal antiinflammatory drugs (NSAIDs) can help control swelling and pain. There are numerous classes of NSAIDs available both with and without a prescription. Their efficacy varies so their usage is based on physician and patient familiarity. All NSAIDs have the potential to cause gastric and renal injury, especially in susceptible patients. Patients with preexisting renal insufficiency or active ulcers should avoid antiinflammatory medications.

It is very difficult to perform a thorough physical examination on a knee with acute-onset pain or trauma. The mechanism of injury, the patient's general medical status, and preinjury ambulatory status should be ascertained. Although not always the case, the ability to bear weight often rules out severe injury. The specific causes and management of various causes of knee pain are discussed below.

Anatomy

There are many structures that have been proposed to cause knee pain. Table 17.1 outlines conditions that can cause knee pain. Figure 17.1 depicts the complex anatomy of the knee.

Innervation

The skin about the knee is innervated in a dermatomal pattern. The largest nerve supplying the knee is the posterior–articular branch of the tibial nerve crossing the posterior capsule. The obturator and saphenous nerves contribute to a lesser degree. In addition, peripheral nerves provide local innervation. Referred pain can stem from hip abnor-

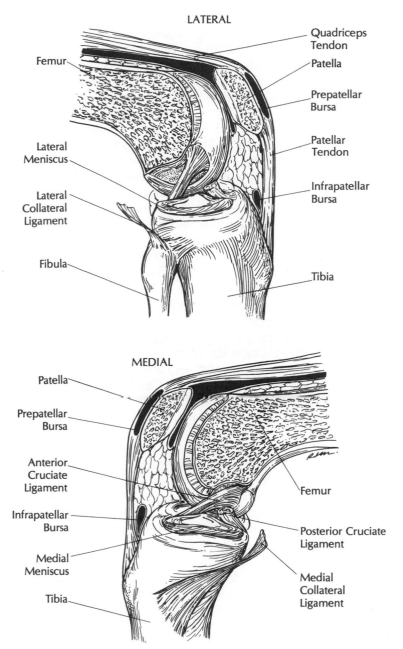

FIG. 17.1. Anatomy of the knee.

malities. Arthritic-hip changes can cause knee pain and can delay diagnosing the true etiology of knee pain. Following a normal evaluation of a painful knee, plain radiographs of the ipsilateral hip can rule out referred hip pain as a cause of the knee pain. Common causes of peripheral neuropathy should be sought in instances of specific patterns of pain and/or sensory changes.

Knee Pain Caused by Acute Injury

The mechanism and severity of injury should be sought to anticipate the type of injury sustained. X-rays taken at right angles to one another represent the minimal amount of views required. Very often, oblique, weight-bearing, and/or patellar tangential ("skyline") views can aid in the evaluation. Despite seeming self-evident, the x-rays need to be of good quality. The distal femur, proximal tibia, and patella should all be well visualized on knee x-rays.

Tendons attach muscles to bones and are relatively resistant to deforming forces. They consist of collagen and proteoglycans derived from fibroblasts. As the tendon inserts onto bone, there are two intervening zones of fibrocartilage and calcified cartilage as the tendon transitions into the bone. Surrounding the tendon is a fluid-filled sac or bursa that allows greatly reduced friction during gliding or movement of the tendon. The collagen fibers of the tendon usually are oriented parallel to the direction of the tensile forces to allow maximal strength in the plane of insertion and maximal load.

Tendinous injuries often occur at their insertion or the muscle-tendon junction. These include overuse and strain (microtrauma) injuries. Tendonitis develops about the insertion sites. Bursitis can occur simultaneously and the clinical distinction often is difficult to make. The iliotibial band (ITB), the quadriceps, patellar, pes anserinus, biceps, and popliteus tendons all can develop inflammation. ITB inflammation often causes pain and occasional snapping located around the lateral part of the knee. It often is seen in runners. Quadriceps and patellar tendonitis causes pain and tenderness at the superior and inferior pole of the patella, respectively. Patellar tendonitis also is known as jumper's knee and the pain can extend to the tibial tuberosity insertion site of the tendon. Pes anserinus (insertion of the sartorius, gracilis, and semitendinosus muscles) tendonitis causes medial knee pain often focused about the proximal aspect of the tibia. Point tenderness can be elicited at its insertion site. These various conditions can be very debilitating injuries and usually respond to rest, activity modification, ice, and NSAIDs. Severe pain, swelling, and often a palpable deformity mark complete tendon ruptures. Injuries that require operative repair should be performed usually within 7 to 10 days of injury.

Differentiating bursitis from tendonitis often is difficult. The physical examination findings may mimic one another. The fluid-filled sac can underlay or overlay the tendon and become part of the injury complex. A physical examination with careful palpation is the best method for diagnosis. Occasionally, the bursa is appreciated as a bulging or ballotable soft-tissue area. Treatment of bursitis parallels that of tendonitis.

If pain continues despite common modalities, a lidocaine and steroid injection into the bursa can be considered. Theoretically, steroid usage can weaken tendons or cause other soft-tissue atrophy. There are no studies documenting a consistent effect of steroid usage, but caution must be exercised. Steroids control local swelling and decrease the pain response from inflamed tissues. As a general guideline, no more than 3 to 5 injections should be used into one site spaced at least 2 to 6 months apart. The tendon sheath or the bursa is entered using a 20- to 25-gauge needle with 6 to 10 mL of lidocaine mixed with a deposition form of steroid. Immediate onset of relief often accompanies the injection because of the presence of the lidocaine. Patients should be warned that 1 to 2 days following the injection, there might be increased soreness but that relief will likely follow thereafter for an undetermined amount of time.

Ligaments, like tendons, are composed primarily of collagen. They contain elastin, which permits more resilience following a deforming force when compared to tendons. At bony insertion sites, the ligament becomes more flexible. Sharpey's fibers connect the ligament to bone. Nociceptive fibers have been documented in the knee ligaments and provide the basis for the pain following injury. Different ligaments of the knee, such as the anterior-cruciate ligament (ACL) and the medial-collateral ligament (MCL), have different properties, including different tensile strengths, articular relationships, surface area of collagen, and structural properties.

Acute injury causes swelling whether the ligament is intraarticular, like the ACL, or extraarticular, like the MCL. Acute swelling of the capsule and surrounding tissues contribute to the pain. Aspiration of a hemarthrosis can be both therapeutic and diagnostic. Aspiration should not be done for all hemarthroses. Tensely swollen knees should be aspirated for pain control, but any invasive procedure can introduce infection, even when done under standard sterile conditions. If fat globules are seen with the aspiration, there is likely the presence of an occult fracture. Ligament healing depends upon the surrounding environment and the presence of adequate vascularity. Ligament sprains are graded by severity from grade 1 to 3—from the tearing of only a few fibers to a complete tear. Immobilization often is effective for sprains but delayed surgical repair occasionally is required.

ACL reconstruction following complete rupture usually is planned after the swelling has receded and physical therapy has restored a full range of motion. An anterior drawer test or Lachman (the anterior drawer test at 30 degrees of knee flexion) will show a marked difference of tibial translation when compared to the normal, uninjured knee. Because of guarding caused by the injury, classically described provocative tests to evaluate specific injured ligaments are difficult to perform acutely.

Muscle strains comprise about half of sports injuries. Where the muscle links to tendon, the muscle units tend to stiffen. This is where most musculotendinous strains occur. Although tendons, rather than muscle fibers, cross the knee joint, muscle injuries can cause knee pain by affecting excursion of the muscle unit. Muscles that span two joints, such as the hamstrings, adductor longus, and gastrocnemius, may be more susceptible to strains. Passive stretching of the muscle at one joint may increase the risk of injury at the other joint. Muscular contusions may lead to heterotopic ossification (HO), which is bone formation in soft tissues that may cause pain or limit function. Surgical excision of radiographically proven HO is undertaken only once the bone tissue is mature (usually 16 to 24 months after its initial development). Treating muscle strains follows the same principles outlined above. "RICE" and avoiding strenuous and provoking activities are the mainstay of treatment.

The menisci are specialized fibrocartilaginous discs that absorb much of the loading impact upon the knee. In flexion, the menisci absorb up to 80% to 90% of the load borne across the knee joint. They have a peculiar pattern of blood supply. The peripheral third of the meniscus that connects to the capsule is the only source of blood supply. The remainder of the nutrition comes from gradient diffusion derived from the synovial fluid. This is why repair attempts are undertaken primarily in this outer rim region that permits healing. The previous method of resection of torn menisci has evolved into partial resections and far less meniscal removal. Studies show that joint degeneration can occur following even partial meniscectomies.

Meniscal injury results in swelling and pain not unlike the acute presentation of many other types of intraarticular knee injuries. Locking of the knee may be a distinguishing characteristic that may onset with a bucket-handle tear because part of the torn meniscus, resembling a bucket handle, displaces into the joint. The locking may resolve, but initially there is a mechanical block to motion. Locked knee is one of the few occasions when urgent arthroscopic debridement may be necessary. A less extreme injury pattern, including smaller tears, may result in similar clinical signs and symptoms but without locking.

Knee pain caused by fractures requires immobilization for pain control. Intraarticular fracture patterns should be surgically addressed because they run the risk of delayed degenerative arthritis. Proximal tibial fractures should be evaluated with CT to rule out "die punch" lesions of the chondral surface. Displaced fractures, including patellar fractures, are treated with open reduction and internal fixation. Because operative intervention may be required, referral to an orthopaedist should be sought.

Painful Pathologic Conditions of the Knee

Degenerative Arthritis

Osteoarthritis (OA) can be idiopathic or posttraumatic. Current research has elucidated specific genetic foci for idiopathic OA. Continued research might permit early diagnosis and treatment and perhaps change the course of the disease process. In either type of arthritis, typical x-ray changes include subchondral sclerosis, peripheral osteophytes (from reactive bone), and joint-space narrowing (from cartilaginous losses) (Fig. 17.2). With progressive loss of joint space, bone can become eburnated (bare of articular cartilage) and cause pain and swelling with any movement. Range of motion becomes limited and physical examination often reveals crepitus. The knee may be the only involved joint but other joints, such as the hand, may show characteristic changes as well.

Inflammatory Arthritis

There are many types of inflammatory arthritis. Some are thought to be autoimmune-mediated and many involve other organ systems in addition to the joint destruction they can cause. Soft-tissue abnormalities may

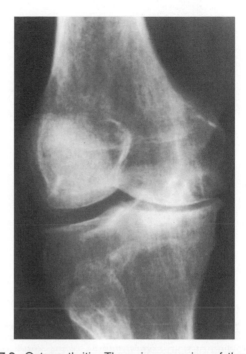

FIG. 17.2. Osteoarthritis. There is narrowing of the medial compartment of the joint space with a large cyst at the articular surface of the distal femur and a small amount of spur formation. (Reprinted from Greenfield GB, Arrington JA, Vasey FB. *Imaging of Arthritis and Related Conditions.* Philadelphia: Lippincott Williams & Wilkins, 2001, with permission.)

lead to more gross deformity of the knee. Rheumatoid arthritis involves synovial inflammation and therefore affects the entire knee joint as well as many other joints of the body (Fig. 17.3). This destructive form of arthritis can be greatly debilitating. Characteristic hand deformities can be seen with ulnar drifting of the digits and progressive disability from spontaneous tendon ruptures. Other inflammatory arthritides include the HLA-associated conditions and reactive arthritis. The arthritic etiologies differ, but the resulting joint destruction remains consistent.

For the inflammatory arthritides, drug therapies play an important role in medical and pain management. Antiinflammatory medications can include steroids and, when severe, chemotherapeutic agents such as penicillamine and methotrexate. These potent agents are disease altering and are thought to potentiate other medical means of management. They are not without potentially severe side-effect profiles. Appropriate referrals to specialists should be made and great caution should be exercised with their usage.

Arthritis Treatment

Initial nonoperative therapy for all knee arthritic conditions includes activity modification, NSAIDs and, often, an ambulatory device. A cane can greatly reduce

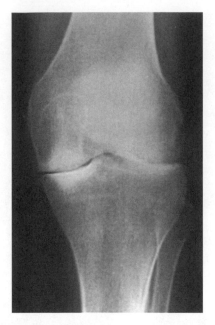

FIG. 17.3. Rheumatoid arthritis. Anteroposterior view showing narrowing of both compartments of the knee joint with subchondral sclerosis (Reprinted from Greenfield GB, Arrington JA, Vasey FB. *Imaging of Arthritis and Related Conditions*. Philadelphia: Lippincott Williams & Wilkins, 2001, with permission.)

the load borne across the knee joint. Proper usage places the cane in the contralateral hand from the affected knee. This permits leaning away from the injured side. At the time of this writing, there are no means by which cartilage can be replaced once the degenerative process accel-

erates. Current research is searching for new ways to preserve and possibly replace the injured cartilage surface.

Cartilage grafts can replace traumatic defects. Minimally invasive pain-control measures include intraarticular deposition of steroid and lidocaine. The mixture and strength of the injection is not different from the description outlined earlier in this chapter. Previously described methods of intraarticular injection often describe a midregion parapatellar approach with needle entrance either medial or lateral to the patella. Occasionally, those sites are not optimal (because of body habitus or overlying cellulitis). An alternative method utilizes the same entry sites as those used in the operating room for arthroscopic surgery.

With the knee flexed to approximately 90 degrees, on either side of the patellar tendon is a triangular-shaped palpable soft-tissue area. The boundaries consist of the tibia, the femur, and the patellar tendon. The needle should be inserted at approximately 45 degrees to both the vertical and the horizontal planes (Fig. 17.4). This directs the needle to the center of the joint thereby assuring entrance into the joint and avoiding cartilaginous injury that other entry sites may risk. Although there are many ways to inject a knee joint, this method may be less painful, especially if the lateral side of the knee is entered.

End-stage OA that is refractory to all nonoperative treatment and medical management can be treated with joint arthroplasty. There are various types of joint replacement, but all replace the damaged articulating surfaces using variable synthetic surfaces ranging from

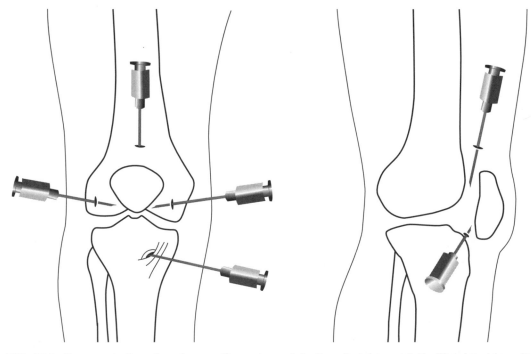

FIG. 17.4. Knee aspiration sites shown with pes bursa injection site inferomedially. (Reprinted from Reilly D. In: May H, ed. *Emergency Medical Procedures*. New York: John Wiley and Sons, 1984, with permission.)

metal alloys to ceramics to polyethylene. The exact timing and indications have evolved over the past decade. Previous contraindications, such as young age, are becoming relative contraindications with component and surgical improvements. Joint arthroplasty is lasting longer. Excellent results have been reported in long-term, follow-up studies of knee arthroplasty. Age, activity level, premorbid medical conditions, and other factors play a role in the planning of this elective surgery.

Infectious Causes of Knee Pain

By far, the most common infectious agents affecting the knee are staphylococcus and streptococcus. Infections can arise from blood-borne pathogens, local extension, or direct inoculation from the soft tissues. There are other infectious agents, such as *Salmonella*, or more opportunistic infections, but they are found in particular cases, such as sickle cell disease or diabetes mellitus. A patient's immune status and the presence of any concomitant disease(s) need evaluation. Joint infections can be quickly destructive to the articular surfaces. A delay in diagnosis can result in devastating and irreversible injury. A high index of suspicion and clinical history and physical examination remain the most effective method of diagnosis. X-rays should be obtained to rule out osteomyelitis. In the acute setting, radiographs do not show bone involvement, which can lag up to 3 weeks behind the clinical setting.

Confirmation of an infected knee joint comes only from aspiration of the joint fluid. There is no definitive synovial white blood cell count that qualifies as sufficient or necessary for the diagnosis. Values over 70,000 to 80,000 are considered grossly positive but a wide range of values can indicate infection as well. The aspiration should utilize the entry sites outlined for injections. Alternative sites may be required to avoid aspiration through cellulitis or suspected superficial infections. A positive diagnosis requires immediate intervention and orthopaedic consultation for irrigation and debridement of the joint.

Gout can closely mimic an infectious process. Its cause has not been firmly established but is thought to result from acute fluctuations in blood uric-acid levels. Higher-than-normal levels are not always associated with gout. One must bear in mind that its presence does not preclude an infectious process. The most common site of gout is at the great toe, called pellagra, but the knee can be a commonly presenting joint. The diagnosis is confirmed by microscopic presence of crystals in the joint fluid. Acute treatment consists of indomethacin or colchicine. Long-term maintenance medications include allopurinol and indomethacin. Calcium pyrophosphate deposition or pseudogout, can mimic gout. Again, the diagnosis is dependent on specific crystals found in knee-joint fluid aspiration.

Other infectious causes of knee pain may include sexually transmitted diseases, such as gonococcal arthritis. It should be suspected in a sexually active person with monarticular transitory or migratory arthritis. Treatment includes antibiotics to eradicate the infection. Joint aspiration does not always yield positive results and treatment can be based on clinical suspicion, especially if coupled to genitourinary symptoms. Other infectious causes of knee pain are treated according to specific joint aspiration sensitivity results.

Tumors Causing Knee Pain

Malignant tumors are relatively rare causes of knee pain. Extremes of age, insidious onset of pain, nocturnal pain, a history of radiation therapy, systemic symptoms such as lethargy, and unexplained weight loss all can raise the suspicion of a malignant lesion. Any suspected malignant lesions should be referred to a medical center trained in evaluating and treating malignant tumors about the knee. Benign lesions are far more common. Tumors such as osteochondromas can cause mechanical knee symptoms because of location and size. Treatment may consist of surgical excision if indicated. All suspected tumors of the knee should minimally have two plain x-ray views obtained at the first clinical visit.

A popliteal-fossa mass or Baker's cyst also can cause knee pain. The fluid in the cyst, which is documented with ultrasound, is thought to accumulate in the sheath of the hamstring musculature (semitendinosus). It can enlarge in size to compress neurovascular structures and cause pain. Spontaneous rupture of the cyst can cause severe pain that radiates down the calf. Rarely is surgical intervention needed.

Patellofemoral Syndrome (Anterior Knee-Pain Syndrome)

The term patellofemoral syndrome (or anterior knee-pain syndrome) has gradually replaced the term "chondromalacia patella," which means softening of the patellar cartilage. Anterior knee-pain syndrome does not implicitly imply the cause of pain. It can be caused by a constellation of contributing factors. Patellar malalignment may play a role, and overuse injuries may contribute. The angle the femur makes with the tibia is, on average, more valgus in females. This may predispose to a higher incidence of patellofemoral syndrome in females with constrained lateral ligaments. Physical examination reveals tenderness with patellar compression. Again, initial treatment is symptomatic. Activity modification and bracing the patella may decrease the pain. Strength training of the vastus medialis obliques and quadriceps muscles may rehabilitate the knee. When all nonoperative modalities fail, surgical realignment possibly including arthroscopy and lateral ligament adjustments may be an option.

Tibial tubercle apophysitis, also known as Osgood–Schlatter disease, can cause knee pain at the insertion of the patellar tendon on the tibia. It affects the adolescent with open apophyses. It can rarely affect the skeletally mature with residual pain. The pain is exacerbated by activities, especially ascending and descending stairs. Activity modification and antiinflammatory medications are the mainstay of treatment. Very rarely, operative intervention may be required.

Other Causes of Knee Pain

Conditions such as complex regional-pain syndrome types I or II, or postsurgical neuromas are also causes of knee pain. Regional pain syndromes are not treated surgically. The diagnosis is primarily a clinical one but supportive tests, such as a positive three-phase bone scan, can aid in the diagnosis. Local modalities, pain medication, and physical therapy are the mainstay of treatment. Sympathetic blockade may be both diagnostic and therapeutic.

All surgically resected nerves cause neuromas. Painful neuromas are caused by the inadvertent overgrowth of nerve endings entrapped in scar tissue. If neuromas occur, they can be treated with injections of lidocaine to confirm the diagnosis. Subsequent denervation with a cryoanalgesia probe can be attempted to ablate the pain. Surgical resection is sometimes indicated.

CONCLUSION

Appropriate treatment relies upon correctly identifying the etiology of the knee pain and utilizing effective treatment modalities. Knee pain can be greatly debilitating. For all patients with knee pain, preventive therapies are initiated to relieve symptoms and slow the articular aging process. Reconstruction of a torn anterior cruciate ligament can relieve knee instability, return the patient to a more active life style, and reduce articular-cartilage deterioration. Surgically filling posttraumatic articular defects with cultured cartilage graft can salvage a knee. Arthroscopically removing, trimming, shaving, and repairing internal derangements such as torn menisci, loose bodies, inflamed plica, and osteochondritis desiccans relieves pain and restores function. Oral chondroitin sulfate or hyaluronic acid preparations injected into the knee joint help to restore cartilage integrity. NSAIDs provide temporary relief for inflammatory processes, and pain medications are helpful for patients with osteoarthritis who are not ready for total knee arthroplasties. Unloader braces that shift weight bearing from an osteoarthritic knee compartment to a lesser-involved side, as well as supports that help align the tracking course of the patella, sometimes are helpful.

Current trends toward exercise and increased physical activity further mandate improving diagnostic and thera-

peutic skills when dealing with knee pain. Physical therapies aimed at maintaining range of motion and building muscular strength can greatly relieve symptoms. Strength and flexibility are maintained by regular exercise and modalities that reduce pain and swelling. Such modalities might include ultrasound, transcutaneous-electrical nerve stimulation (TENS) (Fig. 17.5), massage, compression wraps, leg elevation, and weight loss. Avoidance of obviously harmful and painful activities should be considered part of the treatment protocol. Warming up before and icing down after a specific sport or activity can reduce

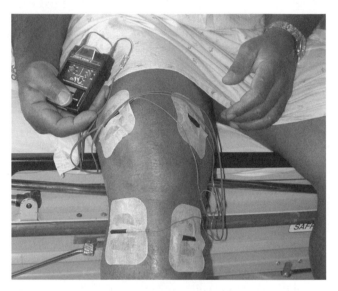

FIG. 17.5. Transcutaneous electrical nerve stimulation is also known as TENS or TNS. It is a passive, noninvasive, nonaddictive modality with no known side effects. TENS works to decrease pain perception and may be used to control acute and chronic pain. Transcutaneous (through the skin) electrical nerve stimulation sends a painless electrical current to specific nerves. The current may be delivered intermittently. The mild electrical current generates heat that serves to relieve stiffness, improve mobility, and relieve pain. The exact mechanism by which TENS relieves pain is unknown. TENS also is used to deliver topical steroid medication through the skin to treat acute episodes of pain. This treatment is called iontophoresis. The mild current causes the medication to migrate into soft tissue serving to reduce inflammation. A physical therapist applies electrode patches to the skin in the area to be treated. The mild current runs from the stationary stimulator through these patches. The portable stimulator is a small battery-operated device that can be worn around the waist. The unit can be turned on or off as needed for pain control. To ensure the patient will benefit from TENS, the portable device is used on a trial basis before the patient takes it home for long-term use. The patient then is taught how to apply the electrodes independently. Unfortunately, TENS is not always an effective treatment. Patients with pacemakers should avoid TENS because the electrical current could interfere with the operation of a pacemaker. This figure illustrates one possible configuration of electrode placement for a patient with knee pain from osteoarthritis.

inflammation. Proprioceptive exercise programs can help prevent further injuries.

SELECTED READINGS

Allum RL, Thomas NP. *Clinical Challenges in Orthopaedics: The Knee.* Isis Medical Media, 2000.

Creamer P, Hochberg MC. Why does osteoarthritis of the knee hurt—sometimes? *Br J Rheumatol* 1997;36:726–728.

Fransen M, Crosbie J, Edmonds J. Physical therapy is effective for patients with osteoarthritis of the knee: a randomized controlled clinical trial. *J Rheumatol* 2001;28:156–164.

Hakkinen A, Sokka T, Kotaniemi A, et al. A randomized two-year study of the effects of dynamic strength training on muscle strength, disease activity, functional capacity, and bone mineral density in early rheumatoid arthritis. *Arthritis Rheum* 2001;44:515–522.

Hannan MT, Felson DT, Pincus T. Analysis of the discordance between radiographic changes and knee pain in osteoarthritis of the knee. *J Rheumatol* 2000;27:1513–1517.

Hastings-Nield, D. *The Hip, Thigh and Knee (The Anatomy Project Series).* The Parthenon Publishing Group, 2001.

Joensen AM, Hahn T, Gelineck J, et al. Articular cartilage lesions and anterior knee pain. *Scand J Med Sci Sports* 2001;11:115–119.

LaValley MP, McAlindon TE, Chaisson CE, et al. The validity of different definitions of radiographic worsening for longitudinal studies of knee osteoarthritis. *J Clin Epidemiol* 2001;54:30–39.

Young L, Katrib A, Cuello C, et al. Effects of intraarticular glucocorticoids on macrophage infiltration and mediators of joint damage in osteoarthritis synovial membranes: findings in a double-blind, placebo-controlled study. *Arthritis Rheum* 2001;44:343–350.

CHAPTER 18

Common Causes of Foot Pain

James Mann

Painful disorders of the leg, ankle, and foot are the third most common reason for a visit to a physician. Only backache and headache are more common.

A wide constellation of disorders may cause these pains, and this chapter will attempt to highlight some of the most common of them. Some topics, while not common, are distinctive enough and useful enough to be commonly considered in one's differential diagnosis. Some of these will be discussed as well. Topics such as complex regional pain syndromes and neuropathic pain are discussed in Chapters 27 and 32 and they will not be covered in this chapter.

TRAUMA

The foot is composed of 26 bones, 19 muscles, and 107 ligaments. All of these structures are involved in weight bearing and propulsion, and all of these structures are vulnerable to traumatic injury.

Fracture and Dislocation

History

The patient should be questioned about a known traumatic event, overuse, sudden onset of pain, a history of diabetes mellitus (DM) (Charcot fractures), and inability to bear weight without significant pain. The pain is usually well localized, and is sharp in nature when the involved structure is exposed to weight bearing or motion.

Lab/Imaging

X-rays may show local soft-tissue swelling and/or deformity. In a fracture, the cortex of the bone may show a defect or a plastic deformity (torus fracture). Some fractures, especially stress fractures, may not be visible on a plain film for 10 to 14 days until a fracture callous forms and becomes visible. Magnetic resonance imaging (MRI) usually can diagnose these fractures immediately if necessary.

Physical Findings

Physical findings include erythema, swelling, bruising, deformity, and point tenderness to palpation.

Treatment

Definitive treatment of the various fractures and dislocations of the foot are beyond the scope of this chapter. The general principles include immediate attention to neurovascular compromise, reduction of the deformity, and some type of immobilization.

Achilles Tendon Ruptures

History

A rupture occurs when the force of a stretch or contraction (or both) exceeds the tensile strength of the tendon. Stretch occurs when the knee is forcefully extended with the foot and ankle fixed in dorsiflexion, or the foot is forcefully dorsiflexed with the knee fully extended. Sudden forceful contraction of the calf muscles such as occurs in basketball, racquetball, tennis, sprinting, and in lifting heavy loads, is the most frequent cause of Achilles-tendon rupture. The patient usually is a somewhat sedentary individual who undertakes intense physical activity without proper training or warm-up. He or she generally remembers the precipitating trauma, and will report the sensation of being shot with a gun or hit with a baseball bat in the calf. Often, a loud pop is heard. The patient may or may not have severe pain initially. It is not unusual for the patient to finish the game he is playing. Within a short time, however, the patient experiences weakness, swelling, and unremitting increasing pain.

Lab/Imaging

Sonography is an excellent way to image the Achilles tendon. If a total rupture has occurred, the continuity and movement of the tendon will not be seen. A dyshomogeneous echogenicity will be seen at the site of injury. Neglected tears are difficult to diagnose with sonography, because the hematoma becomes organized and develops an echogenicity similar to normal tendon.

MRI also is an excellent way to visualize the Achilles tendon, and it has the advantage in delayed diagnosis of easily differentiating damaged tendon with an organized hematoma from normal tendon.

Physical Findings

Physical exam reveals local edema and ecchymosis. One can usually palpate a defect in the continuity of the tendon. With the patient prone, one will see decreased equinus on the injured side. The Thompson test may be performed by squeezing the calf muscle and watching the foot response. Absence of plantarflexion indicates a severely ruptured tendon. Note that patients can actively plantar flex their foot using their posterior and lateral muscle groups even in the case of a complete Achilles tendon rupture. It is important to compare the examination of the injured side to the uninjured side.

Treatment

Treatment may be nonsurgical or surgical, and controversy exists as to which is the best treatment. If the patient is over 50 years old and sedentary, most feel the rupture can be treated by placing the patient in a non–weight-bearing cast with the foot in gravity equinus. The cast is changed every 2 weeks with the foot in decreased equinus with every cast change for a total of 12 weeks. A course of physical therapy and rehabilitation would follow. The other option is surgical repair followed by 10 to 12 weeks of casting to protect the repair. Physical therapy and rehabilitation are required after the casting is discontinued. This method is felt to lower the incidence of rerupture, especially in athletic individuals.

Peroneal Tendon Rupture or Dislocation

History

Injuries of these tendons are rare and usually are from strong tendon contractions against an actively inverting foot, such as occurs in skiing. Pain is quite variable, ranging from minimal to severe. The pain may be located from behind the malleolus to the lateral cuboid region. Many of the dislocations will spontaneously reduce, but the patient may be able to reproduce a snapping dislocation by moving the ankle or toes.

Lab/Imaging

Radiographs may demonstrate impingement from an associated calcaneal fracture. Retrofibular fractures, an enlarged peroneal tubercle, or a fractured os peroneum may be noted. Sonography or MRI will demonstrate tears or discontinuities of the tendons.

Physical Findings

There will be tenderness and edema along the course of the peroneal tendons. Ecchymosis often is present. The patient may be able to reproduce a snapping subluxation of the tendons by movement of the ankle or toes.

Treatment

Conservative treatment consists of 6 weeks of non–weight-bearing casting. This results in about a 60% success rate. Most authorities therefore recommend surgical treatment, especially in acute cases. There are three categories of surgical repair. The first is direct repair of the tendon and retinaculum. The second is creation of a new peroneal retinaculum. The third category is deepening of the retromalleolar sulcus. After surgery, the patient is placed in a below-the-knee cast for 6 weeks, the first 3 weeks nonweight bearing, and the next 3 weeks weight bearing.

Tibialis-Posterior Tenosynovitis

History

This condition is most common in women over 40 years of age. The patient complains of medial arch or ankle pain that progressively worsens. There often is local warmth and edema. A progressive flat-foot deformity may be present. The symptoms are aggravated by weight bearing, but walking may be tolerated better than standing. Some patients may report an incident when they feel a snap and a warm feeling inside the ankle.

Lab/Imaging

X-ray may reveal an increase in the talocalcaneal angle, severe forefoot abduction, and subluxation of the talonavicular joint. MRI is very useful for diagnosing tendon hypertrophy, osseous impingement, and partial ruptures.

Physical Findings

Examination usually will reveal a pes-valgus deformity of varying degree. The heel often is everted, and the forefoot severely abducted. The talonavicular joint may be collapsed and bulging. Warmth, edema, and tenderness to palpation may be found along the course of the tibialis-posterior tendon. If a rupture of the tendon is present, a defect in the tendon may be palpable. Muscle weakness against resistance to inversion can be demonstrated. The patient may demonstrate the "too many toes" sign. When the patient is viewed from behind, the marked forefoot abduction will allow greater than three lesser toes to be seen. The patient also may have a heel-varus sign, i.e., when the patient is asked to stand on his toes, the affected side will fail to exhibit the typical varus position of the heel that is normally present with tibialis-posterior function.

Treatment

Treatment may include shoe modification, orthotics, weight-bearing casts, and nonsteroidal antiinflammatory drugs (NSAIDs). Steroid injection into the area should be avoided because this may increase the risk of total rupture of the tendon. If the tendon has ruptured, there is little in the way of adequate conservative therapy. For those patients who are not operative candidates, the best option is a high-top oxford shoe with a rigid counter, orthotic support, and bracing. There are two approaches to operative therapy. The first is tendon reconstruction. This is best done before arthritic changes have taken place.

The other surgical approach is the use of arthrodesis. Most individuals who have had prolonged tibialis-posterior rupture sustain severe deformity and arthritic changes that only can be adequately addressed with joint fusion.

Neuroma

A Morton's neuroma is a benign enlargement of the third-common digital branch of the medial plantar nerve. It usually is located between and often distal to the third and fourth metatarsal heads. It also may occur in the second intermetatarsal space and rarely in the first or fourth intermetatarsal space. There often is a communicating branch from the lateral planter nerve that also supplies this area.

History

Neuroma usually is diagnosed between the fourth and sixth decades. It is more common in overweight people. A neuroma occurs in women more commonly than in men.

Initially, patients may complain of the sensation of walking on a wrinkle in their stockings, or a lump in their shoe. As the condition worsens, they may complain of a paroxysmal burning sensation, like walking on a hot pebble or having a hot poker thrust between their toes. The pain also may be described as sharp, dull, or throbbing. It is located between the third and fourth metatarsal heads and may radiate distally into the adjacent toes or proximally up the leg to the knee and, in rare cases, as far as the hip. The patient may describe a numb sensation, but there is rarely a sensory deficit. The digits usually are hyperesthetic. Sometimes, patients will complain of a cramping sensation in the arch, forefoot, or toes. The pain is aggravated by walking in shoes and is alleviated somewhat by rest. A classic complaint that is almost pathognomonic is the intense desire to remove one's shoes, rub the forefoot, and flex the toes. This often provides dramatic but temporary relief.

There may be a history of antecedent trauma such as stepping on a rock, twisting an ankle, striking the floorboard of a car in a motor vehicle accident or striking the edge of a curb. There may be a history of new shoes or overuse.

Physical Findings

Tenderness or sometimes the exact reproduction of the pain can be elicited by squeezing each metatarsal space in a dorsoplantar direction at or distal to the metatarsal–phalangeal joint (MPJ), especially with simultaneous transverse compression to the first and fifth metatarsal heads. A palpable and sometimes painful click during this maneuver is a positive Mulder's sign and is very suggestive of a neuroma.

There may be perceptible swelling of the plantar metatarsal surface or the sulcus area when compared to the other side. If the neuroma is large, the adjacent toes may be forced to spread apart on weight bearing.

Lab/Imaging

X-rays should be obtained to rule out other pathologic conditions. MRI can be used to diagnose the neuroma, but because of the expense, this is done rarely. Ultrasound is an excellent test to visualize a neuroma. The typical appearance is an ovoid hypoechoic mass, which is greater than or equal to 5 mm in diameter.

Treatment

Wide shoes with adequate room for the toes and good arch support are appropriate initial measures to try in mild cases. High-heeled shoes should be avoided. Metatarsal padding may be applied just proximal to the second, third, and fourth metatarsal heads to help draw weight away from the neuroma and to splay the metatarsals. A local injection of a corticosteroid plus a local anesthetic is sometimes effective. This may be repeated up to three times on a monthly basis. Conservative measures fail in the majority of cases, and when this happens, surgical excision is the therapy of choice.

Plantar Fasciitis

History

This is the most common of all foot pain complaints. It is common in patients who do a great deal of standing or walking, especially when there is an increase in such activity. It is more common in patients who have a pronated foot. The hallmark is moderate-to-severe tenderness beneath the anterior portion of the heel. The most tender area often is at the medial tubercle of the calcaneus. Often, the entire medial band of the plantar fascia is tender. Patients will often complain of poststatic dyskinesia (i.e., they will complain of increased pain upon getting out of bed in the morning or after having been seated for several hours).

Lab/Imaging

Radiography reveals either nothing or a spur typically arising from the medial tubercle of the calcaneus. The spur often is found in asymptomatic feet and may have no clinical significance.

Physical Findings

There is tenderness to palpation of the plantar–anterior aspect of the heel, especially in the area of the medial tubercle of the calcaneus. The medial band of the plantar fascia also can be tender to palpation.

Treatment

Initial treatment consists of decreased activity and preventing hyperpronation of the foot. Strapping or the use of an orthotic can be very helpful. A 2-week course of NSAIDs often is beneficial. Stretching of the foot muscles is recommended before the patient gets out of bed in the morning. This can be accomplished by having the patient draw the alphabet with the foot, therefore bringing the foot through a full range of motion. If the pain persists, injection of a mixture of local anesthetic and steroid into the painful region can be done. If there is still no relief after three such injections one month apart, splinting the foot at night or the use of a walking cast can be quite helpful as well. In less than 5% of the cases, surgical release of the plantar fascia is necessary.

Posterior Calcaneal Bursitis

History

Painful inflammation of the bursa between the Achilles tendon and skin is caused by friction from ill-fitting shoes. Chronic irritation will thicken the bursa and the overlying skin. Patients complain of exquisite pain and tenderness over the posterior aspect of the heel.

Lab/Imaging

X-ray of the foot may reveal hypertrophy of soft tissues overlying the posterior aspect of the calcaneus. Occasion-ally, the posterior–superior aspect of the calcaneus may be hypertrophied.

Physical Findings

The bursa is tender to palpation and it may be visibly inflamed and distended with fluid. If the condition is chronic, the walls of the bursa and the overlying skin are thickened.

Treatment

Initial treatment consists of proper-fitting shoes with moderately low heels. The use of ice and NSAIDs to decrease inflammation is quite helpful. If the bursitis is severe, the swollen bursa may be drained by needle aspiration followed by an injection of a local anesthetic and steroid into the bursa. Occasionally, excision of the hypertrophied posterior aspect of the calcaneus (Haglund's deformity) is necessary.

Osteochondritis Dissecans

Osteochondritis dissecans is an osteochondral defect in the talar dome, which occurs after an ankle injury. The anterior–lateral talar dome is affected on the lateral side and the posterior–medial aspect is affected on the medial side. This lesion can occur at any age, but it mostly affects adolescents and young adults.

History

Patients complain of chronic mild-to-moderate ankle pain with some catching with motion. When the osteochondral lesion loosens or separates from the underlying talar dome, it can mechanically abrade the joint, producing chronic pain, swelling, and intermittent locking.

Lab/Imaging

Occasionally, a large lesion can be seen on plain radiographs. Often, a computed tomography (CT) or MRI is needed to diagnose the patient.

Treatment

Small, superficial lesions can be treated with casting. Fragments that are displaced from their chondral bed will require surgical curettage and drilling of the subchondral bone to promote ingrowth of more fibrocartilage. This can be done with an open technique or with an arthroscopic technique.

Tarsal Coalition

Tarsal coalition is a fibrous or bony union between two or more tarsal bones that causes restricted motion or absence of motion between these bones. Talocalcaneal and calcaneonavicular coalitions are the most common types, accounting for approximately 90% of all tarsal coalitions.

History

Tarsal coalition may be completely without symptoms, but three symptoms should make the clinician suspicious of tarsal coalition. These are pain, limitation of motion, and muscle spasm. The pain usually is deep and aching in nature and usually is in the area of the tarsal coalition. Rarely, the pain can be neuritic in nature. It often is located in the sinus tarsi, the anterior–lateral part of the ankle, or the dorsum of the midfoot and may encompass the entire rear foot. The onset of the pain usually is insidious, developing after unusual activity or minor trauma. The pain is usually aggravated by activity and relieved with rest and often is related to walking over rough, uneven terrain, prolonged standing, or athletic activity. Limitation of subtalar and midtarsal motion is common. Usually, the subtalar joint is limited in inversion. Tonic muscle spasm may occur. The peroneus brevis is the muscle most commonly involved. Spasm of the tibialis posterior, tibialis anterior, and peroneus longus also may occur. The muscle spasm is precipitated by activity and relieved by rest.

Lab/Imaging

In most cases, routine radiographs will portray a tarsal coalition and will confirm the diagnosis. CT and MRI imaging are useful in fibrocartilaginous coalitions.

A calcaneonavicular coalition can be seen best on the medial oblique view. A bar between the calcaneous and navicular usually can be seen. This bar may be osseous, fibrous, cartilaginous, or mixed. In an incomplete union, the calcaneus and navicular are in close proximity, and their contiguous cortical surfaces appear flattened and irregular like a pseudoarthrosis.

Subtalar coalitions occur predominately in the middle facet. This is seen as the "halo sign," which is decreased visualization of the middle facet and enhancement of the sustentaculum tali. One also sees narrowing of the posterior facet of the subtalar joint with loss of clarity of the subtalar joint. Beaking of the talonavicular joint usually is present, as is flattening of the lateral talar process.

Physical Findings

Firm palpation in the area of the coalition usually is painful. As mentioned previously, there is decreased range of motion of the subtalar and or midtarsal joints. A peroneal spastic flatfoot may be present. A local anesthetic injected into the area of the coalition may·relieve the pain and muscle spasm sufficiently to allow a more

accurate assessment of the quality and quantity of joint motion.

Treatment

Conservative treatment is directed toward restricting midtarsal and subtalar motion. This can be done with shoe modification, padding, orthotics, or casting. Physical therapy and antiinflammatory medications also are helpful. If these treatments are not adequate, surgical treatment to resect the coalition or fuse the involved joint complex is necessary.

ARTHROPATHIES

Gout

Gout is a heterogeneous group of diseases caused by deposition of monosodium-urate crystals in tissues or uric acid in supersaturated solution in extracellular fluids. There are four main clinical manifestations. These are: (a) recurrent attacks of articular and periarticular inflammation; (b) accumulation of crystalline deposits (tophi) in cartilage, bone, joints, and soft tissue; (c) uric-acid calculi in the urinary tract; and (d) gouty nephropathy, i.e., interstitial nephropathy with renal function impairment.

Gout can be caused by overproduction of uric acid, underexcretion of uric acid, or both.

Approximately 10% of patients with gout are "overproducers." This occurs in a variety of acquired and genetic disorders. Causes of primary hyperuricemia include hypoxanthine guanine phosphoribosyl-transferase (HGPRT) deficiency, and phosphoribosylpyrophosphate (PRPP) synthetase superactivity.

Secondary causes of hyperuricemia include excessive dietary purine intake, increased nucleotide turnover such as occurs in psoriasis, myeloproliferative and lymphoproliferative disorders, hemolytic anemias, anemias associated with ineffective erythropoiesis, and Paget's disease of bone. Other causes of secondary hyperuricemia include severe muscle exertion and accelerated ATP degradation as occurs in glycogen-storage diseases.

Most patients with gout (90%) have a relative deficit in renal excretion of uric acid. They may have a primary idiopathic hyperuricemia or a secondary hyperuricemia. Secondary causes include diminished renal function, dehydration, and drugs that alter renal tubular function, (e.g., diuretics, cyclosporine, and low-dose salicylates). Competitive anions such as occur in lactic acidosis and ketoacidosis also can decrease uric acid excretion.

Other mechanisms that are not completely understood include hypertension, hyperparathyroidism, and lead nephropathy.

Combined overproduction and underexcretion occur in ethanol abuse, hypoxemia, tissue underperfusion, glucose-6-phosphatase deficiency, and fructose-1-phosphate-aldolase deficiency.

History

The first attack of acute-intermittent gout usually follows decades of asymptomatic hyperuricemia. In men, the attack usually occurs between the fourth and sixth decades. In women, it usually occurs after menopause. The onset involves faint twinges with rapid development of warmth, erythema, swelling, and exquisite pain that builds to its most intense level over 8 to 12 hours. The initial attack usually is monoarticular and involves the MPJ in half of the cases. The MPJ eventually is involved in 90% of patients. The midfoot, ankles, heels, and knees also are frequently involved in early gout. Less commonly, fingers, wrists, and elbows can become involved.

Fever, chills, and malaise may accompany the acute attack. Pain may be mild and only last a few hours ("petite attacks"), or may be severe and last for 1 or 2 weeks.

Early in acute-intermittent gout, the attacks are infrequent, and the interval between attacks may be years. The mean interval from the initial attack to a subsequent attack is 11 months. The attacks usually become more frequent, involve more joints, and become longer in duration. Between attacks, the involved joints are virtually free of symptoms.

Chronic tophaceous gout usually develops after more than 10 years of acute-intermittent gout. The intercritical periods are no longer free of pain, and the joints become persistently uncomfortable and swollen. Acute attacks continue against this background as often as every few weeks. Visible tophi may or may not be present for the first few years of this stage. Polyarticular involvement becomes much more common during this stage.

Subcutaneous gouty tophi eventually develop and may form anywhere on the body. Common sites include fingers, ears, wrists, knees, olecranon bursa, and the Achilles tendon. Tophi also may occur at other connective-tissue sites such as the renal pyramids, sclera, and heart valves.

Lab/Imaging

In early gout, the only initial finding may be soft-tissue swelling. After many years of disease, one may see bony erosions. These usually are slightly removed from the joint. The erosion has features that are both atrophic and heterotrophic leading to erosions with an overhanging edge (Martel sign). The joint space is preserved until very late in the disease. Juxta-articular osteopenia, which is common in rheumatoid disease, usually is very minimal or nonexistent in gout.

Elevated serum urate levels are not very helpful. The vast majority of patients with elevated serum urate levels never develop gout. Serum urate may be normal during an acute attack.

Definitive diagnosis is only possible by aspiration and inspection of tophaceous material or synovial fluid. Synovial tissue always should be cultured, as infection and gout can coexist.

Osteoarthritis

The American Academy of Orthopedic Surgeons and The National Institutes of Health defined osteoarthritis in the following way:

> Osteoarthritis (OA) is the result of both mechanical and biologic events that destabilize the normal coupling of degradation and synthesis of articular cartilage and subchondral bone. Although it may be initiated by multiple factors including genetic, developmental, metabolic and traumatic, OA includes all of the tissues of the diarthroidal joint. Ultimately, OA is manifested by morphological, biochemical, molecular, and biomechanical changes of both cells and matrix which lead to a softening, fibrillation, ulceration, and loss of articular cartilage, sclerosis and eburnation of subchondral bone, osteophytes, and subchondral cysts. When clinically evident, OA is characterized by joint pain, tenderness, limitation of movement, crepitus, occasional effusions, and variable degrees of local inflammation.

History

The patient usually is middle aged or elderly and complains of pain and stiffness in and around the joint. There usually is a limitation of function. The onset is mild and gradual. The pain initially is mild, worsens with use, and improves with rest. Pain at rest or during the night is unusual and is a feature of severe structural damage or cancer. Morning stiffness is common, but the duration is short (often less than 30 minutes.) Gel phenomenon (stiffness after periods of inactivity) is common and often resolves in several minutes. Pain and stiffness worsens in cool, damp, or rainy weather. Remember to consider vascular insufficiency in patients whose pain is brought on by activity and predictably resolves with rest.

Lab/Imaging

The classic radiologic finding is bony proliferation (osteophytes) at the joint margins. Later in the disease, one sees asymmetric joint space narrowing and subchondral bone sclerosis. Later still, one sees subchondral cysts with sclerotic walls and alteration of the shape of the bone ends secondary to bone remodeling.

Note that periarticular osteoporosis and marginal erosions are not features of OA, and the presence of these findings strongly suggests a diagnosis of inflammatory arthritis.

Routine lab tests are normal and are used to rule out other conditions. Rheumatoid factor is frequently ordered, but a positive rheumatoid factor does not rule out OA as 20% of healthy elderly people have a positive rheumatoid factor. Erythrocyte-sedimentation rate (ESR) also is ordered frequently, but a mildly elevated ESR can be seen in OA. This test is very useful, however, in the case of a markedly elevated level to alert the clinician of possible polymyalgia rheumatica, an underlying malignancy (such as multiple myeloma), and chronic infection.

Synovial fluid analysis usually will show a white blood cell (WBC) count of less than 2,000 cells/mm³. The finding of elevated protein and WBC count suggests a septic arthritis or a superimposed microcrystalline process.

Physical Findings

Bony enlargement is common. This can cause tenderness at the joint margins. Joint motion can be limited because of osteophyte formation. Crepitance, and joint malalignment are found frequently. The joint can be unstable, and one can see excess motion of the joint. Locking secondary to loose bodies in the joint can be seen.

Treatment

Nonpharmacologic therapy includes patient education, physical therapy, occupational therapy, range-of-motion and strengthening exercises, aerobic conditioning, weight loss, and the use of assistive devices, including orthotics and ankle–foot orthoses.

Pharmacologic treatment includes the use of oral nonopioid analgesics (e.g., acetaminophen), NSAIDs, topical analgesics (e.g., capsaicin), opioid analgesics, and intraarticular steroid injections. These injections are limited to three per year because of concern regarding the potential for progressive cartilage damage and pseudo-Charcot's arthropathy.

Surgical treatment includes a large number of osteotomy procedures designed to improve joint alignment and function. Surgical excision or fusion of the joint can provide excellent pain reduction, but decreased function.

Hallux Limitus

Hallux limitus is a special case of osteoarthritis of the first MPJ. This is a commonly seen entity and is a cause of pain and decreased dorsiflexion of the hallux.

Many causes have been proposed for this disorder, most of them biomechanical. A long first metatarsal can create overloading of the first MPJ as the foot enters the propulsive phase of gait, thus leading to degenerative changes. Hypermobility of the first ray is the result of abnormal subtalar joint pronation in the late midstance and propulsive phases of gait. When this occurs, the lateral column of the foot becomes unstable, and the per-oneus longus is deprived of its mechanical advantage, which is needed to provide functional plantarflexion of the first ray. The first metatarsal then will dorsiflex and invert (bunion), and the head of the metatarsal will fail to articulate properly with the sesamoids. This will cause a limitation of hallux dorsiflexion.

Metatarsus primus elevatus is present when the first metatarsal lies above the plane of the lessor metatarsals. When this happens, the first ray cannot plantar flex to a point where hallux dorsiflexion can occur. This condition may be congenital or may be the result of abnormal subtalar joint pronation. The end result is jamming of the proximal phalangeal base into the head of the metatarsal during the propulsive phase of gait.

Hallux limitus also may be associated with a hallux valgus deformity, trauma, systemic arthritides, and infectious arthritis.

History

See osteoarthritis section.

Lab/Imaging

Radiographic signs of hallux limitus include flattening and eburnation of the metatarsal head, narrowing of the joint space, and osteophytes on the dorsal and dorsomedial aspects of the base of the proximal phalanx and of the first metatarsal head. A lateral view may show metatarsus primus elevatus, but clinical correlation is required as this finding may be seen in many asymptotic individuals.

Physical Findings

The first MPJ may be circumferentially enlarged. There usually is a dorsal or dorsomedial prominence. Passive dorsiflexion of the hallux is limited and may be painful. Full plantarflexion usually is present. An associated hyperextension deformity of the interphalangeal joint (IPJ) may be present. A callous may develop under or medial to the IPJ.

The patient may try to compensate for MPJ tenderness by inverting the forefoot, thereby taking weight off of the medial column. This may cause diffuse lesser metatarsal pain and callous formation beneath the fourth or fifth metatarsal.

Treatment

Treatment is directed toward addressing the cause of the deformity. If a hypermobile first ray is the cause, an appropriate orthotic may be very helpful. Another conservative measure is the use of a stiff-soled shoe to decrease motion of the MPJ. A rocker bottom on the sole of the shoe also will relieve stress on the MPJ.

Pharmacologic treatment as outlined in the osteoarthritis section can provide much symptomatic relief.

Numerous surgical treatments for this disorder have been devised. The most simple is a cheilectomy, which is surgical removal of the osteophytic proliferations on the metatarsal head and proximal phalanx. This procedure works best on patients with mild disease.

Many surgical osteotomies have been devised to decompress the MPJ and elevate the metatarsal head. Other approaches include the Keller arthroplasty, implant arthroplasty, and arthrodesis of the joint.

Neuropathic Arthropathy (Charcot's Arthropathy)

Neuropathic arthropathy is defined as severe degenerative arthritis in the setting of neurologic damage to a limb or joint. The most common cause is diabetes, where the prevalence is 1 in 1,680 (Table 18.1).

Two theories have been proposed to explain this phenomenon. Charcot felt that increased blood flow promoted metabolic changes in bone and cartilage leading to bone and joint destruction. This theory is supported by reports of diabetic patients with vascular insufficiency developing neuropathic arthropathy after revascularization procedures. Virchow proposed that the destruction was caused by multiple episodes of minor trauma occurring in the neuropathic setting where normal protective sensation is absent. This theory is supported by the observation that acute neuropathic arthropathy is commonly seen after minor trauma. Both theories may be operative.

History

The patient with neuropathic arthropathy typically presents with an acute or subacute monoarthritis with swelling, erythema, and variable amounts of pain. In the classic diabetic Charcot's foot, the midfoot or ankle is quite warm, swollen, and erythematous. Erythema can involve the entire lower leg. This is easily confused with an infectious process. It is helpful to strongly suspect an acute red, swollen foot in a neuropathic diabetic as being neuropathic arthropathy if there are no openings on the foot that could be a portal of entry for infection. One also

TABLE 18.1. *Conditions Associated With Neuropathic Arthropathy*

Diabetes mellitus	Syringomyelia
Brain trauma	Spinal-cord trauma
Meningomyelocele	Nerve trauma
Alcoholism	Multiple sclerosis
Charcot–Marie–Tooth disease	Riley–Day syndrome
Pernicious anemia	Congenital insensitivity to pain
Amyloidosis	Arnold–Chiari malformation
Leprosy	Yaws
Syphilis	

typically notes that the pain is less than would be expected considering the amount of destruction seen on the x-rays.

The speed of onset, the rate of progression, the amount of pain, and the balance between bone overgrowth and bone destruction is quite variable.

The location of the arthropathy in the foot is in the tarsometatarsal area 60% of the time, the metatarsal phalangeal joints 30% of the time, and in the tibiotalar joint 10% of the time.

There is often a history of relatively minor trauma such as an ankle sprain preceding the onset of the symptoms.

Lab/Imaging

Plain radiographs of early neuropathic arthropathy will show joint-space narrowing, osteophytes, and demineralization. Later, one sees bone fragmentation, periarticular debris formation, and joint subluxation. There is chaotic bony destruction and repair.

In diabetics, most of the fragmentation and loose body formation occurs in the tarsal bones, while absorptive changes predominate in the metatarsals and forefoot.

MRI may be helpful in ruling out osteomyelitis.

Joint effusions can be very large and may contain calcium pyrophosphate dihydrate (CPPD) crystals and calcium-phosphate crystals. It is unknown if these crystals play a part in the pathogenesis of this disease or if they are simply markers of severe joint destruction.

Synovial fluid typically is noninflammatory, with 50% of samples being hemorrhagic or xanthochromic.

Treatment

Initial treatment includes immobilization, elevation, and strict nonweight bearing. Many of these fractures go on to coalesce in a very disorganized and deformed pattern, frequently with a "rocker bottom" sole. Neuropathic patients with this deformity are at high risk for recurrent ulcerations and infections that can become limb threatening. Osteotomy and fusion to correct these deformities can be limb-saving procedures.

Septic Arthritis

Septic arthritis is the bacterial infection of a joint caused by trauma, surgery, injection, spread from contiguous infected tissues, or by way of hematogenous spread from a remote focus of infection.

The joint is damaged by a variety of mechanisms. Bacterial products such as gram-negative endotoxins, exotoxins from gram-positive organisms, cell-wall fragments, and immune complexes stimulate synovial cells to release tumor necrosis factor alpha, and interleukin (IL)-1β, which up-regulates expression of adhesion ligands in synovial-vessel endothelial cells. This results in leukocyte migration and attachment to synovial fluid and articular tissues. The bacteria are phagocytized by polymorphonuclear lymphocytes causing the release of lysosomal enzymes into the joint. This damages synovium, ligaments, and cartilage. Antigen-antibody complexes form, which activate the compliment system. Arachidonic acid metabolism is stimulated resulting in the release of collagenase and proteolytic enzymes. The proteases persist in the cartilage even after the bacteria have been eradicated, causing continuing degradation of the cartilage. More IL-1 also is released, which further amplifies the inflammatory response.

After 48 hours, the cellular immune system begins to play a role. There is an infiltration of T lymphocytes, increased IL-6 levels, and polyclonal B-cell activation resulting in IgG antibody production.

Bacterial products can directly affect chondrocytes causing decreased proteoglycan synthesis and increase protease activity.

Bacterial toxins can activate the coagulation system leading to intravascular thrombosis in the subsynovial vessels and fibrin deposition on the synovium and articular cartilage. The layer of fibrin provides a gelatinous nidus for bacterial replication. The fibrin also activates the fibrinolytic system with formation of plasmin, which destroys the protein core and the polysaccharides in the cartilage matrix. The microvascular obstruction causes ischemia and necrosis.

The inflammatory synovitis causes the synovium to proliferate and form a pannus, which erodes cartilage and subchondral bone. This pannus may persist even after the infection has been eradicated, hypothetically because of alteration of the cartilage from the infection, which causes it to become antigenic.

History

There is an acute onset of moderate-to-severe joint pain, erythema, warmth, tenderness, and decreased painful range of motion of the joint. Eighty percent to 85% of the time, a single joint is involved. Eighty percent of the infections are caused by *Staphylococcus aureus* in adults. 80% of the patients are febrile. The most common organisms found in children 6 months to 2 years of age are *Haemophilus influenzae* and *Kingella kingae*. *Neisseria gonorrhea* is the most common cause of polyarticular septic arthritis.

Approximately one third of septic arthritis cases occur in drug abusers. Most infections are caused by *S. aureus* or gram-negative organisms such as *Enterobacter, Pseudomonas aeruginosa*, or *Serratia marcescens*. Gram-negative joint infections tend to be indolent and difficult to diagnose. 99m-technetium bone scans are helpful in these situations.

Disseminated gonococcal infections present with a 5- to 7-day history of fever, shaking chills, fleeting migratory polyarthralgia, tenosynovitis of the fingers, toes, wrists, and ankles that evolves into persistent monoarthritis or oligoarthritis. These patients have multiple skin lesions that may be petechiae, papules, pustules, hemorrhagic bullae, or necrotic ulcerated lesions. These lesions can occur on the trunk or extremities, including the palms of the hands and the soles of the feet. The oral mucosa is not involved.

Labs/Imaging

Synovial fluid analysis is the most important test with greater than 50,000 WBC/mm^3 in 50% to 70% of cases. The remainder are in the range between 2,000 and 50,000 WBC/mm^3. The differential shows greater than 85% polymorphonuclear leukocytes. Synovial-fluid glucose often is less than one half of the serum glucose, but this also can be seen in reactive arthritis and in rheumatoid arthritis. Lactic acid usually is elevated. Urate and calcium pyrophosphate crystals may be seen because intraarticular deposits may leach out during infection. The presence of crystals should not rule out infection.

Peripheral WBC is elevated in 50% of the cases. C-reactive protein and ESR usually are elevated. Blood cultures are positive one half of the time, and this may be the only way the organism is identified.

Early radiographic signs include soft-tissue swelling and joint effusions. After 10 to 14 days, one can see joint space narrowing and subchondral bony erosion.

Treatment

Antibiotic therapy and adequate drainage are the mainstays of therapy. The initial antibiotic choice is determined by the clinical setting and the initial laboratory studies. Antibiotic choice then can be refined when culture and sensitivity data are available. Duration of therapy is determined by clinical response and usually varies from 2 to 6 weeks.

Nongonococcal septic arthritis must be treated with adequate drainage of the joint, which can be accomplished by surgical arthrotomy, arthroscopic lavage, or by large-bore needle aspiration one or more times daily. Gonococcal infections usually do not require aspirations unless the synovial fluid continues to accumulate.

SELECTED READINGS

Banks AS, Downey MS, Camasta C, Martin DE. *McGlamry's Comprehensive Textbook of Foot Surgery*, 3rd ed. Philadelphia: Lippincott Williams & Wilkins, 2000.

Barrett SJ, O'Malley R. Plantar fasciitis and other causes of heel pain. *Am Fam Physician* 1999;59:2200–2206.

Calabrese LH. Rheumatoid arthritis and primary care: the case for early diagnosis and treatment. *J Am Osteopath Assoc* 1999;99:313–321.

Canale ST, Belding RH. Osteochondral lesions of the talus. *J Bone Joint Surg [Am]* 1980;62:97–102.

Clarke HD, Kitaoka HB, Ehman RL. Peroneal tendon injuries. *Foot Ankle Int* 1998;19:280–288.

Haas DW, McAndrew MP. Bacterial osteomyelitis in adults: evolutionary considerations in diagnosis and treatment. *Am J of Med* 1996;101:550–561.

Hutchinson BL, O'Rourke EM. Tibialis posterior tendon dysfunction and peroneal tendon subluxation. *Clin Podiatr Med Surg* 1995;12:703–723.

Irvine S, Munro R, Porter D. Early referral, diagnosis, and treatment of rheumatoid arthritis: evidence for changing medical practice. *Ann Rheum Dis* 1999;58:510–513.

Johnson KA, Strom DE. Tibialis posterior tendon dysfunction. *Clin Orthop* 1989;239:196–206.

Klippel JH, ed. *Primer on the Rheumatic Diseases*, 11th ed. Atlanta, GA: Arthritis Foundation, 1997.

Kulik SA Jr, Clanton TO. Tarsal coalition. *Foot Ankle Int* 1996;17:286–296.

Lipsky LA. Osteomyelitis of the foot in diabetic patients. *Clin Infect Dis* 1997;25:1318–1326.

Lynch DM, Goforth WP, Martin JE, et al. Conservative treatment of plantar fasciitis. A prospective study. *J Am Podiatric Med Assoc* 1998;88: 375–380.

Mader JT, et al. Update on the diagnosis and management of osteomyelitis. *Clin Podiatr Med Surg* 1996;13;701–723.

Perry CR. Septic arthritis. *Am J Orthop* 1999;28:168–178.

Redd RA, Peters VJ, Emery SF, et al. Morton's neuroma: sonographic evaluation. *Radiology* 1989;171:415–417.

Sammarco GJ. Peroneal tendon injuries. *Orthop Clin North Am* 1994;25: 153–145.

Sobel E, et al. Orthosis in the treatment of rearfoot problems. *J Am Podiatric Med Assoc* 1999;89:220–233.

Vincent KA. Tarsal coalition and painful flatfoot. *J Am Acad Orthop Surg* 1998;6:274–281.

CHAPTER 19

Abdominal Pain

Robert I. Cohen

Significant changes in diagnosis and management of abdominal pain have occurred in the past decade. For example, treating acute abdominal pain in the emergency department with opioid analgesia is no longer considered contraindicated by many. The risk of masking the diagnosis of a surgical abdomen may be outweighed by the value of treating suffering. This change of values is paralleled by increased utilization of sophisticated computed tomography (CT) and ultrasound imaging technologies, which have significantly improved diagnostic accuracy. An increasing number of surgeons and emergency physicians are comfortable titrating potent opioid medication until suffering is relieved. As studies continue to be published demonstrating safety and efficacy, abdominal pain may become as aggressively managed as pain occurring in other locations.

Attitudes of providers and expectations of patients have effected a significant change in culture regarding the aggressive management of pain in other body regions, such as chest pain and acute postsurgical pain. The Agency for Healthcare Research and Quality has successfully educated providers through publication of evidence-based, multispecialty, expert-panel guidelines. More recently, education of hospital administrative personnel has begun as major credentialing agencies such as The Joint Commission on Accreditation of Healthcare Organization has added requirements for documentation of patient pain levels and of effective treatment to biannual facility certification.

While current technology has improved imaging sensitivity and specificity, the diagnosis of acute appendicitis continues to be the most commonly missed diagnosis for patients with abdominal pain. The resulting morbidity and mortality is not trivial. However, appropriate management of this acute pain need not prevent timely diagnosis. One thing that has not changed is that the path to correct diagnosis begins with a careful history. It is worth repeating briefly what every clinician knows: that every

pain history should include a careful description of the multiple dimensions of pain including its intensity, character, timing (onset, duration, pattern), associated aggravating and alleviating factors, location, and radiation.

Abdominal pain may originate from the structures in the abdominal cavity or from outside as a referred-pain syndrome. Referred pain is most frequently from the spine, pelvis, or thorax. It can be of metabolic origin such as lead poisoning or porphyria. Lower-lobar pneumonia may present as pain referred to the upper abdomen that is intense, of acute or subacute onset, and accompanied by guarding. This pain resolves with treatment of the pneumonia.

The abdomen is not exempt from being a manifestation of psychogenic pain, although this is rare and must be a diagnosis of exclusion. True psychogenic pain may respond to psychotherapeutic intervention. It may fail to be blocked by even high concentrations of local anesthetic injected into a thoracic–epidural catheter as part of a graded test with increasing concentrations of local anesthetic.

According to Alon Winnie, a differential neuraxial block can be helpful in identifying the source of pain. According to this theory, somatic and sympathetic pain can be discriminated based upon the concentration of local anesthetic required to block the pain. It was postulated that because sympathetic pain is carried by small, nonmyelinated C fibers, sympathetically maintained pain could be blocked by much lower concentrations of local anesthetics than that required for blocking the larger A-α and A-δ fibers responsible for the transmission of somatic pain. Proponents of this test suggest that patients with psychogenic pain and or malingering can be identified based on the pattern of their response. Failure to block the pain even with high concentrations of local anesthetic that produce profound sensory (somatic) and motor block suggests a central pain syndrome, where pain is modulated at higher centers in the central nervous system than the level of spinal block. Interestingly, Dr. Winnie suggests that malingering patients often report persisting pain when sensory and motor fibers have been fully blocked.

A test for sympathetically mediated pain is resolution of pain following injection of local anesthetic at or near sympathetic ganglia. The sympathetic ganglia lie against the anterolateral aspect of the thoracic and lumbar vertebral bodies, and are anatomically well separated from the somatic nerves that supply sensation to the abdominal wall. With CT or fluoroscopic guidance, they can be blocked selectively, although some blockade of somatic nerves may occur if high volume of local anesthetic is used.

While chronic abdominal-pain syndromes are commonly associated with the report of deep (visceral) pain, other pain syndromes are associated with a more superficial location. In costochondritis, the location often is epigastric overlying the xiphoid, or along the costal margin. The pain frequently is exacerbated by movement or touch. This form of arthritis is responsive to oral antiinflammatory agents or intraarticular injection of corticosteroid. Some patients may even find relief from the simple use of a broad elastic belt splinting costochondral junctions during strenuous activities.

Superficial pain in the soft tissues of the abdominal wall may be caused by a myofascial pain syndrome. In the case of myofascial pain syndrome, palpation of a tender trigger point within the abdominal musculature initiates a pattern of pain radiation characteristic of the muscle group involved. Pain clinics often offer trigger-point injection with local anesthetic, depo-steroid, and even botulinum toxin, in conjunction with a course of physical therapy. These patients frequently report that the pain is worse with exercise. Patients who are able to work through this pain, however, with a gradually increasing intensity of exercise may find they improve with a regular home-exercise program.

Patients with fibromyalgia also may report abdominal-wall pain and tenderness, but usually have tender spots rather than true trigger points. Although none of the classic 18 tender spots associated with this syndrome (see Fig. 24.1 on page 155) involve the abdomen, patients with fibromyalgia syndrome may experience abdominal pain as part of their complaint.

Pain radiating in a bandlike distribution along the dermatomes across the abdomen suggests a radicular origin. Inflammatory changes in a sensory nerve root caused by exposure to even small amounts of extruded disc material may respond to injection of epidural steroid. MRI technology is useful for diagnosing degenerative-disc disease, vertebral-body collapse, and compression by space-occupying lesion or invasive tumor.

Volleys of lancinating pain or constant burning pain radiating along a dermatome may precede herpetic skin eruptions. Prevention of postherpetic neuralgia is best accomplished with aggressive management of pain in combination with antiviral therapy and a tricyclic antidepressant. For patients with severe pain, membrane-stabilizing drugs like gabapentin, as well as opiates, intrathecal steroids, and topical agents have mostly replaced the use of sympathetic nerve blocks. There are no prospective, controlled studies proving the efficacy of sympathetic nerve blockade performed in the acute or subacute period for preventing the pain of postherpetic neuralgia, although sympathetic block remains an effective treatment option.

Nerve irritation from surgical lysis, neural entrapment in healing tissue, or sprouting regeneration with neuroma formation are common postoperative complications. Injection of local anesthetic will assist the diagnosis and may be therapeutic by breaking a pain cycle. The patient may report lessening of symptoms with subsequent injections. Injection of a depo corticosteroid such as triamcinolone also may be worth trying. Withdrawal symptoms from opiates, whether prescribed or a drug of abuse, such as heroin, can produce severe abdominal pain; although this is an uncommon presentation, it may lead a user to seek physician assistance, not realizing its relation to the addiction.

Pain originating in the abdominal wall may be blocked by injecting the painful area or the appropriate intercostal or paravertebral nerves with local anesthetic. Block of the celiac plexus may be helpful in differentiating abdominal wall or genitourinary pain from intraabdominal visceral pain, as the plexus supplies all abdominal viscera except the rectum, sigmoid, bladder, and reproductive organs. Celiac-plexus block is very effective for pancreatic pain. When a lytic substance such as phenol or alcohol in high concentration is used, patients may get prolonged relief. This is a frequently used modality for terminal patients, whose life expectancy is shorter than the several months required for injured nerves to resprout and reconnect, with the subsequent risk of neuropathic pain.

Deep-abdominal pain is either visceral or somatic in origin. Visceral pain often is described as a dull aching or diffuse midabdominal discomfort. Somatic pain originating in the parietal peritoneum and the root of the mesentery is more intense, better circumscribed, and often in close proximity to the area of origin. Referred pain is more often associated with somatic pain.

To determine the source of the pain, it is important to assess not only its intensity, location, and character, but also its onset, whether acute or insidious, and temporal profile. The circumstances that intensify or alleviate the pain are most significant. Relief with eating or antacids is suggestive of gastroesophageal reflux or ulcer disease. Postprandial pain, depending on its location and character, could be of biliary or ischemic origin or associated with a more benign condition, such as lactose intolerance or irritable-bowel syndrome. Seasonal patterns are frequently seen in ulcer disease and occasionally with regional enteritis. The pain of inflammatory-bowel disease and irritable-bowel syndrome may be relieved by defecation, whereas pain accompanied by urgency to defecate suggests an intraabdominal bleed such as ruptured aortic aneurism in the old and ectopic pregnancy in the young. Application of heat or cold may relieve pain of musculoskeletal origin, while pain from peritoneal irritation or spinal origin may worsen with certain postures, sudden movement, coughing, straining, and sneezing.

GASTROINTESTINAL TRACT

The gastrointestinal tract is a common source of abdominal pain. This discussion will address the constellation of findings by anatomic region and include complaints associated with the esophagus, stomach, small intestine, colon, pancreas, liver, and biliary tract.

Esophagus

Heartburn is the most common complaint referable to the esophagus (Fig. 19.1). It has a burning or gnawing character located in the substernum or epigastrium. It usually occurs after eating or on bending or reclining; it rarely occurs after exercise. Whether it is solely a result of discomfort from chemical irritation or whether secondary muscle spasm plays a role is not entirely clear. Pain from an esophageal ulcer or esophageal spasm usually is perceived in the mid chest with a component extending into the back, but it also can be felt in the epigastrium. When an esophageal ulcer is present, the pain usually is steady, burning, or gnawing. That pain syndrome also may represent esophageal spasm, a condition that more typically presents as a heaviness or tightness in the chest.

Stomach

The character of pain from ulcer disease varies widely. Typically, it is located in the epigastrium. It may be a sharply localized, burning, gnawing pain or just a vague discomfort occurring from 1/2 hour to 2 hours after eating or during the night. Food or antacids relieve it. The pain occasionally may be more localized to the right or left upper quadrant (particularly when a gastric ulcer is

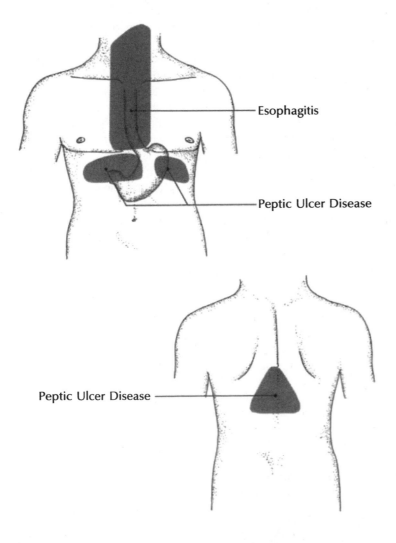

Esophagitis

Peptic Ulcer Disease

Peptic Ulcer Disease

FIG. 19.1. Patterns of esophagitis and peptic-ulcer disease.

present) and may radiate into the back. The concomitant back pain usually indicates a posterior duodenal wall ulcer with irritation of or penetration into the pancreas. That pain usually is deep, boring, persistent, and less well localized; food or antacids usually do not relieve it.

Unlike heartburn, ulcer pain frequently occurs in clusters; daily pain for several weeks may be followed by variably long pain-free intervals. That irregularity, particularly if the pain is somewhat atypical, makes it easy to confuse ulcer pain with the pain of irritable-bowel syndrome. As with heartburn, it is not known whether the discomfort results from irritation of nerve endings by acid or from spasm of antral and duodenal smooth muscle.

Epigastric pain occurring soon after eating, unrelieved by antacids and with lack of periodicity, does not necessarily rule out ulcer disease. Pyloric channel ulcers may present in such a manner, and unless there is associated postprandial vomiting, the diagnosis may not be made until frank gastric-outlet obstruction develops.

Pain associated with the entrapment of a portion of the stomach within a defect in the diaphragm may produce pain radiating into the epigastrium or substernal region. Although hiatal hernia is common and is present in more than 50% of patients over 60, pain from this anatomical defect is thought to be much less common.

Small Intestine

As a rule, pain originating in the small intestine is periumbilical, crampy, and colicky in nature (Fig. 19.2). It may result from abnormal motility patterns or from a lowered threshold to the pain of bowel distension. It usually is caused by a lesion obstructing the lumen of the bowel (e.g., regional enteritis, metastatic or primary adenocarcinoma, endocrine tumor, or lymphoma). Chronic malabsorption states are not generally associated with pain, unless a complication, such as a lymphoma, develops in a patient with celiac sprue.

The pain of irritable-bowel syndrome usually is chronic. It is not always accompanied by a change in bowel habits, although constipation is common. Nausea, bloating, and dyspepsia frequently occur and may simulate peptic ulcer or biliary-tract disease. The pain may be localized or may migrate over time. It is most commonly described as a knotting sensation or as a sharp pain but may present as a burning discomfort. Eating usually pre-

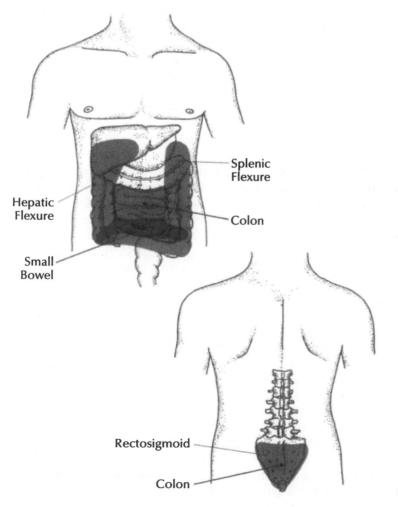

FIG. 19.2. Patterns of small bowel and colonic pain.

cipitates it; defecation or fasting relieves it. Although classically it is an episodic complaint, pain in the lower abdomen may occasionally be described as constant.

Pain from a partial bowel obstruction also commonly occurs 1 to 2 hours after meals; the closer the lesion is to the stomach, the sooner the pain presents. It commonly manifests as crampy pain. It comes in a wave and abates over the next hour and may be associated with nausea and vomiting. Regional enteritis is suggested by localization of the pain to the right lower quadrant and associated diarrhea, chills, fever, weight loss, or extraintestinal manifestations such as arthritis and mouth ulcers.

Significant weight loss and cachexia may suggest an underlying lymphoma or metastatic disease of the bowel. It may be several months before complete obstruction develops, at which time the diagnosis becomes considerably more obvious. As in the case of appendicitis, the initial pain may be nonspecific, periumbilical discomfort, but as the obstruction becomes nearly total or the mass enlarges and irritates the overlying peritoneum, the pain localizes and approximates the site of the underlying lesion.

Postoperative adhesions frequently are blamed for chronic or recurrent abdominal pain. Definitive CT or kidney–ureter–bladder (KUB) image showing evidence of small-bowel obstruction with angulation and proximal dilation of small bowel on a contrast study should be documented prior to exploration. For those patients with positive findings who go to the operating room without delay, the risk of acid-aspiration syndrome can be decreased by the use of nonparticulate contrast materials. Poor outcome following aspiration is associated with a large volume, low pH, and the presence of particles in the aspirated material. The diagnosis of intermittent small-bowel or colonic volvulus also will be greatly aided with CT or KUB imaging done during an episode of pain.

Lactose intolerance may cause chronic abdominal cramping that is not always associated with bloating or diarrhea. Because dairy products are so ubiquitous, 30% to 40% of patients will not make the association.

Abdominal pain is a frequent complaint associated with food-born illness. Again, timing is helpful in suggesting the etiology. For pain associated with the upper gastrointestinal tract, the onset of nausea, vomiting, and abdominal pain usually occurs within minutes following mushroom poisoning and poisoning resulting from ingestion of antimony, cadmium, copper, lead, tin, and zinc.

The scenario usually is a very acid food cooked or stored in a utensil containing the metal. Rapid onset of abdominal pain may result from fluoride poisoning when powdered pesticides are mistaken for food ingredients.

Incubation of one to several hours is associated with bacterial agents such as the exoenterotoxins of *Staphylococcus aureus*. Dinoflagellate (red tide) toxins from contaminated shellfish usually produce abdominal pain within a few hours of ingestion. The cyclopeptides and gyromitrin from mushrooms (certain species of amanita, andgyromitra, galerina) may take 6 to 24 hours to produce characteristic abdominal pain, fullness, protracted vomiting, thirst, weak rapid pulse, drowsiness, dilated pupils, even coma and death.

The pain associated with food-born illness affecting more the lower gastrointestinal tract often has a longer incubation. A 7- to 12-hour incubation is associated with pain resulting from the enterotoxin of *Bacillus cereus* and the endoenterotoxin from *Clostridium perfringens*. Longer incubation in the range of 12 to 72 hours suggests *Campylobacter*, cholera, pathologic diarrhea producing *Escherichia coli*, salmonellosis, shigellosis, *Vibrio parahaemolyticus*, and *Yersinia*. Incubation periods greater than 72 hours suggest parasitic agents such as amebiasis (3 to 4 weeks), giardiasis (1 to 6 weeks), taeniasis (beef tapeworm, 3 to 6 weeks/pork tapeworm, 3 to 6 months), and diphyllobothriasis (fish tapeworm, 5 to 6 weeks).

Colon

Pain from the colon tends to be localized to the lower abdomen. Pain from the cecum and ascending colon localizes to the right lower quadrant and that from the descending colon to the left lower quadrant. A rectosigmoid lesion may cause discomfort in the left lower quadrant and suprapubic and sacral areas. Adenocarcinomas or diverticula of the colon with microperforation may cause clearly localized lower-abdominal pain. Diverticulitis usually presents acutely but may occasionally cause chronic left-sided, lower-abdominal discomfort, particularly if complications such as pericolonic abscess, sigmoid stricture, or fistulas develop.

Pancreas, Liver, Biliary Tract

Because the pancreas, liver, biliary tree, stomach, and duodenum share some of the same neuropathways, it is easy to understand the difficulties involved in the differential diagnosis of chronic epigastric pain (Fig. 19.3). Disorders of the pancreas, mainly pancreatitis and pancreatic cancer, are among the most difficult to diagnose. The pain of chronic pancreatitis may be intermittent but, when present, lasts for days or weeks. It may vary in intensity and usually is epigastric, unless the tail of the pancreas is involved. Eating and movement may aggravate it, and there may be associated nausea and vomiting. Classically, relief of pain is obtained when a patient sits with his trunk flexed and his knees drawn up. With time, the pain-free intervals are shorter and eventually the pain may become constant. Persistent inflammation of the organ may be responsible for some of the pain, but it is most likely to be traceable to pancreatic duct obstruction and secondary ductal distention. Sympathetic blockade by infusion of very dilute local anesthetic through a thoracic epidural catheter is a highly effective method for managing this pain state. Celiac-plexus blockade appears

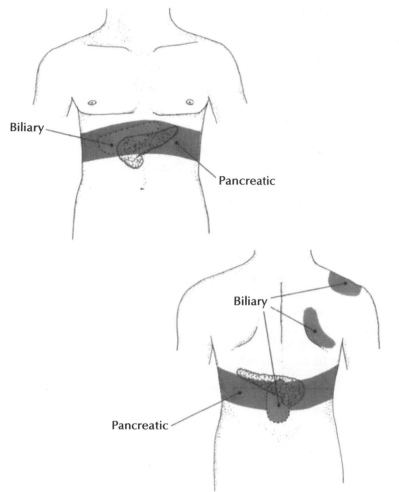

FIG. 19.3. Patterns of pancreatic and biliary pain.

to provide better pain relief for pancreatic cancer than for alcoholic pancreatitis, although this commonly held belief has not been studied.

The pain of pancreatic cancer is very similar to that of chronic pancreatitis. It is initially episodic and related to eating but soon becomes constant with radiation into the back. Severe pain suggests infiltration of the retroperitoneal area and celiac axis with its neural plexus. Tumors in the head of the pancreas tend to produce pain in the right epigastrium, those in the body localize to the midline, and those in the tail localize to the left-upper quadrant. Weight loss, jaundice, thrombophlebitis, and depression are more commonly seen with pancreatic cancer than with chronic pancreatitis. Neurolytic coeliac-plexus block is very effective for management of pain resulting from pancreatic cancer, while it is considered controversial for management of pain from chronic pancreatitis because nerve regrowth makes this a "permanent block" only for patients with a short life expectancy. Use of a long-acting/mechanical release formulation of the local anesthetic butamben has produced responses similar to neurolytic block when injected into the epidural space.

Biliary pain usually is caused by a passing stone or by biliary-tree dilatation secondary to an obstruction. Pain is characteristically localized to the right, upper quadrant and may radiate into the right shoulder and shoulder blade, and may last from 2 to 12 hours. After an acute attack, residual soreness in the right, upper quadrant or epigastrium may persist for several days. Epigastric or back discomfort, initially after meals but eventually becoming constant, may signal common bile-duct obstruction from a stone or a carcinoma. Right upper-quadrant pain accompanied by fever and jaundice suggests cholangitis.

The liver parenchyma is insensitive to pain, but relatively rapid distention of the liver capsule will initiate well localized, right, upper-quadrant pain; rapidly expanding lesions in the liver are more likely to be painful. Acute hepatitis may present with right, upper-quadrant pain, although this rarely becomes chronic. Chronic, active hepatitis may present with a history of recurrent attacks of right upper-quadrant pain. The pain usually is dull, well localized, and associated with worsening liver function tests.

Liver neoplasm, benign or malignant, also may cause pain in the right upper quadrant. Benign focal–nodular hyperplasia or adenomas associated with the use of birth-control pills may present with recurrent right upper-quadrant discomfort or, occasionally with a dramatic crisis of severe abdominal pain and hypotension from a bleed into the capsule or peritoneum. Recurrent "warning" pains may be caused by small bleeding episodes in the lesions. Primary or metastatic liver neoplasms cause pain secondary to capsular stretching, either by growth of the tumor or by intermittent swelling resulting from bleeding or necrotic changes. The episodes usually are associated with fever and jaundice. The pain is well localized, sharp, steady, and exacerbated by movement producing friction between the liver surface and the chest wall. A bruit may be identified in as many as 25% of cases.

Liver abscesses commonly follow an episode of intraabdominal sepsis and present with malaise, fever, and right upper-quadrant pain. The pain may be dull and vague or sharp and well localized. It may be relieved when the patient lies on their right side. Right-shoulder pain, cough, hiccups, and pleuritic components indicate diaphragmatic irritation by the abscess.

VASCULAR DISEASES OF THE BOWEL

Although mainly asymptomatic, occlusive vascular disease (usually atherosclerotic and affecting at least two of the three main splanchnic vessels) may present with chronic, intermittent, dull periumbilical, or epigastric pain. Classically, this relatively uncommon syndrome has been termed abdominal angina. It occurs approximately 1/2 hour after eating and lasts while digestion and absorption of the ingested meal are occurring; because the collateral vascular supply is insufficient to meet the increased need a that time, a state of relative ischemia and consequent pain is created. The recurrent pain may precipitate a fear of eating, with subsequent weight loss. When patients are questioned retrospectively, one finds that the sudden presentation of bowel ischemia or infarction has often been preceded by postprandial abdominal discomfort for weeks or months.

Abdominal–aortic aneurism usually presents more acutely, but a slowly expanding or leaking aneurism may be associated with recurrent, dull midepigastric or back pain over several months. This pain, like pancreatic pain, may occasionally be relieved by sitting up or leaning forward. The pulsating, sometimes tender mass can be palpated and a bruit may be heard.

The authenticity of the superior mesenteric artery syndrome has been discussed and debated over many years. The epigastric right upper-quadrant postprandial pain was thought to be caused by compression of the duodenum between the superior mesenteric artery and the retroperitoneal structures. It usually followed significant weight loss when the loss of fat would accentuate the anatomic angle of the superior mesenteric artery.

The vasculitis of polyarteritis nodosa and systemic lupus erythematosus occasionally may be responsible for attacks of abdominal pain.

PERITONEUM

Because there are no pain receptors in the visceral peritoneum, pain may be generated only from the parietal peritoneum. In that setting, chronic pain is most frequently traceable to a malignancy such as mesothelioma, metastatic bowel tumors, sarcoma, teratoma, ovarian cancer, or lymphoma. Although diffuse abdominal aching is the major complaint, occasionally a more localized pain may develop. The diffuse discomfort is frequently compounded by the presence of ascites, which further distends the peritoneum and also impairs respiratory function. Spontaneous bacterial peritonitis, as seen in alcoholics and in patients with ascites, usually presents acutely but may be associated with chronic malaise and diffuse abdominal discomfort. Tuberculous, fungal, and other types of infectious peritonitis are rather uncommon but should be considered in the immunosuppressed patient. Endometriosis also may produce abdominal pain and should be considered in the differential diagnosis of abdominal pain in women, especially if the timing is related to menses.

In young patients of Mediterranean decent who have chronic, recurrent attacks of sudden diffuse or localized peritoneal pain, familial Mediterranean fever should be entertained as a possible diagnosis. Abdominal tenderness, fever, and arthritis frequently coexist. The symptoms mimic those of acute surgical abdomen and may provoke a negative laparoscopic examination. The patient usually feels well within 2 to 3 days and is entirely asymptomatic until the next attack.

MESENTERY AND OMENTUM

Mesenteric diseases are rare but should be considered in patients with chronic abdominal pain, particularly when the diagnosis is elusive. It usually is the older patient who presents with either a localized or diffuse, crampy abdominal pain. There may be fever, nausea, vomiting, and weight loss. A mass may be palpable in 60% of the patients with localized tenderness but no peritoneal signs. Mesenteric panniculitis or retractile mesenteritis are found upon surgical exploration. Occasionally, a mesenteric or omental tumor, such as a fibroma, lipoma, or neurofibroma may be present.

GENITOURINARY TRACT

Perinephric abscess and renal-cell carcinoma are quite difficult to diagnose (Fig. 19.4). The classic triad of

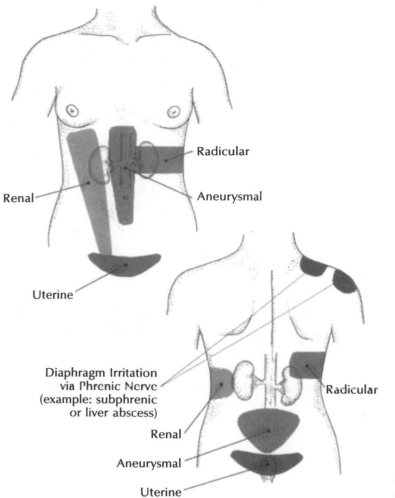

Renal

Radicular

Aneurysmal

Uterine

Diaphragm Irritation
via Phrenic Nerve
(example: subphrenic
or liver abscess)

Radicular

Renal

Aneurysmal

Uterine

FIG. 19.4. Pain patterns of nongastrointestinal abdominal origin.

hematuria, flank pain, and palpable mass is highly suggestive of renal-cell carcinoma, yet it is seen infrequently. Instead, patients often present with a dull sensation of pain in the upper quadrant or flank and with intermittent fever, anemia, and weight loss. Mildly elevated liver function values may distract the investigators unless a urinalysis is done and hematuria is noted. Perinephric abscess, although uncommon, should be considered in a patient with a history of urinary-tract infections or pyelonephritis. Typically, dull upper-quadrant or flank discomfort is present and is accompanied by malaise and low-grade fevers. For patients hospitalized with ureteral colic, this intense pain may respond well to management with epidural analgesia where a dilute solution of local anesthetic is infused into a thoracic epidural catheter.

The pain of pelvic inflammatory disease (PID) usually is acute but may become chronic if the condition is undiagnosed or inadequately treated. In that event, the discomfort is localized to one of the lower quadrants. The pain can be associated with a change in the patient's defecation pattern or with urinary-bladder irritation. Pain

from an expanding ovarian cyst usually is well localized, persistent, and sharp. The crampy pain of endometriosis usually is associated with menses, although its variable location can mimic other complaints if the timing with menses is not appreciated. Chronic PID and ovarian pathology together with regional enteritis and irritable-bowel syndrome should be considered in the differential diagnosis of chronic lower-abdominal pain in a woman of childbearing age.

METABOLIC CAUSES OF PAIN

The three hepatic porphyrias (hereditary coproporphyria, variegate porphyria, and acute intermittent porphyria) have many features in common, mainly recurrent attacks of abdominal pain. The pain probably results from an autonomic neuropathy causing disturbed gastrointestinal motility. Spasm and dilatation may cause severe pain, which is frequently associated with fever and leukocytosis, causing the condition to mimic an inflammatory process. The pain usually is sharp and may be localized or diffuse. On examination, the abdomen is commonly soft and not tender. The attacks may last from days to weeks. Infection, deliberate fasting, and ingestion of barbiturates, anticonvulsants, alcohol, estrogens, or oral contraceptives are known to precipitate events.

Lead poisoning is most frequently encountered in children. Although anemia, neuritis, and encephalopathy complete the picture, a patient may present with only lead colic, or "painter's cramps." Associated with severe migrating, poorly localized, crampy abdominal pain, there may be accompanying guarding and rigidity of the abdominal wall; this may be so dramatic as it may raise the suspicion of an acute intraabdominal event. The lightning-sharp abdominal pain of tabes is mainly associated with syphilis but also may occur with diabetes and meningeal tumors. This is a radicular syndrome, resulting from damage to the large posterior lumbosacral roots. When in a hemolytic crisis, a patient with paroxysmal nocturnal hemoglobinuria may have substernal, lumbar, or abdomen pain in addition to generalized weakness. The pain may be colicky and last for several days. The abdominal may be tender with some guarding and even rebound tenderness on examination.

Hyperparathyroidism has been called the syndrome of "bones, stones, and groans." The abdominal pain usually is from the associated peptic ulcer disease or pancreatitis. The abdominal pain of hyperlipidemia also is generally related to associated pancreatitis.

CONCLUSION

The diagnosis of abdominal pain can often be quite challenging. With an understanding of pain patterns, the history and physical examination will often yield the diagnosis. New technology in MR, CT, and ultrasound, coupled with nerve blocks or laboratory tests can help to further elucidate the etiology of a patient's discomfort. Although the cause of abdominal pain may be obvious, a thorough search and analysis may be warranted to uncover and rule out more obscure painful syndromes. While management varies with diagnosis, a willingness to believe the patient is essential and can be conveyed by the provider's efforts to carefully help the patient communicate the details of the painful condition in terms of intensity, character, timing (onset, duration, pattern), associated aggravating and alleviating factors, location, and radiation.

SELECTED READINGS

Duarte MA. Pressure pain threshold in children with recurrent abdominal pain. *J Pediatr Gastroenterol Nutr* 2000;31:280–285.

Hotopf M. Why do children have chronic abdominal pain, and what happens to them when they grow up? Population based cohort study. *BMJ* 1998;316:1196–1200.

Lee JS. Adverse outcomes and opioid analgesic administration in acute abdominal pain *Acad Emerg Med* 2000;7:980–987.

Lo Vecchio F. The use of analgesics in patients with acute abdominal pain. *J Emerg Med* 1997;15:775–779.

Olden KW. Rational management of chronic abdominal pain. *Compr Ther* 1998;24:180–186.

Silen W. *Cope's Early Diagnosis of the Acute Abdomen.* New York: Oxford University Press, 2000.

CHAPTER 20

Pancreatic Pain

Vijayasree Arvind

Abdominal pain is a major clinical problem in patients suffering from pancreatitis and pancreatic cancer. The pancreas is a retroperitoneal organ lying posterior to the stomach between the spleen and the duodenum.

The autonomic fibers from the celiac plexus innervate the pancreas. Preganglionic fibers from T5 to T10 form greater splanchnic nerve and end in corresponding celiac ganglia. The lesser splanchnic nerve (T10 to T11) and least splanchnic nerve (T11 to T12) also synapse at the celiac ganglia. The celiac ganglia lies anterior to the diaphragmatic crura and anterior and slightly lateral to the aorta. Fibres arise from the preganglionic splanchnic nerves, preganglionic nerves from the vagus, and some sensory fibers from the phrenic and vagus nerves.

The postganglionic fibers arising from the celiac ganglion innervate pancreas and other abdominal organs derived from the embryonic foregut. They accompany the blood vessels supplying these organs.

The nociceptive information from the pancreas is mainly carried by the celiac plexus, which is mostly made of sympathetic fibers with some parasympathetic contribution. The visceral pain transmitted reaches the spinal cord and thalamus and is perceived by the cortex as pain. Pain from pancreas is mainly visceral and is characterized as a deep, dull, epigastric pain, which is poorly localized. The pain also radiates to the upper thoracic and lower lumbar regions in the back in view of the origin of the splanchnic fibers from T5 to T12 segments of the spinal cord. The pancreas also is located so closely to the spinal vertebrae and the lumbar sympathetic fibers that any pathology spreading to this highly innervated region results in great pain and suffering to the patient.

The etiology of pain can be from mechanical or chemical stimuli. Local release of digestive enzymes could result in the loss of the perineural sheath in these small nerve fibers innervating the pancreas. The resultant hypersensitivity to prostaglandins and bradykinin may account for the pain in patients with acute and chronic pancreatitis. Increased intraductal pressures also can cause ischemic pain as a result of decreased blood supply in patients with chronic pancreatitis. Surgical decompression by the way of pancreaticojejunostomy or other decompression procedures could help alleviate the pain in these patients.

Repeated peripheral nociceptive input results in widening of receptive area with decreased thresholds, increased sensitivity, and prolonged firing of the peripheral nerves, which in turn then results in central sensitization at the level of the spinal cord. Hence, early aggressive treatment of pain becomes very important in patients suffering from recurrent attacks of pancreatitis.

ACUTE PANCREATITIS

The causes of acute pancreatitis can be multiple. Chronic alcohol abuse can lead to repeated attacks of acute pancreatitis. The other causes include hypercalcemia, gallstones, and certain drugs such as furosemide, azathioprine, and steroids. But alcoholism remains the most common cause.

Clinical symptoms include severe epigastric pain radiating to the back, with nausea, vomiting, and fever. It can be associated with severe adult respiratory-distress syndrome (ARDS) and septicemia. Serum amylase is elevated in 90% of the patients and computed tomography (CT) scan of the abdomen confirms the diagnosis.

Treatment includes stopping all oral intake. Patients will need intravenous fluids not only to replace insensible loss, but also to account for tremendous third-space loss of fluids. Trypsin inhibitors, anticholinergics, and H2 blockers can be used to reduce the secretions of the pancreas. Continuous epidural analgesia and celiac-plexus block with local anesthetic and steroid should be also be considered for adequate pain relief.

The above might help provide better pain relief without systemic side effects associated with the use of opioid patient-controlled analgesia. Repeated celiac-plexus block with local anesthetic and steroid done every day seems to reduce morbidity and mortality associated with an acute attack of pancreatitis in some patients.

CHRONIC PANCREATITIS

Alcoholism is the most common cause of chronic pancreatitis. Other rare causes include biliary stones. The most common clinical finding in chronic pancreatitis is dull, boring, epigastric pain that radiates to the back. It also is accompanied by exocrine insufficiency of the pancreatic enzymes, which lead to chronic malnutrition, steatorrhea, weight loss. The endocrine insufficiency of chronic pancreatitis manifests as glucose intolerance or overt diabetes mellitus.

Pancreatic calcification observed by routine abdominal x-ray or chronic fibrosis with intraductal dilation observed in CT of the abdomen is diagnostic. The enzymes of pancreatic origin are not elevated in the chronic pancreatitis.

Conservative treatment includes long-acting opioids, tricyclic antidepressants (TCA) or perhaps a selective serotonin reuptake inhibitor (SSRI). Physical dependence to opioids is a real problem in these patients who usually have repeated attacks of abdominal pain. It is advisable to initiate the opioid treatment after careful psychological evaluation, and after informing the patient of the addictive nature of the opioid drugs. Some practitioners advise the use of only long-acting opioids as opposed to short-acting opioids. The long-acting opioids achieve more steady levels of drug in the blood and avoids the peaks and troughs observed with the short-acting opioids. Anticholinergics, cimetidine, and pancreatic enzyme therapy all reflexly inhibits secretions and alleviates pain from ductal dilatation.

Invasive therapy could include neurolytic celiac-plexus block though the risk probably outweighs the benefits in treating nonmalignant pancreatic pain. Because the central sensitization of the spinal cord results from repeated afferent nociceptive input, long-term benefit could be achieved by placing a catheter near the celiac plexus, thus avoiding the creation of a neuropathic pain syndrome. Local anesthetic infusion of bupivacaine continuously through the catheter can give prolonged pain relief and perhaps limit the likelihood of central sensitization.

The other modalities of treatment include the epidural catheter placement and intrathecal opioid pump.

PANCREATIC CANCER

Pancreatic adenocarcinoma is a rapidly lethal disease where 90% of the patients are dead within 1 year of diagnoses. Poorly controlled pain leading to major depression and poor quality of life is prevalent in more than one half of the patients. Hence, to effectively tackle the challenge of providing adequate pain relief, the pain specialists should integrate early conservative and interventional therapies.

Pain is one of the early presenting symptoms in patients with pancreatic cancer. Obstructive jaundice also is present in patients with carcinoma of the head of the pancreas. The pain is present in the epigastric region, and can radiate to the back. In addition, the patient also feels back pain in lower-thoracic and lumbar segments. The close proximity of the celiac plexus and other rich aortic renal plexus of nerves to the pancreas results in very severe pain early on in the disease.

Diagnosis is made by CT scan, endoscopic retrograde cholangiopancreatogram, or percutaneous biopsy. Most of the patients undergo laparotomy either for curative or palliative surgery. Radiation and chemotherapy have very little role in providing palliation.

Analgesic regimen for mild-to-moderate pain could include a nonsteroidal antiinflammatory drug (NSAID), and chronic opioid therapy may be warranted. Though the NSAID does not help with the visceral pain, it may help with somatic abdominal-wall pain or bone pain resulting from vertebral spread. It should not be used as sole analgesic in patients with severe pain.

The opioid analgesic chosen should be a long-acting opioid with round-the-clock pain relief and short-acting opioids for break-through pain only. The disease warrants a liberal use of opioids early on without undue concern about habituation or physical dependence. A clonidine patch can be used along with the opioids to help slow the development of tolerance and improve efficacy.

Because depression also plays a major role early on in the disease, starting the patients on tricyclic antidepressants or SSRI is very well warranted. The sedative effect of TCAs such as amitriptyline can be best utilized to ensure adequate sleep in these patients. The patients should be closely monitored for adverse effects of these drugs including postural hypotension, xerostomia, urinary retention, and occasional cardiovascular arrhythmias.

Anxiety should be treated with benzodiazepine along with other above-mentioned drugs. Combination therapy of the above drugs should be tailored to the clinical picture in each individual patient.

CELIAC PLEXUS BLOCK

Celiac plexus block with local anesthetic should be done initially to evaluate the degree of pain relief in patients suffering from pancreatic cancer. This could be followed by neurolytic block with alcohol or phenol if more than 50% pain relief was obtained with the local anesthetic block.

It is contraindicated in patients who suffer from coagulopathy, sepsis, or local intraabdominal infections. It could be technically difficult or impossible to perform in patients where the malignancy or lymphadenopathy severely distorts the anatomy in the vicinity of celiac ganglia.

Posterior Approaches to the Celiac Plexus

Classic retrocrural technique is most commonly used. After careful hydration, two 22G needles are inserted about 8 cm from the midline, just beneath the 12th ribs, as shown in Figure 20.1.

The needles are advanced to contact the body of the L1 vertebral body by directing them 45 degrees medially and 15 degrees cephalad. Once the depth is noticed, the needle is withdrawn and redirected to lie anterior to the L1 vertebral body. The left needle is positioned just posterior to the aorta and the right needle is positioned anterolateral to the aorta. Initial dye confirmation should show spread confined to the anterior aspect of the L1 body around the aorta. Care must be taken to prevent posterior spread of local anesthetics or neurolytics to prevent involvement of somatic nerve roots. Initial confirmation of the block can be done by giving 1% lidocaine or Marcaine, and 80 mg of methylprednisolone can be added for treating patients with pancreatitis. Fluoroscopic or CT-guided placements are recommended for neurolytic blocks.

Transcrural technique using fluoroscopic and CT guidance is advocated by some, where the needles are advanced further anteriorly thus allowing smaller volumes to be used with improved efficacy.

Transaortic technique is done by using a single, 22G needle, which under fluoroscopic or CT guidance, is directed anterolateral to the L1 vertebral body on the left side only. The needle is carefully advanced through the posterior wall of the aorta, through the lumen, and then through the anterior walls of the aorta to directly lie close to the celiac plexus. Dye confirmation should be done to show anterior midline and preaortic location of the needle. Again, a careful aspiration and slow injection of the local anesthetic or neurolytic agent is done.

The major disadvantage of using a posterior approach is that the prone position might be very uncomfortable for patients with severe abdominal pain. Lateral approach also can be used in patients who are unable to tolerate a prone position in spite of sedation. There is also increased risk of posterior spread of neurolytic agents, which result in severe, sensory nerve-root involvement. The risk of epidural or subarachnoid spread also exists. The posterior approach also tends to be more uncomfortable, requiring more sedation because the needle traverses the paraspinous muscles.

Anterior Approach to Celiac-Plexus Block

Anterior abdominal approach to the celiac plexus can be used in patients who are unable to remain prone for

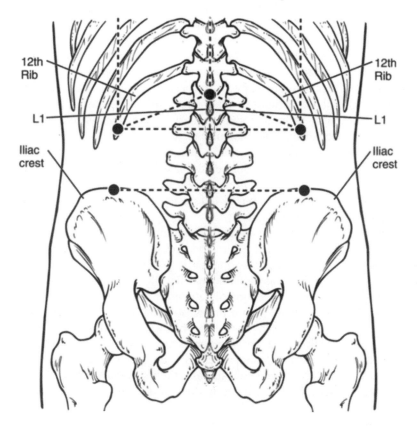

FIG. 20.1. Landmarks for celiac-plexus block.

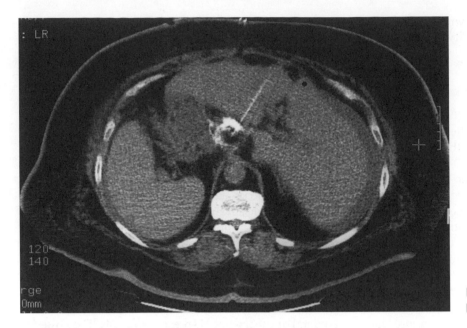

Fig. 20.2. Anterior approach to celiac-plexus block.

prolonged periods of time. It also avoids the possibility of local anesthetic or neurolytic spread in the retrocrural space and involvement of the nerve roots. A 22G needle is advanced 1.5 cm below and lateral to the xiphoid process. A CT-guided or ultrasound-guided approach is used to advance the needle through liver, stomach, and intestine to ultimately lie anterior to the aorta as shown in Figure 20.2.

Again, after dye confirmation of the preaortic location of the needle, the local anesthetic is injected first, followed by 6% phenol or 50% alcohol.

The major disadvantage of using an anterior approach includes increased risk of infection, hemorrhage, abscess, or fistula formation. The use of CT guidance and the use of very fine needles to perform this block have greatly reduced the incidence of these complications.

CATHETER TECHNIQUES

There have been reports of periaortic catheter placement in patients with chronic pancreatitis. Local anesthetic infusion was performed through the catheter continuously. A CT-guided approach to the catheter placement provides good, accurate placement. Intraoperative placement of the catheter also has been tried successfully. The catheter techniques hold great promise to treat patients with chronic pancreatitis and recurrent acute flare up leading to severe abdominal pain and repeated hospital admissions for pain control.

Most common complications of celiac-plexus block include hypotension and increased gastrointestinal motility. Hypotension is a result of splanchnic vasodi-

latation. This can be treated effectively by prehydrating the patient and also by careful monitoring of blood pressure to rule out orthostatic hypotension before the patient is allowed to assume a standing posture. The increased gastrointestinal motility in these patients could potentially be a blessing and might regulate the bowel habits in these patients who tend to be constipated as a result of opioids, but severe diarrhea has occasionally been observed. This is a result of unopposed parasympathetic activity.

The incidence of epidural and subarachnoid puncture is extremely rare, and is even reduced more by using fluoroscopy. Retrocrural techniques, though performed using fluoroscopy, can occasionally still lead to neurolytic agents spreading posteriorly and causing involvement of lumbar somatic nerve roots. This is reduced by performing a transcrural technique.

Accidental vascular injury can lead to retroperitoneal hematoma or rarely epidural hematoma. Careful aspiration to rule out intravascular or subarachnoid placement of needle is advised before injecting local anesthetic or neurolytic agents.

Rarely, pneumothorax or renal injury also can result. Careful aseptic technique should prevent fistula formation or abscess formation in patients who have anterior celiac-plexus block done.

Careful selection of patients and repeated confirmation of adequate pain relief with local anesthetic would prevent a failed neurolytic block. Though celiac-plexus block with neurolytic agents also has been done for various nonmalignant diseases such as chronic pancreatitis and ischemic bowel disease, the risks and benefits should be carefully weighed in these situations.

INTRAOPERATIVE CHEMICAL SPLANCHNICECTOMY

Intraoperative chemical splanchnicectomy can be performed during the time of laparotomy in patients with pancreatic cancer. The retroperitoneal covering is left intact over the celiac axis so that the neurolytic agent is contained in the space. Accurate volume and placement of the needle obtain good results. Though direct transection of splanchnic nerves and celiac ganglia has been tried, the results are no more gratifying than a chemical splanchnicectomy. Direct placement of neurolytic agents during laparotomy saves these patients from undergoing an additional procedure.

Transthoracic Splanchnicectomy

A thoracoscopic approach to transect greater splanchnic nerves bilaterally has greatly reduced morbidity and improved or obtained total pain relief in more than 75% of the patients in some studies.

Case Report

A 68-year-old man was referred to our chronic pain management service for evaluation and treatment of abdominal pain. The patient was diagnosed to have gastric cancer and had undergone palliative surgery. He was experiencing chronic epigastric pain radiating to the back. He had been tried on combination of long-acting opioids, NSAIDs, and TCAs without adequate pain relief. He was experiencing severe drowsiness and constipation as a result of the opioids with poor pain relief.

A thorough physical examination revealed a malnourished gentleman who was drowsy. He also appeared to be in great pain with a VAS score of 7 out of 10. His vital signs were stable. His clotting studies were performed including prothrombin time, partial thromboplastin time, and platelet count, which all were within normal limits. CT of the abdomen was discussed with the radiologist to assure that the anatomic configuration of the celiac-plexus area was not distorted tremendously either from the disease or lymph adenopathy.

After a detailed discussion with patient and his primary-care physician, a decision was made to do a diagnostic celiac-plexus block in the pain clinic. The patient was kept NPO overnight and good prehydration was done in the clinic. Mild anxiolytic and opiate was given to enable the patient to tolerate prone position and the procedure.

Under fluoroscopic guidance, two needles were placed 8 cm from the midline just below the border of the 12th rib. They were advanced until they lay just anterior to the body of the L1 vertebral body. The left needle is positioned just posterior to the aorta, and the right needle is positioned just anterolateral to the abdominal aorta. Dye spread should be observed to prevent posterior spread of the local anesthetic and to confirm retroperitoneal placement of the needle.

After careful aspiration, 15 cc of 0.5% bupivacaine was injected through each needle. The patient was turned supine and the vital signs were closely watched to avoid sudden precipitous drop in the blood pressure. The patient got 75% pain relief within the next 30 minutes and this continued for the next 6 hours.

After detailed discussion with the patient and his primary-care physician, the patient was brought the next day to the radiology suite. A CT-guided, left-sided, celiac-plexus block was performed using 20 cc of 50% alcohol. This again was done after dye confirmation of periaortic spread of the dye and careful negative aspiration. An initial local anesthetic block was done with 1% lidocaine because injection of alcohol for neurolytic block is very painful. Liberal use of sedative and analgesics such as fentanyl also is advisable.

The patient once again was monitored carefully for hypotension, epidural, or subarachnoid block and for pain relief. The patient obtained 80% pain relief and needed very little opiate analgesia for the rest of his life span. His mental status improved significantly and the patient also enjoyed better pain control than he did before with just systemic opioids.

CONCLUSION

Treatment of pain in acute and chronic pancreatitis is a major challenge. Given the history of alcoholism in most of these patients and tendency towards drug dependence, careful psychological evaluation and close monitoring should be done if these patients are prescribed chronic-opioid therapy. Alternate medical regimen including NSAIDs, and psychotropic drugs also should be tried. Interventional procedures such celiac-plexus block with local anesthetic and steroid improves pain relief in these patients. Neurolytic celiac-plexus block usually is reserved for malignant abdominal-pain syndromes. Implantable epidural or subarachnoid pumps has been tried with variable results in this patient population.

Pain in pancreatic cancer is a major clinical problem faced by pain-specialist physicians. Because the life span is very short in these patients, liberal use of long-acting opioids along with TCA and anxiolytic agents should be tried. Early, aggressive treatments including neurolytic celiac-plexus blocks along with medical management is warranted to ensure good quality of life in these very unfortunate patients. Consideration also should be given to doing either chemical ganglionectomy or thoracoscopic splanchnicectomy if above-mentioned procedures fail to obtain good results.

SELECTED READINGS

Matamala AM, Sanchez JL, Lopez FV. Percutaneous anterior and posterior approach to the celiac plexus: a comparative study using four different techniques. *Pain Clinic* 1992;5:21–28.

Raj PP. Autonomic nerve blocks. In: Raj PP, ed. *Pain Medicine. A comprehensive review*. St. Louis: Mosby, 1996:237–246.

Waldman SD. Avoiding complications when performing celiac plexus block. *Pain Clinic* 1993;6:62–63.

Waldman SD, Winnie AP. Celiac plexus and splanchnic nerve block. In: Waldman SD. *Interventional Pain Management*. Philadelphia: WB Saunders, 1996:360–372.

Wong GY, Sakorafas GH, Tsiotos GG, et al. Palliation of pain in chronic pancreatitis. *Surg Clin North Am* 1999;79:4.

CHAPTER 21

Interstitial Cystitis and Urologic Pain

Jong M. Choe, Benjamin S. Battino, and David R. Staskin

INTERSTITIAL CYSTITIS

Interstitial cystitis (IC) is one of three painful disease complexes of the lower urinary tract. Others include urethral syndrome (US) and pelvic pain syndrome (PPS). It is important to note that these entities are diagnoses of exclusion. Symptom complex of IC, US, and PPS often overlap, making an accurate diagnosis difficult. Urine cultures typically are negative. Methodical evaluation coupled with appropriate diagnostic tests remain the cornerstone of diagnosis and therapy.

Patients with urethral syndrome experience urinary frequency, urgency, and dysuria. Suprapubic pain typically is absent. Patients with IC and PPS have suprapubic pain associated with irritative voiding symptoms. Women with PPS experience suprapubic pain radiating to back and lower extremities that is unrelated to bladder volume.

Typical patients with interstitial cystitis present with suprapubic pain, urinary frequency, urgency, and nocturia. Dyspareunia also may be present. The degree of suprapubic pain is proportional to the bladder volume. Patients report exacerbation of pain with bladder filling and relief of pain upon voiding. Symptoms not associated with IC include urge incontinence or suprapubic pain that becomes worse with voiding. Patients with IC do not have symptoms of dysuria, fever, or menstrual difficulties. Quality of life for an affected patient is worse than being on chronic hemodialysis. Interestingly, the National Institutes of Health (NIH) only requires two symptoms (suprapubic pain and urgency) to meet the criteria for IC.

Epidemiology

IC most often occurs in women. Although IC can occur in men, it is rare. Approximately 90% of patients with IC are women. Middle-aged Jewish women are most commonly affected. Peak incidence of IC occurs during 30 to 40 years of age. Women with IC are ten to 12 times more likely to have a history of childhood bladder problems.

Average onset of symptoms to diagnosis of IC is 2 to 4 years. Stabilization of symptoms during the early phase of the disease is typical, and late deterioration is unusual. Approximately 50% of these cases undergo spontaneous remission. However, 10% of these cases may progress to cause worsening symptoms.

Etiology

The cause of IC is unknown and several theories have been proposed. One theory is insufficient glycosaminoglycan (GAG) layer lining the bladder mucosa. The GAG layer is a heparinlike substance that has a protective mechanism for the bladder wall. When this protective layer is damaged, urine can diffuse across the mucosa and into the bladder wall to produce symptoms of IC. Toxic-urine theory holds that toxins in the urine produce IC symptoms. Autoimmune theory supposes IC is the result of autoimmune-collagen dysfunction. Some investigators propose that the release of neurotransmitters by mast cells within the bladder wall result in IC, while others feel that release of neuropeptides from C fibers causes bladder inflammation to cause symptoms of IC. Whatever the cause, the end result is a small-capacity bladder with a fibrotic wall that produces pelvic or suprapubic pain with bladder distention.

Diagnosis

The cornerstone of diagnosing IC remains a good history and physical examination. Supplemental tests are helpful but not necessarily diagnostic. Medical history consistent with IC include urinary frequency, urgency, and nocturia. Time to diagnosis from onset of symptoms is usually more than 9 months. Affected patients often complain of having to urinate more than eight times per day. Suprapubic pain and sense of urgency relieved during or after voiding is characteristic of IC. Dyspareunia during sexual relations is a common complaint.

Findings not associated with IC include urinary frequency that occurs less than eight times per day during waking hours. If voiding symptoms are relieved by antibiotics or if the duration of symptoms is less than 9 months, the diagnosis of IC is questionable.

During the physical evaluation, it is critical to perform a detailed bimanual examination to rule out gynecological disorders such as cervicitis, labial/vaginal wall disorders, uterine fibroids, endometriosis, ovarian cysts, Mittelschmerz, or pelvic-inflammatory disease. A focused neurological exam such as bulbocavernosus reflex, anal wink, rectal tone, deep-tendon reflexes, and sensory-motor assessment is an important part of the physical examination.

A voiding log is a valuable adjunct to history and physical. It is an important record of the patient's voiding habits. The voiding log allows both patient and physician to objectively evaluate the severity of voiding dysfunction.

Laboratory Tests

Routine lab tests such as urinalysis and urine culture should be part of the basic evaluation of any patient with voiding dysfunction. Urinary-tract infection is a simple problem that is easy to treat but sometimes is overlooked. Symptoms of IC mimic those of urinary-tract infection or bladder tumor (carcinoma–in-situ). It is critical to send urine cytology as part of the basic evaluation to rule out bladder carcinoma.

Specific Tests

Intravesical Potassium Chloride Test

In the past, the intravesical potassium chloride (KCl) test was felt to be a diagnostic test for IC. In this test, KCl is directly instilled into the bladder, and the diagnosis of IC is made if the patient experienced pain. However, due to the lack of sensitivity and specificity, the routine use of this test is controversial.

Urodynamics

Urodynamic studies such as uroflow, postvoid residual urine, and filling cystometrogram are not diagnostic for IC. However, these tests offer information regarding bladder capacity, compliance, motor instability, and sensory urgency. Findings not associated with IC are bladder capacity greater than 350 mL or presence of phasic contractions. When the bladder is filled at a medium fill rate (30 to 100 cc/minute), patients with IC experience intense urgency at 150 mL bladder capacity. Absence of intense urgency at this capacity is not consistent with IC.

Cystoscopy Under Anesthesia

Because bladder tumor is in the differential diagnosis of irritative voiding symptoms and bladder pain, cystoscopy is an important part of urologic work-up. During cystoscopy, bladder washings should be sent and bladder biopsies should be performed to rule out carcinoma–in-situ. Mast cells often are found on bladder biopsy but are not diagnostic of IC.

Presence of Hunner's ulcer has been reported to be pathognomonic for IC, but these lesions are seen rarely. NIH criteria for making the diagnosis of IC is by distending the bladder under general anesthesia (bladder hydrodistention). During bladder hydrodistention, the bladder is filled to capacity at a pressure of 80 to 100 cm H_2O. Bladder capacity less than 300 to 400 cc at 100 cm H_2O is indicative of severe IC. Patients with IC typically have terminal hematuria and exhibit glomerulations after hydrodistention. NIH has decreed that the presence of glomerulations after hydrodistention is indicative of IC.

Management of Interstitial Cystitis

Management of IC ranges widely from dietary modification to surgical extirpation. Treatment is tailored to each individual, as the degree of suffering and the impact on quality of life varies from person to person. This must be taken into account when making treatment recommendations.

A dietary modification involves eliminating or decreasing the amount of bladder stimulants consumed. Bladder stimulants that exacerbate symptoms of IC include alcohol, smoking, caffeine, carbonated beverages, acidic juices, spicy foods, and excessive fluid intake.

Oral medications used to treat IC include pentosan polysulfate sodium, amitriptyline hydrochloride, hydroxyzine hydrochloride, and nifedipine.

Hydrodistention involves stretching the urinary bladder under anesthesia with intravesical pressure of 80 to 100 cm H_2O for 10 minutes. Hydrodistention renders 30% of patients symptom-free for 3 to 6 months. Often, hydrodistention must be repeated because of recurrence of symptoms.

Intravesical treatments involve instilling drugs into the bladder and allowing local absorption to take effect. The drugs used include dimethylsulfoxide (DMSO), $AgNO_3$, heparin, DMSO cocktail, and chlorpactin. DMSO is placed in the bladder once a week for 6 weeks followed by monthly maintenance doses. $AgNO_3$ (silver nitrate) is instilled into the bladder once a week for 6 weeks with monthly maintenance dose. Heparin [10,000 units in 10 to 20 mL normal saline (NS)] is self administered every other day for 8 to 10 weeks. DMSO cocktail is a combination of DMSO (50 cc), heparin (5,000 to 10,000 units), triamcinolone (10 mg), and bicarbonate (44 mg). DMSO cocktail is administered once a week for 6 to 8 weeks followed by a monthly maintenance dose. Chlorpactin is instilled in the bladder when the patient is symptomatic and maintenance therapy is not required. The subjective response/cure rate for intravesical therapy ranges 30% to 60% and relapses are common.

Alternative therapies include the use of transcutaneous-electrical nerve stimulation, biofeedback, and acupuncture. There has been anecdotal reports that sacral-nerve modulators (InterStim, Medtronics, Minneapolis, MN, U.S.A.) appear to have a promising role for treatment for IC. There are no prospective, randomized studies at this time however, preliminary data appear encouraging.

Surgical management of IC includes transurethral resection of Hunner's ulcer, augmentation cystoplasty, and total cystectomy. If Hunner's ulcer is present, the lesion may be resected to improve voiding symptoms. As discussed above, Hunner's ulcers are rare. Patients who have failed maximal medical therapy are candidates for augmentation cystoplasty. Most investigators recommend supratrigonal cystectomy with augmentation. When augmentation cystoplasty is contemplated, indication for surgery must be strictly defined. For example, the bladder capacity under anesthesia must be less than 300 cc at 100 cm H_2O and the patient should have complete, albeit transient, relief of suprapubic pain with voiding. Cystectomy is only mentioned to be condemned. It is important to realize that cystectomy is not a permanent cure for IC and symptoms of IC have been noted to recur after cystectomy.

UROLOGIC PAIN

Patients with chronic urologic pain often are difficult to treat. In many cases, the diagnosis is elusive and specific therapies are difficult to apply. Often, the patients are frustrated and angry, making medical intervention difficult. However, systematic and methodical evaluation with empathic attitude will lead to an accurate diagnosis and effective intervention.

Neuroanatomy

The somatic nerve supply to the genital area arises from L1–L2 and S2–S4 nerves. The parasympathetic nerves arrive from the sacral segments S2–S4 and the sympathetic nerves from T10–L2 segments. The cutaneous innervation of the inguinal region is served by the ilioinguinal and the iliohypogastric nerves (L1–L2). The anatomy of these nerves is shown in (Figs. 21.1 and 21.2). The iliohypogastric nerve provides sensation to the suprapubic region; the ilioinguinal nerve provides sensory innervation to the skin over the inguinal ligament, base of the scrotum, and labia majora.

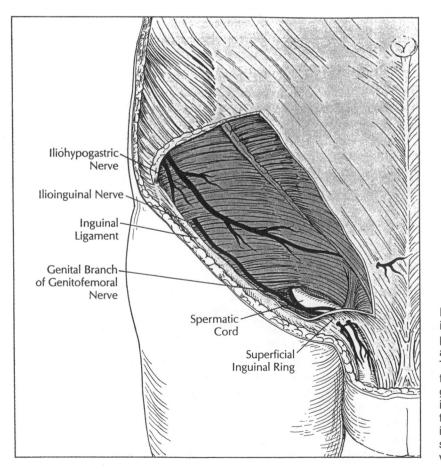

FIG. 21.1. The skin over the inguinal region is served by three nerves from the lumbar plexus: the iliohypogastric, the ilioinguinal, and the genital branch of the genitofemoral. The iliohypogastric nerve provides sensation to the suprapubic region. The ilioinguinal nerve supplies the skin over the inguinal ligament and possibly also part of the base of the scrotum (or labia). The genital branch of the genitofemoral nerve serves the lateral part of the scrotum (or vulva).

Iliohypogastric Nerve

Ilioinguinal Nerve

Inguinal Ligament

Genital Branch of Genitofemoral Nerve

Spermatic Cord

Superficial Inguinal Ring

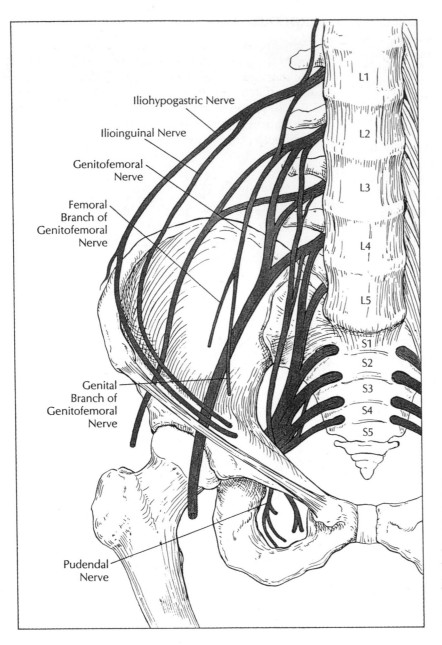

Iliohypogastric Nerve

Ilioinguinal Nerve

Genitofemoral Nerve

Femoral Branch of Genitofemoral Nerve

Genital Branch of Genitofemoral Nerve

Pudendal Nerve

FIG. 21.2. Somatic nerve supply to the genital region comes predominantly from the lumbar (*L1–L2*) and sacral (*S2–S4*) vertebrae. In general, the parasympathetic nerves arrive from the sacral segments, whereas the sympathetic nerves arrive from the lumbar segments (as well as from more distant thoracic segments, not shown here). The end branches of the pudendal nerve (S2–S4) supply the skin of the penis (or the lower part of the vagina).

The penile skin is innervated by the dorsal nerve of the penis [end branches of the pudendal nerve (S2–S4)]. The perineum and anal sphincters derive their nerve supply from the inferior rectal and perineal nerves (branches of the pudendal nerve).

The afferent nerve supply of the upper vagina and cervix is via the pelvic splanchnic (parasympathetic) nerves (S2–S4), but the lowest part of the vagina is supplied by the pudendal nerve.

The testes are supplied by sympathetic nerves from T10–T12; the vas and epididymis are supplied by sympathetic fibers from T10–L1; and the cremaster, cord structures, and tunica vaginalis are supplied by somatic fibers from L1–L2 (genital branch of the genitofemoral nerve). Essentially, the whole of the skin of the scrotum (not just

the posterior aspect) is innervated by S2–S3 (posterior scrotal nerves).

Kidneys

Kidney stones produce renal colic when they obstruct the urinary-tract system. Typical symptoms include flank pain that radiates to the abdomen or to the genital area. Hematuria, nausea, and vomiting are commonly associated symptoms. Patients with kidney stones have a difficult time being comfortable in any one position and often are restless. The most common stone type is calcium oxalate. Other stone types include struvite, calcium phosphate, uric acid, and cystine. The diagnosis of kidney stone is made by intravenous pyelogram (IVP) or computed tomography (CT). The treatment is medical or surgical or both, in combination.

Renal carcinoma or angiomyolipoma can produce flank pain when an acute bleeding episode occurs. The triad of symptoms (flank pain, mass, and hematuria) usually ascribed to renal carcinoma occurs in less than 10% of patients with renal carcinoma. Hematuria or flank pain are by far more commonly isolated symptoms. The diagnosis of renal carcinoma is suspected by CT and confirmed by radical nephrectomy. Angiomyolipoma is a benign renal mass composed of blood vessels, muscle, and fat. Because of preponderance of angiogenesis, angiomyolipoma has a tendency for spontaneous bleeding and resultant flank pain. The diagnosis of angiomyolipoma is made by CT and confirmed by surgery. Because of the nonmalignant nature of this disease, nephron-sparing surgery is advocated.

Infections of the kidney such as pyelonephritis, renal–cortical abscess, perinephric abscess, and xanthogranulomatous pyelonephritis present with varying degrees of flank pain, fever, and urinary-tract infection. Pyelonephritis is a complication of bacterial cystitis that has ascended to the renal parenchyma. Treatment is intravenous antibiotics. Renal–cortical abscess develops as a result of hematogenous spread of *Staphylococcus aureus* from a distant site. Patients present with chills, fever, and flank tenderness. The radiologic study of choice is CT. Treatment is intravenous antibiotics in combination with percutaneous or open surgical drainage. Perinephric abscess is contiguous extension of intrarenal abscess into the perirenal space. The diagnosis is made by CT. Treatment is intravenous antibiotics in combination with percutaneous drainage. If percutaneous drainage is unsuccessful, prompt, open drainage or nephrectomy is warranted. Xanthogranulomatous pyelonephritis is an unusual form of chronic bacterial infection often associated with a staghorn calculus. The most common offending bacteria is *Proteus mirabilis*. The diagnosis is made by CT, and surgical extirpation is the mainstay of therapy.

Ureters

Diseases of the ureter produce flank pain when the ureters become obstructed. Obstructing lesions unique to the ureter include stones, tumors, blood clots, sloughed papilla, infection, congenital obstruction, ureteral trauma, and retroperitoneal fibrosis.

Obstructing stones in the ureter cause pain in the flank referred to the genital area because the distention of the ureter stimulates the pain fibers specific to those areas. In addition, nausea and vomiting ensue as a result of stimulation of visceral splanchnic nerves. Stones localized to the ureter have greater than 90% probability of passing spontaneously if the stone is less than 4 mm in diameter. The likelihood of stone passage decreases with an increase in stone size and the proximal location of the stone. The diagnosis is made by IVP or CT. The treatment is medical or surgical.

Presence of transitional-cell carcinoma of the ureter or the renal pelvis can cause ureteral obstruction, hydronephrosis, and flank pain. The diagnosis is made by IVP or CT in combination with tissue biopsy or ureteral cytology. The gold standard treatment is nephroureterectomy with excision of bladder cuff.

Bloods clots obstructing the ureter must be suspected in those patients with a history of bleeding diathesis or clotting disorder. Blood clot obstructing the ureter is a diagnosis of exclusion. If the patient is asymptomatic, no treatment is necessary as the blood clot will spontaneously dissolve.

Sloughed papilla from the kidney can produce ureteral obstruction in patients with pyelonephritis, obstructive nephropathy, sickle cell disease, tuberculosis, cirrhosis of the liver, analgesic nephropathy, renal-tubular necrosis, and diabetes mellitus (POSTCARD). The diagnosis usually is made by IVP. Bacterial infections are treated promptly with appropriate antibiotics. Obstructing symptoms are relieved by placement of an indwelling ureteral stent.

Infection such as tuberculosis can cause stricture and scars anywhere along the urinary tract. Most commonly, distal–ureteral strictures occur. Obstruction of the ureter produces renal colic. The diagnosis is made by IVP and urine cultures specific for acid-fast bacilli. Management of tuberculosis-induced strictures include antituberculosis medication [isoniazad (isonicotinic acid hydrazide, or INH), rifampin, pyrazinamide], balloon dilation, or the ureter, steroids, or ureteral reconstruction.

Congenital entities that can cause ureteral obstruction include fibroepithelial polyp of the ureter and ureteropelvic junction obstruction (UPJO). Fibroepithelial polyp is a benign tumor of the ureter that can produce obstructing symptoms. The diagnosis is suspected on IVP or CT and confirmed at surgery. The treatment of choice is ureteral excision and primary spatulated anastomosis.

Congenital UPJO usually is a childhood disease. In the adult population, UPJO commonly has a secondary cause such as a crossing vessel. Regardless of the underlying cause, affected patients complain of renal colic especially after imbibing large quantities of fluid or drinking alcohol. UPJO has characteristic radiographic findings on IVP but nuclear renal scan is diagnostic. The treatment for UPJO include Anderson–Hynes dismembered pyeloplasty or antegrade or retrograde endopyelotomy.

Ureteral trauma after ureteroscopy or ureteral manipulation may result in ureteral obstruction causing renal colic. When this occurs, a percutaneous nephrostomy tube should be placed to decompress the obstructing urinary system. Although retrograde stent placement may be attempted, it is difficult to do after a ureteral trauma has occurred.

Retroperitoneal fibrosis (Ormond's disease) is also known as idiopathic retroperitoneal fibrosis. Fibrosis or scarring of the retroperitoneum envelops and draws both ureters in medially to the great vessels. This results in bilateral ureteral obstruction and chronic flank pain. Identifiable risk factors for retroperitoneal fibrosis include drugs such as methysergide, inflammatory disorders such as aortic aneurysm, and tumors such as retroperitoneal carcinoma. However, the underlying cause is unknown for the majority of patients with retroperitoneal fibrosis hence, idiopathic retroperitoneal fibrosis. For symptomatic patients, a temporizing measure is placement of internal stents or percutaneous nephrostomy tubes. The diagnosis is made by deep biopsy of the retroperitoneal mass. The definitive treatment is ureterolysis and intraperitonealization with omental wrapping of both ureters.

Bladder

Diseases of the urinary bladder that cause bladder pain include bladder-outlet obstruction, bacterial cystitis, bladder tumor, and IC. Bladder-outlet obstruction may occur in the setting of benign prostatic hyperplasia, urethral tumor, or after antiincontinence surgery. Acute urinary retention secondary to bladder-outlet obstruction results in overdistension of the detrusor muscle and activation of pain fibers. The diagnosis is made by assessing for post-void urine volume. Bladder infection causes symptoms of urinary frequency, urgency, urge incontinence, hematuria, and dysuria. The diagnosis is made by urine culture. Carcinoma–in-situ of the bladder also presents with irritative voiding symptoms and pain on urination. The diagnosis is made by urine cytology, cystoscopy, and bladder biopsy.

Prostate

Three major diseases of the prostate that produce perineal pain include inflammation, cancer, and prostadynia. Inflammation and infection of the prostate can be lumped under the heading of prostatitis. Prostatitis is defined as inflammation of the prostate. Symptoms of prostatitis include urinary frequency, urgency, hematospermia, terminal hematuria, perineal pain, and pain with urination or defecation. Prostatitis is subdivided into bacterial and nonbacterial prostatitis. Nonbacterial prostatitis is the most common form of prostatitis. The specific pathogen for nonbacterial prostatitis is unknown, but *Ureaplasma* and *Mycoplasma* have been implicated. *Escherichia coli* is the most common pathogen causing bacterial prostatitis. Patients with acute bacterial prostatitis typically present with fever, obstructive voiding symptoms, and perineal pain. Often they appear septic and urine cultures always are positive. In the setting of acute bacterial prostatitis, coexisting urinary retention must be ruled out. Chronic bacterial prostatitis present with symptoms that are more nagging in nature. Patients with chronic-bacter-

ial prostatitis have been noted to have prostatic calcifications. Harbinger of bacteria within the prostatic calculi have been theorized to be a risk factor for chronic-bacterial prostatitis. Afflicted patients complain of perineal pain and discomfort associated with irritative and obstructive voiding dysfunction. The mainstay of treatment involves antibiotics (sulfa derivative or quinolone), nonsteroidal antiinflammatory drugs (NSAIDs), and sitz baths. Generally, 6 to 12 weeks of antibiotics are indicated and relapses are common. Localized prostate cancer typically does not produce clinical symptoms. Prostate cancer is screened by a combination of prostate-specific antigen (PSA) and prostate examination. Invasion of pelvic organs or metastasis to bone may cause perineal pain, dysuria, and pelvic pain. Metastasis to other parts of skeleton will manifest bone pain specific to the area of involvement. When the spinal column is involved, one must be wary of impending spinal-cord compression as neurologic function may become compromised. Prostadynia is a diagnosis of exclusion. Clinical symptoms mimic those of chronic prostatitis; however, urinary leukocytosis is characteristically absent. Affected patients are often young men with a stressful personality. The mainstay of therapy involves α blockers and Sitz baths.

Urethra

Pain arising from the urethra may be attributed to urethritis, tumor, diverticulum, and stricture. Symptoms resulting from urethritis often are nonspecific and mimic urinary-tract infection. Urethritis from sexually transmitted disease include gonorrhea, syphilis, and chlamydia. Sexually transmitted urethritis often produces characteristic urethral discharge. Urethral tumor presents with obstructive voiding symptoms, hematuria, and dysuria. The diagnosis of urethral tumor is made by urethroscopy and urethral biopsy. Symptomatic urethral diverticulum occurs more often in women than in men. Female urethral diverticulum produces a triad of symptoms — dysuria, urinary dribbling, and dyspareunia. The diagnosis is made by voiding cystourethrogram (VCUG). When the diagnosis is in doubt, double-balloon retrograde urethrogram or magnetic resonance imaging may be performed. Urethral strictures occur more commonly in men than in women. Symptomatic urethral strictures cause obstructive and irritative voiding. Hematuria and urethral pain also may be present. When recurrent stricture is present, urethral carcinoma should be suspected.

Penis

Penile pain may arise from Peyronie's plaque, penile prosthesis, priapism, or penile carcinoma. Peyronie's disease is an abnormal development of penile plaque on the penis with associated penile curvature. The plaque most often is found on the dorsum of the penis. Impotence and pain during intercourse may occur. Treatment has included paraaminobenzoate, vitamin E, and steroid injections into the plaque. The most effective oral agent is vitamin E. Surgical removal of the plaque and the use of dermal grafts have been successful.

Severe penile pain can develop many months or years after the insertion of a penile prosthesis. Patients with diabetes mellitus are more susceptible to prosthetic-penile pain. Usually, no other associated physical findings are present. Presence of penile pain in a prosthetic patient usually heralds an impending infection. Unremitting pain is relieved by removing the prosthesis. Presence of pain and infection mandates prosthetic explantation.

Priapism is persistent erection in the absence of sexual stimulation that has lasted for more than 4 hours. Two types of priapism exist — high-flow priapism and low-flow priapism. High-flow priapism occurs from an arteriovenous shunt and is painless. High-flow priapism most often occurs as a result of a blow to the perineum. Low-flow priapism occurs as a result of poor venous outflow. Risk factors for low-flow priapism include drugs, leukemia, and sickle cell disease. Stagnation of blood in the erectile bodies causes localized ischemia and resultant penile pain. Diagnosis of priapism is made by history and physical examination. The distinction of high flow and low flow is made by arterial blood gases (ABGs) of corporal blood. Treatment of high-flow priapism involves embolization of the fistula. Treatment of low-flow priapism includes intracorporeal injection of alpha agonist, saline irrigations, and shunting procedures. For sickle cell-induced priapism, medical therapy with oxygenation, transfusion, and alkalinization are the initial methods for detumescence.

Penile carcinoma typically presents as a maculopapular lesion (erythroplasia of Queyrat or Bowen's disease) or an exophytic mass of the foreskin or the penis. Usually, penile carcinoma does not produce pain unless the tumor is disturbed. Penile carcinoma most often affects uncircumcised men. Retraction of the foreskin is the mainstay of clinically diagnosing penile cancer. Treatment is most often surgical and involves partial or total penectomy followed by ilioinguinal lymph-node dissection.

Testis

Testicular pain may arise from infection, hydrocele, tumor, torsion, vasectomy, and varicocele. Epididymitis is inflammation of the epididymis. Epididymitis presents with progressive enlargement of the affected hemiscrotum associated with testicular pain. Often, reactive hydrocele is present. In epididymitis, the pain site is localized to the tail of the epididymis. If the testis also is involved (orchitis), the entire testicle is tender. On examination, epididymal pain will lessen when the scrotum is elevated (positive Plehn's sign).

Hydrocele is a large fluid sac surrounding the testicle. Hydrocele causes testicular pain because its weight drags the spermatic cord in a more dependent position. Although hydrocele is a benign condition, presence of acute hydrocele should raise the suspicion of testicular carcinoma. Incarcerated bowel hernia also may be mistaken for hydrocele. If clinical diagnosis of hydrocele cannot be made on physical examination, scrotal ultrasound should be obtained.

The most common presentation of testicular tumor is asymptomatic testicular lump. However, testicular tumors can present with pain, especially after intratesticular bleeding. Large testicular tumors may present with scrotal or testicular discomfort from dragging on the spermatic cord. The diagnosis of testicular tumor is best made by scrotal ultrasound and tumor markers AFP and bhCG. Testicular torsion results in acute scrotal pain associated with nausea and vomiting. Testicular torsion is a urologic emergency. Emergency scrotal exploration with orchiopexy is a corrective measure. Torsion of appendix testis or epididymis is a benign and self-limited process. However, clinical symptoms of testicular torsion and torsion of testicular appendages often overlap. In this situation, scrotal ultrasound with Doppler studies or nuclear testicular scan will be diagnostic.

Chronic testicular pain is a vexing problem after vasectomy. Vasectomy is the leading cause of urologic litigation in this country. Chronic testicular pain is not something that should be taken lightly or dismissed. Affected patients complain of constant testicular pain that waxes and wanes. The pain becomes worse during sexual intercourse, sports, and ejaculation. It has been hypothesized that chronic testicular pain arises from vasal obstruction and/ or perivasal nerve entrapment during the healing process. Treatment for chronic testicular pain involves scrotal support and NSAIDs. Failure of medical therapy often warrants vasectomy reversal, epididymectomy, orchiectomy, or spermatic cord stripping.

Varicoceles are dilated internal spermatic veins. They invariably occur on the left side and cause chronic testicular pain that becomes worse later in the day. Varicocele also is the most common surgically correctable cause of male infertility. A right-sided varicocele is unusual and should lead to suspicion of possible retroperitoneal disease such as renal-cell carcinoma with renal vein or vena cava involvement. The cornerstone of treatment for varicocele is surgical ligation of the internal spermatic vein. Other rarer causes of local testicular pain are polyarteritis nodosa, Henoch–Schönlein purpura, and thrombosis of the testicular arteries in cases of repeated trauma.

Pelvic-Floor Tension Myalgia

Pelvic-floor tension myalgia is a syndrome that causes pain in the levator ani musculature and their areas of attachment — the sacrum, pubic rami, ischial tuberosity, and coccyx. Symptoms include perineal pain, pelvic pain, and chronic low-back pain. Variable urinary symptoms are present. A vicious cycle of pelvic-floor tension leading to pain, and pain leading to an increase in tension results. This syndrome is more common in women and is often associated with dysuria and dyspareunia. A characteristic finding is pain or tenderness of the levator ani musculature on rectal examination. Treatment is aimed at inducing temporary relief of pain using deep heat (rectal diathermy), sitz baths, pelvic-floor muscle massage, biofeedback, and patient education to keep the pelvic floor muscles relaxed.

SELECTED READINGS

Addison RG. Chronic pain syndrome. *Am J Med* 1984;77:54.

Anderson, J. Prostate disease: an overview. *Hosp Med* 1999;60:698–699.

Chambers GK, Fenster HN, Cripps S, et al. An assessment of the use of intravesical potassium in the diagnosis of interstitial cystitis. *J Urol* 1999;162:699–701.

Choe JM. Diagnostic work up. *Freedom Regained: Female Urinary Incontinence Can Be Overcome*. Columbus: Anadem Publishing, 1999: 87–116.

Forbes P. Diagnosis and treatment of chronic pelvic pain. *Practitioner* 1998;242:120–123, 125.

Henderson LJ. Diagnosis, treatment, and lifestyle changes of interstitial cystitis. *AORN J* 2000;71:525–530, 533–536, 538.

Nocks BN. Pain in the male genitalia. In: Aronoff GM, ed. *Evaluation and Treatment of Chronic Pain*. Baltimore: Urban & Schwarzenberg, 1985: 393–405.

Peeker R, Fall M. Treatment guidelines for classic and non-ulcer interstitial cystitis. *Int Urogynecol J Pelvic Floor Dysfunct* 2000;11:23–32.

Propert KJ, Schaeffer AJ, Brensinger CM, et al. A prospective study of interstitial cystitis: results of longitudinal followup of the interstitial cystitis data base cohort. *J Urol* 2000;163:1434–1439.

Ratner V, Taylor N, Wein AJ, et al. Re: Epidemiology of interstitial cystitis: a population based study. *J Urol* 1999;162:500.

Smaki M, Merritt JL, Stillwell GK. Tension myalgia of the pelvic floor. *Mayo Clin Proc* 1977;52:717.

Teichman JM, Nielson-Omeis BJ. Potassium leak test predicts outcome in interstitial cystitis. *J Urol* 1999;161:1791–1796.

Walsh PC, Retik AB, Stamey TA, et al. *Campbell's Urology*, 6th ed. Philadelphia: WB Saunders, 1992.

Zermann DH, Wunderlich H, Schubert J, et al. Re: The diagnosis of interstitial cystitis revisited: lessons learned from the National Institutes of Health Interstitial Cystitis Database Study. *J Urol* 1999;162:807.

CHAPTER 22

Chronic Pelvic Pain

David S. Chapin

DEFINITION

Chronic pelvic pain (CPP) in women usually is defined as noncyclic pain that is present for more than 3 to 6 months, and may include cyclic pain present for more than 6 months. Although long considered a gynecologic disease, CPP is more likely one manifestation of the chronic-pain syndrome, where the patient's perception of pain is localized to the pelvis. The more generic Chronic Pain Syndrome definition includes pain for more than 6 months, incomplete relief from standard treatments, impaired function at home and/or work, signs of depression, pain out of proportion to pathology, and altered family roles. This chapter will discuss some of the causes of CPP, discuss the evaluation and treatment with an emphasis on the multifactorial nature of the syndrome, and the integrated approach necessary to help the patients who have it.

SCOPE OF THE PROBLEM

Ten percent of referrals to gynecologists are for CPP. Forty percent, or about 400,000, of all laparoscopies, and 15%, about 70,000, of all hysterectomies are performed each year for CPP.

CAUSES OF CHRONIC PELVIC PAIN

The Physical Versus Mental Dichotomy

Traditional medical approaches to pain have involved finding a pathophysiologic cause for the pain and then treating it pharmacologically or surgically. If diagnostic methods failed to reveal the cause, the pain was assumed to be psychosomatic, and the patient was told, or made to feel, that "it is all in your head." Recent research and experience have indicated that this dichotomous way of categorizing chronic pain is not helpful in evaluating or treating these patients. Rather, an integrated approach appreciating physical, psychologic, and social factors will be more rewarding.

The Integrated Approach

Figure 22.1 diagrams a model of the circular interaction among biologic stimuli capable of causing pain, alterations of lifestyles and relationships, and anxiety and affective disorders results in CPP. Keeping this model in mind during the evaluation of the patient facilitates diagnosis and selection of therapy.

Gynecologic Causes of Chronic Pelvic Pain

Endometriosis, pelvic-inflammatory disease (PID), pelvic adhesions, adenomyosis, and leiomyomata (fibroids) of the uterus are the most common gynecological conditions implicated in or associated with CPP.

Endometriosis, a bizarre and unpredictable disease, is characterized by endometrial tissue growing outside the

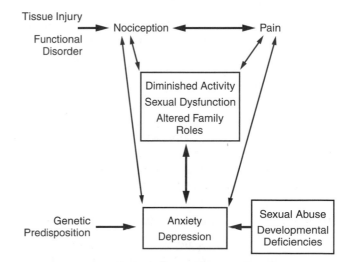

FIG. 22.1. Integrative model for chronic pelvic pain. (Reprinted from Steege JF, Stout AL, Somkuti SG. Chonic pelvic pain in women: toward an integrated approach. *Obstet Gynecol Survey* 1993;48:95–110, with permission).

uterus. The ectopically placed tissue continually waxes and wanes under the influence of the hormones of the menstrual cycle. Its most common symptoms are menstrual pain and dyspareunia, but chronic full-time pain also can result. Definitive diagnosis must be made by laparoscopy or biopsy.

Chronic PID, a more unusual entity, is the long-term result of repeated infection and is most often manifested by CPP. Most of these conditions, especially endometriosis and pelvic adhesions, can exist without any pain being present, making the correlation between pain and demonstrable anatomic pathology difficult and unreliable.

Fibroids, adenomyosis, and adhesions, although they may be present, rarely account for CPP.

Nongynecologic Causes of Chronic Pelvic Pain

Psychologic factors associated with, predisposing to, or possibly at the root of CPP include depression, history of sexual abuse, and opioid-seeking behavior.

Neurologic conditions contributing to pelvic pain include fibromyalgia and other syndromes of abnormal pain processing by the nervous system.

Gastrointestinal syndromes known to cause CPP include irritable bowel syndrome, inflammatory bowel diseases (ulcerative colitis and Crohn's), cancer, and chronic diverticulitis.

Genitourinary conditions such as interstitial cystitis and chronic urethral syndrome also can underlie the CPP syndrome.

Musculoskeletal diseases to be considered are spinal-disc degeneration or stenosis and levator-muscle spasm.

EVALUATION OF THE PATIENT WITH CHRONIC PELVIC PAIN

The Role of the Gynecologist

The gynecologist is commonly the first consultant for the patient with CPP. He or she must first separate the dysmenorrhea and Mittelschmerz patients from those with CPP. Pain always coincident with periods or midcycle (ovulation) is more likely to have a remedial gynecologic cause than full-time or randomly occurring pain. A calendar may prove helpful. These cyclic pain patterns are best treated empirically with oral contraceptives and/or nonsteroidal antiinflammatory drugs. Those patients with random or full-time pain patterns require the evaluation and treatment outlined here.

History and Physical Examination

The history should include the severity, duration, location, and timing of the pain. Ask the patient to quantify the pain on a one-to-ten scale. The examiner should specifically inquire about dyspareunia. The psychologic history should include psychoactive medications, hospitalizations,

previous diagnoses (especially depression), and sexual abuse. A careful review of gastrointestinal symptoms such as diarrhea, constipation, painful bowel movements, and bloody stools is in order. Urinary symptoms including painful urination, urinary frequency, poor bladder emptying, and incontinence also need exploration.

On general physical examination, abdominal tenderness may signal intestinal problems, and generalized tenderness in multiple sites may raise the suspicion of fibromyalgia. On pelvic examination, careful inspection of the vulva and evaluation of pelvic support are the first steps. Then, vaginal examination should take note of any discharge. A gentle bimanual examination follows, noting any tender areas, cervical-motion tenderness, pelvic masses, and *cul-de-sac* nodularity. Evaluate levator tone and/or sensitivity by directly palpating the levator muscle and asking the patient to squeeze.

Ancillary Testing

To evaluate the possibility of pelvic inflammatory disease, perform complete blood count, erythrocyte sedimentation rate, C-reactive protein, urinalysis, urine culture, cervix culture, and urine chlamydia test. Ultrasound, abdominal and transvaginal, can point out or rule out adnexal pathology and leiomyomata, but magnetic resonance imaging may be necessary to demonstrate adenomyosis or small implants of endometriosis in the *cul-de-sac*.

Laparoscopy

Laparoscopy quickly became a favorite tool for the evaluation of pelvic pain shortly after the introduction of the procedure in the United States in the late 1960s. Its success was so great, that it quickly became the first procedure of choice in the evaluation of CPP. But the value of laparoscopy is not clear at this time. Many studies have shown that more pelvic pathology can be identified in CPP patients than in pain-free controls, but whether or not the identified pathology is the cause of the pain is debatable. In particular, visualization of endometriosis does not guarantee that endometriosis is the cause of the pain, and failure to visualize endometriosis does not rule it out. Adhesions found at laparoscopy rarely correlate with pain, but they can be lysed during the procedure, with occasional good results. A new technique of laparoscopy under conscious sedation allows the surgeon and patient to map the areas of pain; this may improve the diagnostic and therapeutic efficacy of laparoscopy in the future.

Empiric Therapy Prior to Laparoscopy

Many specialists now believe that gynecologic causes of CPP can be treated empirically prior to any invasive procedure. Nonsteroidal antiinflammatory drugs can be effective, especially for dysmenorrhea. If any suspicion of infection is present, i.e., cervical motion tenderness or elevated sedimentation rate, doxycycline and/or metronidazole may be tried. Suppressing ovulation for 3 months with oral contraceptives also may be tried in the hopes of avoiding laparoscopy. There is growing enthusiasm for empiric leuprolide (Lupron, TAP Pharmaceuticals Inc., Deerfield, IL, U.S.A.) therapy. This gonadotropin-releasing hormone agonist, given by monthly injection for 3 months, effectively treats minor endometriosis and may obviate the need for laparoscopic diagnosis and/or treatment.

TREATMENT OF CHRONIC PELVIC PAIN

Treatment of Specific Diagnoses

Patients with specific nongynecologic diagnoses should be treated as indicated by the disease. Irritable-bowel syndrome likely will respond to fiber, tricyclic antidepressants, and/or antispasmodics. Interstitial cystitis, although difficult to diagnose and treat, may respond to tricyclics, intravesical dimethyl sulfoxide, or bladder overdistension. Urethral syndrome usually can be treated with antibiotics. Levator massage, pelvic floor exercise, and other physical-therapy techniques can relieve levator spasm. Fibromyalgia, a controversial entity, usually is managed with tricyclics and gabapentin.

Because the most common gynecologic entity likely to be at the root of CPP is endometriosis, aggressive treatment is in order if this diagnosis is made. Once PID, leiomyomata, and adenomyosis have been ruled out, medical treatment with leuprolide is the treatment of choice. A 6- to 12-month treatment period is common, using a monthly injection of 3.75 mg of the depot form of the drug. Randomized trials have shown excellent relief of pain with this regimen. If more than 6 months is required, a small dose of estrogen can be added to the Lupron to prevent osteoporosis and treat vasomotor symptoms. If the endometriosis is extensive, surgical therapy is indicated. There has been unreliable response to laparoscopic laser or electrical ablation of endometrial implants, and most experts believe total excision of the endometriosis is necessary, either by laparoscopy or laparotomy.

Pain Unit Referral

When empiric therapy has failed and there has been no definitive singular diagnosis, referral of the CPP patient to a pain unit is indicated. The patient then can receive the benefit of the multidisciplinary approach. All modalities of therapy available can be utilized to address the patient's needs. The value of this approach has been demonstrated in at least one randomized trial. Pain-unit referral before extensive workup may be beneficial in some cases where suspicion is high for a chronic pain syndrome and low for extensive gynecologic disease.

SELECTED READINGS

Barbieri RL. Primary GnRH a therapy for suspected endometriosis: a non surgical approach to the diagnosis and treatment of chronic pelvic pain. *Am J Managed Care* 1997;3:285–290.

Ling FW, for the Pelvic Pain Study Group. Randomized controlled trial of depot leuprolide in patients with chronic pelvic pain and clinically suspected endometriosis. *Obstet Gynecol* 1999;93:51–58.

Peters AA, van Dorst E, Jellis B, et al. A randomized clinical trial to compare two different approaches to women with chronic pelvic pain. *Obstet Gynecol* 1991;77:740–744.

Steege JF, Metzger, DA, Levy BS. *Chronic Pelvic Pain: An Integrated Approach*. Philadelphia: WB Saunders, 1998.

Steege JF, Stout AL, Somkuti SG. Chronic pelvic pain in women: toward an integrated approach. *Obstet Gynecol Survey* 1993, 48:95–110.

Walker EA, Katon WJ, Harrop-Griffiths J, et al. Relationship of chronic pelvic pain to psychiatric diagnosis and childhood sexual abuse. *Am J Psychiatry* 1988;145:75–80.

PART III

Common Painful Syndromes

CHAPTER 23

Arthritis

Hilary J. Fausett

When evaluating the patient with pain in one or more joint, a complete history and physical examination must be performed. As "arthritis," or inflammation of a joint, may be part of a localized condition or a systemic disease.

Many conditions are misinterpreted as arthritis by the patient, such as the stiffness of Parkinson's disease, a stress fracture, or fibromyositis. The presence of extraarticular findings can be helpful in identifying the type of arthritis (such as the tophi in gout, the classic nodules in rheumatoid arthritis, or the pustular rash associated with gonococcemia). Often, arthritis is transient and may resolve without diagnosis. Certain problems require immediate attention and prompt treatment, such as acute monarthritis, which could be infectious and proper diagnosis is essential.

Blood tests are useful in diagnosing some specific types of arthritis. For example, an elevated erythrocyte-sedimentation rate (ESR) or C-reactive protein suggests inflammatory disease. Elevated serum uric-acid levels may suggest gout, although this is a nonspecific marker. Latex fixation tests for rheumatoid factor often are highly positive in rheumatoid arthritis (RA) but may also be positive in hepatitis and cirrhosis, as well as infections and collagen vascular diseases. Antinuclear factors may be positive in RA, Sjögren's syndrome, progressive-systemic sclerosis, systemic lupus erythematosus (SLE), hepatitis, and other diseases. Therefore, after preliminary screening tests, patients usually are referred to a specialist.

Once joint involvement is established, inflammatory (for example, RA) and noninflammatory processes (e.g., osteoarthritis) must be differentiated.

OSTEOARTHRITIS

Degenerative joint disease, also called hypertrophic osteoarthritis (OA) is an arthropathy with altered hyaline cartilage. OA is characterized by the loss of articular cartilage and by hypertrophy of bone, which produces osteophytes.

Osteoarthritis is the most common rheumatologic disorder. Almost all persons by age 40 have some pathologic change in weight-bearing joints, although most people are asymptomatic until their 70s.

OA is classified as primary (idiopathic) or secondary to some known cause. Secondary OA appears to result from conditions such as congenital joint abnormalities and genetic defects, any disease that alters the normal structure and function of hyaline cartilage (as with RA, gout, chondrocalcinosis); and trauma (including fracture) to the hyaline cartilage or surrounding tissue (such as from prolonged overuse of a joint or group of joints associated with occupations such as years of heavy lifting or fine joint overuse as with a seamstress).

Normal joints have a low coefficient of friction and do not wear out with typical overuse and trauma. Hyaline cartilage is 95% water and extracellular cartilage matrix and only 5% chondrocytes. The pathophysiologic process of OA is progressive. Triggered by a change in the microenvironment, some type of interaction between chondrocytes and osteoblasts results in increased bone formation in the subchondral area. The degree of formation of these spurs varies among joints in proportion to the underlying cause. Finally, bony cysts (pseudocysts) form in the marrow below the subchondral bone. By the time symptoms appear, synovial proliferation and some mild synovitis are virtually always present.

Symptoms and Signs

Onset is gradual, usually involving one or only a few joints (Table 23.1). The classic presentation is "stiffness" in the morning or after inactivity that then lessens with normal activity. Pain usually is worsened by exercise and relieved by rest. Proliferation of cartilage, bone, liga-

TABLE 23.1. *Common Symptoms of Osteoarthritis and Rheumatoid Arthritis*

Symptom	Osteoarthritis	Rheumatoid arthritis
Tenderness	Rare	Common
Swelling	Bony irregular, spurs	Synovial, capsular, soft tissue
Distal phalangeal joints	Usually affected	Rarely affected
Proximal phalangeal joints	Frequently affected	Usually affected
Metocarpal phalangeal involvement	Rare	Usually affected
Wrist involvement	Rare	Common

ment, tendon, capsules, and synovium, along with varying amounts of joint effusion, ultimately produces the joint enlargement characteristic of OA. Tenderness on palpation and pain on passive motion are relatively late signs. Muscle spasm and contracture of surrounding muscles are often pain generators for the patient.

Diagnosis

Diagnosis usually is based on symptoms and signs or on x-ray in asymptomatic patients. Although diagnosis usually is straightforward, other common rheumatic diseases must be considered. The ESR is normal or only moderately increased. Blood studies may help rule out identifiable causes of arthritis (e.g., gout or RA). X-ray generally reveals narrowing of the joint space, but may reveal osteophytes or pseudocysts in the subchondral bone marrow.

Prognosis and Treatment

The pathophysiologic process of OA usually is progressive. The mainstay of treatment is to prevent deformity and maintain function. Treatment must include patient education regarding the nature of the problem and need for optimal physical fitness. Exercise helps to maintain healthy cartilage and range of motion. Daily stretching exercises are of utmost importance. Referral to physical therapy or a class for proper education about healthcare maintenance usually is warranted.

Medications are for symptom management. The nonsteroidal antiinflammatory drugs (NSAIDs) are analgesics. It is doubtful that their antiinflammatory activity has any effect on the course of OA. Muscle relaxants (usually in low doses) occasionally provide temporary benefit when pain arises from muscles strained by attempting to support OA joints. Oral corticosteroid therapy usually is not indicated. Intraarticular depot corticosteroids are helpful when effusions or signs of inflammation are present; these drugs usually are needed only intermittently and should generally be used as infrequently as possible. The repeated injection of steroids into joint spaces is not recommended.

Hyaluronic acid, a normal physiologic component of synovial fluid, has proven effective in the management of OA of the knee. Commercial preparations, such as Hyalgan

Solution (Sanofi–Synthelabo, Inc., New York, NY, U.S.A.) by injection, have been shown to result in measurable improvement using clinical, radiologic, and laboratory criteria. Many orthopedic specialists now offer injection therapies aimed at improving functions and not just easing pain.

Laminectomy, osteotomy, and total joint replacement should be considered when conservative therapy fails. In spinal, knee, or first carpometacarpal OA, various supports can provide relief, but they should be followed by specific exercise programs. Other adjuncts to therapy are transcutaneous-electrical nerve stimulation and local rubs with medications like capsaicin. Experimental therapies that may preserve cartilage or allow chondrocyte grafting are being studied.

INFECTIOUS ARTHRITIS

Inflammation in a joint resulting from bacterial, fungal, or viral infection of synovial or periarticular tissues is referred to as infectious arthritis. Onset of acute infectious arthritis is rapid (a few hours to a few days) with moderate to severe joint pain, warmth, tenderness, and restricted motion. The patient may have no other symptoms of serious infection, which can delay diagnosis, thereby reducing the likelihood of a successful outcome

Risk factors for infectious arthritis include advanced age, alcoholism, diabetes, and immunosuppression. Risk of joint infection is substantially increased in patients with a past history of joint infection or with a prosthetic joint implant.

Acute infectious arthritis (95% of cases) is caused by bacteria or viruses. *Neisseria gonorrhoeae* is the most common bacterial cause in adults. It spreads from infected mucosal surfaces (cervix, rectum, pharynx) to the small joints of the hands, wrists, elbows, knees, and ankles, but rarely to axial skeletal joints.

Nongonococcal arthritis is usually caused by *Staphylococcus aureus* , but also may result from gram-negative bacterial infection. Anaerobic infections are less common, and factors predisposing to anaerobic infection include penetrating trauma, arthrocentesis, recent surgery, joint prosthesis, contiguous infection, diabetes, and malignancy.

Viral causes of acute arthritis are many, including hepatitis B, hepatitis C, and rubella virus (active infection

TABLE 23.2. *Type of Effusion Aspirated from Joint*

Characteristic	Normal	Inflammatory	Non-inflammatory	Septic
Color	Clear	Yellow	Yellow	Varies, cloudy
White cell count	Very low	Moderate	Low	High
% PMN	<25%	50%	50%	>75%
Culture	Negative	Negative	Negative	Positive

PMN, polymononuclear cell.

and after immunization). Varicella virus, mumps (in adults), and Epstein–Barr virus mononucleosis also are associated with arthralgias and arthritis. Viral infections are more likely than bacteria to cause polyarthritis.

Infection in a joint produces an inflammatory reaction (arthritis) that is an attempt to kill the infecting organisms but that damages joint tissues. The infecting organisms multiply in the synovial fluid and synovial lining tissue. Joint infections may be acute, with sudden onset of joint pain and swelling, or chronic, with insidious development of milder symptoms.

Diagnosis

Diagnosis may be suggested by the clinical picture and by recovering an organism from a remote site of infection. A blood sample usually reveals elevation of the patient's white blood cell (WBC) count. It often is necessary to aspirate the joint, as laboratory analysis of the synovial fluid confirms the diagnosis (Table 23.2).

Treatment

Treatment with antibiotics is initiated aggressively. In addition to antibiotics, more invasive treatment for proper drainage may be indicated, and is best managed by a specialist. Joints may be splinted for the first few days to reduce pain, followed by passive and active range–of–motion exercises with muscle strengthening as soon as tolerated. Prosthetic joint infections require prolonged treatment, and these patients are best managed by an orthopedic surgeon.

There is no specific treatment of viral arthritis. Mycobacterial and fungal joint infections require prolonged treatment, usually with multiple antibiotics, depending on sensitivity testing of the isolated organism.

GOUT

A recurrent, acute or chronic arthritis of peripheral joints that results from deposition in and about the joints and tendons of monosodium urate crystals from supersaturated hyperuricemic body fluids is commonly referred to as "gout."

In patients with gout, the plasma is saturated with uric acid, and because urate solubility is low, needle-shaped monosodium urate (MSU) crystals are deposited in avascu-lar tissues like cartilage or relatively avascular tissues such as tendons and ligaments; these crystals are found around cooler distal peripheral joints and cooler tissues, such as ears. Tophi are MSU crystal aggregates. They are large enough first to be seen on x-rays of the joints as punched-out lesions and later seen or felt as subcutaneous nodules.

Acute gouty arthritis starts without warning. It may be precipitated by minor trauma; overindulgence in purine-rich food or alcohol; surgery; fatigue; emotional stress, or the medical stress associated with infection; or vascular occlusion. Acute, monarticular, nocturnal pain usually is the first symptom. The pain becomes progressively more severe and often is excruciating. The joint may appear to be infected with swelling, warmth, redness, and exquisite tenderness. The metatarsophalangeal joint of the great toe is most often involved *(podagra)*, but the instep, ankle, knee, wrist, and elbow also are common sites. Fever, tachycardia, chills, malaise, and leukocytosis may occur.

The first few attacks usually affect only a single joint and last only a few days, but later attacks may affect several joints simultaneously or sequentially and persist for weeks if untreated. Without prophylaxis, several attacks may occur each year, and chronic joint symptoms may develop with permanent joint deformity.

Acute gouty arthritis has such distinctive clinical features that it usually can be tentatively diagnosed by history and physical examination. Elevated serum urate [more than 7 mg/dL (more than 0.41 mmol/L)] supports the diagnosis but is not specific. About 30% of patients have a normal serum urate at the time of the acute attack. Demonstration in tissue or synovial fluid of needle-shaped urate crystals that are free in the fluid or engulfed by phagocytes is pathopneumonic.

Treatment

Objectives are (a) termination of the acute attack with NSAIDs, (b) prevention of recurrent acute attacks (if frequent) with daily colchicine, and (c) prevention of further deposition of MSU crystals and resolution of existing tophi by lowering the urate concentration in extracellular body fluid. A preventive program should aim to avert both the disability resulting from erosion of bone and joint cartilage and the renal damage. Specific treatment depends on the stage and severity of the disease. Coexisting conditions such as hypertension, hyperlipidemia, and obesity should be treated.

Treatment of the acute attack is important, as is starting prophylactic therapy if the attacks are frequent. The response to colchicine usually is dramatic. Joint pains generally begin to subside after 12 hours of treatment and cease within 2 days. The NSAIDs are effective in acute attacks of established gout. Gouty attacks also may be treated by aspiration of affected joints, followed by instillation of a corticosteroid esters.

In addition to specific therapy, rest and abundant fluid intake to combat dehydration and to decrease urate-crystal precipitation in the kidneys are indicated. To control pain, opiates (perhaps oxycodone 5 to 10 mg p.o. every 4 to 6 hours) may be needed. Splinting of the inflamed joint to limit inadvertent movement and diminish pain may be helpful. Patients should be referred to a rheumatologist or other person familiar with the disease to initiate chronic therapy.

RHEUMATOID ARTHRITIS

Rheumatoid Arthritis (RA) classically presents with symmetric inflammation of the peripheral joints. This inflammation may progress to the destruction of articular and periarticular structures (Figs. 23.1, 23.2). There may be other, generalized symptoms as well. The cause of RA is unknown, although a genetic predisposition has been identified. Environmental factors also may play a role. Although RA most often affects women between 25 and 50 years old, onset may be at any age.

In chronically affected joints, the synovium develops many villous folds. The increased number and size of synovial lining cells, as well as colonization by lymphocytes and plasma cells causes the synovium to thicken. Rheumatoid nodules are nonspecific granulomas that have a necrotic core surrounded by lymphocytes and plasma cells. Rheumatoid nodules occur in up to 30% of patients. The nodules are found subcutaneously at sites of chronic irritation such as the extensor surface of the forearm.

Symptoms and Signs

Onset usually is insidious, with progressive joint involvement. Although abrupt inflammation in multiple joints may occur. The inflamed joints are tender and have synovial thickening. Involvement usually is symmetric, and usually affects the small hand joints (especially proximal interphalangeal and metacarpophalangeal), and foot joints (metatarsophalangeal.) But initial manifestations may occur in any joint.

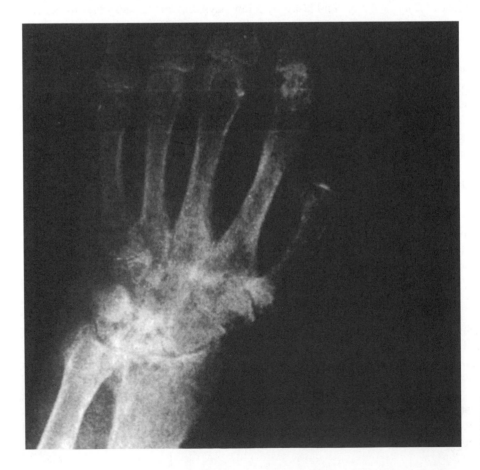

FIG. 23.1. Erosive disease at the wrist and metacarpophalangeal joints is seen on x-ray of patient with severe rheumatoid arthritis.

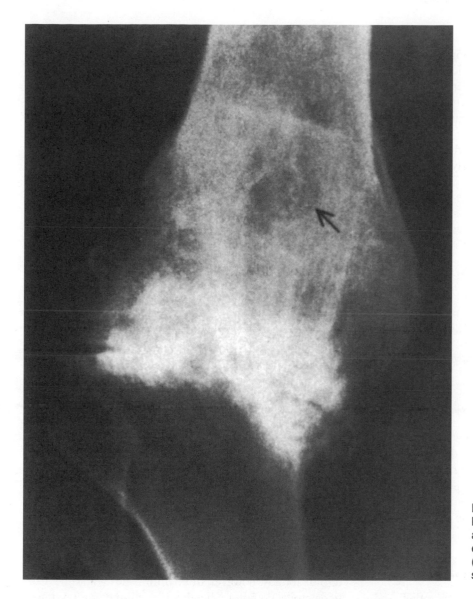

FIG. 23.2. Obliteration of joint space, in knee of patient with severe rheumatoid arthritis, is associated with advanced disease. Large cysts in subchondral areas (*arrow*) may contribute to the loss of joint space.

Many patients describe stiffness lasting greater than 30 minutes when they arise in the morning or after prolonged inactivity. Many patients also complain of early-afternoon fatigue and malaise. Deformities, particularly flexion contractures, may develop rapidly. The "swan neck" deformity of ulnar deviation of the fingers with slippage of the extensor tendons off the metacarpophalangeal joints is a typical late result. Subcutaneous rheumatoid nodules usually are not an early manifestation. Fever may be present and usually is low-grade, and other generalized, nonspecific symptoms may occur.

Laboratory Findings

The ESR is elevated in 90% of cases. Antibodies to altered -globulin, so-called rheumatoid factors (RFs), as detected by agglutination tests that show IgM RF, occur in about 70% of cases. Although RFs are not specific for RA and are found in many diseases (including granulomatous diseases, chronic infections, hepatitis, sarcoidosis, and subacute-bacterial endocarditis), a high RF titer helps confirm the diagnosis. A very high RF titer suggests a worse prognosis and often is associated with progressive disease, nodules, vasculitis, and pulmonary involvement. The titer can be influenced by treatment and often falls as inflammatory joint activity decreases.

The synovial fluid should be examined by an expert to confirm the absence of crystals or of infectious agents. On x-ray, only soft-tissue swelling is seen in the first months of disease. Subsequently, periarticular osteoporosis, joint-space narrowing, and marginal erosions may be present. The rate of deterioration, seen on x-ray and clinically, is highly variable, but erosions as a sign of bony damage may occur within the first year.

Diagnosis

The American College of Rheumatology has developed simplified criteria for the classification of RA. Primarily intended as a communication aid for those in clinical research, these criteria also can help suggest the clinical diagnosis. Almost any other disease that causes arthritis still must be considered.

SLE may mimic RA. Polyarteritis, progressive systemic sclerosis, dermatomyositis, and polymyositis may have features that resemble RA. Ankylosing spondylitis usually involves the spine and more often affects men than women. Osteoarthritis often involves the proximal and distal interphalangeal joints, first carpometacarpal and first metatarsophalangeal joints, and often the large joints such as knee joints, and spine.

Treatment

As many as 75% of patients improve symptomatically with conservative treatment during the first year of disease. Some patients, however, become severely disabled despite full treatment.

Rest and Nutrition

Regular rest for the patient as well as the affected joints should be prescribed. Some practitioners do believe that fish or plant oil supplements may partially relieve symptoms because they can decrease production of prostaglandins. A search of the internet reveals many sites that tout certain diets or food items as provocative or curative for RA.

Nonsteroidal Antiinflammatory Drugs and Salicylates

NSAIDs provide important symptomatic relief and may be adequate as simple therapy for mild RA, but they do not appear to alter the long-term course of disease.

Salicylates are relatively safe and inexpensive analgesics that have antiinflammatory activity. Aspirin (acetylsalicylic acid) is started at a dose of 0.6 to 1.0 g four times a day with meals and with a bedtime snack. Dosage is increased until the effective dose is reached or the patient exhibits evidence of mild toxicity, such as tinnitus.

Other NSAIDs are available for patients who cannot tolerate sufficient aspirin to obtain a good effect. Usually, only one such NSAID should be given at a time. The dose of the drug can be increased every 2 weeks until response is maximal or maximum dosage is reached. A drug should be tried at a sufficient dose for 2 to 3 weeks before assuming the drug is not working.

Although often less irritating to the gastrointestinal (GI) tract than high-dose aspirin, these other NSAIDs also can produce gastric symptoms and GI bleeding.

Because of the effect of NSAIDs on renal function, these drugs often are avoided in patients at risk for renal insufficiency.

Gold compounds are given in addition to salicylates or other NSAIDs if needed to sufficiently relieve pain or suppress active joint inflammation. In some patients, gold may produce clinical remission and decrease the formation of new bony erosions. Preparations of gold compounds are given intramuscularly at weekly intervals in gradually increasing doses until comfort is achieved or to a maximum dose of 1 g. Gold compounds are contraindicated in patients with significant hepatic or renal disease. Because patients may have an untoward reaction to gold compounds, these agents must be used only under the supervision of a trained professional. An oral-gold compound also is available. Auranofin is started at a low dose and slowly titrated up. The most prominent side effects of the oral-gold compounds are gastrointestinal.

Hydroxychloroquine also can control symptoms of mild or moderately active RA. Toxic effects usually are mild and include dermatitis, myopathy, and generally reversible corneal opacity. However, irreversible retinal degeneration has been reported. Ophthalmologic testing of visual fields using a red test object is recommended before and every 6 months during treatment. *Sulfasalazine* also may be used. The patients must be monitored carefully for side effects. Oral *penicillamine* is an alternative to gold therapy. Side effects are common, and the patient's care must be closely supervised.

Corticosteroids

Corticosteroids are the most effective short-term antiinflammatory drugs. The clinical benefit of corticosteroids for RA, however, often diminishes with time. Corticosteroids do not predictably prevent the progression of joint destruction, although there is evidence to suggest that they may slow erosions. Severe rebound, with marked increase in symptomatology, follows the withdrawal of corticosteroids in active disease. The long-term use of corticosteroids is associated with multiple side effects. Therefore, most specialists recommend that corticosteroids should be given only after a careful and usually prolonged trial of less-hazardous drugs. Relative contraindications to corticosteroid use include peptic-ulcer disease, hypertension, untreated infections, diabetes mellitus, and glaucoma. Occult infection with tuberculosis should be ruled out before initiating treatment with corticosteroids.

Corticosteroids promptly suppress clinical manifestations for many patients and may be used for disease exacerbations to maintain joint function and to allow continued performance of customary duties, but the patient should be cautioned about complications with long-term use. Prednisone dosage should not exceed 7.5 mg/day, except in patients with severe systemic manifestations of RA (e.g., vasculitis, pleurisy, pericarditis).

Intraarticular injections of corticosteroid esters may temporarily help control local synovitis in one or two particularly painful joints. Triamcinolone hexacetonide may suppress inflammation for the longest time; other depot corticosteroids, including prednisolone tertiary-butylacetate, also are effective. The soluble 21-phosphate preparations of prednisolone or dexamethasone are not recommended because of rapid clearance from the joint and very short duration of action. Overuse of the recently injected, less painful joint may accelerate joint destruction. Because corticosteroid esters are crystalline, local inflammation transiently increases within a few hours in about 2% of injections.

Cytotoxic or Immunosuppressive Drugs

These drugs (e.g., methotrexate, azathioprine, cyclosporine) are increasingly used in management of severe, active RA. They can suppress inflammation and may allow reduction of corticosteroid doses. However, major side effects can occur, including liver disease, pneumonitis, bone-marrow suppression, and, after long-term use of azathioprine, malignancy. Patients should be fully informed of these potential side effects, and supervision of immunosuppressive therapy by a specialist is suggested.

Combinations of slow-acting drugs may be more effective that a single drug. Recent experience suggests that hydroxychloroquine, sulfasalazine, and methotrexate together are more effective that methotrexate alone or the other two together.

Exercise, Physiotherapy, and Surgery

Flexion contractures can be prevented and muscle strength restored most successfully after inflammation begins to subside. Joint splinting reduces local inflammation and may relieve severe local symptoms. Before acute inflammation is controlled, passive exercise to prevent contracture is given carefully and within the limits of pain. Active exercise (including walking and specific exercises for involved joints) to restore muscle mass and preserve the normal range of joint motion is important once the inflammation subsides but care to avoid fatiguing is important. Established flexion contractures may

require intensive exercise, serial splinting, or orthopedic measures. Orthopedic or athletic shoes with good heel and arch support can be modified using inserts to fit individual needs and frequently are helpful; metatarsal bars placed posteriorly to painful metatarsophalangeal joints decrease the pain of weight bearing.

Although synovectomy only temporarily relieves inflammation, arthroscopic or surgical synovectomy may help preserve joint function if drugs have been unsuccessful. Arthroplasty with prosthetic replacement of joint parts is indicated if joint damage severely limits function. Both total hip and knee replacements have been offered with great success, although prosthetic hips and knees cannot be expected to tolerate resumption of vigorous activities, they can restore mobility to impaired patients. Excision of subluxated painful metatarsophalangeal joints may greatly aid walking. Thumb fusions may be needed to provide stability for pinch and grasp. Individuals with RA are at risk for cervical subluxation at C1-2. This may cause cord compression as well as severe pain.

Surgical procedures always must be considered in terms of the total disease. Deformed hands and arms limit use of crutches and other assist devices during rehabilitation. By correcting an antalgic gait, hip surgery may provide relief for knee and foot pain. Reasonable objectives for each patient must be determined, and function usually is considered before appearance. Surgery may be safely performed while the disease is active. The goal is to promote independence as well as comfort.

SELECTED READINGS

Campbell R, Evans M, Tucker M, et al. Why don't patients do their exercises? Understanding non-compliance with physiotherapy in patients with osteoarthritis of the knee. *J Epidemiol Community Health* 2000; 55:132–138.

Hanninen O, Kaartinen K, Rauma AL, et al. Antioxidants in vegan diet and rheumatic disorders. *Toxicology* 2000;155:45–53.

Klippel JH, Dieppe PA. *Rheumatology*. St. Louis: Mosby–Year Book, 1998.

Moskowitz RW, Howell DS, Goldberg VM. *Osteoarthritis: Diagnosis and Medical/Surgical Management*. London: WB Saunders, 1992.

O'Reilly SC, Muir KR, Doherty M. Effectiveness of home exercise on pain and disability from osteoarthritis of the knee: a randomised controlled trial. *Ann Rheum Dis* 1999;58:15–19.

Palmer ML, Epler MF, Adams M, et al. *Fundamentals of Musculoskeletal Assessment Techniques*. Philadelphia: Lippincott Williams & Wilkins, 1998.

Rau R, Wassenberg S, Zeidler H. Low dose prednisolone therapy (LDPT) retards radiographically detectable destruction in early rheumatoid arthritis—preliminary results of a multicenter, randomized, parallel, double blind study. *Z Rheumatol* 2000;59(suppl 2):90–96.

CHAPTER 24

Fibromyalgia

José M. Hernández-García

Fibromyalgia is a condition of widespread pain and tender points, predominantly involving muscles. It is associated with persistent fatigue, sleep disturbances, and generalized stiffness. Frequently it is part of a syndrome that may involve multiple symptoms, such as headaches, irritable bowel and bladder, dysmenorrhea, cold sensitivity, Raynaud's phenomenon, restless legs, atypical patterns of numbness and paresthesias, exercise intolerance, and weakness.

These patients also may experience significant depression or anxiety that may worsen the symptoms and may be a result of having chronic pain.

The concept of fibromyalgia was introduced in the 1970s after the symptoms had been described under different names, including neurasthenia, fibrositis, fibromyositis, or chronic myofascial-pain syndrome. Yunus and colleagues suggested in 1981 to label the constellation of symptoms with the name of "Fibromyalgia," which was accepted in an editorial by the Journal of the American Medical Association in 1987. A Multicenter Criteria Committee was formed with the purpose of refining the definition. In 1990, the American College of Rheumatology published the classification criteria for fibromyalgia: widespread pain in the four body quadrants lasting 3 or more months, with the finding of at least 11 of 18 tender points on digital palpation (Fig. 24.1).

The committee recommended abolishing the previous distinction between primary, secondary, and concomitant fibromyalgia (for example, when diagnosed with systemic lupus erythematous or rheumatoid arthritis) because they could not determine differences in either symptoms or physical examination findings among them.

EPIDEMIOLOGY

The prevalence of fibromyalgia varies from 0.7% to 3.2% in the general adult population, according to health surveys in different countries. According to a U.S. study by Wolfe, among 3,006 persons at random, the estimated prevalence is 2%. It is more frequently found in women, who are affected 6 to 10 times more often than men. There are reports that describe the frequency of fibromyalgia in the primary-care setting from 2% to 6% and in rheumatology clinics it ranges from 10% to 20%.

The onset of symptoms is most frequently in patients in their 20s and 30s, with the highest prevalence in women above age 50, although it has been reported in all ages, including childhood. The prevalence in children varies from 1.2% to 6.2%, according to two studies available from school-children population.

There is little known about risk factors for fibromyalgia in the general population, although some studies describe a higher rate of fibromyalgia in family members. Physical as well as emotional trauma is involved in some cases. Infections and connective-tissue disorders also appear related to cases of fibromyalgia. Another common factor in these patients is a low level of aerobic fitness and physical conditioning.

PATHOPHYSIOLOGY

Fibromyalgia was thought initially to be a muscle disorder but over the last several years there is evidence of other abnormalities involving not only muscle but also the neuroendocrine system, sleep disturbances, autoimmune dysfunction, immune regulation, and more recently, abnormalities of the cerebral blood flow.

Muscle Abnormalities

Fibromyalgia was described initially as fibrositis and was considered for long time to be a muscle disorder, as muscle pain was the most significant symptom. Initial histological studies demonstrated some abnormalities, such as increased "moth eaten" and "ragged red" muscle

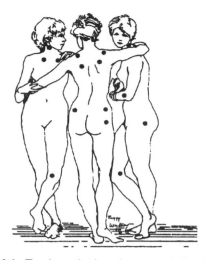

FIGURE 24.1. Tender point locations are shown for the 1990 American College of Rheumatology classification criteria for fibromyalgia. Pain is considered widespread when it is present in the left and right sides of the body and above and below the waist. In addition, axial skeletal pain (cervical spine or anterior chest or thoracic spine or low back) must be present. Shoulder and buttock pain is considered as pain for each involved side. "Low back" pain is considered lower-segment pain. Pain, on digital palpation, must be present in at least 11 of the following 18 tender point sites: occiput (bilateral, at the suboccipital muscle insertions), low cervical (bilateral, at the anterior aspects of the intertransverse spaces at C5–C7), trapezius (bilateral, at the midpoint of the upper border), supraspinatus (bilateral, at origins, above the scapula spine near the medial border), second rib (bilateral, at the second costochondral junctions, just lateral to the junctions on upper surfaces), lateral epicondyle (bilateral, 2 cm distal to the epicondyles), gluteal (bilateral, in upper outer quadrants of buttocks in anterior fold of muscle), greater trochanter (bilateral, posterior to the trochanteric prominence), and knee (bilateral, at the medial fat pad proximal to the joint line). Digital palpation should be performed with an approximate force of 4 kg. For a tender point to be considered "positive," the subject must state that the palpation was painful. "Tender" is not to be considered "painful." For classification purposes, patients will be said to have fibromyalgia if both criteria are satisfied. Widespread pain must have been present for at least 3 months. The presence of a second clinical disorder does not exclude the diagnosis of fibromyalgia. (Reproduced from Wolfe F, Smythe HA, Yunus MB, et al. The American College of Rheumatology 1990 criteria for the classification of fibromyalgia. *Arthritis Rheum* 1990;38: 160–172, with permission.)

fibers at sites of tenderness, like trapezius muscle. Other studies described abnormalities in muscle-energy metabolism, muscle-tissue oxygenation, and decrease in high-energy phosphate compounds at tender areas. From these findings, it was thought that local hypoxia could be responsible for the pain and weakness associated with fibromyalgia.

However, these studies have been criticized from the methodological point of view. More recently, and using techniques such as phosphorus-31 magnetic resonance spectroscopy, which allows the study of muscle metabolism *in vivo*, no differences were found between fibromyalgia patients and sedentary controls matched for aerobic fitness levels. This is particularly true when a significant number of fibromyalgia patients are below the average level of aerobic fitness, which may suggest that muscle deconditioning could be responsible for some of the abnormalities previously described.

In summary, well-controlled studies of muscle tissue in fibromyalgia have failed to demonstrate that this is the primary cause of the disorder.

Neuroendocrine Abnormalities

Several reports have suggested that there is evidence of primary adrenal insufficiency in fibromyalgia: there is an exaggerated adrenocorticotropin hormone (ACTH) response to corticotropin-releasing hormone (CRH) and a decrease production of cortisol in response to CRH or ACTH. There are also blunted diurnal variations in cortisol levels and low 24 hours urinary-free cortisol.

It also has been described as blunted secretion of TSH and thyroid hormones in response to TRH in patients with fibromyalgia. Furthermore, the growth hormone axis has been found to be hypoactive in patients with fibromyalgia. Insulinlike growth factor-1 (IGF-1) or somatomedin C has been shown to be low in fibromyalgia. (This is a way to measure the activity of growth hormone resulting from the inability to be measured because of its short half life.)

In summary, there is evidence of blunted stress response in fibromyalgia patients, although similar findings can be found in other disorders such as chronic-fatigue syndrome or posttraumatic stress disorder. These anomalies most likely are not the primary problem but may be responsible for symptoms as fatigue and mood disorders.

Sleep Abnormalities

One of the common complaints of patients with fibromyalgia is nonrestorative sleep.

They describe early-morning awakening, sometimes insomnia, and even when they sleep 6 to 8 hours, they describe stiffness, aching, or fatigue upon awakening.

There are several polysomnographic findings in patients with fibromyalgia, including lower amounts of slow-wave sleep, rapid eye movement sleep, and total sleep as well as a higher number of arousals and awakenings. Other characteristic finding include α waves into all stages of nonrapid eye movement sleep, and this has been correlated with both experiencing less restorative sleep, when compared with healthy individuals, and an increase in the pain scores.

Neurotransmitters in Fibromyalgia

The process of pain transmission is thought to be altered in fibromyalgia. Pain perception is normal but there is a decrease in pain tolerance, which may be related to alterations of central nociceptive mechanisms, and perhaps in different transmitters and neuromodulators that are responsible for pain amplification in fibromyalgia. The substances that are antinociceptive act as inhibitory neurotransmitters, including serotonin, norepinephrine, and endogenous opioids.

Among the neurotransmitters, serotonin has been found to be low in patients with fibromyalgia. The role of serotonin as a neurotransmitter is to inhibit the release of substance P in the afferent neurons of the spinal cord that transmit signals from peripheral receptors. Substance P (S.P.) has been found to be elevated in the cerebrospinal fluid of fibromyalgia patients, although it also has been measured normal in serum and urine. S.P. is released by A-δ and C fibers into laminae I, V, and II of the spinal cord dorsal horn. The mechanism of action of S.P. is not clear but it seems to facilitate activation of nociceptors.

Functional Brain Activity Studies

There is a characteristic decrease of regional cerebral blood flow (rCBF) in the caudate nucleus of patients with fibromyalgia. In contrast, patients with chronic pain showed consistently a decrease of rCBF in the thalamus, as described in studies using single photon-emission computed tomography (SPECT) and positron-emission tomography (PET).

When patients with fibromyalgia were exposed to an acute-pain stimulus, they had low activation of the thalamus, contrary to healthy subjects, who experienced increases in rCBF. The significance of this, as described by the authors, is probably an excessive nociceptive input that is transmitted to the brain by spinal-horn neurons, which produce a decrease in thalamic and caudate rCBF and may be responsible for the abnormal pain perceptions of patients with fibromyalgia.

DIAGNOSIS

The ACR criteria, since its publication in 1990, are used by most clinicians to diagnose fibromyalgia. More recently, in the Vancouver Consensus Report, new recommendations were made that included the diagnosis of fibromyalgia with less than the required number of tender points, as long as the patients had other symptoms (e.g., sleep disturbance, fatigue, stiffness, etc.) or with tenderness at sites different from the ACR criteria.

Most patients experience diurnal and seasonal variations of the symptoms. Typically, the symptoms are worse during cold or damp weather, at the beginning and the end of the day, and during periods of emotional distress.

In a prospective U.S. study, most fibromyalgia patients had symptoms that persisted for as long as 15 years after onset.

Physical examination in patients with fibromyalgia is significant for a normal neurological exam, and it shows no signs of muscle weakness, despite the patient's subjective description of it. Joint examination also is normal, except for signs secondary to a related condition. There may be muscle spasms and diffuse soft-tissue swelling.

Laboratory evaluation of complete blood count, chemistry profile, and urinalysis usually is normal. There may be unspecific findings. Other laboratory testing like autoimmune serologies, thyroid function, or creatine phosphokinase also are normal.

Fibromyalgia is a syndrome that can be seen in the absence or presence of other conditions such as rheumatoid arthritis or systemic lupus erythematosus, which may present with alterations in laboratory findings.

Fibromyalgia can be confused with regional myofascial-pain syndrome. These patients have localized pain distribution and a limited number of tender points. They usually are responsive to specific myofascial therapy. Occasionally, these patients develop a typical fibromyalgia syndrome.

Other conditions that may mimic fibromyalgia are hypothyroidism, widespread malignancy, polymyalgia rheumatica, osteomalacia, generalized osteoarthritis, early Parkinson's disease, connective-tissue disease, or chronic-fatigue syndrome.

There are reports that relate fibromyalgia to various infectious disorders, including coxsackievirus, parvovirus, and human immunodeficiency virus, although there is no evidence that these agents are responsible for the symptoms of fibromyalgia.

TREATMENT

Fibromyalgia patients must be told that it is a chronic disorder, which requires long-term and usually multidisciplinary treatment, including pharmacological, as well as nonpharmacological approach, such as exercise and cognitive-behavioral interventions.

Pharmacological Treatment

Among all the medications used in patients with fibromyalgia, there are only few that have been described to be of some benefit. Amitriptyline (Elavil, Zeneca Pharmaceuticals, Wilmington, DE, U.S.A.) was found to be better than placebo both in reduction of pain, as well as in improvement in sleep quality and fatigue in several studies, although these effects tend to diminish over time. Fluoxetine (Prozac, Dista Products Company, Indianapolis, IN, U.S.A.) is effective in fibromyalgia patients, but only when used with cyclobenzaprine (Flexeril, Merck &

Co., Inc., West Point, PA, U.S.A.), according to another study. Furthermore, fluoxetine (20 mg) used with amitriptyline (25 mg) may be more beneficial than when used alone. Reports with other selective serotonin reuptake inhibitors did not find the same improvement.

The only anxiolytic found to be beneficial in is alprazolam (Xanax, Pharmacia & Upjohn Company, Bridgewater, NJ, U.S.A.), when used in combination with ibuprofen (Motrin, McNeil Consumer Products Company, Fort Washington, PA, U.S.A.), which is the only NSAID proven to be effective in patients with fibromyalgia.

Interestingly, intravenous lidocaine (starting with 250 mg and increasing by 50 mg daily for 6 days) was shown to improve levels of pain and mood scores for 30 days.

Other medications used frequently in patients with fibromyalgia but without evidence of benefit are opioids and prednisone. Another common practice, but without support, is the use of trigger-point injections with local anesthetics and/or corticosteroids, or the use of topical capsaicin.

Growth hormone (GH) therapy has been evaluated in patients with low levels of IGF-1, and compared to placebo was found to improve myalgic scores and quality-of-life ratings over a 9-month period.

Nonpharmacological Treatments

Nonmedicinal approaches to fibromyalgia have included exercises, physical therapy, and cognitive-behavioral techniques, although it is more difficult to perform well-controlled studies with these techniques. When examining cognitive-behavioral interventions such as electromyogram biofeedback, relaxation training, and training in cognitive coping strategies, there was no superior improvement than in patients treated with attention-placebo techniques.

But what is more significant, among studies based on exercise programs, a 20-week cardiovascular-fitness training program was more effective than a program based on flexibility exercises in fibromyalgia patients.

Other techniques like hypnotherapy and frontal electromyogram biofeedback have produced some positive results, although the effectiveness still is unclear.

Despite the good results with some of the treatments described above, finding a therapy with benefit for patients with fibromyalgia often is an elusive goal.

Working with patients with a chronic disorder can be frustrating, but improvement in function is an attainable goal. Diminution in symptoms is a triumph for both the patient and the practitioner.

SELECTED READINGS

Clauw DJ. The pathogenesis of chronic pain and fatigue syndrome. *Med Hypotheses* 1995;44:369–378.

Fibromyalgia Symposium. *Am J Med Sci* 1998;315:6.

Jacobsen S, Lund B, Danneskiod-Samsoe D. Proceedings from the second world congress on myofascial pain and fibromyalgia. *J Musculoskeletal Pain* 1993;1:3–4.

Simms RW. The Fibromyalgia Syndrome. *Arthritis Care Research* 1996;9:3 15–328.

Wallace D. The Fibromyalgia Syndrome. *Ann Med* 1997;29:9–21.

Wolfe F. The fibromyalgia syndrome: a consensus report on fibromyalgia and disability. *J Rheumatol* 1996;23:534–539.

Wolfe F, Smythe HA, Yunus MB, et al. The American College of Rheumatology 1990 criteria for the classification of fibromyalgia. *Arthritis Rheum* 1990;38:160–172.

CHAPTER 25

Myofascial Syndrome

John C. Makrides

Since the dawn of antiquity, mankind has been at the mercy of pain, a perception inherent in the spectrum of cognition. Ancient healers discovered that techniques like massage could reduce the suffering of certain painful states. Myofascial syndrome or MPS is a painful condition in which distinct trigger point (TP) areas, generally within muscles or fasciae, become abnormally active and produce local and referred pain. Diagnosis and treatment of myofascial pain syndrome (MPS) has advanced only slightly beyond the boundaries of knowledge in traditional medicine. MPS can affect all ages, commonly increases with age, and peaks during the "middle years." It still is not understood what type of patient is susceptible to MPS. As the patient ages with decreasing activity, muscle stiffness and decreased range of motion (ROM) often are noted secondary to previously undetected TPs. With today's societal fascination with herbal remedies and the increasing popularity in "nontraditional" therapies, the physician is faced with the daunting task of unraveling the mysteries of MPS in the 21st century.

In the prevailing preoccupation in the quest for pathology of a more technologically demonstrable nature, the condition often is initially overlooked. At present, no blood markers are available for use by a physician, and the diagnosis of myofascial syndrome is a clinical one often mired in a quagmire of other patient complaints. Myofascial TP pain is most frequently muscle in origin with tender nodules and taut bands (Table 25.1). The

TABLE 25.1. *Clinical Characteristics of Myofascial Trigger Points*

Localized tenderness in a taut band of muscle
Local twitch response to the contracted taut band
Referred pain
Symmetry of pain or trigger points
Restricted movement at muscle or nearby joint
Weakness
Autonomic dysfunction

trapezius muscle is one of the most commonly affected muscles in MPS; however, TPs also have been found in skin, scars, tendons, ligaments, and even periosteum.

In the work-up of back pain, a physician might mentally compose a differential diagnosis, including nerve-root compression, herniated disc, inflammatory myopathies, obstructive or inflammatory abdominal conditions, rheumatoid arthritis, ankylosis, spondylosis, idiopathic scoliosis, osteoporosis, or dissecting aortic aneurysms. Skeletal abnormalities such as leg-length discrepancy, a small hemi-pelvis, or scoliosis should be noted on the physical examination. Systemic disease also is a possibility, and the patient should be investigated for vitamin B deficiencies, diminished thyroid function, low calcium, hypoglycemia, chronic bacterial infection, or undo emotional stress. Malignancy also should be considered as a precipitating factor in MPS. The patient may present to a pain clinic as a referral from numerous specialists without a definitive diagnosis, but with a "laundry list" of treatments. In the diagnosis of myofascial pain, the importance of the history and physical (H/P), palpation of taut band, and identification of a TP with referred pain cannot be overemphasized (Table 25.1). When palpating a trigger point and the pain is referred elsewhere, an important clue to the diagnosis has been made (Figs. 25.1–25.3). Inconsistencies even of well-trained examiners in the diagnosis of myofascial pain have been noted. As a result, several authors have proposed essential criteria for myofascial TPs (Table 25.2). The combination of spot tenderness in a palpable muscle band and recognition of referred pain are minimal acceptable criteria for the diagnosis of a myofascial TP.

MPS must not be confused with fibromyalgia. These two syndromes are very different although the two often can overlap clinically (Table 25.3). The American College of Rheumatology has established classification criteria for fibromyalgia; furthermore, these criteria must be adhered to and not confused with MPS. There are no

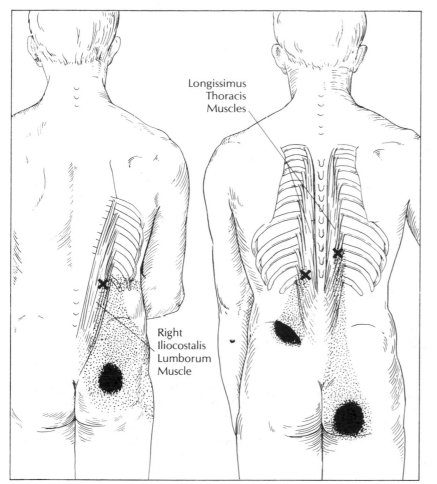

FIG. 25.1. Referred-pain patterns associated with trigger points (*Xs*) at different levels of the superficial paraspinal muscles are shown. The essential reference zones are depicted in *solid black* and the spillover areas in *stippled black*.

definable abnormalities of skeletal muscles yet known as a "cause" of fibromyalgia; however, myofascial TPs are a readily discernible muscular dysfunction that could lead to spinal-cord level changes with a resultant chronic-pain syndrome. Approximately 20% of myofascial pain patients also have fibromyalgia, and approximately 70% of patients with fibromyalgia also have myofascial TPs.

Myofascial TPs could be defined as hyperexcitable foci in skeletal muscle or fascia. Over the years, there have been numerous synonyms for this syndrome: interstitial myofibrositis, myalgic spots, muscular rheumatism, myogelosis, muscle hardenings, and myofascial pain-dysfunction syndrome. A condition termed "posttraumatic hyperirritability syndrome" refers to a patient experiencing myofascial pain, with sensory nervous-system irritability and enhanced TP associated pain after-physical trauma. This patient experiences and complains of constant pain, worsened by what would be considered nonnoxious stimuli.

Unfortunately, there is no specific laboratory test to definitively diagnose MPS. X-rays are useful for ruling out other pathologies. Electromyograms generally are normal in uncomplicated MPSs. However, nerve-root compression syndromes yielding abnormal electromyogram findings may activate a TP and cause pain long after the compression has been relieved—a sequence thought to be a common source of the "postlaminectomy syndrome." The physiologic mechanisms underlying the myofascial syndrome are not entirely understood. No consistent anatomical change has been identified using light microscopy, electron microscopy, or histochemistry. No inflammatory response has been noted yet at the TP site, and prostaglandins do not mediate TP pain. Thus, blocking the cyclooxygenase pathway would be of little benefit for TP pain, and nonsteroidal antiinflammatory drugs merely provide general analgesia in the treatment of myofascial pain. It is yet unclear how calcium, actin-myosin, troponin, or the ATP-dependent calcium pump interact at the level of the TP. Is the contracted taut muscle band the result of depleted adenosine triphosphate (ATP) stores? It is postulated that local physiologic changes, such as muscle tension and vasoconstriction produce local ischemia (decreases ATP) or increased vascular permeability. This, in turn, causes derangement of the immediate extracellular environment, which increases the sensitivity or activity of the nociceptive

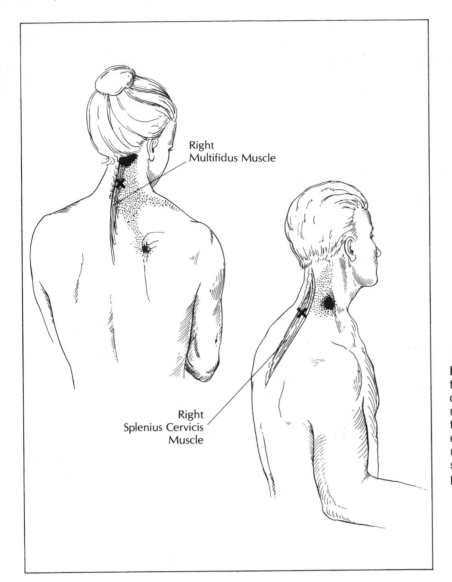

Right
Multifidus Muscle

Right
Splenius Cervicis
Muscle

FIG. 25.2. Trigger point (*X*) above the base of the neck (left) is the most common posterior–cervical location and often leads to entrapment of the greater occipital nerve. Pain and tenderness are referred upward to the suboccipital region and sometimes downward to the upper vertebral border of the scapula. Lower splenius cervicis trigger point (right) refers pain to the angle of the neck.

releases of algesic, or pain-producing agents (such as bradykinins). Next, an increase in sympathetic activity could occur, thereby perpetuating the painful TP cycle. It is sometimes noted, but not known why temperature differences of a TP-affected extremity can occur. Are sympathetically mediated components present? Electromyography studies describe spontaneous electrical TP activity when the remainder of a muscle remains quiescent. Neuromuscular blocking agents abolish voluntary muscle activity but not the spontaneous TP activity. Specific sympathetic blocking agents such as phentolamine have been shown to abolish the TP electrical activity but not the voluntary muscle activity. Does norepinephrine play a role in muscle-spindle activity, because the muscle-spindle fibers are sympathetically mediated? It is thought that a single event may initiate a trigger point and that subsequent conditions perpetuate it: both systemic and mechanical stresses may be the underlying factors.

The most prominent feature of MPS is, of course, pain (Table 25.1, Figs. 25.1–25.3). In addition, patients often complain of stiffness (usually in the morning), fatigue, decreased ROM, weakness, and increased sensitivity to cold. The weakness without muscle atrophy that commonly occurs in patients with myofascial pain is by an unknown mechanism. Myofascial TPs frequently affect symmetrical muscle groups. It is unclear how and why with even a "single" TP, this symmetrical pattern of pain occurs in muscle groups, and sometimes affects different muscles. Are there TPs that we cannot detect? Secondary psychological reactions, such as depression and disturbances in sleep patterns, further muddle the diagnosis. If a myofascial syndrome is of extremely long duration, other areas of the body may become involved (as in a pelvic-pain syndrome).

Trigger points are thought to be either active or latent. An active TP is tender and has a spontaneous painlike component, and upon direct compression, always causes

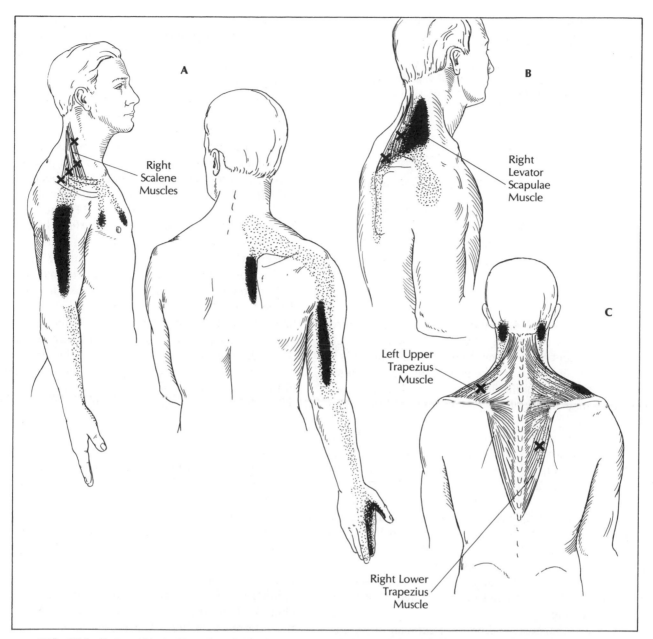

FIG. 25.3. Referred pain from the trigger points (*Xs*) in right scalene muscles **(A)** extends down the front and back of the arm (over the biceps and triceps). Pain skips the elbow and reappears in the radial side of the forearm, the thumb, and the index finger. Other reference zones are in the back and chest. Trigger points in right levator scapulae muscle **(B)** produce consolidated pain pattern shown. Trigger points in left upper trapezius and right lower trapezius refer pain ipsilaterally **(C)**.

TABLE 25.2. *Typical Differences Between Myofascial Trigger Point Syndrome and Fibromyalgia*

Myofascial (TP)	Fibromyalgia
Male:female @ 1:1	Male:female @ 1:7
TPs	Tender areas/points
Tense, taut muscle bands	Soft "doughy" muscle
Decreased ROM	Increased ROM
Focal tenderness	Diffuse tenderness
Local-referred pain	General malaise, widespread pain
"Immediate" response to TP injection	Poor response to injection of TP

ROM, range of motion; TP, trigger point.

referred pain elsewhere in the body (Figs. 25.1–25.3). Additionally, the muscle demonstrates a taut band, decreased ROM and reduced strength, with possible referred autonomic phenomena (Tables 25.1, 25.2). Active TPs mediate a local twitch response of muscle fibers when adequately stimulated. A latent TP also shows muscular evidence of those changes but with only a local twitch response. Latent myofascial TPs do not present with spontaneous pain, like active TPs do; however, they are painful when palpated, and may have all the other characteristics of active TPs. A latent TP also is located within a taut muscle band, increases muscle ten-

TABLE 25.3. *Recommended Criteria for Myofascial Trigger Point Identification*

Essential criteria
  Palpable, taut muscle band (if accessible)
  Intense spot tenderness of a nodule within taut band
  Patient recognition of current pain complaint upon
    pressure on nodule (active TP)
  Painful limit to full stretch ROM
Confirmatory observations
  Visual/tactile identification of local twitch response
  Twitch response elicited by needle penetration of tender
    nodule
  Pain or altered sensation in distribution expected from a
    TP in that muscle
  EMG spontaneous electrical activity in the tender nodule
    of a taut band (active locus)

EMG, electromyogram; ROM, range of motion; TP, trigger point.

sion, and restricts ROM. Leaving a muscle in the "shortened" position can activate a latent to an active TP. Palpation of a latent TP may cause no referred pain—this is sometimes referred to as a tender point. Tender points are not TPs. Tender points have no referred pain component and may be found in patients with fibromyalgia (Table 25.3).

The initiating event in the formation of TPs is believed to be an acute strain caused by a sudden overload or over stretching of muscle. With adequate rest, and in the absence of perpetuating factors, and active TP may spontaneously revert to a latent state. It often repairs itself spontaneously if demands are sufficiently reduced, but immobilization is undesirable. Pain symptoms may disappear, but occasional reactivation of the TP by exceeding the muscle's tolerance may explain the history of recurrent episodes of the same pain persisting over several years. On the other hand, once activated, a TP can be self-perpetuating.

The key to diagnosis and proper treatment of myofascial syndrome is identification of the TPs (Tables 25.1, 25.2). A TP is not necessarily where all the pain is. The pattern of referred pain does not typically follow normal peripheral nerve or dermatomal pathways. A muscle that contains a TP contains taut fibers that can be identified as a palpable band that tightens and shortens the muscle—this has sometimes been termed a "ropiness" or "nodularity" of the muscle. Suspect muscles should be compared with the contralateral muscle group, because of the symmetrical pattern of muscle involvement often found in MPS. The affected muscle will exhibit decreased ROM and decreased strength. When a TP is present, a brisk rolling of the taut band with one's fingers can stimulate a local twitch response. TPs and taut bands are best appreciated when the examiner's fingertips move perpendicular to muscle fibers. The local twitch response is considered to be unequivocal evidence of a myofascial

syndrome (Tables 25.1, 25.2). Placement of a needle within the TP, or application of sustained pressure generally will evoke its referred pain pattern. Examination should be conducted with muscles in both the relaxed and stretched positions.

Proper treatment generally involves inactivation of the TP, with resultant return of muscle strength and full ROM. Eliminating the TP muscle focus relieves the TP pain. Long-lasting relief also requires resolution of the perpetuating factors as well as visits to a physical therapist. Different treatment sequences have been proposed and utilized. Muscle stretching, passive massage, physical therapy, and digital pressure on TPs should initially be tried to alleviate the discomfort. Heat, biofeedback, and ultrasound vibrations all have been tried with varied success. One method is the passive-muscle stretch with application of a vapor-coolant spray. Alternatively, some authors recommend immediate, precise injection of a TP with dry needling, saline, or a local anesthetic. Perhaps the least-invasive method is an attempt to deactivate a superficial TP by direct compression similar to that used in acupressure or shiatsu. Adjunctive modalities then could include deep massage, low-intensity ultrasound, electrical stimulation, intermittent cervical or lumbar traction, and relaxation training (biofeedback).

The spray and stretch method has gained popularity because of its simplicity, and can be used to treat several TPs at one time. A topical, vaporous coolant is applied to prevent muscle reflex responses, and the muscle then is passively stretched through its entire ROM. The stretching can be envisioned as "pulling out" the taut fibers: the muscle must be relaxed, and the stretching must be passive (without use of sudden force). A fluoromethane spray consisting of 15% dichlorodifluoromethane and 85% trichloromonofluoromethane is applied in several parallel sweeps, initially to cover the skin overlying the affected muscle and then to include the referred pain area. The muscle then is firmly but passively brought through its full ROM. The spray-and-stretch treatment generally is followed by the application of moist heat, and the muscle then is actively moved through its ROM. Ultrasound treatments could be tried at this time.

Injection of trigger points requires dexterity. The target for injection (TP) is the most tender spot within the taut, palpable band. TP injection with a local anesthetic (or saline), and even "simple" mechanical manipulation by a needle in the TP (dry needling) are the most effective myofascial TP treatment modalities. Generally, the needle penetration of an active TP will elicit a local, brief twitch response accompanied by both local and referred pain. Dry needling or normal saline injections can be extremely painful and thus potentially detrimental. A near miss of the TP might actually aggravate the condition. Typically, 25- or 30-guage needles are used.

Some clinicians advocate making several passes of the needle through the TP in order to "break up" the muscle fibers within it even if one injects solution. It is unclear if it is the manipulation of the needle itself, the injection of a fluid, or the injection with needle manipulation of a TP that offer the best results for relief of pain. Acupuncture needles can and have been used for mechanical TP manipulation; however, acupuncture points must not be confused with myofascial TPs. "Classical" acupuncture points are not myofascial TPs. Acupuncturists often can include TP needling in their treatments, and most are aware of TP-associated pain. Some proponents of local anesthetic solutions advocate the use of procaine because its vasodilatory (antiis-chemic) properties outlast its anesthetic action. Injection of 0.5 to 2 mL of 0.5% procaine per TP generally is effective; however, 0.25% bupivacaine, 1% and 2% lidocaine, and other local anesthetics have been used with success. Depo-steroids are sometimes added to the solution but with questioned efficacy. Myofascial pain patients with fibromyalgia who then have TPs treated with injections showed a delayed to poor response as compared to patients who solely had MPS without fibromyalgia.

In conclusion, when a patient presents with back pain or shoulder pain, one must not overlook the possibility of MPS as a potential source of the aggravated state. Even the most skilled and experienced examiners can overlook the condition. A thorough history and physical is paramount, and one must eliminate both skeletal, biochemical, and systemic possibilities for the pain condition. When palpated, TPs with referred pain are the *sine qua non* for MPS. The TP is the "source" of pain, and its precise location and its injection or mechanical manipulation will eliminate the pain focus. Yes, not all pain is myofascial pain. If TPs are found and then treated, both the patient and caregiver will be gratified with the almost instantaneous relief; however, the importance of eliminating perpetuating factors is obvious. If the underlying factors creating the myofascial TP condition are not alleviated, frequent visits to the caregiver are inevitable, and a chronic pain state could ensue.

CASE REPORTS

Typical cases might present as follows:

Patient 1

A 63-year-old woman had a 4-month history of non-radicular, low-back discomfort. She recalled that onset occurred when she spent a week caring for her grandchildren. One afternoon, after having scrubbed the kitchen floor, she felt what she believed to be a muscle spasm in her right lower back. She continued her daily activities. Nightly warm soaks did not significantly relieve her discomfort. Her primary physician suggested bed rest and aspirin. That regimen did not produce a major change in her symptomatology, and she had x-rays taken. The x-rays suggested diffuse osteoarthritic changes in her lumbosacral spine without obvious hip pathology. Her discomfort persisted, and when she came to the pain center, she described low-back discomfort with additional pain over her right iliac crest and greater trochanter. Walking, rising from a sitting position, twisting of her torso, spine flexion and extension, and coughing exacerbated her pain. Examination revealed extreme tenderness at points above her right iliac crest and below her 12th rib. With the patient lying at her right side, her right arm elevated above her head to elevate the rib cage, and her pelvis tilted to depress the iliac crest, superficial TPs were easily identified within the quadratus lumborum muscle. After marking the TPs with a felt-tip pen, the skin surface was cleaned with a sterile skin-preparatory solution. The TPs were injected with 1 mL of 0.5% procaine using a 30-guage needle, single-pass technique. Hot packs were applied to the area, and ROM maneuvers were performed. The patient obtained complete relief. Physical therapy training ensued over the next several weeks, and she was able to resume normal activities. No further follow-ups were necessary.

Patient 2

A 43-year-old male executive had a 3-month history of left-sided occipital headaches with neck stiffness. He had been involved in a minor motor-vehicle accident without serious sequelae 1 month prior to his symptoms. Cervical-imaging studies and cranial CT had not demonstrated a visible etiology for his persistent pain. No changes in hearing or vision were reported, and he did not have a history of migraine headaches. A soft cervical collar was used intermittently but abandoned because he felt it offered him no relief, and that it limited his ability to work at his office. He had been referred to your office by a neurosurgeon for consideration of a greater occipital nerve block (presumed occipital neuralgia). Prior to visiting your office, he had made visits to a chiropractor, yoga instructor, and herbalist. He eliminated coffee from his diet, has been drinking willow-bark tea, and taking St. John's Wort each day for the last 2 months without relief. He denied bleeding problems. He presents to you with a list of what he feels are potential diagnoses that he had obtained from various searches on the internet and from a fibromyalgia web site. On examination, he was found to have limited extension, flexion, and rotation of his neck; furthermore, he was found to have muscle bands with focal points of tenderness within the superior aspect of the trapezius muscle as well as above the base of the neck (to the right and left of C5). Palpation at these points produced intense focal pain as well as worsened the occipital distribution of his present pain. These were thought to be TPs, and their locations were marked with a felt-tip pen. Direct digital pressure to the points of tenderness combined with a passive neck-flexion technique were initially tried, but with limited relief. A vapor-coolant then was sprayed on the areas of pain, and the same passive neck-flexion technique used, but with minimal effect. Finally, while still noting the pen markings of the TPs, the TP areas were cleaned with a sterile skin-preparatory solution swab. A 30-gauge needle was used to inject 2 mL of 0.25% bupivacaine into each TP (several passes with the needle also were made at each TP after injection). The patient reported immediate relief of his symptoms. Visits to a physical therapist were scheduled for neck flexion-extension techniques. At his 6-week follow-up, he returned to the clinic for one more TP injection, and has not returned to the clinic since that time.

SELECTED READINGS

Bennett RM. Contribution of muscle to the generation of fibromyalgia symptomatology. *J Musc Pain* 1996;4:35–39.

Gerwin R. *Ballier's Clinical Rheumatology*, 1994;8.

Gerwin RD. 96 Subjects examined for both fibromyalgia and myofascial pain. *J Musc Skeletal Pain* 1995;3(suppl 1):A121.

Gerwin RD, Shannon S, Hong CZ, et al. Inter-rater reliability in myofascial trigger point examination. *Pain* 1997;69:65–73.

Hong C-Z. Persistence of local twitch response with loss of conduction to and from the spinal cord. *Arch Phys Med and Rehab* 1994;75:12–16.

Hong C-Z, Hsueh TC. Difference in pain relief after trigger point injections in myofascial pain patients with and without fibromyalgia. *Arch Phys Med Rehab* 1996;77:1161–1166.

Hong C. Lidocaine injection verses dry needling trigger points: the importance of the local twitch response. *Am J Phys Med Rehab* 1994;73:256–263.

Simons D, Travell J, Simons L. *Travell & Simon's Myofascial Pain and Dysfunction, The Trigger Point Manual*, vol. 1, 2. 2nd ed. Philadelphia: Williams & Wilkins, 1999.

Wolfe F, Smythe HA, Yunus MB, et al. American College of Rheumatology criteria for the classification of fibromyalgia: report of the Multicenter Criteria Committee. *Arthritis Rheum* 1990;33:160–172.

CHAPTER 26

Cancer Pain

Stephanie Cooper Kochhar

The challenge of treating cancer pain is evident. Statistics support cancer's widespread effects and associated pain. Each year, there are millions of new cases of cancer diagnosed worldwide. It is estimated that one third of cancer patients in active treatment will have pain. With disease progression, 60% to 90% of cancer patients with advanced disease will have pain. It is well known that cancer pain is undertreated but it is believed that cancer pain can be controlled in up to 90% of cases. Pain management has become a prominent focus for many physicians as pharmacological and invasive treatments for cancer pain continue to evolve.

CAUSES OF CANCER PAIN

Treatment of cancer pain begins with determining the etiology of the pain. Obtaining a complete history of the patient's pain complaint accompanied by a careful medical and neurological exam is of extreme importance. A patient's description of the type of pain may assist in the diagnosis or may categorize the pain into a cancer-pain syndrome caused by therapy or the tumor itself (Table 26.1). The types of pain are classified as nociceptive (somatic and visceral) and neuropathic. Nociceptive, somatic bone pain is the most common type of cancer pain. Somatic nociceptors are activated in cutaneous and/or deep tissues and is of myofascial or musculoskeletal origin. It can be caused by metastasis to bone or a postsurgical incision. Patients may describe the pain as aching, well-localized, sharp, gnawing or dull. Visceral pain nociceptors are activated by infiltration, compression, extension, or stretching of sympathetically mediated organs in the abdomen, pelvis, or thorax. The third most common pain complaint is from tumor infiltration of hollow viscus. Visceral pain (i.e., pancreatic cancer) is described as crampy, colicky, less well-localized, vague, aching, deep, dragging, squeezing, dull, or pressure pain. Neuropathic pain nociceptors are activated by nerve damage secondary to chemical injury, tumor compression, or infiltration of a component of the nervous system such as peripheral nerves or the spinal cord. Tumor infiltration of nerve is the second most common cancer pain complaint. Neuropathic cancer pain syndromes include chemotherapy-induced peripheral neuropathy and brachial or lum-

TABLE 26.1. *Common Cancer Pain Syndromes*

Postsurgical
   Thoracotomy
   Mastectomy
   Neck disection
   Amputation-phantom limb pain
   Nephrectomy
Post chemotherapy
   Polyneuritis
   Mucositis/pharyngitis/esophagitis
   Peripheral neuropathy
Post radiation
   Neuritis
   Osteoradionecrosis
   Plexopathies
   Enteritis/mucositis
Metastasis: Bone
   Vertebral body
   Base of skull
   Pelvis
   Long bones
   Multiple sites
Direct tumor involvement: Viscera
   Obstruction causing distention of hollow viscus
   Obstruction of duct of solid viscus
   Rapid tumor growth in solid viscus
Direct tumor involvement: Nerves/plexus/spinal cord
   Peripheral neuropathy
   Plexopathies (cervical/brachial/lumbosacral)
   Complex regional pain syndrome
   Leptomeningial carcinomatosis
   Epidural spinal cord compression
Direct tumor involvement: Blood vessels
   Necrosis
   Ulceration of mucous membrane (mucositis)

Modified from Bonica JJ, *The Management of Pain,* Vol II, Philadelphia: Lea & Febiger, 1990.

bosacral plexopathy. This type of pain may be described as burning, itching, dysesthetic, numbness, tingling, pressure, shooting, electrical shocklike, lancinating, or squeezing. Cancer patients may have one or a combination of the above-mentioned pain types. Most cancer patients have somatic and visceral pain and 15% to 20% may have neuropathic pain.

Radiographic studies can be useful in determining the etiology. Plain films or conventional radiographs are the easiest and most cost-effective in demonstrating the overall picture and showing the structural alignment and compression fractures. However, tumor detection may require a 40% to 60% change in bone density while pain can be present with less pathology. Bone scan is widely used for detection of bony metastasis. Myelography is effective in showing the components of the spinal canal including the spinal cord and nerve roots. A computed tomography (CT) following a myelogram is helpful in visualizing the spinal-canal contents and surrounding tissues. CT is very effective in visualizing bony structures, disc herniations, and with intravenous (i.v.) dye vascular structures as well. Magnetic resonance imaging (MRI) has greater tissue contrast resolution and is better for visualizing multiple tissue types especially brain, spine and contents, bone, and most of the musculoskeletal system. MRI may demonstrate smaller abnormalities as compared to CT. In the past, MRI's limitation has been due to claustrophobia of the patient, however, now there are open MRI scanners to assist with this problem. Once the etiology of the pain has been determined, a well-directed, multidisciplinary pain management plan may be initiated.

MANAGEMENT OF PAIN

Pain is subjective but in cancer patients it most often means a pathological process. Therefore, assessment and reassessment is necessary to rule out reoccurrence or advancement of disease. Primary goals of cancer pain management are to provide adequate pain relief within a reasonable amount of time with minimal side effects and to ensure that patients can tolerate their anticancer therapy. These goals also would include maintenance of pain control in the simplest and least invasive manner possible so that patients would be able to function during the remainder of their life and die relatively pain free.

Pain management of the patient as a whole person would be most effective under the direction of a multidisciplinary team. Important members would include internist, oncologist, surgeon, anesthesiologist, neurologist, psychiatrist or psychologist, nurses, physiatrist, physical therapist, social worker, spiritual counselor, family, and possibly hospice. Psychiatrist and/or psychologists are valuable in giving the patient mental tools to help combat the pain such as: guided imagery, biofeedback, and behavioral modification. They also could help the patient with their inevitable depression as they deal with pain, suffering, and possible death.

An ideal plan would be generated utilizing anticancer therapy to limit or eliminate the neoplasm or cause of the pain coupled with specific treatment of the pain. Anticancer therapy includes radiation, chemotherapy, radioisotope therapy, surgery, and endocrine therapy. Should the neoplasm persist or be widely metastasized, neuroablative techniques to interrupt the pain pathways, therapeutic nerve blocks, pharmacologic therapy, and intraspinal narcotics may remain viable alternatives.

PHARMACOLOGIC THERAPY

Pharmacologic goals include achieving adequate pain control within a reasonable time frame and with minimal side effects. The World Health Organization (WHO) in addition to many other organizations have published guidelines to assist in the treatment of cancer pain. Therapy must always be individualized, however, the WHO guidelines have been tested and shown to be effective for the pharmacologic control of cancer pain in 71% to 75% of patients studied. Under these guidelines, medications used for pain control have been classified as nonopiate, opiate, and adjuvants. Choice of medication will depend on the individual patient's severity of pain and type of pain. Each type of pain responds differently to medical management.

The first line of medications for mild cancer pain includes nonopiates. Nonopiate medications such as nonsteroidal antiinflammatory drugs (NSAIDs) and acetaminophen are most beneficial for pain of musculoskeletal or bone origin and of inflammatory nature. The analgesic effects of NSAIDs are believed to be from the inhibition of prostaglandin synthesis. The use of NSAIDs is limited by a ceiling effect in which above a certain dose, a patient will not receive any further pain relief. NSAIDs are very useful as coanalgesics with their synergistic, opioid-sparing properties. Ketorolac has provided an intramuscular and intravenous route for the administration of NSAIDs and has been shown to give effective pain relief comparable to morphine. Contraindications of NSAIDs in patients with histories revealing gastrointestinal bleeding or coagulopathies may be avoided by the use of the new Cox-2 inhibitors.

Adjuvants may be added for certain types of pain problems (Table 26.2). Adjuvants are directed towards analgesia and relief from side effects of therapy and medications. Neuropathic pain can be treated with anticonvulsants, antidepressants, oral and cutaneous local anesthetics, clonidine, baclofen, and NMDA antagonists. Somatic bone pain tends to respond well to radiation, corticosteroids and NSAIDS but also can be treated with bisphosphonates (pamidronate) and calcitonin. Bisphosphonates and calcitonin are believed to have their effects by

TABLE 26.2. Indications for Adjuvant Therapy

Adjuvant Medication	Indication
Anticonvulsants	Neuropathic pain
Gabapentin	
Carbamazepine	
Valporic acid	
Phenytoin	
Antidepressants	Neuropathic pain
Amytriptyline	
Nortriptyline	
Desiprimine	
Imipramine	
Antiarrhythmics/membrane stabilizers	Neuropathic pain
Lidocaine	
Mexilitine	
Clonidine	Neuropathic pain
Baclofen	Neuropathic pain/muscle relaxation
Corticosteroids	Bone pain
Dexamethasone	Antiinflammatory
Methylprednisolone	Mood elevation
	Antiemetic/appetite stimulation
Bisphosphonates	Bone pain
Pamidronate	
Calcitonin	Bone pain
Benzodiazepines	Anxiolysis
Diazepam/lorazepam	Muscle spasm
Antiemetics	Chemotherapy or narcotic-induced nausea/emesis
Ondansetron/dolasetron/granisetron	
Metoclopromide	
Cannabinoids: dronabinol	
Cisapride	
Procloperazine	
Promethazine	
Scopalamine	
Meclizine	
Antihistamines	
Benzodiazepines	
Haldoperidol	
Anticholinergics: atropine/hyoscine	
Laxatives	Constipation, narcotic induced
Bowel stimulant: Ducosate	
Stool softener: Senna/peri-colace	
Bulk forming: Metamucil/bran	
Saline or osmotic cathartics: Milk of magnesia, magnesium citrate	
Phosphate enema (Fleets)	
Lactulose	
Bisacodyl	
Stimulants	Sedation, narcotic induced
Dextroamphetamine	
Methylphenidate	
Antihistamines	Nausea/pruritis/allergic reactions

Modified from Mahaney GD, Peeters-Asdourian C. Cancer pain management. In: Abram SE, ed. *Atlas of Anesthesia, Volume VI: Pain Management*. Philadelphia: Churchill Livingstone, 1998:9.1–9.14.

inhibiting osteoclastic activity on bone. Benzodiazepines and muscle relaxants may be helpful with muscle spasms. Corticosteroids have antiinflammatory properties to assist in pain control of headache from brain metastasis, back pain from spinal-cord compression, and bone pain from prostate metastasis. Appetite stimulation, mood elevation, and antiemetic properties of corticosteroids also are very useful.

Should a cancer patient be in moderate to severe pain, the nonopiate and adjuvant trial would be bypassed and opiates would be initiated. Nonopiate and adjuvant agents may be coadministered for synergistic and opiate-sparing effects. Opiates remain the foundation of treatment for moderate to severe cancer pain. Unlike NSAIDS, opiates do not have a ceiling effect. They may be titrated to pain relief and are only limited by side effects. Side effects include constipation, nausea, vomiting, sedation, myoclonus, pruritus, cognitive impairment, and hallucinations. Adjuvants can be used prophylactically to treat these side effects (Table 26.1). Constipation should be an expected side effect and treated aggressively. Dose-limiting toxicity warrants a change to another narcotic.

It is believed that 90% to 95% of cancer pain should be controlled by opiate and adjuvant treatment. Somatic and visceral pain tends to respond to opiates, and neuropathic pain has been known to be less responsive to narcotics. Choice of opiate is influenced by route of administration available, severity of pain, and patient history of intolerances. Advantages of narcotics are their efficacy in a variety of pain states and the availability of preparations for administration by a multitude of routes. Patients may receive opiates by transmucosal, transdermal, epidural, intrathecal, intraventricular, parenteral, and oral routes, with oral being the preferred method of administration.

Morphine remains the opioid of comparison and is utilized for designations of equianalgesic doses (Table 26.3). Transdermal fentanyl is effective and long acting for constant pain but requires monitoring because of the delay in both peak effect with application and termination of effect when removed. Demerol (Sanofi Pharmaceuticals, Inc., New York, NY, U.S.A.) is not recommended for cancer pain secondary to short duration of action and side product accumulation of normeperidine causing central nervous system stimulation and seizures. Agonist-antagonist opiates such as pentazocine, butorphanol, and nalbuphine are not recommended because they have limited analgesia and may cause acute withdrawal symptoms in patients accustomed to receiving opiates. Tramadol is a synthetic analog of codeine and works through weak opioid receptor agonism and blocks reuptake of serotonin and norepinephrine. Tramadol is not recommended to be coadministered with tricyclic antidepressants. Routes of parenteral administration of opiates include patient-controlled analgesia devices, continuous intravenous infusions, and continuous subcutaneous infusions. With these routes, pain medication requirements can be self-administered and amount used tabulated and used for adjustments or changes to different routes. These methods also may be used for opioid administration in a home hospice setting.

The pain pattern (constant versus intermittent) would dictate dosing. The most common cancer pain pattern is constant pain with acute exacerbations. Around-the-clock dosing of a long-acting opiate is recommended for constant pain in conjunction with intermittent or rescue dosing of a shorter-acting opiate for the acute exacerbations or breakthrough pain. The initial rescue dose should be approximately 5% to 10% of the total 24-hour dose given every 1 to 2 hours, and it is useful in determining a patient's pain requirements and the necessity of adjusting the long-acting opiate. The long-acting opiate may be adjusted every 24 hours until pain relief or intolerable side effects are attained. Commonly used long-acting opiates include MSContin/Kadian (Purdue Pharma L.P./Purdue Frederick Company, Stamford, CT, U.S.A.), OramorphSR (Roxane Laboratories, Ontario, Canada), OxyContin (Purdue Pharma L.P.), and Duragesic Fentanyl Patch (Jansen Pharmaceutica Inc., Titusville, NJ, U.S.A.). Frequently used, short-acting narcotics are oxycodone, codeine, hydromorphone, Morphine Sulfate Immediate Release/Roxanol/Roxanol-T/Roxanol 100 (Roxane Laboratories), and other opiate–analgesic combination medications. Should opiates need to be changed secondary to side effects, calculations will need to be made to an equianalgesic dose and then reduced by one third to one half secondary to incomplete cross tolerance. Patients need to be reassessed frequently for dose adjustments due to progression of disease or successful therapeutic treatments. The most common cause of dose escalation in cancer-pain patients is from disease progression.

TABLE 26.3. *Routes and Equianalgesic Doses of Selected Opiates*

Opiate	Routes available	Equianalgesic doses
Morphine	i.v./i.m./subQ/short and long-acting p.o./rectal	i.v./i.m.: 10 mg p.o.: 30–60 mg
Methadone	i.v./i.m./p.o.	Rectal: 5 mg
Levorphanol	i.v./i.m./subQ/p.o.	i.v./i.m.: 2 mg p.o.: 4 mg
Fentanyl	Transdermal/i.v.	Transdermal: 0.1 mg/i.v. 0.1 mg
Oxycodone	Short and long-acting p.o.	p.o.: 20–30 mg
Hydromorphone	i.v./i.m./subQ/p.o./rectal	i.v./i.m.: 1.5 mg p.o.: 7.5 mg Rectal: 7.5 mg
Oxymorphone	i.v./i.m./p.o./rectal	i.v./i.m.: 1 mg p.o.: 6 mg Rectal: 5–10 mg
Meperdine	i.v./i.m./p.o.	i.v./i.m.: 75 mg p.o.: 300 mg
Diamorphine/heroin	i.m./i.v./p.o.	i.v./i.m.: 5 mg p.o.: 60 mg
Propoxyphine	p.o.	p.o.: 65–130 mg
Codeine	i.v./i.m./p.o.	i.v./i.m.: 130 mg p.o.: 200 mg

Modified from Patt RB, *Cancer Pain.* Philadelphia: JB Lippincott Co., 1993.
i.m., intramuscular; i.v. intravenous; p.o., per os (orally).

Invasive Techniques

Should patients experience unacceptable side effects to narcotics, unrelieved intractable pain, or localized pain, invasive techniques may be indicated. It is believed that only 10% to 20% of cancer-pain patients need invasive therapy. In more advanced disease, the risk-to-benefit ratio is shifted to favor invasive techniques. A trial blockade of local anesthetics into the area of nerves supplying a specific lesion can be useful in diagnosis of the pain etiology and may possibly be prognostic of an effect that may be obtained with a more permanent technique such as chemical neurolysis, cryotherapy, radiofrequency lesioning, or neurosurgical options. Because of central nervous system plasticity, the neuroablative procedures are not reliably permanent. Therefore, blocks are frequently repeated within 3 to 6 months. Neuritis may be an unwanted side effect of a lesion and cause increasing pain for an extended time period beyond the procedure.

Most nerve blocks and neuroablative techniques are limited in that they would be most useful in those patients with localized pain. Patients with generalized bone pain may benefit from pituitary ablation. Other generalized pain has been treated with deep-brain stimulation, bilateral cordotomy, and epidural or intrathecal opioids with or without local anesthetics. A list of several of the available procedures for pain relief has been compiled (Table 26.4). Many procedures would require a neurosurgeon. A few of the procedures listed that have been shown to be very effective for cancer pain will be discussed briefly.

One of the most valuable blockades is the celiac-plexus block. This block is known to be very effective for abdominal malignancies, especially pancreatic cancer. The pain of pancreatic cancer is typified by severe mid-epigastric pain that radiates to the midback. Most relief is gained in the fetal position with exacerbation of pain with recumbency. A meta-analysis of 24 papers reported that 70% to 90% of the cancer patients receiving a neurolytic celiac-plexus block had partial to complete pain relief long enough to last their lifetime, which in some patients extended beyond 3 months.

CASE REPORTS

Patient 1

An 88-year old woman was referred to the pain management unit for evaluation and treatment of abdominal pain. Eight months earlier, she had begun to experience abdominal pain and nausea accompanied by jaundice. Ultrasound revealed a pancreatic mass, and a transhepatic

TABLE 26.4. *Selected Procedures Available and Their Indications*

Procedures	Indications
Local anesthetic (i.v., subcutaneous, transdermal)	Neuropathic pain site of hyperesthesia/allodynia
Trigger-point injections	Myofascial pain
Trigeminal/gasserian ganglion blocks	Facial pain
Cervical ganglion/plexus blocks	Neck pain
Stellate ganglion block	Sympathetically mediated pain, Face/upper ext
Cervical/thoracic/lumbar epidural block	Radiculopathy
Epidural/intrathecal neurolysis	Chemical rhizotomy
	Pelvic/perineal pain if no bowel/bladder function
Epidural/intrathecal narcotics +/− opioids	Many applications; side effects appear less severe than p.o./i.v.
Intercostal nerve blocks	Radicular pain (postthoracotomy/mastectomy rib fracture)
Celiac plexus	Abdominal pain syndromes (pancreatic cancer)
Superior hypogastric plexus block	Pelvic/Perineal visceral pain syndromes
Lumbar sympathetic	Sympathetically mediated pain, lower extremities
Rhizotomy	Somatic/neuropathic pain: tumor infiltration head/neck/arms/legs/pelvis/perineum
	Lesion: Nerve root sectioned surgically
Cordotomy	Unilateral pain in trunk or lower extremity
	Lesion: spinothalamic tract sectioned contralateral side after cross-over
Dorsal-Root entry zone lesioning (DREZ)	Unilateral neuropathic pain (brachial/intercostal/lumbosacral
Percutaneous: radiofrequency	plexopathies and postherpetic neuralgia)
Open: surgery	Lesion: Ipsilateral nucleus caudalis
Pituitary ablation	Diffuse bone pain/endocrine-dependent tumors
Surgical excision	
Chemical ablation: alcohol	
Cryoablation	
Spinal-cord stimulation	Neuropathic pain/painful dysesthesias
Cryoablation	Peripheral nerve block: pituitary ablation
Radiofrequency lesioning	Peripheral nerve blocks/cordotomy/rhizotomy
Deep brain stimulation	Generalized pain

i.v., intravenous; p.o., per os (orally).

cholangiogram was consistent with a lesion at the pancreatic head. Exploratory laparotomy revealed an unresectable pancreatic carcinoma. Postoperatively, she continued to experience a constant, deep, dull abdominal pain in the epigastrium, radiating to the umbilicus and increasing in intensity over the next several months. Narcotics induced lethargy and disorientation and failed to relieve her pain completely.

On physical examination, the patient appeared pale and chronically ill but well hydrated. Her abdomen was obese and somewhat distended, and the epigastrium was diffusely tender to deep palpation. Clotting studies were within normal limits. The patient underwent diagnostic celiac-plexus block under fluoroscopic guidance. A bilateral approach was used, and the patient received a total dose of 25 mL of lidocaine 1%, which produced complete relief of her pain. Her vital signs were monitored frequently, and there was a mild decrease in her blood pressure and a very minor increase in heart rate. Several days later, she underwent successful neurolysis of the celiacplexus with 20 mL of absolute alcohol, after first anesthetizing the celiac-plexus with 10 mL of lidocaine 1%. She remained pain-free for three months, after which modest doses of opiates were used as needed until her death 4 months after the procedure.

Intercostal nerve blocks can be very helpful for pathological rib fractures or metastasis, post-thoracotomy pain, and postmastectomy pain. Disadvantages of these blocks include temporary relief, associated neuritis, and risk of pneumothorax.

Intolerance to oral or i.v. opiates may warrant a trial of epidural or intrathecal narcotics. Less drug is necessary with the direct delivery of opioid to spinal-cord opioid receptors that mediate analgesia and inhibit pain transmission. Side effects may be less with these routes with an added benefit of efficacy in multiple pain states.

Patient 2

A 29-year-old woman was referred to the pain management unit for treatment of pelvic pain. Three years earlier, chondrosarcoma of the sacrum was diagnosed, and she was given chemotherapy and treated with radiation. She subsequently became pregnant and her pain increased as the uterus enlarged, necessitating large doses of methadone for pain relief. She delivered a healthy infant, who required gradual narcotic withdrawal, but otherwise did well. Unfortunately, the mother's tumor metastasized, and her pain did not diminish after delivery despite large doses of oral, intramuscular, and intravenous narcotics in addition to a tricyclic antidepressant. She wished to return home with her baby; therefore a course of epidural local anesthetics was instituted and her other narcotics were gradually

withdrawn over a period of 3 days. At that time, 7 mg of preservative-free morphine was injected into the epidural catheter, which provided her with excellent pain relief. A subcutaneous epidural morphine reservoir was implanted, with a catheter tunneling into the epidural space. On this regimen, she was discharged without pain or drowsiness and was instructed to inject morphine into the reservoir twice daily at home.

In summary, the challenge of cancer-pain treatment continues despite the development of new medications, therapies, and additional understanding of cancer-pain mechanisms. With pain management increasing in popularity, hopefully there will be a strong impetus to seek more effective pain control in cancer-pain patients.

SELECTED READINGS

Abramowicz M, ed. Celecoxib for arthritis. *The Medical Letter* 1999;41: 11–12.

American Pain Society. *Principles of analgesic use in the Treatment of Acute Pain and Cancer Pain*, 3rd ed. Skokie, Illinois: American Pain Society, 1992.

Benzon HT, Raja SN, Borsook D, et al. *Essentials of Pain Medicine*. New York: Churchill Livingstone, 1999.

Bonica JJ, Ventafridda V, eds. *Advances in Pain Research and Therapy*. New York: Raven Press, 1979:59.

Bonica JJ. *The Management of Pain*, Vol. II. Philadelphia: Lea & Febiger, 1990:400–460.

Brown C, Mazzula JP, Mok MS, et al. Comparison of repeat doses of intramuscular ketorolac tromethamine and morphine sulfate for analgesia after major surgery. *Pharmacotherapy* 1990;10:45S–50S.

Coyle N, Adelhardt J, Foley KM, et al. Character of terminal illness in the advanced cancer patient; pain and other symptoms during the last 4 weeks of life. *J Pain Symptom Manage* 1990;5:83.

DeVita VT Jr., Hellman S, Rosenberg SA, eds. *Cancer: Principles and Practice of Oncology*, 5th Edition. Philadelphia: Lippincott–Raven Publishers, 1997:2807–2841.

Eisenberg E, Carr DB, Chalmers TC. Neurolytic celiac plexus block for treatment of cancer pain: a meta-analysis. *Anesthesia Analgesia* 1995;80: 290.

Foley KM. Advances in cancer pain. *Arch Neurol* 1999;56:413–417.

Foley KM, ed. *Advances in Pain Research and Therapy*, Vol. 16. New York: Raven Press, Ltd., 1990.

Kaiko RF, Foley KM, Grabinski PY, et al. Central nervous system excitatory effects of meperidine in cancer patients. *Ann of Neurology* 1983;13: 180–185.

Mahaney GD, Peeters-Asdourian C. Cancer pain management. In: Abram SE, ed. *Atlas of Anesthesia. Volume VI: Pain Management*. Philadelphia: Churchill Livingstone, 1998:9.1–9.14.

Patt RB. *Cancer Pain*. Philadelphia: JB Lippincott Company, 1993.

Portenoy RK. Cancer pain: pathophysiology and syndromes. *Lancet* 1992; 339:1026.

Raj PP. *Pain Medicine, A Comprehensive Review*. St. Louis: Mosby, 1996; 502–516.

Stouten E, Armbruster S, Houmes RJ, et al. Comparison of ketorolac and morphine for postoperative pain after major surgery. *Acta Anaesthesiol Scan* 1992;36:716–721.

Ventafridda V, Tamburini M, Caraceni A, et al. A validation study of the WHO method for cancer pain relief. *Cancer* 1987;59:850–856.

Ventafridda V, Ripamonti C, DeConno F, et al. Symptom prevalence and control during cancer patient's last days of life. *J Palliat Care* 1990;6:7.

Waldman SD, Winnie AP. *Interventional Pain Management* Philadelphia: WB Saunders, 1996.

Warfield CA. *Manual of Pain Management*. Philadelphia: JB Lippincott, 1991.

World Health Organization. *Cancer Pain Relief*. Geneva: WHO, 1986.

CHAPTER 27

Complex Regional Pain Syndromes (Reflex Sympathetic Dystrophy and Causalgia)

Anna G.A. Sottile and Hilary J. Fausett

The history of this group of diseases provides not only important information about them, but also is very helpful in understanding the reasons behind the recent changes in taxonomy.

HISTORY

In 1864, S. Weir Mitchell, a Civil War "surgeon" was quite intrigued by a series of pain syndromes affecting some wounded soldiers. The majority of the wounded young men underwent an initial series of acute pain and inflammation, followed by a fast recovery. Others continued to suffer persistent pain associated with other symptoms and, with time, they got worse, rather than better. The syndrome was characterized by a prior trauma, mostly affecting the limbs, followed by a persistent burning pain in the injured limb. The burning pain was accompanied by local autonomic and trophic changes. Eventually, these changes resulted in the inability to use the limb and persistent, intractable pain. Mitchell used the word *causalgia*, meaning "burning pain" to label the disorder. All of the soldiers affected by this condition had a similar presentation: a previous trauma with nerve injury and persistent pain. Later, the pain changed in *character* becoming more of burning in nature. This burning pain was worsened by light touch, and once initiated, persisted over time, despite the removal of the stimuli. These qualities now are referred to as *allodynia* (perception of pain caused by otherwise non-noxious stimulus, such as light touch or cold) and *hyperesthesia* (increased sensitivity to stimulation). This crescendo effect progressed up to the point where the pain became spontaneous and constant. Moreover, the location of the pain *spread* to a much larger and proximal area.

Along with these subjective symptoms, the patient started to develop some objective and local autonomic changes, such as swelling and skin-color abnormalities as well as changes in sudomotor activity and increased temperature. Months later, a series of trophic changes such as deformities from contractures, fibrosis, and muscular atrophy occurred. Eventually, the patient was left with partial or total inability to use the affected limb and constant pain.

Other physicians noticed similar clinical presentations, but although the patients affected were almost all exposed to injury, true nerve damage could not be consistently found associated with the other symptoms. Also, the painful sensation wasn't necessarily described as "burning." The term "causalgia" did not fit the phenomenon. A new entity without nerve injury was challenging the medical world.

In 1939 and 1943, Lerich and Livingston advanced the hypothesis that the disorders were caused by a vicious circle where an abnormal firing of stimulation to the spinal cord was taking place.

In 1946, Evans proposed the possibility that the sympathetic nervous system was responsible for this cycle. Until recently, the term "reflex sympathetic dystrophy" has been used to describe this syndrome. Let's analyze this term word by word.

"Dystrophy," meaning abnormal appearance, is an unspecified term. The word "sympathetic" suggests that a disturbance of the sympathetic system is always present, and this may not be completely true during all phases of the disease. Finally, the word "reflex" implies the rapidity of the development of the condition, again, not necessarily correct all the time. Moreover, this definition was based on a postulated pathophysiologic disturbance, which is still unproved. Thus, the term "reflex sympathetic dystrophy" is not only vague, but also misleading. Subsequently, this disorder has been described by a number of terms such as Sudeck's atrophy, sympathetically maintained syndrome, shoulder–hand syndrome, atypical post-traumatic pain syndrome, sympathetic dystrophy, and others.

DEFINITION

In 1993, a meeting was held in Orlando, Florida to review the issue and propose a new name. As a result of that meeting, in 1994 the International Association for the Study of Pain officially announced the new taxonomy, which classifies the two distinct conditions based upon a *descriptive* method, rather than a pathophysiological one.

It was decided to use the term *complex regional pain syndrome* (CRPS). Under this umbrella is now included a full spectrum of diseases characterized by a previous injury to the affected area, followed by persistent and disproportional pain and accompanied at some point by autonomic changes, not necessarily seen at the time of the physical examination and not following any dermatomal distribution. The difference between type I and II is based upon the lack (type I) or presence (type II) of nerve injury. A proven sympathetically mediated mechanism of the pain may or may not be present, but does not have a role in the definition of the disorder.

INCIDENCE

The incidence of CRPS, both types I and II, is assumed to be similar to the previous definition of reflex sympathetic dystrophy and causalgia, respectively. The abovementioned confusion about the definitions could have made the data regarding the incidence less accurate.

For CRPS type I (former reflex sympathetic dystrophy), the incidence is 0.05% to 15% of the population. CRPS type II (former causalgia) has a smaller range of 2% to 5%.

Peak occurrence is between the fifth and seventh decade. The syndrome also appears in children; however, it seems to be self-limiting. It is more prominent in the female population, with a female-to-male ratio of 2.9:1. It also seems to be more likely among Caucasians. Cigarette smoking may play a role. Cultural implications may be present. A genetic predisposition for the condition is under investigation.

STAGES, SIGNS, AND SYMPTOMS

In the so called classic presentation of both CRPS types I and II, the clinical presentation has been divided into three stages. A prior trauma is almost always identified. In type I, it can be as minor as a strain injury. Reported instigators of CRPS type I include arterial puncture, bursitis, impacted teeth, radiotherapy, and myocardial infarction.

In CRPS type II, a nerve injury must be present. Days later, a more intense burning pain may start to affect a larger area. As a result of the nerve injury, possible sensory and motor loss are present along a dermatomal distribution, while the pain, the autonomic changes, and the atrophy do not follow any dermatomal nerve distribution.

This initial stage is quite subtle and variable and it may not always be apparent. Very rarely is the disease diagnosed at this early stage.

Stage 1 or Acute Phase

The hallmark is symptoms of underactivity of the sympathetic system, which cause the hyperemic, hyperthermic, vasodilated appearance of the affected area. The increased blood flow also is responsible for the overgrowth of nails and hair. The burning pain is constant and worsens by light touch, emotional stress, cold, a breeze in the environment, loud sounds, and even bright light. Patients guard the affected area, protecting it from direct physical contact with the environment. A quiet surrounding may somewhat alleviate the constant pain.

In some cases, the disease is recognized at this early stage, which allows relatively early treatment and a higher chance of success.

Stage 2 or Dystrophic Phase

Two or 3 months later, the vasoconstrictive phase starts. It is thought to be the result of hyperactivity of the sympathetic nervous system. The area appears pale, sweaty, and cold. Nails and hair become brittle and cracked. Because the pain increases with motion, the patient holds the affected part still, leading to a stiff and immobile posture of the limb. Contractions and muscle atrophy begin. It is in this stage that we can observe osteoporosis on x-ray (Sudeck's atrophy or patchy atrophy).

Stage 3 or Atrophic Phase

This phase begins months or years after the initial presentation. Pain spreads proximally and may even involve the contralateral limb, perhaps by way of central nervous system activation.

Atrophy involves the skin, subcutaneous tissue, fat, muscles, and pericapsular tissue. The affected limb is pale, thin, contracted, and stiff. This stage is irreversible.

In some severe cases, the disease progression results in severe depression, malnutrition, sleep disorders, pain behavior, and fixation, and even suicidal ideation.

TREATMENT

Early intervention is essential. The disease must be approached aggressively with psychological interventions, physical-therapy pharmacological interventions, and regional blocks. The goal is to return to function.

PHYSICAL-THERAPEUTIC ALGORITHM

Stanton-Hicks, et al. composed a "consensus report" after the Orlando meeting of 1994. The authors offer a suggested treatment strategy, which will be used to guide our discussion. It is important to realize that, while no studies have proven the validity of the proposed management, clinical experience suggests the algorithm is helpful.

Ideally, the algorithm should be completed within 2 weeks, but for chronic or complicated cases, the timeframe may need to be adjusted. For any case requiring more than 3 weeks of therapy, a more aggressive treatment and psychological reassessment is highly suggested.

The first step is the assessment of a complex therapeutic regimen including active mobilization. The goal is to restore normal, sensory function and desensitize the painful limb. This may involve the use of pharmacological support to reduce the pain, together with the increased use of non-nociceptive stimulation. The program may need to be tailored to each patient's need. In some cases, heat stimuli, and in others, cold can be used. In general, massage, vibration, pressure, and movement can be utilized to try to normalize the sensory activity (light touch felt as such). For this to succeed, it is very important to address the "touch and movement phobia" most commonly present.

The second step involves movement. It may start with isometric strengthening accompanied by electrode stimulation. The presence of any secondary pain, such as myofascial pain, should be addressed and treated.

The third step involves more isometric strengthening with stress loading, such as walking, if the inferior extremity is involved or carrying weights if the upper extremity is involved. Maintenance of a constant but gradual increase in the range of motion, avoiding any aggressive or passive movements also is important.

The fourth step aims at reconditioning for full functional recovery and return to the preinjury activity. Any psychological difficulties should be addressed and managed by an appropriate specialist.

PSYCHOLOGICAL INTERVENTIONS

Depression, anxiety, and anger are common companions of chronic-pain syndromes in general. This condition is not an exception.

A full psychological assessment with the goal of adjusting the patient's expectations, producing self-motivation, and proposing self-control often is necessary. The involvement of other family members is recommended. Behavioral techniques, relaxation techniques, hypnosis, and coping skills all are advocated.

PHARMACOLOGICAL MANAGEMENT

Despite a conspicuous amount of research on the subject, the management of this disease is still quite difficult and most times, the use of "trial and error" technique is valid.

Sequential or combined techniques are appropriate and may be chosen depending on the circumstances. Medical treatment has proven to be beneficial in most cases. Some drug classes are part of the routine management, while some are more often seen as adjuvants. In general, drugs used for the treatment of neuropathic pain are commonly used to treat these disorders.

Nonsteroidal Antiinflammatory Drugs

These agents appear to provide some pain relief by inhibition of the cyclooxygenase pathways. They tend to be most effective during the early stages of the disease, when inflammatory signs are evident. The goal is not necessarily good pain relief from them, but simply a reduction of the possible inflammation of tissues around the injury. This is especially important if tendons and joints happen to be involved.

Opioids

The use of opioids is quite controversial. Opioids have been thought to be ineffective for neuropathic pain, but more recent studies strongly suggest an important role. No controlled opioids studies for CRPS have been conducted yet, making this an open issue to be researched in the future. Some experts like to think of opiates as the last resort.

Antidepressant

Unlike the opioids, the role of the norepinephrine and serotonin reuptake inhibitors has been shown to be successful in the treatment of neuropathic pain in several studies. The best models studied have been diabetic neuropathy and postherpetic neuralgia, where these agents have been shown to improve symptomatology.

Their dual action in both pain perception and mood modulation is recognized.

It may well be that a multifactorial effect is achieved by the use of this class of drugs. Their capacities to improve sleep patterns, decrease anxiety, and modulate mood are all beneficial effects of both the tricyclic antidepressant and the selective serotonin reuptake inhibitors (SSRIs). It seems, though, that the SSRIs are more effective in the presence of a coexisting picture of depression, and the older class of the tricyclics may be more useful without clinical signs of depression.

Amitriptyline is the most studied antidepressant in the field of neuropathic pain. Several clinical trials demonstrate an analgesic effect at lower doses than the one used for the treatment of depression. An initial low dose of 10 mg 12 hours before the morning awaking time is suggested. This will help to decrease the drowsiness during working hours. A gentle incremental dose then is started until either development of side effects or a moderate dose is reached. No maximal dose is defined, but usually, there is no need to dose higher than 100 mg. If no significant improvement is obtained, the first antidepressant can be gently weaned down to none, and a new one can be started, using again a low dose, followed by a gentle increment. Similarly, nortriptyline and desipramine, which may have less anticholinergic side effects, can be used.

Evidence of the effectiveness of SSRIs in the treatment of neuropathic pain per se is not as strong as it is for tricyclics. Still, they are recommended especially in the cases of coexisting clinical depression. The lack of anticholinergic side effects and the often absence of drowsiness allows these patients to feel and be more alert and functional while on SSRI as opposed to tricyclics. Venlafaxine (Effexor, Wyeth–Ayerst Laboratories, Philadelphia, PA, U.S.A.) 150 to 375 mg/day in the morning seems to have a good mood-modulating effect, but side effects can be a problem, such as excessive mood swings, gastrointestinal problems, and others.

Occasionally, some patients are already on one antidepressant for treatment of conditions other that neuropathic pain. In this case, the addition of a different class of antidepressant for the treatment of the pain syndrome may be helpful. In these cases, drug-blood levels are good guide toward the correct dose.

Alpha Agonist

The role of clonidine for pain modulation is well documented. The efficacy of it in CRPS treatment, though, is estimated to be low. It seems that a successful pretrial with sympathetic blocks or phentolamine infusion can be used as a "predictor" of the pain relief effect from clonidine. This α agonist has been used orally as well as neuro axially, but its side effects, especially orthostatic hypotension and dry mouth, limit its use. Clonidine also is available as a 0.1 mg patch to be changed every week. Application of the patch on the area affected by the pain is a common recommendation.

Calcium-Channel Blockers

Many studies have found a role for calcium-channel blockers such as nifedipine and verapamil in treating CRPS. Careful monitoring of cardiovascular parameters is important, initially. A small initial dose of nifedipine of 10 to 20 mg a day or verapamil sustained release of 240 mg is recommended as starting dose, and increased if there are no side effects.

Antiarrythmics

Some promising studies have focused attention on the use of sodium-channel blockers such as mexiletine. An intravenous lidocaine infusion (3 to 5 mg/kg over 45 to 60 minutes) with monitoring of pain level is used to screen for patients who will be a good candidate for p.o. mexiletine. A negative history of cardiac arrhythmia as well as a baseline electrocardiogram to rule out prolonged QT interval pathology or other contraindications first is obtained. When in doubt, a consultation with a cardiologist is suggested.

Anticonvulsants

This class of drugs seems to have a role in the pharmacopoeia of the CRPS. Carbamazepine is one of the most studied. The recommended starting dose is 200 mg B.I.D, and it can be slowly increased. Careful monitoring of complete blood count and liver-function tests (LFTs), both before and every 3 months after starting, may complicate patient compliance.

LFT monitoring is required for other anticonvulsants often used for neuropathic pain, such as valproic acid. Starting dose usually is 15 mg/kg/day, with a maximal recommended dose of 60 mg/kg/day. The same liver-function monitoring is recommended with the use of phenytoin usually started at 300 mg qd.

Newer anticonvulsants such as gabapentin and topiramate are becoming more and more popular, as they do not require blood monitoring. Gabapentin has a very safe profile. Initial recommended dose is 100 mg three times a day if the patient is young and healthy. For elderly patients or patients with coexisting cardiovascular pathologies, the recommended initial dose is 100 mg once a day, slowly increased to effect. If the patient tolerates the initial dose without major problems, a gentle increment is started. A 3,600-mg/day dose is considered the ceiling dose. Topiramate is started at 50 mg qd. and can be increased weekly up to 200 mg b.i.d.

Corticosteroids

Although this was one of the first and widely used medications during the 1970s and 1980s, more recent studies have failed to validate a role for steroid therapy. Some authors, though, seem to believe that corticosteroids may have a role in treating possible coexisting inflammation, especially in the joint in patients who experience pain relief at rest and persistent pain with motion. Most of the time, steroids are not recommended.

REGIONAL ANESTHETIC TECHNIQUES

There are at least two good reasons to use regional blocks: their potential pain-relieving effect and their role in the diagnosis of sympathetically mediated pain.

Blocks alone usually are insufficient to treat the condition, but the analgesia obtained helps the suffering patient to tolerate more physical therapy, which allows more functional recuperation, the real goal of treatment.

Blocks can divided into the following four major categories:

1. Direct and exclusive sympathectomy, no sensory or motor involvement.
2. Sympathectomy by way of neuroaxial administration of local anesthetics with sensory and potential motor involvement.
3. Peripheral blocks, with sensory and possible motor effect.
4. Intravenous and infiltration blocks.
5. Blocks can be repeated or a catheter can be placed for daily repeated injections or even continuous infusion.

Sympathetic blocks can be achieved by way of direct injection of local anesthetics around the sympathetic chain. Advantages of these blocks include their lack of motor involvement. Stellate-ganglion block is used if the upper extremities are affected. Lumbar-sympathetic blocks are used if the lower extremities are affected. It is possible to try to leave a catheter to the vicinity of the appropriate sympathetic ganglion. This is mainly performed for the lumbar blocks, especially for children, to avoid repetitive procedures under general anesthesia (unnecessary for adults), but such catheters appear to have a very high incidence of displacement. To avoid this inconvenience, a sympathectomy also can be achieved by way of epidural or intrathecal administration of local anesthetics. Motor involvement then is more likely, and therefore epidural is preferred to spinal. A catheter can be threaded very easily and used for continuous infusion of local anesthetics, or even daily injections. Physical therapy then can be performed during the period of blockade.

Under appropriate monitoring, opiates can be added or used as solo treatment for analgesia. If they are added to the anesthetic solutions to enhance analgesia, the sympathectomy is still achieved. If used without anesthetics, no sympathectomy will be present. In general, if the upper extremities are affected, sympathetic blocks are more dangerous because of the risk of accidental vascular or high-intrathecal injection of local anesthetics. The major risk for a lumbar-sympathetic block is puncture of the kidney, aorta vena cava, and nerve damage.

Peripheral nerve blocks, such as brachial plexus, interscalene, and axillary blocks can be performed if the upper limb is affected and sciatic, 3-in-1 blocks if the lower limb is affected.

Another type of block is the intravenous block or Bier block. It can be performed easily, with the same benefit and even less risk. In Europe, the use of phentolamine and guanethidine are quite common, but are not approved for the use in the United States where bretylium currently is used for these blocks.

These type of blocks are quite safe in the right hands and they are able to produce good or even excellent pain relief. Bier blocks also can be performed on the lower extremities. In general, the Bier block may be technically more difficult than expected because of the coexisting allodynia as well as possible vasoconstriction resulting from sympathetic activity.

Spinal-cord stimulators or peripheral stimulators have been used successfully. Spinal-cord stimulation should be considered after failure of other techniques.

SUMMARY

Early recognition and multidisciplinary intervention are the secrets for the increase of successful treatment of these challenging disorders. Ongoing pain research in this field will reveal more of the unknown mechanisms of a disease that has fascinated as well as frustrated many physicians and scientists for over one century all over the world.

SELECTED READINGS

Kingery WS. A critical review of controlled clinical trials for peripheral neuropathic pain and complex regional pain syndrome. *Pain* 1997;73: 123–139.

Loeser JD, Butler SH, Chapman CR, et al., eds. *Bonica's Management of Pain*, 3rd ed. Philadelphia: Lippincott Williams & Wilkins, 2000.

McLesky C, Balestrieri F, Weeks D. Sympathetic dystrophies. In: Warfield C, ed. *Principles and Practice of Pain Management*. New York: McGraw-Hill, Inc. Health Profession Division, 1993.

Stanton-Hicks M, Baron R, Boas R, et al. Consensus report. Complex regional pain syndrome: guidelines for therapy. *Clin J Pain* 1998;14: 155–166.

Warfield C. Sympathetic dystrophy. In: Warfield C, ed. *Manual of Pain Management*. Philadelphia: JB Lippincott Company, 1991.

CHAPTER 28

Pain Management in Peripheral Vascular Disease

Kyung Won Park

PAIN FROM PERIPHERAL VASCULAR DISEASE

Peripheral vascular disease (PVD) is a multifactorial syndrome that progressively gives rise to ischemic pain of the affected limbs. Common causes of PVD include arteriosclerosis, often in connection with diabetes; Raynaud's disease, involving exaggerated vasoconstrictor reflex response during exposure to cold, most commonly in the upper extremities; Buerger's disease, also known as thromboangiitis obliterans, caused by inflammation of small vessels in the legs and occasionally in the arms; and embolic-occlusive disease. Less common causes of peripheral-vascular pain include popliteal artery entrapment, adventitial cystic disease of the popliteal artery, and compartment syndromes. Whereas arteriosclerotic PVD involves obstruction of the large arteries with compensatory dilation of the distal small arteries, Raynaud's disease and Buerger's disease are diseases of the smaller vessels.

Ischemic pain from arteriosclerotic PVD progresses through predictable stages, as described originally by LaReich and Fontaine (Table 28.1).

Claudication is cramping pain that occurs when blood flow to a limb is inadequate to meet its metabolic demands. Severity of claudication is inversely proportional to muscle activity in the limb and, in the early stages of the arteriosclerotic disease, will be minimized by rest. However, as the disease progresses, blood flow will become inadequate even for resting metabolic demands and rest pain will ensue. Blood flow to the affected limb is commonly followed by measuring the ankle-brachial index (ABI). A cuff is placed around the ankle and the threshold pressure for Doppler detection of flow over the dorsalis pedis or posterior tibial artery is noted. This pressure then is divided by the blood pressure in the arm to obtain the ABI. A normal ABI is 1.1 to 1.2.

Raynaud's syndrome may be precipitated by cold or stress. It is much more common in females than in males and is associated with a connective-tissue disease in 50% to 80% of cases. It also may be associated with a variety of other diseases and drugs (Table 28.2). The pain, which initially is episodic, may become constant and severe with progression of the disease. An attack of Raynaud's syndrome has three components: (a) an initial arterial blanching, with relative numbness secondary to arterial constriction, (b) cyanosis resulting from arterial desaturation, and (c) a reactive hyperemia. Raynaud's syndrome is diagnosed by the ice-water immersion test. Following a measurement of baseline digital-tip temperature, the patient's digits are immersed in ice water for 30 seconds and then tip temperatures are recorded every 5 minutes

TABLE 28.1. *LaReich and Fontaine's Stages of Arteriosclerotic Peripheral Vascular Disease*

Stage	Symptomatology	Physical changes
0	None	None
1	Intermittent claudication with moderate exercise (such as walking >1 block)	None
2	Severe claudication with minimal exercise (such as walking <½ block)	Dependent rubor
3	Rest limb pain	Atrophy, cyanosis, rubor
4	Worsening rest limb pain	Nonhealing ischemic ulcer or gangrene

TABLE 28.2. *Raynaud's Syndrome: Associated Diseases, Drugs, and Occupational Causes*

Immunologic and connective-tissue disorders
   Scleroderma
   Mixed connective-tissue disease
   Systemic lupus erythematosus
   Rheumatoid arthritis
   Dermatomyositis
   Polymyositis
   Hepatitis B antigen-induced vasculitis
   Drug-induced vasculitis
   Sjögren's syndrome
   Undifferentiated connective-tissue disease
Obstructive arterial diseases without immunologic
    disturbance
   Arteriosclerosis
   Thromboangiitis obliterans
   Thoracic-outlet syndrome
Miscellaneous
   Vinyl-chloride exposure
   Chronic renal failure
   Cold agglutinins
   Cryoglobulinemia
   Neoplasia
   Neurologic disorders
   Endocrinologic disorder
Occupational Raynaud's syndrome
   Vibration injury
   Direct arterial trauma
   Cold injury
Drug-induced Raynaud's Syndrome without arteritis
   Ergot
   β-blocking drugs
   Cytotoxic drugs
   Birth-control pills

for up to 45 minutes. Prolonged return to baseline temperature (more than 10 minutes) signifies a positive test.

Buerger's disease involves inflammation of the neurovascular bundle of the limb small vessels. It classically manifests as intermittent claudication of the arch of the foot and can progress to frank gangrene. The disease also may affect the arms and be responsible for recurrent superficial thrombophlebitis. A typical patient is a young man who smokes heavily. Angiograms will reveal multiple small-artery occlusions, with tapering proximal to the occlusions and an absence of plaques. Pathological features include a pan-angiitis with preservation of vessel architecture and infiltration of vessel walls with lymphocytes and giant cells.

Embolic-occlusive disease leads to ischemic pain secondary to acute arterial insufficiency. Emboli tend to lodge where arteries branch (Fig. 28.1). Muscle necrosis is expected if blood flow is not reestablished within 4 to 6 hours. The pain from embolic occlusion is sudden in its onset, well localized, and is distinguished by the five P's: pain, pallor, paresthesias, paralysis, and pulselessness. In addition, there may be a decrease in skin temperature distal to occlusion.

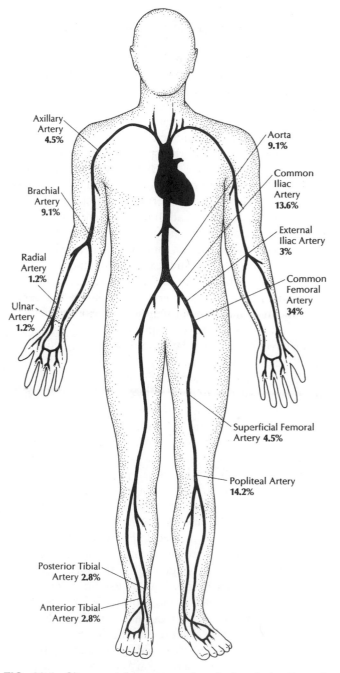

FIG. 28.1. Sites and frequency of embolic obstruction of peripheral arteries are indicated on body map. Leg arteries are involved in the majority of cases.

NONSURGICAL MANAGEMENT OF PAIN FROM PERIPHERAL VASCULAR DISEASE

Management of pain from PVD is directed at treating the underlying causes and modifying any risk factors. In case of arteriosclerotic PVD, smoking cessation, exercise and weight loss, meticulous foot care, and, in diabetics, tight control of blood-glucose levels are suggested to slow the progression of PVD. A flow-enhancing medication such as pentoxifylline often is prescribed as well. However, these conservative measures invariably fail to halt the progression of the disease and a more definitive therapeutic measure becomes necessary.

"Nonsurgical" pain management modalities for lower-extremity PVD include neurolytic lumbar sympathetic block, radiofrequency lumbar sympathetic block, and spinal-cord stimulators. In general, these modalities tend to be effective in and indicated for ischemic conditions in which there is a major vasospastic component such as from Raynaud's disease or Buerger's disease. In arteriosclerotic PVD with a fixed stenosis in a conduit artery with compensatory distal arteriolar dilation, sympathetic block usually does not lead to any further dilation of the small arteries and there is little improvement in flow. Therefore, although a few authors such as Huber and Kumar have advocated the use of sympathetic block as the first-line therapy even in the early stages of LaReich and Fontaine, in practice sympathetic block is reserved for patients in the terminal stages of arteriosclerotic PVD who are not considered surgical candidates either because of the advanced PVD or because of severity of coexisting cardiovascular problems.

The lumbar-sympathetic chain and ganglia lie near the anterolateral surface of the first through fifth lumbar vertebral bodies and anterior to the psoas sheath. Lumbar-sympathetic block is performed under fluoroscopic guidance with the patient prone. A skin wheal is raised three to four finger breadths lateral to the caudal tip of the L2 spinous process and a 10- to 15-cm 22-gauge block needle is advanced at approximately a 30-degree angle toward the body of the vertebra. Once the body of the vertebra is met, this is confirmed by fluoroscopy in two planes. A loss of resistance is sought as the needle penetrates the psoas fascia into the groove between the muscle and the vertebrae where the sympathetic ganglia lie. At this time, 0.5 to 1 cc of radio-opaque dye may be injected to demonstrate a characteristic linear spread in the groove. Before proceeding with the neurolytic block, a diagnostic block with a small volume (2 cc) of a local anesthetic should be performed. A successful diagnostic block would be indicated by (a) relief of symptoms for a time period consistent with the estimated duration of action of the local anesthetic used, (b) more than 50% increase in the amplitude of the digital plethysmographic tracing, and (c) a negative ice-water challenge. For definitive neurolysis, phenol 5% to 10% dissolved in a radiopaque substance is injected slowly until the dye spreads three vertebral bodies. Complications include intravascular injection of local anesthetics or neurolytic agents and allergic or anaphylactic reactions to the contrast material. Resuscitation equipment always should be immediately available.

Radiofrequency sympathetic neurolysis is similarly performed under fluoroscopic guidance at L2, L3, and L4 levels. At each level, a test block is performed with 2 cc of a dilute local anesthetic (e.g., 1% or less of lidocaine).

An important part of the test is to ensure that there is sympathetic block (evidenced by a temperature rise of 2°C), but no somatic block. Major complications of this procedure are related to unintended coagulation of the lumbar-somatic nerves, the ureters, and the sidewall of the aorta or the inferior vena cava. If there is any motor or sensory block with the test dose, the procedure should be postponed to another date and restarted with a repeat test. With a negative test block, the radiofrequency cannula is positioned under fluoroscopic guidance so that it is directly behind the facet-joint line while in contact with the anterior/anterolateral aspect of the vertebral body. The cannula position is further confirmed by injection of 1 cc of water-soluble contrast and noting its spread directly behind the facet-joint line. Resistance to the spread of the dye may indicate incorrect positioning. After injecting 1 cc of 2% lidocaine through the cannula, a thermal lesion is created for 60 seconds at 80°C. Although the patient may have local back discomfort for about 3 days, the ischemic pain relief usually is immediate. The radiofrequency procedure produces a more controlled neurolysis than phenol and is associated with a lower incidence of neurovascular or ureteral damage or of anaphylactic or allergic reactions.

Spinal-cord stimulators are surgically placed in the operating room. The leads and electrodes are introduced into the epidural space at the level of T10–T12 and connected to a screening pulse generator. Various stimulating patterns are applied and a pattern that results in paresthesia covering the ischemic leg is sought. With a good pattern, a feeling of warmth may accompany the paresthesia. Once such a pattern is found, a 3- to 7-day trial is begun. Onset of pain relief may not occur for 48 to 72 hours. Important prognostic indicators during the trial period include (a) more than 50% pain relief on a visual analog scale and (b) transcutaneous oxygen tension that is initially over 30 mmHg and increases measurably with spinal-cord stimulation. If the patient reports over 50% pain relief during the trial period, a permanent implant is placed. The most common complication of the procedure is related to mechanical disruption of the leads and consequent cessation of pain relief. Epidural abscesses or hematomas and meningitis are rare complications.

To date, there have been no controlled, randomized studies comparing different nonsurgical techniques of pain management in PVD. Often, availability of technology and operator experience and comfort level are the determining factors in selection of one of these techniques. Each of the techniques is expensive and nonpayment by certain third-party payers has been another limiting factor.

SURGICAL MANAGEMENT OF PAIN FROM PERIPHERAL VASCULAR DISEASE

Acute ischemic pain from embolic-occlusive disease or compartment syndrome requires prompt surgical attention and tends to be relieved immediately with appropriate surgery. Surgical management of pain from other types of PVD may not lead to as clear-cut benefits, however. In patients with Buerger's disease, the role of a bypass surgery has been controversial because of a relatively high incidence of graft failure. In the series reported by Sasajima et al., graft patency rate was 49% at 5 years and 43% at 10 years, which improved to 63% and 56%, respectively, with revisional surgery. Nearly 60% of the patients were considered to have had successful revascularization and were returned to full-time work. Cessation of smoking contributes to patency of grafts.

Surgical revascularization is the standard therapy for Fontaine stage III or IV patients in arteriosclerotic PVD. Even in diabetic patients with arteriosclerotic PVD, in whom the disease may involve distal arterioles as well as large conduit arteries, recent improvements in surgical techniques have demonstrated that extreme distal arterial reconstruction is not only possible, but also carries high success rates. Logerfo et al. have demonstrated the benefit of grafts to the pedal arteries not only for limb salvage, but also for pain relief and functional recovery of the patients. They have reported 36-month limb salvage rates of over 90% in all diabetics; the rate was lower at 84% at 2 years for juvenile-onset diabetics, but still was considered acceptable. With successful operations that improve blood flow to the extremities, most patients report symptomatic relief and functional improvement.

MANAGEMENT OF PERIOPERATIVE PAIN FOR PATIENTS UNDERGOING PERIPHERAL VASCULAR SURGERY

Surgical pain in the immediate postoperative period may be managed with various combinations of analgesics delivered orally, parenterally, or near the neural axis. It generally is agreed that epidural analgesia is more effective in relieving postoperative pain than parenteral analgesia delivered by way of a patient-controlled analgesia (PCA) regimen or by a healthcare provider. However, there is no consensus on whether the use of epidural anesthesia and analgesia is additionally associated with a lower incidence of major morbidities such as graft failure, myocardial infarction, congestive heart failure, and death.

During the revascularization procedure, the patient is systemically heparinized. In addition, the surgeon may often use angioscopy intraoperatively to verify the patency of grafts as well as using a Doppler to qualitatively measure graft flow. Therefore, it is unlikely that regional anesthesia that does not extend to the postoperative period can be demonstrated to differ in incidence of graft failure from general anesthesia. In theory, epidural analgesia used postoperatively may decrease stress responses and hypercoagulability and may therefore be surmised to be associated with a lower incidence of graft

failure. In practice, however, the use of epidural analgesia generally is not associated with reduction in the rate of reoperation for graft failure during the immediate postoperative period. Surgical technique may be the most important determinant of graft success. For example, anecdotally, graft thrombosis often is seen near an untied branch of an *in-situ* vein graft where a type of arteriovenous fistula ensues and leads to thrombosis.

In the largest prospective, randomized trial to date to evaluate the effect of anesthesia type on perioperative cardiovascular morbidity and mortality in vascular surgery, Bode et al. failed to demonstrate that there is any clinically significant difference in cardiovascular outcome between anesthetic techniques. Even when epidural anesthesia was extended to postoperative epidural analgesia, Christopherson et al. did not see any difference in cardiovascular morbidity and mortality. Other smaller studies have produced contradictory results. The advantage of epidural analgesia in the postoperative period may be in providing superior pain relief with relative safety, rather than in concomitant reduction of cardiovascular morbidities.

SELECTED READINGS

Bode RH, Lewis KP, Zarich SW, et al. Cardiac outcome after peripheral vascular surgery: comparison of general and regional anesthesia. *Anesthesiology* 1996;84:3–13.

Broseta J, Barbara J, deVera JA. Spinal cord stimulation in peripheral arterial disease. *J Neurosurg* 1986;64:71–80.

Christopherson R, Beattie C, Frank SM, et al. Perioperative morbidity in patients randomized to epidural or general anesthesia for lower extremity vascular surgery. *Anesthesiology* 1993;79:422–434.

Gevirtz C. Pain management in peripheral vascular disease. *Semin Cardiothor Vasc Anesth* 1999;3:182–190.

Gibbons GW, Burgess AM, Guadagnoli E, et al. Return to well-being and function after infrainguinal revascularization. *J Vasc Surg* 1995;21:35–45.

Go AS, Browner WS. Cardiac outcomes after regional or general anesthesia. Do we have the answer? *Anesthesiology* 1996;84:1–2.

Haynesworth RF, Noe CE. Percutaneous lumbar sympathectomy: a comparison of radiofrequency denervation versus phenol neurolysis. *Anesthesiology* 1991;74:459–463.

Huber SJ, Vaglienti RM, Midcap ME. Enhanced limb salvage for peripheral vascular disease with the use of spinal cord stimulation. *WV Med J* 1996;92:89–91.

Kahn RA. Pain management after vascular surgery. *Semin Cardiothor Vasc Anesth* 1999;3:177–181.

Kempczinski RF. The differential diagnosis of intermittent claudication. *Pract Cardiol* 1981;7:53.

Kempczinski RF. The management of chronic ischemia of the lower extremities. In: Miller DC, Roon AJ, eds. *Vascular Surgery*. Menlo Park, California: Addison-Wesley Publishing Co, 1982:135–149.

Kumar K, Toth C, Nath RK, et al. Improvement of limb circulation in peripheral vascular disease using epidural spinal cord stimulation in prospective study. *J Neurosurg* 1997;86:662–699.

Kwolek CJ, Pomposelli FB Jr, Tannenbaum GA, et al. Peripheral vascular bypass in juvenile-onset diabetes mellitus: are aggressive revascularization attempts justified? *J Vasc Surg* 1992;15:394–401.

Logerfo FW, Gibbons GW, Pomposelli FB Jr, et al. Trends in the care of the diabetic foot. Expanded role of arterial reconstruction. *Arch Surg* 1992;127:617–621.

Noe CE, Haynesworth RF. Lumbar radiofrequency sympatholysis. *J Vasc Surg* 1993;17:801–806.

Pernak J. Percutaneous radiofrequency thermal lumbar sympathectomy. *Pain Clin* 1995;1:99–106.

Pierce ET, Pomposelli FB Jr, Stanley GD, et al. Anesthesia type does not influence early graft patency or limb salvage rates of lower extremity arterial bypass. *J Vasc Surg* 1997;25:226–233.

Rosenfield BA, Beattie C, Christopherson R, et al. The Perioperative Ischemia Randomized Anesthesia Trial Study Group: the effects of different anesthetic regimens on fibrinolysis and the development of postoperative arterial thrombosis. *Anesthesiology* 1993;79:435–443.

Sasajima T, Kubo Y, Inaba M, et al. Role of infrainguinal bypass in Buerger's disease: an eighteen-year experience. *Eur J Vasc Endovasc Surg* 1997;13:186–192.

Tannenbaum GA, Pomposelli FB Jr, Marcaccio EJ, et al. Safety of vein bypass grafting to the dorsal pedal artery in diabetic patients with foot infections. *J Vasc Surg* 1992;15:982–990.

Tuman KJ, McCarthy RJ, March RJ, et al. Effects of epidural anesthesia and analgesia on coagulation and outcome after major vascular surgery. *Anesth Analg* 1991;73:696–704.

CHAPTER 29

Phantom Limb Pain

Stephen A. Houser

Look ye, carpenter, I dare say thou callest thyself a right good workmanlike workman, eh? Well, then, will it speak thoroughly well for thy work, if, when I come to mount this leg thou makest, I shall nevertheless fell another leg in the same identical place with it; that is, carpenter my old lost leg; the flesh and blood one, I mean. Canst thou not drive that old Adam away?

Truly, Sir I begin to understand somewhat now. Yes, I have heard something curious on that score, Sir; how that a dis-masted man never entirely loses the feeling of his ol spar, but it will be still pricking him at times may I humbly ask if it really be so, Sir?

It is man. Look, put thy live leg here in the place where mine once was; o, now, here is only one distinct leg to the eye, yet two to the soul.

—Melville, Herman; *Moby Dick*

A phantom limb is a sensory illusion of a limb that occurs after its sensory roots have been destroyed. It was first described by the French military surgeon Ambrose Paré, in 1551. However, Civil War surgeon Silas Weir Mitchell invented the term "phantom limb" to detail the unalterable consequence of amputations he saw in Civil War veterans: the incessant ghostly representations of the missing limbs. Phantom limbs were thought only to be associated with trauma. Sensations were almost always felt most prominently in the distal parts of the limb. Then gradually, the phantom foot or hand is felt to be closer to the stump than one would anatomically expect in a phenomenon known as telescoping. The sensation of the phantom limb often is associated with a painful amputation stump and progresses to the development of phantom-limb pain.

Phantom-limb pain is pain referred to a surgically removed limb or portion thereof in the absent body part. Phantom-limb pain occurs in up to 50% of all amputees. Studies have shown that preamputation pain greatly increases the development of stump pain and phantom-limb pain (up to 70%). The pain usually appears within the first few days after amputation. The quality of the pain has been described as tingling, numbness, itching, "feeling asleep," tickling. Most of these sensations are short in duration lasting mostly seconds or minutes and rarely hours or days. They occur at least once a day in up to one half of patients. In 10% to 20% of patients, the pain persists and worsens over time, although in the vast majority of cases, the phantom-limb pain usually becomes less intense and frequent after 6 months.

Interestingly, pain in other areas of the body occurs in conjunction with phantom-limb pain. Stump pain usually coincides with the development of phantom-limb pain. All phantom-limb pain patients show areas of abnormal sensitivity in the stump, whether or not they complained of pain at the time of amputation. Phantom-limb pain is associated with headaches (35%), pain in joints (35%), sore throat (28%), stomachaches (18 %), and backaches (13%). Obvious pathology is not necessarily related to the development of phantom-limb pain.

Psychological and physiological input has a large role in the manifestation of phantom limbs and phantom-limb pain. Melzack showed that amputation is not necessary for the development of a phantom. He noted that children born without a limb still experience phantom sensations. He also observed that a brachial-plexus block or spinal block of the lower extremity produces a phantom in most patients. These patients report vivid phantoms of extremities unrelated to the position of the real extremity. Moreover, in studies of war veterans, physically and mentally active amputees have fewer problems with phantom sensations and phantom-limb pain. In addition, phantom-limb pain is aggravated by cold, dreams, illness, exercise, anxiety, not wearing a prosthesis, and an object approaching the perceived limb. Furthermore, patting the posterior thigh over the sciatic nerve, stroking, tapping, or squeezing the stump, or simply ignoring it sometimes can relieve the pain.

PATHOGENESIS

Despite numerous attempts to formulate a theoretical basis for phantom limb pain beginning with Mitchell's study of Civil War veterans in 1872, the pathogenesis of the phantom limb phenomena remains unknown. Initially considered to be a learned behavior, attempts to define and deal with phantom limb pain in psychoanalytical terms, have been unsuccessful. Although controversial, current theories of phantom limb pain focus on central nervous system stimulation.

In one such theory, persistent transmission of noxious afferent input from the periphery to the spinal cord induces a prolonged state of central neural sensation, which amplifies subsequent input. Yaksh described this state as hyperalgesia: a state in which afferent sensory input is processed in such a way that this input evokes a greater then expected response for any given input. Following cutaneous injury, the increased generation of nerve terminals permits the volume of input to nociceptors to increase. Large-diameter nerve fibers, normally low-threshold mechanoreceptive afferents, become sufficient to evoke pain via the activation of central pain signaling neurons. Central changes can also occur in higher centers.

A study using neuroelectrical source imaging examined a relationship between cortical representation and phantom limb pain produced by brachial plexus block. It found a high correlation between phantom limb pain and phantom limbastic changes in the contralateral hemisphere of the primary somatosensory cortex of upper extremity amputees, but could not establish a functional relationship between the two. Further studies measuring regional cerebral blood flow in amputees with phantom limb pain using technetium-99 and single photon emission control tomography before and after pain was relieved suggest reorganization of cortical blood flow occurs in amputees. The study did not address causation: did the amputation stump anesthesia erase the preexisting cortical reorganization which in turn eliminated the phantom limb pain; or, conversely, did the stump anesthesia dispose of the phantom limb pain and cause the obliteration of the cortical reorganization?

DIAGNOSIS

The approach to the patient with phantom limb pain must begin as with any clinical problem, with a careful history and a thorough physical examination. Careful attention must also be paid to the mental status examination, especially with regard to recent psychological stresses and depression. In the treatment of phantom-limb pain, the general rules of individualization of therapy, the titration of drugs to balance therapeutic and side effects with attention to the psychologic and physical substrates of the problem apply.

TREATMENT

Early attempts at the treatment of phantom-limb pain focused on blocking stimulation. Because intraoperative pain is presumably covered by general or regional anesthesia, attention first was directed to postoperative analgesia with continuous infusions of local anesthetics. This proved effective in eliminating postoperative pain, but not phantom-limb pain. Therefore, others looked at preemptive analgesia to avoid central nervous system (CNS) stimulation and reduce the incidence of postoperative phantom-limb pain. Randomized prospective studies using neural blockade for preemptive analgesia have shown mixed results. Bach used lumbar-epidural anesthesia for 3 days prior to amputation and found after 1 year of follow up none of the blockade group reported phantom-limb pain. However, Nikolajsen found that perioperative epidural blockade started a median of 18 hours before the amputation and continued into the postoperative period does not prevent phantom or stump pain. Because there is no satisfactory explanation of the pathogenesis of phantom-limb pain, it is not surprising that there is no satisfactory therapy.

Sympathetic blocks inhibit the actions of endogenous catecholamines in the CNS or in the peripheral nervous system (PNS). The role of the sympathetic nervous system in phantom-limb pain is controversial. Preemptive analgesia, which blocks both somatic and sympathetic nervous systems, shows promise in the treatment of phantom-limb pain. However, sympathetic blocks may result in substantial relief in only some patients. Diagnostic sympathetic blocks, used to elucidate a sympathetically mediated component of pain are valuable tools in the treatment of phantom-limb pain.

Transcutaneous electrical stimulation is used to characterize phantom phenomena and to treat it. In many cases, it is the most successful treatment regimen when no reversible cause is found. Initially, electrodes are fixed to the skin on opposite sides of the stump in the office. Duration of stimulation, frequency, pulse width, and amplitude are determined on an individual basis. Patients are instructed in the use of the device at home. The advantages of peripheral-nerve stimulation are the lack of adverse side effects and easy reproducibility.

Tricyclic antidepressants (TCAs) inhibit the reuptake of monoamines. Through this mechanism, they are believed to augment the effects of amines in inhibitory descending spinal pathways. The TCAs are effective in neuropathic pain syndromes. Amitriptyline, a commonly used TCA, has been shown to achieve analgesic effects within 2 weeks of its initiation. The newer agents fluoxetine, paroxetine, fluvoxamine, and sertraline, although effective in the treatment of depression, have shown little or no efficacy in the treatment of neuropathic pain.

The antiarrhythmics lidocaine, mexiletine, and tocainide also are effective in relieving some pain syndromes. They act on sodium channels to stabilize membranes and thereby inhibit ectopic activity of afferent nerve fibers. Clinically, mexiletine has been shown to alleviate diabetic neuropathy. Recent trials have shown some promise in treating phantom-limb pain. It is important to note that despite the success of these drugs in the treatment of neuropathic pain, some of these drugs are not yet approved by the Food and Drug Administration (FDA) for this indication.

Antiepileptics such as carbamazepine and the newer gabapentin act by reducing repetitive, high-frequency discharges. Carbamazepine has proven very effective in the treatment of trigeminal neuralgia. Its use in phantom-limb pain has been less conclusive. If phantom-limb pain is associated with spasms of pain, however, a trial with antiepileptics may be warranted.

Nonsteroidal antiinflammatory drugs inhibit the formation of proinflammatory arachidonic-acid metabolites and reduce pain. These drugs usually are very effective in the treatment of acute inflammatory or cancer pain. However, they generally are ineffective in the treatment of phantom-limb pain.

Opiate analgesics interact with μ-opioid receptors in the spinal cord. They inhibit central nociceptive neurons producing a hyperpolarized state. Opiates have proven effective in acute postoperative, inflammatory, and cancer pain. Recent studies indicate that they may also be effective in neuropathic pain. Nevertheless, because phantom-limb pain often has no clearly identifiable aggravating factor, they should be used with caution. There are no studies to support the effectiveness of opiates in treating phantom-limb pain. Nevertheless, many practitioners have found their patients achieve good relief of some component of their pain with the judicious use of opiates. Because the chronic nature of phantom-limb pain renders dependence inevitable if opiates are used as primary therapy, patients and their practitioners should discuss the risks and benefits of this class of medications before initiating therapy.

Experimental and newer treatment options are being actively investigated. Recent efforts have turned to unique therapies such as the use of *calcitonin*. Binding sites for calcitonin have been found in the CNS. Calcitonin was first used as an antinociceptive agent in rabbits where it increased B endorphin levels. The mechanism through which calcitonin blocks pain is unknown; however, research directed at calcitonin blockade of serotonin reuptake, prostaglandins, and cytokines synthesis is progressing. Recent anecdotal reports on the use of calcitonin in phantom-limb pain seem promising. Still, many controversies about its use remain; including optimum dose and route of administration.

Another class of drugs that might be useful is *N*-methyl-D-aspartate (NMDA) antagonists. NMDA antagonists block the glutamate receptors in the CNS. Glutamate is an excitatory neurotransmitter thought to propel the CNS after noxious stimuli. There are four clinically available drugs in the United States with NMDA receptor-blocking properties: ketamine, dextromethorphan, amantadine, and memantine. It is important to note that these drugs have not been approved by the FDA for use as analgesics. Therefore, these drugs should be prescribed with caution. Adverse side effects of these drugs include sedation, nausea, dysphoria, and even hallucinations.

Phantom-limb pain is a challenging and complex syndrome. Its successful treatment requires patience from both the physician and the patient, as there is no standard therapy to be offered, only alternatives to be tried. As research into the mechanism of phantom-limb pain is ongoing, perhaps a definitive cure will be found. Until then, it is encouraging for both clinicians and patients to recognize that this condition is likely to improve with the passage of time.

SELECTED READINGS

Bach S. Phantom limb pain in amputees during the first 12 months following limb amputation, after preoperative lumbar epidural blockade. *Pain* 1988;33:297–301.

Baron R. Optimal treatment of phantom limb pain in the elderly. *Drugs Aging* 1998;12:361–76.

Hill A. Phantom limb: a review of the literature on attribute and potential mechanisms. *J Pain Symptom Manage* 1999;17:125–142.

Jensen TS. Immediate and long term phantom pain in amputees: incidence, clinical characteristics, and relative relationship to pre-amputation limb pain. *Pain* 1985;21:267–278.

Nikolajsen L. Randomized trial of epidural bupivacaine and morphine in the prevention of stump and phantom limb pain in lower limb amputation. *Lancet* 1997;350:1353–1357.

Pinzur MS. Continuous postoperative infusion of a regional anesthetic after an amputation of the lower extremity. A randomized clinical trial. *J Bone Joint Surg* 1996;78-A:1501–1505.

CHAPTER 30

Pain in AIDS

Anna G.A. Sottile and Kimberly A. Cox

Human immunodeficiency virus (HIV) infection is a malignant and debilitating disease and has an alarmingly increasing incidence. It is strongly associated with chronic and acute pain of various etiologies, which require appropriate treatment. Modern antiviral and chemotherapies have been used successfully to prolong the lives of patients with HIV/acquired immunodeficiency syndrome (AIDS). This leads to continued growth of the total number of HIV patients who are getting older with added risk factors. This results in an increased need to attend to this problem.

Pain is the second most common reason for hospitalization of AIDS patients. In the last decade, many studies have been conducted to learn more about the real dimensions of the HIV-associated pain problem to try to identify the various etiologies and to provide successful treatments to improve the quality of life of these suffering patients.

Despite all these efforts, several studies demonstrate that the work, which has been done, is still far from being sufficient and much is still to be done. As with any chronic pain syndrome, HIV-associated pain has multiple dimensions. Physical, psychological, and social aspects coexist, adding complexity. The issue is even more complicated in patients whose disease was the result of intravenous drug abuse.

EPIDEMIOLOGY

The World Health Organization estimates that over 1.5 million human HIV infections have occurred to date in South and Southeast Asia, meaning that in the next decade, this will be a major global health problem. The Centers for Disease Control estimates that 1.2 million Americans are infected with HIV. Now that the life span of HIV-infected patients is being prolonged by early antiviral therapy and prophylaxis for opportunistic infections, quality of life issues are increasingly important. Several studies show that more than 50% of HIV patients suffer from pain, requiring treatment and even hospitalization.

In 1989, Lebovits et al. reviewed 96 AIDS patients' charts. The results showed that 54% contained at least one notation of nonprocedural pain or analgesic prescription. Other subsequent studies confirmed this or found an even higher incidence of pain.

Several studies show that pain has been underrepresented and suboptimally managed in HIV-infected patients. Singer et al. reported one or more HIV-related pain in HIV-seropositive patients. Of those patients who reported HIV-related pain, 28% were asymptomatic for AIDS-related infections, 55% were considered to have AIDS-related complex (ARC) disease, and 80% were considered to have full-blown AIDS.

In 1994, another review study by Lebovits et al. demonstrated that both opioids and antidepressants were underutilized, suggesting the need for a more aggressive approach. In one study, women appeared at twice the risk of men to be undertreated for their pain. Patients with less education and with a history of intravenous drug abuse also are likely to be undertreated.

CLINICAL PRESENTATION

HIV patients suffer from pain originating from a number of sources. It appears that chest pain secondary to *Pneumocystis carinii* and peripheral neuropathy are the most common sources of pain.

The systems most commonly affected by pain are the central and peripheral nervous system, respiratory system, gastrointestinal system including the oral cavity and rectal area, and the immune system. Up to 30% of patients with AIDS present with gastrointestinal problems, 6.7% of HIV-infected hospitalized patients complain of persistent arthralgia, and another portion will have other rheumatological manifestations with associated pain.

CENTRAL NERVOUS SYSTEM

Headache is the most common pain complaint with central nervous system (CNS) involvement. Infection, inflammation, and tumor with mass effect are the three most common etiologies. Aseptic meningitis syndrome with a triad of fever, headache, and meningism occurs not uncommonly. Infection can involve the entire surface of the meninges, giving a picture of fever, headache, seizure, and changes in mental status. A focal, intracerebral infectious process can result from a confined intracerebral abscess, which causes localized symptoms, seizures, and fever. Multiple abscesses are not rare. Herpes virus infection is a common cause of encephalitis, which can be acute or subacute. Tumor involvement usually is caused by primary lymphoma of the CNS, but Kaposi's sarcoma also has been described.

Headache accompanied by CNS changes in HIV patients requires further evaluation including lumbar puncture and computed tomography. Brain biopsy may be indicated. Treatment may include analgesics, chemotherapeutic agents, antiseizure drugs, radiation therapy, and drainage.

PERIPHERAL SENSORY NEUROPATHY

Peripheral sensory neuropathies are among the most common sources of pain in patients with HIV infection. Several peripheral neuropathies have been described. Their incidence has increased proportionally with prolongation of life for HIV patients, which concurs with the hypothesis that these may be late signs of the disease. These neuropathies may be the result of nutritional deficiencies or associated with antiviral and chemotherapy drugs.

The most common type, the sensory neuropathy, presents in 10% to 30% of patients with AIDS. The usual complaint is of a stocking distribution of painful dysesthesia starting on the soles of the feet and spreading proximally to involve the entire foot and lower extremities. The ankle reflexes are diminished or even absent. The upper extremities also may be affected. Distal axonal degeneration (dying-back neuropathy) has been suggested by electrophysiological studies revealing abnormal sensory and motor conduction.

Peripheral sensory neuropathies require prompt recognition and treatment. The use of tricyclic antidepressants starting with a small dose and slowly increasing to effect often is successful. Antiepileptics also have been shown to be effective. Among them, gabapentin has the safest profile and does not require blood testing. If not successful, other antiseizure medications, such as phenytoin and carbamazepine, can be carefully tried with periodic screening for toxicity by monitoring white blood cell count and liver-function tests.

RADICULITIS

The most common cause of radiculitis in the HIV patient is herpes zoster infection. It most commonly involves the ophthalmic branch of the trigeminal nerve or the chest wall. Other nerve roots can be involved as well. The acute onset of severe pain along a nerve distribution should raise suspicion of herpes zoster in this population of patients. The appearance of vesicles along the distribution of the pain makes diagnosis almost certain.

The success rate of treatment with antiviral agents, steroids, and peripheral or sympathetic blocks increases with the immediate recognition and initiation of treatment. These therapies can also decrease the incidence of postherpetic neuralgia. Therefore, early referral to a pain specialist for blocks is crucial and treatment with topical capsaicin, nonsteroidal antiinflammatory drugs (NSAIDs), antidepressants, or antiepileptic medication often is useful in the postherpetic phase. Radicular symptoms also may be caused by impingement by masses on a nerve root. After a careful neurological exam, magnetic resonance imaging (MRI) evaluation is suggested. Recommended treatment includes analgesics, steroids, and, if necessary, surgery.

DEMYELINATING NEUROPATHY

Although rare, there is a striking association between HIV and inflammatory demyelinating polyneuropathy (IDP). In fact, 50% of patients infected by Guillain–Barré (an acute form of IDP), also are affected by HIV. The onset can be acute or slow. It may present with major motor weakness and minor sensory abnormalities, usually in the form of painful dysesthesia. It is thought to be the result of immune-mediated disease.

No specific treatment is used, but some good results have been achieved with steroids and plasmapheresis. Epidural analgesia also may be helpful when pain is a major issue.

RESPIRATORY SYSTEM

The second most common presenting symptom for *P. carinii* pneumonia is chest pain. Very commonly it is described as severe, burning, pleuritic, and retrosternal. In some cases, pneumothorax can occur. Other forms of opportunistic respiratory infection, such as *Mycobacterium tuberculosis*, atypical mycobacteria, fungi, cytomegalovirus and others, also may present with pleuritic chest pain.

Treatment for pleuritic chest pain includes NSAIDs, analgesics, and antiviral or antibiotic medication as indicated.

GASTROINTESTINAL SYSTEM

Oral-Cavity Pain

Oral-cavity pain is experienced by 28% of HIV-infected individuals. Thrush or oral candidiasis is the most common cause of oral pain. Herpes simplex stomatitis, herpes zoster, radiculitis, recurrent aphthous ulcers, and Kaposi's sarcoma can cause oral pain. Treatment includes antimicrobial therapy in conjunction with local anesthetic oral solutions. Kaposi's sarcoma can be treated with intralesional vinblastine, radiotherapy, and/or laser. Maintenance therapy with ketoconazole can be used to control recurrent candidal infections.

Esophageal Pain

Esophageal pain in HIV-infected individuals is a common occurrence. Esophageal pathology also may be the source of chest pain, which often is reported in HIV-infected patients. Esophageal candidiasis and its resultant ulcerations account for more than 75% of the cases of odynophagia. Cytomegalovirus (CMV), herpes simplex virus (HSV), and HIV also can cause esophageal ulcers. Esophageal cancer, reflux esophagitis, and achalasia occur in this group of patients as they do in the immunocompetent patient. Treatment often is on an empiric basis. Initial treatment usually is an antifungal agent such as ketoconazole and amphotericin B. Herpes simplex virus is treated with acyclovir, and CMV is treated with ganciclovir.

Abdominal Pain

The incidence of abdominal pain is as high as 12% in HIV-infected individuals. Cello et al. reported the commonest single cause of abdominal pain in HIV-infected patients was sclerosing cholangitis. The cause of pain in AIDS-related sclerosing cholangitis remains unknown and is difficult to treat successfully. However, there has been a reported association with cryptosporidial and cytomegaloviral infections, this finding having been partially supported by recent data by Thuluvath et al.

Cholecystitis can occur as a result of CMV, *Campylobacter*, or from infection of the bile by candidal species. Cholecystitis also can occur as a coincidental finding in an HIV-infected patient with gallstones. *Mycobacterium avium* intracellular (MAIC) and Kaposi's sarcoma can produce pain from extrahepatic biliary obstruction. The second most common cause of abdominal pain was cytomegalovirus colitis. Thuluvath et al. reported that toxic megacolon affected five to 27 patients with death occurring in one-third of the study patients resulting from colonic perforation.

Appendicitis and enteritis also may produce abdominal pain. Appendicitis can be coincidental or can result from obstruction by HIV-related neoplasm. Infectious diarrhea in HIV-infected patients usually is caused by *Shigella*, salmonella, *Campylobacter*, *Entamoeba histolytica*, or cryptosporidium, and is associated with crampy abdominal pain and fever. Pancreatitis appears to be a common complication of HIV infection. Pancreatitis also may occur as a result of pentamidine, an agent used in the treatment of *P. carinii* pneumonia (PCP) or the antiretroviral agent dideoxyinosine.

Organomegaly from CMV hepatitis, tumor involvement of intraabdominal organs and *M. avium* intracellular (MAIC) infiltration of the liver and/or spleen are causes of abdominal pain in HIV-infected patients.

One should always keep in mind that HIV-infected patients may develop illnesses not unique to AIDS or the immunosuppressed state. For example, peptic-ulcer disease can be seen in the AIDS patient. Treatment of abdominal pain is directed by etiology. Antimicrobial therapy, antispasmodic agents, and/or antidiarrheal agents may be used. It also should be noted that many HIV-infected individuals may have one or more pain syndromes for which opioid analgesics are part of the treatment. Thus, constipation as a result of opioid analgesic therapy may be the source of abdominal pain. It should be remembered that the HIV-infected patient with diffuse or lower-abdominal pain is likely to have an infectious cause for pain and should be treated accordingly.

Anorectal Pain

In a large series of predominantly homosexual AIDS and ARC patients, Wexner and coworkers reported that 34% had disease of the anorectal area, almost half of whom required surgery. Infections, anal and rectal cancers, lymphoma, Kaposi's sarcoma, trauma, fissures/fistulas/abscesses, and hemorrhoids are common causes of anorectal pain. Healing of anorectal diseases in AIDS patients is poor. It has been recommended that patients with recurrent anorectal sexually transmitted disease, herpes zoster, colonic enteritis, oral candidiasis, weight loss, fever, diarrhea, fatigue, lymphadenopathy, or leukopenia be treated without nonsurgical means.

RHEUMATIC MANIFESTATIONS ASSOCIATED WITH HUMAN IMMUNODEFICIENCY VIRUS INFECTIONS

In patients with HIV infection, it appears that the immune system is not only suppressed but also deregulated. Immunological laboratory data frequently associated with autoimmune disease and connective-tissue disorders have been observed in HIV-infected patients. Much of the clinical presentation of rheumatological disease appears in the HIV-infected patient. The HIV-associated variety may mimic the idiopathic form [e.g., systemic lupus erythematosus (SLE) and Sjögren's syndrome (SS)] while some may represent new nosologic entities that need to be recognized (i.e., AIDS-associated arthritis and vasculitis). Arthralgia appears to be the most common musculoskeletal manifestation. In a prospective study, Berman et al. described arthralgia in 45 (44.5%) of 101 consecutive HIV-1 seropositive patients. Freine et al. reported arthralgia in 33 (27.5%) of 120 HIV-1 seropositive patients studied. In a study performed on 24 HIV-1-seropositive patients with arthralgia, 15 (62.5%) were polyarticular and were 37.5% oligoarticular.

Simms et al. have suggested that fibromyalgia associated with mental depression might be a common cause of chronic arthralgia in HIV-infected individuals. Others have suggested that arthralgia may be a subclinical form of arthritis. This view is supported by the observation of a good response to NSAIDs in HIV-infected patients with large-joint oligo or polyarticular arthritis. It is unclear as to why HIV-infected patients are more prone to arthritis. Its has been suggested that HIV-1 infection itself leads to direct joint inflammation. Some have suggested that HIV infection could enhance immunological mechanism or maybe synovial immune-complex deposits are the causative agents.

Sjögren's Syndrome

Patients with HIV infections can develop a syndrome that closely resembles idiopathic Sjögren's syndrome (SS). However, HIV-infected patients typically do not have the characteristic antibodies such as anti-Ro/SS-A, anti-La/SS-B, and rheumatoid factor.

Polymyositis

Recent reports have described HIV-infected individuals with a myopathy that appears indistinguishable from clinical polymyositis. There is no definitive therapy for HIV-associated myopathy. Most physicians would be reluctant to use immunosuppression in an immunocompromised host.

Lupuslike Syndrome

HIV infection may mimic idiopathic SLE and my be difficult to diagnose in patients with a known history of SLE. deClerck et al. described a 37-year-old woman with SLE-like syndrome who had false-negative serology for HIV. There have been reports that demonstrate false-positive reaction particularly by enzyme-linked immunoassay (ELISA) technique. It may not be uncommon for a patient to have a false HIV test in the presence of connective-tissue disease.

HIV-Associated Vasculitis

Four cases have been described as a polyarteritis nodosalike vasculitis of medium-sized vessels involving skin, muscle, and nerves. In immunohistochemical studies, at least one patient was identified as having viral proteins within the vascular walls.

Reiter's Syndrome

Winchester et al. reported an association between 13 patients with AIDS or ARC and Reiter's syndrome. In that series, four patients had a nearly simultaneous onset of Reiter's syndrome and AIDS. In that group, nine of the 12 tested were HLA-B27 positive. These patients were refractory to conventional therapy. Of note, two patients developed full-blown AIDS after low-dose methotrexate therapy.

Psoriatic Arthritis

Patients with psoriasis and HIV infection generally have severe cutaneous disease. The frequency of psoriasis in HIV-infected individuals has ranged from 13 per 1,000 in Texas to ten in 50 in New York City.

Acquired Immunodeficiency Syndrome–Associated Arthritis

Rynes et al. described a subacute oligoarticular arthritis occurring in four patients with HIV infection. They had severe pain and disability. The joints involved were mainly of the lower extremities. NSAID treatment was almost ineffective in two, with both patients responding to intraarticular steroid injections.

Septic Arthritis

There have been only a few reported cases of septic arthritis occurring in HIV-infected individuals. Cryptococcus neoformans, *Histoplasma capsulatum*, *Sponothrix schenkii*, and HIV all have been isolated from synovial fluid.

Reactive Arthritis

Causative agents in reactive arthritis in HIV-infected patients are similar to those seen in other patients. The most common causative organisms are *Chlamydia*, *Salmonella*, *Shigella*, *Campylobacter*, and *Yersinia* species. Some authors consider HIV itself the most common causative agent. The arthritis usually presents with asymmetric oligoarthritis typically in the lower extremities. It is usually more persistent and severe in the HIV-infected patient. Some of the manifestations include enthesopathy, plantar fasciitis, Achilles tendonitis, dactylitis, and sacroiliitis. The reactive arthritides are the most common rheumatic syndromes in the HIV patient.

POSSIBLE MECHANISM OF PAIN IN HIV INFECTED PATIENTS

Facilitation (hyperalgesia) has been extensively studied. Recent work suggests that the immune system does more than recognize and remove invading pathogens and tumors. It is now known that the immune system functions as a diffuse sense organ that signals the brain about events occurring in the periphery. For HIV-infected individuals, this may represent a significant source of their symptoms and may represent an explanation for multiple pain syndromes in HIV-infected individuals. It is well known that inflammation caused by various agents will induce the release of cytokines. It is also known that cells other than macrophages can initiate a proinflammatory process. Keratinocytes and fibroblasts in skin constantly produce an inactive precursor form of intervention interleukin (IL)-1. These cells store this pro-IL-1 intracellularly as well as tonically release it into the skin. When tissue damage occurs (mechanical, thermal, ultraviolet radiation, inflammatory, or in response to parasites) the intracellular stores of pro-IL-1 are released. Mast cells that reside in the skin plus those attracted by skin damage degranulate releasing a variety of inflammatory mediators including tumor necrosis factor (TNF), IL-1, IL-6, and an enzyme (chymase) that cleaves the keratinocyte and fibroblast-derived IL-1 precursor in the skin to its active form. IL-1 in skin induces the release of substance P from peripheral nerve terminals. Substance P degranulates mast cells producing yet more TNF, IL-1, and IL-6, and stimulates macrophages to release TNF, IL-1, and IL-6. Watkins et al. noted that lipopolysaccharide injected intraperitoneally produced hypoalgesia presumably by immune activation in the liver. It was noted that disruption of Kupffer cells and transection of the hepatic vagus abolished this response. It was also noted that cytokines do not only bind to sites within the liver. Cytokines were observed to exert a more diffuse effect by activating vagal fibers throughout the abdominal cavity. This may lead one to postulate that in HIV-infected individuals with gastrointestinal symptomatology, their pain may be enhanced by this constant immune activation. It also may explain why some patients who are HIV-1 seropositive with no discernible abdominal pathology complain of severe abdominal pain. Morphine blocks immune-cell responses to TNF and substance P, suppresses immune-cell migration from blood, inhibits chemotaxis of immune cells to the sight of injection, and inhibits phagocytosis. Thus, blockade of hyperalgesia by these agents in HIV-infected patients may be the result of their action on the immune system. Immune cells have been implicated repeatedly in both human arthritis and animal models of arthritis. Levine et al. have concluded that mast cells are important mediators of neurogenic inflammation in the synovium. Within joints, these cells are in proximity to terminals of both unmyelinated afferent fibers and sympathetic postganglionic nerves, both of which have been implicated in the etiology of arthritis. Substance P also promotes chemotaxis of immune cells into joints; activates neutrophils, synoviocytes and macrophages; simulates lymphocyte proliferation; induces proinflammatory cytokine release; and stimulates phagocytosis. Levine et al. reported that arthritis can be effectively alleviated by treatments that either disrupt postganglionic sympathetic (e.g.,

guanethidine), or disrupt substance P-containing afferent nerve endings. (e.g., capsaicin pretreatment or gold sodium-thiomalate compounds). This may lead to increasing treatment options for HIV-infected patients who are suffering from severe arthritic pain. Consequently, there is a need for studies looking at nociceptive alterations during chronic viral infections, such as HIV infection. Maybe it is merely a cytokine-induced immune system-to-brain communication that occurs during an infection that leads to intense and prolonged hyperalgesia.

SUMMARY

Pain is a common symptom of HIV infection. With increasingly more effective treatment, patients with HIV infection are living longer, making palliative care and quality of life increasingly more important issues.

Over the last decade, several HIV-related pain syndromes have been described and effective symptom management ranging from oral analgesics to AIDS hospice care can and must be offered to provide adequate pain relief.

SELECTED READINGS

Barone JE, Wolkomir AF, Muakkassa FF,et al. Abdominal pain and anorectal disease in AIDS. *Gastroenterol Clin North Am* 1988;17:631–638.

Berman A, Espinoza LK, Diaz JD, et al. Rheumatic manifestations of human immunodeficiency virus infection. *Am J Med* 1988;85:59–64.

Breitbart W, Lefkowitz M, Levin J.et al. Pain management in AIDS. *BETA* 1995:68–77.

Glare PA. Palliative care in acquired immunodeficiency syndrome (AIDS): problems and practicalities. *Ann Acad Med Singapore* 1994;23:235–243.

Lebovits AH, Smith G, Maignan M, et al. Pain in hospitalized patients with AIDS: analgesic and psychotropic medications. *Clin J Pain* 1994;10:156–161.

Lebovits AH, Lefkowitz M, McCarthy D, et al. The prevalence and management of pain in patients with AIDS: a review of 134 cases. *Clin J Pain* 1989;5:245–248.

Lebovits AH, Lefkowitz M. Pain in patients with AIDS. *Int Conf AIDS* 1989;4–9:255 (abstract no. M.B.P. 202).

Levin JD, Codenne TJ, Covinsky K, et al. Neural influences on synovial mast cell density in rat. *J Neurosci Res* 1990;26:301–307.

Lewis MS, Warfield CA. Management of pain in AIDS. *Hosp Pract* 1990;25:51–54.

Maier SF, Watkins LR, Fleshner M. Psychoneuroimmunology: the interface between behavior, brain and immunity. *Am Psychol* 1994;49:1004–1018.

Prithvi Raj P. Pain management of AIDS patients. In: Janisse T, ed. *Current Management of Pain*. Boston Dordrecht London: Kluwer Academic Publishers, 1991:8,40,91–92,100.

Potter DA, Danforth DN Jr, Macher AM, et al. Evaluation of abdominal pain in the AIDS patient. *Ann Surg* 1984;199:332–339.

Singer JE, Zorilla C, et al. Painful symptoms reported by ambulatory HIV-infected men in a longitudinal study. *Pain* 1993;54:15–19.

Solomon G. Rheumatic disease associated with human immunodeficiency virus infection. *Clin Guide Rheumatol* 1991;1:1–6.

Stefano GB, Kushnerik B, Rodriques M, et al. Inhibitory effect of morphine on granulocyte stimulation by tumor necrosis factor and substance P. *Int J Immunopharmacol* 1994;6:329–334.

Watkins L, Maier S, Goehler LE. Immune activation: the role of proinflammatory cytokines in inflammation. *Pain* 1995;63:289–302.

Yanni G, Nabil M, Farahat MR, et al. Intramuscular gold decreases cytokines expression and microphage numbers in the rheumatoid synovial membrane. *Ann Rheum Dis* 1994;53:315–322.

CHAPTER 31

Central Pain

Wilma Wasco and Hilary J. Fausett

Central-pain syndrome is a neurological condition caused by damage specifically to the central nervous system (CNS) — brain, brainstem, or spinal cord. The damage to the CNS may be caused by stroke, if the area of involvement includes the thalamus or brainstem. Spinal-cord injury, especially traumatic transection or following treatment for syringomyelia, can result in the creation of chronic pain as well. A number of systemic diseases are associated with central pain, most notably multiple sclerosis and acquired immunodeficiency syndrome (AIDS). A number of conditions may cause damage to peripheral nerves. Peripheral neuropathy can lead to central sensitization and syndromes that mirror central pain in many ways. Such systemic diseases include diabetes, ischemic-peripheral vascular disease, and limb amputation. A number of medications such as chemotherapeutic agents and some of the antiviral agents prescribed for patients with human immunodeficiency virus (HIV) infection are known to cause damage to peripheral nerves and the creation of central sensitization.

Central pain also is known as thalamic-pain syndrome, Dejerine–Roussy syndrome, posterior-thalamic syndrome, retrolenticular syndrome, central poststroke syndrome, and often is described as a neuropathic-pain syndrome. The famous French neurologists Dejerine and Roussy reported it as the "thalamic syndrome" near the turn of the century. Riddoch named it "central pain" in a 1938 writing in the *Lancet*. His description of a "pain worse than pain" and of patients with burning agony still is considered one of the best descriptions of central pain to appear in the literature. Some researchers make a distinction between central pain, meaning resulting from CNS pathology and central sensitization in which the recurrent input of an injured peripheral nerve leads to chronic changes in the CNS. For the patient who is suffering, however, the terminology is less important as the treatment options are similar.

Central pain syndrome is most often caused by a stroke, usually an occlusive insult, accounting for around 90% of cases. Because the pain usually is delayed in onset, the patient has started to recover from the motor impairment of the stroke when the pain starts. As many of 15% of patients with central pain following stroke report having been pain free for the first year following their injury.

DIAGNOSIS

The history of the pain syndrome and description of the pain by the patient often is all that is needed to make the diagnosis. The classic triad of symptoms is: burning pain in a fixed location, abnormal sensory processing of cold stimulation, and worsening of pain with touch. The pain is steady and usually is described as a burning, aching, or cutting sensation. Occasionally, there may be brief, intolerable bursts of sharp pain. Central pain is characterized by a mixture of pain sensations, the most prominent being constant burning. Mingled with the burning are sensations of cold and "pins and needles" tingling. The steady burning sensation is increased significantly by any light touch.

Physical examination may reveal evidence of prior cerebral infarction or other stigmata of disease. The patient usually guards the affected part from inadvertent touch and may seem remarkably immobile. There may be evidence of muscle weakness, which may be from the known neurologic injury or from disuse of the affected site. Patients are somewhat numb in the areas affected by this burning pain ("anesthesia dolorosa"). The burning and loss of touch appreciation usually are most severe on the distant parts of the body, such as the feet or hands. Pain may be moderate to severe in intensity and often is exacerbated by movement and temperature changes, usually cold temperatures.

It is worth reviewing the terms pain clinicians use to label the sensations as described by the patient. Most somatic pain can be well localized and described; the burning of central pain often is difficult for the patient to describe. *Dysesthetic* refers to an unpleasant sensation, whereas *anesthetic* refers to an absence of sensation. A patient who perceives light, innocuous touch as a painful or noxious stimuli has *allodynia*. *Hyperpathia* or *hyperalgesia* refers to the exaggerated response of the nervous system to a painful or noxious input. Pain is amplified.

Slow summation refers to evoked burning. A patient may experience light touch for a few moments without pain, but at some point an unbearable sense of dysesthetic burning develops. This is different from *spatial summation*, which refers to an increase in magnitude of the pain as the perimeter of the area of applied stimulus increases. It is not pain over a greater area, rather it is greater magnitude of the pain wherever felt.

Patients with central pain have painful sensations that endure. *Durable* refers to the persistence of burning after the stimulus is discontinued, also termed "afterburn." The burning is slow to appear but is slow to leave. Depending on the level reached the burning may last from a few seconds to 20 minutes or more. Subtle cooling, pleasant distractions, or some other phenomenon may accelerate the quieting of the skin. It is possible, however, that any external stimulation may increase the pain as well.

PATHOPHYSIOLOGY

The exact mechanism by which certain conditions create central pain is not known. Although subtle cord damage associated with central pain often can be detected by electrophysiologic testing or by measuring for cord flattening, patients with damage severe enough to be seen on magnetic resonance imaging usually are completely numb rather than in pain. Central pain thus may represent incomplete damage to pain tracts. This is consistent with what is known about peripheral-nerve injury, where incomplete severing of a nerve will lead to over-firing.

Positron emission tomography of patients with neuropathic pain suggests a theoretical model of how central pain develops. These sophisticated scans reveal that the thalamus, the pain processor in the brain, tries to shut down in the face of overwhelming pain impulses to avoid cellular death of its neurons. In cases of peripheral-nerve injury, there is a constant barrage of impulses to the CNS. An injured motor nerve simply carries less current. Injured pain nerves, paradoxically, do exactly the opposite, they increase their signal. It is not a simple increase,

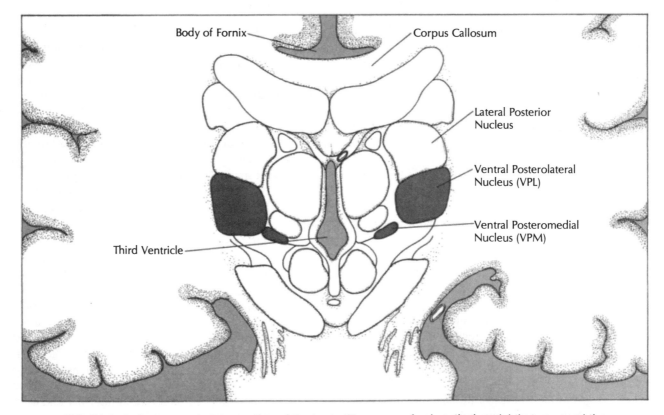

FIG. 31.1. A diagrammed cross-section of the brain. The group of subcortical nuclei that surround the third ventricle makes up the thalamus. The thalamus functions as a transmission and integration system for impulses to the cortex. The ventricular-posterior nuclear complex, consisting of the ventral posteromedial and the ventral posterolateral nuclei, is responsible primarily for somatosensory processing.

however. They eventually gain the power to humorally influence uninjured neighbor neurons, which begin autonomous firing. The process can become so vigorous that "bursts" of impulses from these injured nerves can be recorded in the thalamus in animals. The theory is that after sufficient bombardment threatens neuron death in the thalamus, it "shuts down." (Fig. 31.1) There is a case report of a patient who had a deep-brain stimulator implanted into his thalamus to control a movement disorder. Following successful cardioversion for an arrhythmia, the patient developed a dysesthetic-pain syndrome. The induced thalotomy, although associated with a life-saving maneuver, resulted in the creation of a chronic-pain syndrome. Central pain apparently occurs at this point. In its disabled state, the thalamus is thought to allow unfiltered throughput of pain on into the conscious brain and the emotional centers. Normally, painful events cause increased pain for these patients, upgrading discomforts into demoralizing crises. This state is termed central-neuropathic pain, or central pain. For patients with a thalamic stroke or other lesion to the thalamus, the outcome will be the same.

TREATMENT

Generally, pain medications provide little or no relief for those affected by central-pain syndrome. Opiates provide sedation more than analgesia for these patients. Most of these patients will quickly tire of the side effects and stop taking the opiate. Some clinicians believe that patients with central pain should be mildly sedated so that the nervous system can be kept quiet and as free from stress as possible.

Some patients may have partial relief with the anticonvulsant medications used to treat neuropathic pain. It is certainly worth trying, and all agents should be titrated until side effects limit further dose escalations before deciding that an agent provides no relief.

Patients with central pain should be referred to a neurologist. The patient may wish to discuss possible new medications or clinical trials available for experimental treatment. A referral also should be made to a neurosurgeon. Although, there does not appear to be a role for spinal-cord stimulation or intrathecal opiate pumps for these patients, some proponents offer deep-brain stimulation as a treatment option. deep-brain stimulation is not Food and Drug Administration approved for the treatment of chronic pain, however, these patients are so debilitated that often it is offered on a compassionate-use basis.

Case Report

A 72-year-old man was referred to the pain management center with a complaint of burning pain over most of the left side of his body. He had suffered a small cerebral infarct 18 months earlier and had initially made very good neurologic recovery. Over the past few months, however, he was not eating very much and had become wheelchair bound. Upon questioning, he revealed that he felt "burning ants" and "shooting icicles" along his left arm and occasionally in his left leg as well. His left trunk and abdomen were hyperpathic and once he was undressed for the examination, he was reluctant to get dressed again out of fear of provoking his symptoms. He had been prescribed a number of medications, including a fentanyl patch, which he discontinued as it caused drowsiness without pain relief. He was started on clonazepam 0.5 mg at bedtime, which was eventually increased to clonazepam 0.5 mg in the morning and 1.0 mg at bedtime. This improved his ability to sleep and his appetite, but did not improve his pain. A series of anticonvulsants were tried, each dose being titrated upwards until side effects necessitated a halt to the increase in dosage, but to no avail. He discussed deep-brain stimulation with a neurosurgeon, but he and his family were too afraid of the potential for another stroke to try.

Central-pain syndrome is not a fatal disorder. But for the majority of patients, the syndrome causes intractable pain. Patients must be treated with compassion and understanding. Supportive services should be offered, as current medical care has very little else to offer.

SPINAL-CORD INJURY

Over two thirds of patients who have had spinal-cord injuries report pain of some sort. One third of patients with spinal-cord injuries describe their pain as severe. As more patients survive trauma such as gunshot wounds and motor-vehicle accidents, the incidence of postspinal-injury pain rises.

Pain is associated with incomplete lesioning. Gunshot wounds and the rapid transection that occurs with high-speed automobile accidents seem to predispose to the development of spinal-injury pain. Most patients have a delay in the development of pain of about 6 months following the initial injury. If patients develop pain after more than 6 months or if there is a rise in the level of sensory loss, the possibility of syringomyelia should be investigated.

Patients with spinal-cord injuries develop several types of pain. Musculoskeletal pain is common. Sites close to the level of injury, the bones, ligaments, tendons, or discs often are damaged as well. Because these patients have some level of paralysis, often there is overuse and overcompensation of the muscle groups that can be controlled. If there is damage to the dorsal-nerve roots above the site of injury, the patient will have radicular pain. Pain that radiates in a dermatomal distribution may respond, at least temporarily, to nerve blocks.

Segmental pain occurs at and right above the level of sensory loss. Usually, one to three segments are involved. This pain may be described as burning, a deep aching, or even burning and shooting. There usually is hyperalgesia over the involved area, although some patients may have allodynia as well.

Visceral pain is seen most often with quadriplegics or patients with very high thoracic levels. It is always important to rule out abdominal pathology and bowel or bladder problems. If the transection is above the fourth thoracic vertebral level, patients will have alterations in their autonomic response. To avoid autonomic hyperreflexia, it is important that patients with high spinal-injury levels not be allowed to have pain, such as with bladder distension or an unanesthetized minor surgical procedure.

Dysesthetic pain often is called central pain, as it is the result of the deafferentation injury. This is a spontaneous, burning, shooting, or stabbing pain that is distal to the site of injury. It is often felt in areas of the body where the patient has no other sensation. This pain is caudal to the sensory level experienced by the patient.

Managing spinal-cord injury pain is a challenge. It first is necessary to determine the cause of the pain. Myofascial pain syndromes and overuse injuries must be appropriately diagnosed and treated. Occasionally, something as simple as altering a wheelchair or providing better assist devices in the home can help. For other patients, medications can be tried.

Tricyclic antidepressants (TCAs) often are effective at diminishing dysesthetic pain. The anticonvulsants have been used successfully to help with lancinating or shooting pain, and with radicular pain. Some patients may get relief after a trial with intravenous lidocaine. If the pain relief is good but of short duration, mexiletine on a daily basis may be of benefit. The opiates usually are ineffective for dysesthetic pain, even when given epidurally or intrathecally. The opiates may be more effective, however, when combined with intrathecal clonidine. There currently are no good N-methyl-D-aspartate antagonists commercially available for intrathecal use, but the success of intrathecal ketamine in European trials suggests that there may be the possibility of someday treating or even limiting the creation of pain following spinal-cord injury.

Case Report

A 28-year-old man was referred to the pain management center with shooting pain into his legs and buttocks. He had suffered a dirt-bike accident 3 years previously, which left him with a T4 level. Six months prior to the referral, he had been diagnosed with syringomyelia, which had been successfully treated by a neurosurgeon. The current pain was quite disabling and interfering with his abilities as a wheelchair racer, for which he received corporate sponsorship. He was started on gabapentin and slowly titrated to a dose of 400 mg p.o. t.i.d. He reported "fair" pain control and said if he missed a dose of medication he had an increase in the frequency and severity of his shooting pain. He requested further intervention. Opiates did not relieve his pain, and made him too drowsy to race. Nevertheless, after investigating possibilities on the Internet, he requested an intrathecal opiate trial. He received Dilaudid (Knoll Laboratories, Mount Olive, NJ, U.S.A.) 0.1 mg intrathecally and was monitored for the next 24 hours. He reported no change in his symptoms. He was offered an intrathecal trial of clonidine, but he refused because he needed to participate in a wheelchair "iron man" competition.

Surgical procedures have been offered to patients with spinal-cord injuries, with mixed results. Dorsal-root entry zone lesions have been reported to be effective for radicular pain, but are associated with many complications. Cordotomy may provide up to 50% of patients with relief of pain symptoms, however, for a significant number, the pain recurs. To be effective, cordectomy must be performed two to three levels above the site of injury. This will result in a greater motor and sensory loss and the potential for greater autonomic fiber involvement as well.

The best treatment for spinal-cord–injury pain is prevention.

SELECTED READINGS

Bromm B, Sandkuhler J, Gebhart GF. *Nervous System Plasticity and Chronic Pain*. New York: Elsevier Science, 2000.

Edwards CL, Sudhakar S, Scales MT, et al. Electromyographic (EMG) biofeedback in the comprehensive treatment of central pain and ataxic tremor following thalamic stroke. *Appl Psychophysiol Biofeedback* 2000;25:229–240.

Gonzales GR, Lewis SA, Weaver AL. Tactile illusion perception in patients with central pain. *Mayo Clin Proc* 2001;76:267–74.

Siddall PJ, Taylor DA, Cousins MJ. Classification of pain following spinal cord injury. *Spinal Cord* 1997;35:69–75.

Siddall PJ, Taylor DA, McClelland JM, et al. Pain report and the relationship of pain to physical factors in the first 6 months following spinal cord injury. *Pain* 1999;81:187–197.

Somers MF. *Spinal Cord Injury: Functional Rehabilitation*. Upper Saddle River, New Jersey: Prentice Hall, 2001.

Tiengo M. *Neuroscience: Focus on Acute and Chronic Pain (Topics in Anesthesia and Critical Care)*. New York: Springer–Verlag, 2001.

Yamamoto T, Katayama Y, Fukaya C, et al. Thalamotomy caused by cardioversion in a patient treated with deep brain stimulation. *Stereotact Funct Neurosurg* 2000;74:73–82.

CHAPTER 32

Neuropathic Pain

Hilary J. Fausett

Neuropathic pain results from injury to the nervous system. One of the hallmarks of neuropathic pain is that the individual perceives pain in the absence of noxious stimuli, and occasionally in the absence of any stimuli. Neuropathic pain is defined as damage to the central or peripheral nervous system. The treatment of neuropathic pain is challenging and often daunting: the nerve injury cannot be reversed or "cured," and so symptomatic management of pain and physical dysfunction are the only goals. Symptom treatment often is less than ideal, and for many patients and their clinicians, a source of continued frustration. As more is learned about the pathophysiology of neuropathic pain syndromes, more treatment strategies can be devised.

ETIOLOGY

Peripheral neuropathy is the result of an injury or insult to one or more peripheral nerves. The term peripheral neuropathy usually is used to refer to the insult to small nerve fibers and may be secondary to a variety of etiologies (Fig. 32.1). Common causes of peripheral neuropathy include endocrine abnormalities (such as diabetes mellitus and hypothyroidism), metabolic disorders (renal insufficiency, alcohol abuse, nutritional deficiencies), infectious and postinfectious causes [human immunodeficiency virus (HIV), lyme disease, postherpetic neuralgia], and drug-induced or toxin-induced causes (chemotherapies such as vincristine and cisplatin, and heavy metals). There are immune-mediated disease causes (vasculitis, Guillain–Barré syndrome), hereditary causes (hereditary sensorimotor neuropathies), and paraneoplastic and cryptogenic causes.

Neuropathic pain has an estimated prevalence ranging from 0.6% to 1.5% of the general population of the United States. The most common etiology is diabetic neuropathy. Postherpetic neuralgia also is a very common cause. The term diabetic neuropathy is used most commonly to refer to a peripheral sensorimotor polyneuropa-

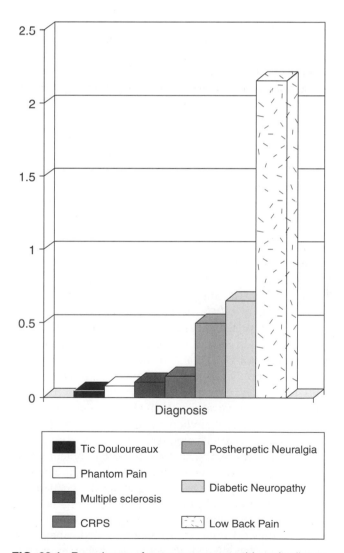

FIG. 32.1. Prevalence of common neuropathic pain diagnosis in the United States, estimated in millions of cases.

thy that may have autonomic involvement. The incidence of neuropathy in patients who have had diabetes for more than 25 years is about 45% to 60%.

Postherpetic neuralgia is a late sequelae of infection with the varicella-zoster virus. Reactivation of latent infection by the varicella-zoster virus results in shingles or herpes zoster. The annual incidence of herpes zoster is about 0.3%, with an estimated prevalence of 800,000 cases currently in the United States.

PATHOPHYSIOLOGY

The pathophysiology of neuropathic pain is an area of intense interest and controversy. It is likely that the mechanisms of injury may be as diverse as the etiology. Initial interest focused on the role of peripheral nerve injury. It is now clear that central mechanisms are of importance as well.

Peripheral sensitization is caused by a lowering of the threshold to fire of the nociceptors and is accompanied by an increased sensitivity of the nociceptor endings. Primary *hyperalgesia*, which is the phenomenon of the enhancement of a previously mild noxious stimuli, is the result. Deafferentation results from the destruction of nerve fibers. The involved area has a complete loss of function and so exhibits anesthesia (the lack of normal sensation) while being painful to the patient. This is called *anesthesia dolorosa*. In these patients, further transection of the nerve proximally does not change the symptomatology. Hyperactivity of the target neurons in the spinal cord and the brain has been demonstrated in animals following nerve transection and this is presumed to be responsible for persistent pain in humans.

Central sensitization is the result of hyperexcitability of spinal-cord neurons in response to repeated peripheral stimulation. These spinal neurons thus are spontaneously active, appear to have a widened receptive field, and become hypersensitive to a variety of stimuli. This may account for the symptom of *allodynia*, in which previous innocuous stimuli is interpreted as pain. A number of mechanisms are likely involved in central sensitization, including activation of excitatory amino acids at N-methyl-D-aspartate (NMDA) receptors. One theory holds that peripheral-nerve injury leads to the destruction of inhibitory interneurons at the spinal cord by a barrage of NMDA-mediated effects and this loss of normal inhibition results in an increase in the transmission of noxious impulses.

In certain syndromes, such as diabetic polyneuropathy and following local nerve injury, the body attempts to repair the destroyed axon. This attempt at regeneration results in a proliferation of hyperexcitable regenerating fibers. A tangle of immature axons sprouts following the regeneration of a transected nerve is called a neuroma. Neuromas are spontaneously active and hypersensitive to mechanical stimuli. Patients with an entrapment neuropathy also may develop neuromas.

In patients with phantom-limb pain, there is the continuation of sensations in the absence of any obvious source. Some patients describe itching, pressure, or tingling in addition to painful burning or throbbing. It has been suggested that there is a central representation of the body that relies upon ongoing peripheral input to function optimally. The loss of this normal input then results in the creation of pain.

CLINICAL PRESENTATION

A variety of terms is used by patients to describe their symptoms. The pain may be "electrical" and travel along a dermatomal distribution (lumbar radiculopathy), or "burn" through the feet (diabetic neuropathy). Neuralgias, such as trigeminal neuralgia, typically have periods of quiescence, followed by "spasms" or "jolts" of "shooting," "knifelike," or "electrical" pain. The individual may describe the involved area as "numb" and the site of exquisite, tortuous pain.

Patients may describe the pain as "squeezing" or "cramping" or "like a sunburn" or "broken glass." Pain may be "jabbing" or a "deep aching." What is remarkable is the range of terminology used and the colorful imagery evoked. The descriptors of the pain are not in themselves diagnostic: myofascial pain syndromes may "burn" and somatic pain often is described as "throbbing."

Patients often have symptoms such as hyperalgesia (severe pain resulting from mildly noxious stimuli) and allodynia (pain produced by innocuous stimuli.) The patient with postherpetic neuralgia may not wear a bra because of the pain evoked from the contact. It is not uncommon for patients with trigeminal neuralgia or postherpetic neuralgia to not brush their teeth, clean their ears, or chew on the side of the pain.

DIAGNOSIS

Because the etiology of the pain is so diverse, proper diagnosis is difficult but important: if the cause is from an ongoing process, it may be possible to limit future damage. It is important to rule out treatable causes.

A thorough history and physical exam are very important. Special attention to the past medical history is important to elicit concurrent illnesses, such as diabetes mellitus or hypothyroidism. A review of the patients past employment and social history may reveal exposure to toxins (such as heavy metals or alcohol use.) It often is necessary to review the patient's medical record or talk with his other treating physicians to learn if diseases such as multiple sclerosis are suspected or to learn the names of any chemotherapeutic agents. A review of medications also is vital.

The physical exam is important to note the patient's general health, and to look for signs of systemic illness. Evidence of skin changes, discoloration, and temperature abnormalities, and trophic changes are important to document. Careful documentation of the neurologic exam is important not only to determine whether a motor-neuron component is present, but also to help guide future therapies. The extent of any altered sensations as well as the area of pain should be documented. This will help in assessing the efficacy of therapy. Often, progress is made slowly and reminding the patient that the area of involvement has shrunk can be very beneficial.

It also is important to elicit any symptoms of psychological distress or social stress. Appropriate referrals should be made promptly. As these types of pain syndromes can be devastating to patients and their families, every effort should be made to make certain the patient feels supported during treatment and understands the resources for psychosocial support that are available.

TREATMENT

The treatment of neuropathic-pain syndromes remains a source of frustration for patients and for pain specialists. Very few treatments have been shown to be effective in well-designed studies, and some syndromes have not had a consistent response to any treatment. Much of the therapy now offered to patients is based on the personal experience of the physician or the bias of a particular institution. Patients often are desperate for relief and so will try anything the equally desperate physician will consider.

The mainstay of therapy is medication (Table 32.1). Nerve blocks, physical therapy, neurosurgical procedures,

TABLE 32.1. *Medication Suggestions for Treating Peripheral Neuropathic Pain*

First-line therapies	
Tricyclic antidepressants	Amitriptyline
	Imipramine
	Nortriptyline
	Desipramine
	Clomipramine
Anticonvulsant	Gabapentin
	Topiramate
Second-line therapies	
Anticonvulsant	Carbamazepine
Analgesic	Tramadol
	Nonsteroidal, antiinflammatory, Cox-2 agents
Topical	Capsaicin
	Lidocaine
Third-line therapies	
Antiarrhythmic	Mexiletine
Anticonvulsant	Phenytoin
	Lamotrigine
Fourth-line therapies	
Selective serotonin reuptake inhibitors	Fluoxetine
	Paroxetine
Opiates	Oral agents

and a variety of electrical-stimulating devices have been tried with mixed success.

MEDICATIONS

Tricyclic antidepressants (TCAs) are the primary treatment medication for most patients. The antinociceptive properties of TCAs are independent of any antidepressant effects. TCAs traditionally are classified by their chemical structure as either secondary amines (nortriptyline, desipramine, and maprotiline) or tertiary amines (amitriptyline, imipramine, and clomipramine.) The medications are successful in treating patients with and without depression. Diabetic neuropathy and postherpetic neuralgia are two syndromes that have shown responsiveness to TCAs. Some of theses studies reveal a decrease in pain scores of 20% to 30% after a 6- to 8-week trial. Although this is clinically significant, it can be disheartening for a patient to have to wait over a month for relief. Patients may notice an almost immediate improvement in sleep, however, and thus an improvement in quality of life with these medications.

Studies and clinical practice reveal that TCAs are associated with a number of side effects, such as sedation, dry mouth, and constipation. Weight gain may be troubling for some patients. The anticholinergic side effects may result in dizziness and postural hypotension, which may predispose to falls, with a risk of injury in frail or elderly patients. For older men with mild symptoms of urinary hesitancy, it may be worsened with amitriptyline and thus desipramine is a better choice for these individuals.

Starting doses of a TCA should be 10 mg to 25 mg, given 1 to 2 hours before sleep. The dose then can be increased by 10 mg to 25 mg each week as tolerated and as necessary. Treatment dosing must be individualized. For a few patients, TCAs result in activation, not sedation. These patients should take the medication in the morning.

Selective serotonin reuptake inhibitors (SSRIs) are better tolerated than TCAs but are not as effective in providing pain relief. The SSRIs are very good in treating depression and thus may have a role in treating the depressed patient with chronic pain. Extreme caution must be exercised if attempting to use both a TCA and an SSRI concurrently, as the combination will boost the bioavailability of both drugs, increasing the likelihood of side effects and excessive serotonin.

The *antiarrhythmic* mexiletine is an oral lidocaine analog that is a sodium-channel blocker. It has been shown to alleviate neuropathic pain, but usage often is limited by gastrointestinal side effects. Because of its effects on the cardiac conduction system, all patients should have a screening electrocardiogram. Any patient with evidence of ischemia or a conduction abnormality should be evaluated carefully and seen by a cardiologist or internist for medical clearance prior to starting treatment with mexiletine. Also, blood tests need to be drawn and monitored every few months for abnormalities in blood count or liver function.

Anticonvulsants are used frequently to treat neuropathic pain. These medications have been used traditionally to treat "lancinating pain," although no study has be performed to test the validity of that usage. Carbamazepine is approved by the Food and Drug Administration (FDA) for the treatment of trigeminal neuralgia and glossopharyngeal neuralgia. Carbamazepine modulates voltage-dependent sodium channels and appears to depress transmission of pain impulses. Carbamazepine has been shown to be effective in providing relief for patients with trigeminal neuralgia, diabetic neuropathy, and postherpetic neuralgia. Phenytoin also modulates voltage-dependent sodium channels, and has been shown in some studies to provide relief of diabetic neuropathy. But, because phenytoin may inhibit insulin secretion and therefore worsen hyperglycemia, it is not considered a first-line drug for the symptomatic treatment of painful diabetic neuropathy.

Lamotrigine and valproate both have been shown to provide some relief of neuropathic pain. Valproate has been used extensively to treat patients with migraines.

Gabapentin is widely prescribed because of its perceived safety and efficacy, and there are many recent trials looking at its usage for clinical pain syndromes. It seems likely that gabapentin binds to a voltage-dependent calcium channel, and does not exert its influence by way of a γ-aminobutyric-acid (GABA)–mediated effect. Gabapentin is unlikely to interact with other drugs, because it does not bind to plasma proteins or induce hepatic enzymes.

Topiramate recently has been approved by the FDA for the treatment of the peripheral neuropathy associated with diabetes. The recommended starting dose is 25 mg at night and is then slowly increased, to avoid excessive sedation, to 50 mg twice a day. Higher doses can be used if needed.

Opioids are used frequently to treat patients with neuropathic pain, despite the traditional wisdom that neuropathic pain is, by definition, "opioid nonresponsive." Controversy exists as to whether neuropathic pain merely increases the dosing requirement for neuropathic pain patients, or whether some of the other effects of the opiates (sedation, mild anxiolysis, perhaps even euphoria) may account for the relief. Practitioners in the United States tend to be very concerned about the potential for addiction and psychological dependence inherent with the use of opiates. Most practicing physicians will prescribe opiates on a case-by-case basis to patients if the individual appears to benefit from use. Long-acting oxycodone (OxyContin, Purdue Pharma L.P., Stamford, CT, U.S.A.) has been shown to provide good pain relief for patients with postherpetic neuralgia, but 76% of these patients reported a side effect with treatment, including nausea, constipation, and sedation.

Opiates also may be delivered transcutaneously, epidurally, and intrathecally. For many patients who get very good pain relief but have intolerable side effects, choosing an alternative route of administration may provide the solution. Because some patients can get relief from intrathecal opiates even when they have not had relief from oral opiates, it may be worth considering a trial of spinal opiates.

Tramadol has low binding affinity to opioid receptors and is a weak inhibitor of norepinephrine and serotonin reuptake. It has been shown to provide pain relief to patients with diabetic neuropathy. Tramadol must be used with caution, however, as it can have significant side effects including nausea, constipation, and sedation. Furthermore, it is not recommended that the drug be used with a TCA or an SSRI unless the patient is watched very closely, as tramadol will increase the effective dose of a variety of drugs, increasing the likelihood of unwanted effects.

Topical Agents

Topically applied medications can be of tremendous benefit, for some patients. *Capsaicin* is an extract of chili peppers that causes the localized depletion of substance P from the terminals of unmyelinated C fibers. Because substance P is one of the primary neurotransmitters of nociceptive stimuli, its depletion should result in a decrease of transmission of noxious impulses. Several studies have shown very good response to the application of capsaicin for patients with diabetic neuropathy and it has been reported to be helpful for patients with other neuropathies, including postherpetic neuralgia. Capsaicin comes as a cream that must be applied to the affected area three to five times a day. Because it can cause intense burning, and because it must be used so frequently to provide any benefit, its practical applications are few: very few patients will be compliant with its proper usage.

Lidocaine is a local anesthetic that comes as a cream, but which also has been studied as a patch for patients with postherpetic neuralgia. In clinical trials, patients found tremendous benefit with the lidocaine patch and it recently has been approved by the FDA for use in patients with postherpetic neuralgia. EMLA Cream (AstraZeneca, London, U.K.) is a mix of local anesthetics that also can be applied to provide localized pain relief. The risk is that of local anesthetic overdose, as suffering patients may apply too much or reapply the medication too frequently to get adequate relief. Nevertheless, for the right patient, topical anesthetics can be a helpful adjuvant.

Antispasticity Agents

Baclofen has been used to treat trigeminal neuralgia with good success. The starting dose of baclofen was 10 mg three times a day and it was increased by 10 mg every other day in a small, double-blind study. Patients reported a reduction in the paroxysms of pain when using the baclofen.

Other Drugs

A variety of other agents have been used with reported success. *Clonidine* is an α-adrenergic blocking agent that has been used both as an oral adjuvant and as a patch applied directly to the damaged area. Clonidine is known to act synergistically with opiates, but its pain-relieving action in neuropathic pain may be a more direct effect on the damaged fibers. Clonidine may result in orthostatic hypotension and should be used with caution in patients on diuretics or other antihypertensive medications.

Botulinin toxin has no effect on sensory nerves. Botox (Allergan, Inc., Irvine, CA, U.S.A.) is used to treat muscle spasticity. Some pain practitioners have used the muscle-relaxing effects to decrease one potential instigation of stimuli, which in this manner may result in pain relief. The role of Botox in treating neuropathic pain is very narrow and the medication should only be used by someone familiar with the risks involved.

NERVE BLOCKS

A variety of nerve-block techniques have been tried, with mixed success. Published reports of the use of nerve blocks tend to be of series of patients, not case-controlled, blinded studies. Early reports are very promising, however few authors have published long-term follow-up results. Most pain practitioners will acknowledge that despite often miraculous responses to the first injection, long-term relief is elusive and very rare.

Some practitioners routinely follow local anesthetic trials with neuroablative techniques. Phenol and alcohol have been reported to provide good, moderate-term relief. The nerve, whether peripheral or at the nerve-root level, does regenerate, however after 4 to 6 months the pain usually recurs in even greater magnitude. For this reason, most pain specialists do not perform neuroablative procedures on patients without malignancies and who are expected to live a normal life span. The risks of phenol and alcohol are great, and other structures, such as blood vessels may be damaged with disastrous effect.

Radiofrequency somatic denervation was once touted as a cure-all. Further experience, however, has lead most specialists to be very cautious about applying this technology to a peripheral nerve. Some highly regarded academic-pain specialists have come out strongly against the use of radiofrequency denervation of peripheral nerves. *Cryoanalgesia* is another technique of providing semi-permanent pain relief. Because the nerve appears to be "stunned" rather than permanently severed, this technique has more acceptance.

Sympathetic blocks are used when there is an element of sympathetically maintained pain, such as with com-plex regional pain syndrome, types I and II. Some practitioners argue forcefully for the preemptive use of sympathetic nerve blocks for patients with herpes zoster to reduce the likelihood of the development of postherpetic neuralgia. This practice has not been extensively studied, but is widespread.

PHYSICAL THERAPY

Studies have demonstrated that being physically fit and participating in physical activity in older women, such a gentle weight lifting, can decrease depression and improve pain scores. No study has demonstrated a superiority of a particular type of physical therapy, massage therapy, or manipulative technique for the treatment of neuropathic pain. Many practitioners have found that encouraging the patient to use the affected limb in as "normal" a manner as possible seems to lessen the progression of pain and disability. It is important that patients get evaluated by a licensed physical therapist, when appropriate, and someone who can determine whether a particular physical-therapy program will be of benefit to the individual.

ELECTRICAL STIMULATION

Electrical stimulation as a method of pain relief has been tried for many years. *Transcutaneous-electrical nerve stimulation* (TENS) is a noninvasive method of stimulating a peripheral nerve. The use of TENS to treat neuropathic pain has not been extensively studied, but it is a method frequently used by pain specialists because it is relatively easy to use and has no serious side effects, if the device is used properly. It is possible to try the device and if it is of no benefit, the patient suffers no harm. For many practitioners, a trial of TENS is amongst the first treatments offered.

Spinal-cord stimulation (SCS) has been extensively studied, and for the right patient may provide excellent relief. A trial of SCS is arranged for a several-day period. Only patients who get very good relief from the trial should be considered candidates for a permanent device. A poor response to the trial is a contraindication for a permanent device. Response to a TENS unit is not an indication for a permanent spinal-cord stimulator.

Peripheral-nerve stimulation (PNS) differs from spinal-cord stimulation in that the site of lead placement is not in the epidural space, but unlike a TENS unit, it is placed under the skin and over a particular nerve root. Many specialists find peripheral-nerve stimulators easy to place and simple to use for a trial. The complication rate, primarily of lead migration and infection, are higher than with modern spinal-cord stimulators and the quality of pain relief is not improved.

Deep-brain stimulation (DBS) is still an experimental technique for the treatment of chronic pain. Although it is being used more frequently and with great success for patients with movement disorders, the FDA has not endorsed its use for chronic-pain syndromes. Only a qualified neurosurgeon should place the device, and patients should not be lead to believe that such a device will "cure" them. Rather, the neurosurgeon should be sent a request for a consultation and make all further decisions as to whether there is any utility in pursing DBS.

SELECTED READINGS

Apfel SC, Kessler JA, Adornato BT, et al., and the NGF (Nerve Growth Factor) Study Group. Recombinant human nerve growth factor in the treatment of diabetic polyneuropathy. *Neurology* 1998:51:695–702.

Bennett GJ. Neuropathic pain: new insights, new interventions. *Hosp Pract (off Ed)* 1998;33:95–114.

Fromm GH, Terrence CF, Chattha AS. Baclofen in the treatment of trigeminal neuralgia: double blind study and long-term follow-up. *Ann Neurol* 1984;15:240–244.

Kingery WS. A critical review of controlled clinical trials for peripheral neuropathic pain and complex regional pain syndromes. *Pain* 1997;73: 123–139.

Kost RG, Strausee SE. Post-herpetic neuralgia: pathogenesis, treatment, and prevention. *N Engl J Med* 1996;335:32–42.

Max MB, Lynch SA, Muir J, et al. Effects of desipramine, amitriptyline, and fluoxetine on pain and diabetic neuropathy. *N Engl J Med* 1992;326: 1250–1256.

Rowbotham MC, Davis PS, Verkempinck C, et al. Lidocaine patch: double-blind controlled study of a new treatment method for post-herpetic neuralgia. *Pain* 1996;65:39–44.

Wright JM, Oki JC, Graves L III. Mexiletine in the symptomatic treatment of diabetic peripheral neuropathy. *Ann Pharmacother* 1997;31: 29–34.

CHAPTER 33

Postherpetic Neuralgia

Hilary J. Fausett

One of the most common and frustrating pain complaints is the neuropathic pain of herpes zoster or shingles. Acute herpes zoster can cause severe pain during its active phase, and in some unfortunate individuals, the pain does not resolve with the infection and postherpetic neuralgia develops.

ACUTE HERPES ZOSTER

Etiology

The varicella zoster virus is the cause of herpes zoster. Otherwise known as shingles, acute herpes zoster is the result of reactivation of the latent varicella zoster virus. Varicella zoster virus usually is contracted in childhood and causes chickenpox. Most healthy children overcome the initial infection within a few weeks, although infection in some children and in many adults may lead to serious complications such as pneumonia, meningitis, and death.

Although the clinical course of chickenpox is soon completed, the varicella zoster virus usually is not gone, but has merely retreated. The virus is thought to become dormant in nerve cells, most often of the sensory ganglia, and then is reactivated at some later date. Shingles represents the reactivation, multiplication, and subsequent transport along sensory nerves of the virus. The incidence of reactivation increases with age, with an overall incidence in the population of about 1 in 10,000. Triggering factors are unknown, but appear to include stress and a decline in immune function, as the incidence is greater in individuals with suppressed immune function following major infections or as with acquired immunodeficiency syndrome, malignancy, and iatrogenic immune suppression, as following organ transplantation. Patients with lymphoproliferative malignancies seem to be particularly vulnerable to infection; this is thought to be a result of the aggressive chemotherapeutic agents and radiation ther-

apy used, as well as from the immunosuppressive actions of the malignancy.

Clinical Presentation

Patients will complain of pain in a dermatomal distribution that may precede the characteristic rash by 7 to more than 100 days. The pain usually accompanies the rash, and may become more prominent. The rash usually becomes pustular in 4 to 7 days, develops a "crust" for 10 to 21 days, and then usually resolves. The acute rash stage of herpes zoster will last from 14 to 28 days, but may result in scarring and pigmentation changes that do not resolve. Many patients seek medical care for the severe pain before the characteristic rash develops. The differential diagnosis of the pain is broad and patients have been thought to be suffering from myocardial ischemia, acute cholecystitis, appendicitis, and disc herniation.

In some patients, a rash never develops, and yet the pain may linger. These patients are presumed to have "zoster-sine herpete," which is a diagnosis of exclusion, meaning no other explanation for the symptoms can be discovered. The only way to make the definitive diagnosis of zoster-sine herpete is by pathologic examination of the dorsal-root ganglion (DRG). This diagnosis has been made at autopsy.

Most cases of herpes zoster develop in the thoracic dermatomes (Table 33.1). Over 50% of cases involve the thoracic dermatomes, most commonly in the T5 distribution. In most patients, only one dermatome is involved, and the infection is unilateral. One sign of immunocompromise is the development of zoster in two or more dermatomes or in a bilateral distribution. The first division of the trigeminal nerve also is commonly involved, with facial involvement in about 25% of cases. This results in a risk of injury to the eye. Ophthalmic involvement is particularly horrendous as the individual may lose sight in the involved eye. There is some suggestion that development of zoster in the

TABLE 33.1. *Pattern of Distribution*

Location of Zoster, in descending order of frequency
Thoracic: T5 (most common)
Trigeminal: V1 (second most common)
Thoracic
Cervical
Lumbar
Sacral (rare)

TABLE 33.2. *Medications for Acute Herpes Zoster*

Antiviral agents
  Acyclovir 800 mg p.o. every 4 h (five times a day) for 7 to
10 days
  Famciclovir 750 mg p.o. every 8 h for 7 days
  Valacyclovir 1 g p.o. t.i.d. for 7 days
Analgesics
  Acetaminophen 1,000 mg p.o. every 6 h for 7 days,
    then as needed
  Ibuprofen 600 mg p.o. every 6 h for 7 days,
    then as needed
  Oxycodone 5–10 mg p.o. every 4 h as needed for pain
    [also available as a preparation that includes oxycodone
    5 mg and acetaminophen 325 mg per tablet, such as
    Percocet (Endo Laboratories, Chadds Ford, PA) and
    Roxicet (Roxane Laboratories, Columbus, OH)]
Steroids
  If no contraindication, for patients over the age of 50
  Prednisone 60 mg per day, taper over 21 days
Tricyclic antidepressant
  Amitriptyline 25 mg p.o. each day for 90 days
  Nortriptyline 10 mg p.o. each day (as alternative if above
    not tolerated)

trigeminal distribution most likely is to result in residual pain and the development of postherpetic neuralgia (see below).

The disease may involve motor neurons as well from spread of infection to the anterior horn of the spinal cord, with the facial nerve being the most commonly affected. Myelitis or encephalitis also may develop. It is uncommon for sympathetic neurons to be primarily infected, although it has been reported. This would lead to the development of complex regional pain syndrome.

Pathogenesis

Reactivation of the virus seems to start in the DRG. Microscopic examination of the DRG of the affected nerve reveals inflammatory changes, which precede the characteristic rash the patient usually experiences. The DRG undergoes degenerative changes and may become replaced by scar tissue. Wallerian degeneration may affect the nerve, which becomes demyelinated, and the changes of fibrosis may affect the dorsal horn and the posterior columns. Local meningitis may be seen as may anterior horn involvement, which, although rare, may result in motor impairment.

Treatment

The mainstay of therapy is early use of an antiviral agent (Table 33.2). Because of the expense and side effects of these drugs, controversy exists as to whether all patients with acute herpes zoster should be treated or only those individuals at most risk for developing chronic pain from postherpetic neuralgia (see discussion below). Nevertheless, even the healthiest patient will still benefit from analgesics, and the addition of a tricyclic antidepressant also should be discussed.

Mild analgesics such as acetaminophen and non-steroidal antiinflammatory drugs used on a fixed-dose regimen (not on an as-needed basis) will suffice for some patients. Opiate analgesics should be used for any patient who is unable to sleep or tolerate normal activity because of severe pain. The benefits of a tricyclic antidepressant are multifold: not only do these agents relieve pain and promote sleep but also early addition of amitriptyline (25 mg p.o., q.d.) may actually decrease the likelihood of developing postherpetic neuralgia.

Systemic steroids may provide pain relief by ameliorating some of the manifestations of infection. The fear that the steroid would induce immune suppression and thus worsen the infection has not been seen. But the hope that the early use of steroids would decrease the likelihood of developing postherpetic neuralgia has not been seen. Topical solutions of local anesthetics and various traditional remedies can be tried, provided the area treated is not so large as to risk overdose from systemic absorption.

The use of nerve blocks to provide pain relief is widespread. Some practitioners have suggested the early and aggressive blockade may reduce the incidence of long-term pain, but this has not been proven. Subcutaneous infiltration at the site of the zoster with local anesthetic and steroids can provide immediate but temporary pain relief. Pain relief also can be accomplished with somatic nerve blocks or epidural blockade with local anesthetic and steroids. The use of semipermanent epidural catheters has been advocated as a means of providing nonsedating pain relief to allow the suffering patient to be comfortable at home.

Sympathetic blockade also is routinely used. Some specialists theorize that by preventing the sympathetic response to pain and by inhibiting vasospasm, the long-term sequelae of the herpetic infection also will be diminished. Lumbar-sympathetic block is used for the lower extremities. For truncal distribution, thoracic-epidural blockade has been used, as has fluoroscopic-guided ganglion blocks at T3 and T4. These blocks run the risk of cardiovascular effects as well as a high incidence of pneumothorax. The mainstay of treatment for zoster of the face, neck, and upper extremity is a stellate-ganglion block (Fig. 33.1). Blocks should be performed with a mix

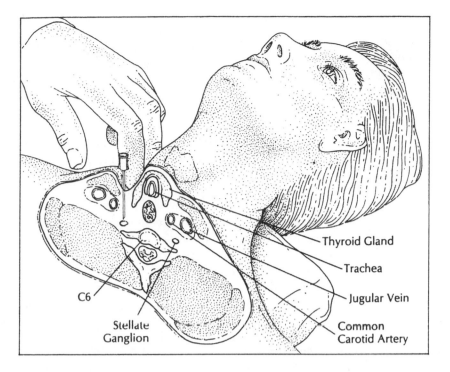

FIG. 33.1. Stellate-ganglion block is effective for acute herpes zoster pain in the head, neck, and arms. Paratracheal approach is used for injection at level of C6 while patient is supine with a pillow below shoulder and neck slightly hyperextended.

of local anesthetic and steroid. The frequency is best determined by the individual case, with many experts suggesting daily or weekly injections.

POSTHERPETIC NEURALGIA

Patients who develop herpes zoster may find that their pain lingers after the rash has regressed. For some patients, the pain disappears or abates and then recurs. Residual scarring with changes in pigmentation is common, and the pain the patient experiences often is in the distribution of the scarring. Some patients describe the classic lancinating, dermatomal pain and yet insist they never had any vesicular eruptions, rash, or skin discoloration. Zoster sine herpete is the term used to describe this less-common condition. All of these patients may present with dysesthesia, hypesthesia, or anesthesia along the dermatomal distribution.

Patients complain of burning, aching pain, which may be constant. Electrical shocks of pain or paroxysmal shooting sensations are common. The jolt of pain may awaken the patient from sleep. For some, the discomfort fades with time, but for most patients, it becomes a constant companion with occasional exacerbations of severe pain. Incidents of increased pain may be evoked by physical or emotional stressors.

Patients commonly report alterations in sensation in the affected area. There may be an area of "numbness" (anesthesia) or "strange sensation" (dysesthesia.) Light touch may be interpreted as pain (allodynia) and mildly noxious stimuli produce excruciating pain (hyperalgesia).

There is no reliable means of determining who will develop postherpetic neuralgia. Although the incidence is clearly increased after 55 years of age , there are other predicting factors as well (Table 33.3). Because "severe pain" appears to be predictive of the development of postherpetic neuralgia, there is tremendous interest in treating the acute infection aggressively and minimizing the discomfort experienced by patients.

Pathogenesis

Postherpetic neuralgia occurs when permanent damage has been done to the sensory pathways by the virus from the evoked immune response. The site of permanent alteration may be the peripheral nerve or the DRG, the dorsal horn, or even the sensory cortex. Thus it is possible for pain impulses to be generated entirely independently from the peripheral nervous system. The development of "central pain" makes treating postherpetic neuralgia a challenge.

TABLE 33.3. *Factors Associated with Persistent Pain*

Severe pain
Severity of skin lesions (may reflect severity of infection)
Presence of scarring after resolution of rash
Degree of sensory loss
Immune response to infection
Not taking antiviral agent
Painful prodrome prior to rash
High fever during acute phase

Treatment

Because treating the syndrome of postherpetic neuralgia is such a challenge, prevention is the best option. For patients in whom postherpetic neuralgia develops, despite antiviral medication and aggressive treatment, the course of therapy may be protracted. Patients need to be educated about the disease process and both the practitioner and patient must have realistic goals for therapeutic options.

Medications are the mainstay of treatment. The goal is not only to alleviate pain, but also to help patients cope with any insomnia. Many patients may become depressed and also have episodes of anxiety as the duration of their pain lengthens. Any treatment plan must address all the patient's needs, including physical, psychological, and social impairment. Proper referrals to social workers (e.g., for the patient who is in too much discomfort to prepare his own meals) or psychologists should be done promptly. Any treatment plan needs to be individualized for the patient.

It is common for patients to express frustration that they must take "so many pills." If this occurs, the pain practitioner becomes psychological support person to help the patient express his anger and also cheerleader to offer encouragement and remind the patient of any improvements in function. For this reason, it often is helpful to document the size of the patient's area of pain as well as a "pain score" and also to document markers of activities of daily living, such as hours slept. The realization that progress is being made is very reassuring.

Medications often used include the tricyclic antidepressants and anticonvulsants (Table 33.4). There is no

TABLE 33.4. *Medications for Postherpetic Neuralgia*

Tricyclic antidepressant
  Amitriptyline 25 mg p.o. q.d. (Titrate upwards as tolerated)
  Notriptyline 10 mg p.o. q.d. (Titrate upwards as tolerated)
  Desipramine 10 mg p.o. q.d. (Titrate upwards as tolerated)
Antiseizure medications
  Phenytoin 15–20 mg/kg i.v. infusion as trial (do not exceed 50 mg/min)
  Phenytoin[a] 300 mg p.o. q.d. continue as needed
  Lidocaine[b] 2–5 mg/kg i.v. infusion over 45–60 min as trial
  Mexilitene[a] 100 mg p.o. q.d. (increase by 100 mg every 3 days up to 200 mg t.i.d.)
  Clonazepam 0.5 mg p.o. q.h.s. (up to 1–2 mg p.o. t.i.d.)
  Carbamazepine 100 mg p.o. b.i.d. (up to 400–600 mg p.o. b.i.d./t.i.d.)
  Gabapentin 100 mg p.o. t.i.d. (up to 3,600 mg/day)
  Valproate[a] 100 mg p.o. b.i.d. (up to 250–500 mg b.i.d./t.i.d.)

[a]Must monitor blood tests before starting medications and every 60–90 days.
[b]Check electrocardiogram for conduction abnormalities.

role for the antiviral agents or for oral steroids in treating postherpetic neuralgia. The anticonvulsant gabapentin was shown to be effective in a randomized control trial. Participants noted a decrease in pain scores after 2 weeks, and after 6 weeks the gabapentin group had a 33% reduction in pain scores, compared with an 8% reduction in the placebo group.

Many patients continue to need analgesics, including opiates. The use of opiate analgesics should be determined on a case-by-case basis, with the goal being to optimize function and independence. Some practitioners prefer to prescribe opiates for use on an as-needed basis only. Other specialists have had excellent results with patients on low-dose opiates given at a fixed-interval dosing schedule. Proper education about the side effects and limitations of opiate medication must be given to all patients before prescribing the drug.

Medications also may be delivered transcutaneously. This includes medications that have a transdermal drug-delivery system, such as fentanyl and clonidine. Researchers have been developing a local anesthetic patch that a patient applies over the area of greatest pain. Clinical trials have reported tremendous success, and the system is both well tolerated and well received by patients. This transdermal preparation of lidocaine has been approved recently for use in patients with postherpetic neuralgia by the Food and Drug Administration. Some pain experts have attempted to duplicate the system by prescribing local anesthetic creams and adhesive dressings to patients, who then are instructed to create their own system at home. This approach runs the risk of having a layperson in charge of dosing, and may have an increase risk of overdose by systemic absorption.

Nerve blocks have been tried with mixed success. Some experts advocate sympathetic blocks on a frequent basis to break the neuropathic-pain cycle. Repeated stellate-ganglion blocks done with local anesthetic, and steroid are used for the upper extremity and face and neck symptoms (Fig. 33.1). More specific blockade at the gasserian ganglion can be done for pain in the trigeminal distribution. Some experts suggest that gasserian ganglion blocks be done under fluoroscopic guidance to minimize any risk to the patient, although the classic approach relies on palpable bony landmarks. The risk of nerve blocks includes bleeding, infection, and seizure, as well as failure to relieve pain. Some patients report an "increase" in their pain following a nerve block. This may occur as the local anesthetic effects are wearing off, and the patient suddenly goes from having no pain to the recurrence of symptoms. An area of pain that is not relieved by an otherwise successful block may seem to be magnified in its intensity, as the surrounding area now is pain free.

Transcutaneous electrical nerve stimulation (TENS) may provide some patients with relief. The electrodes

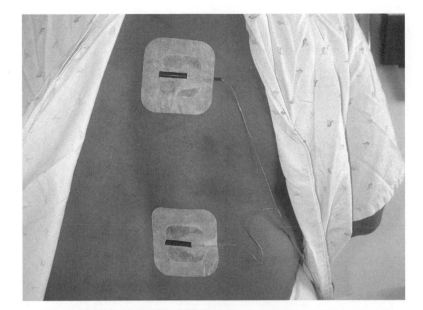

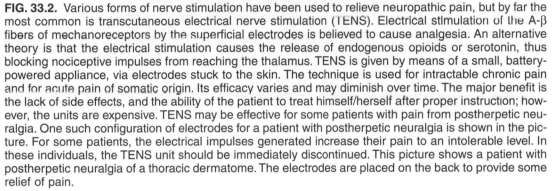

FIG. 33.2. Various forms of nerve stimulation have been used to relieve neuropathic pain, but by far the most common is transcutaneous electrical nerve stimulation (TENS). Electrical stimulation of the A-β fibers of mechanoreceptors by the superficial electrodes is believed to cause analgesia. An alternative theory is that the electrical stimulation causes the release of endogenous opioids or serotonin, thus blocking nociceptive impulses from reaching the thalamus. TENS is given by means of a small, battery-powered appliance, via electrodes stuck to the skin. The technique is used for intractable chronic pain and for acute pain of somatic origin. Its efficacy varies and may diminish over time. The major benefit is the lack of side effects, and the ability of the patient to treat himself/herself after proper instruction; however, the units are expensive. TENS may be effective for some patients with pain from postherpetic neuralgia. One such configuration of electrodes for a patient with postherpetic neuralgia is shown in the picture. For some patients, the electrical impulses generated increase their pain to an intolerable level. In these individuals, the TENS unit should be immediately discontinued. This picture shows a patient with postherpetic neuralgia of a thoracic dermatome. The electrodes are placed on the back to provide some relief of pain.

should be placed to straddle the area of pain (Fig. 33.2). If the patient experiences more pain, the treatment should be discontinued immediately.

More invasive modalities also have been tried, with mixed success. Although several classic works suggest that nerve ablation techniques can be highly successful, most current specialists do not advocate these procedures. Because there is remodeling at the spinal cord and more rostral structures as well, cutting a peripheral nerve will not lessen the pain perceived and may actually increase the pain, if there were some viable fibers left that then are damaged. Most modern specialists understand that the neurophysiologic effects of local-anesthetic blockade are not the same as that of nerve ablation. There are as many strong opponents to radiofrequency lesioning of the gasserian ganglion as there are advocates. Most academic centers and research-oriented pain specialists strongly caution against the procedure, which is never the less still performed by reputable experts in the community.

Spinal-cord stimulation may provide some patients with relief. The advantage of spinal cord stimulation is that it may be performed as a reversible trial first with minimal discomfort to the patient. The risk of postdural-puncture headache and nerve damage must be explained to the patient first, so that the individual can make an informed decision. Spinal-cord stimulation is not a commonly performed procedure, and is done best by a trained expert.

Intrathecal drug trials also are a possibility. The technology to deliver continuous intrathecal medications exists and some pain specialists report very good results with intrathecal delivery of opiates or clonidine, or even very low dose local anesthetic. Because these procedures also are very risky, they should only be done by a trained expert. And a proper trial of the medication must be performed first. Because these patients may be so desperate for any relief, to minimize the likelihood of a positive trial but unsuccessful relief from permanent pump delivery, the trial should include the patient's response to a "placebo."

Because the incidence of herpes zoster in our society is so great, there is a great deal of interest in finding modalities of better pain relief. New drugs and new drug-delivery systems may be available soon.

SELECTED READINGS

Bowsher D. The effects of pre-emptive treatment of postherpetic neuralgia with amitriptyline: a randomized, double-blind, placebo-controlled trial. *J Pain and Symptom Manage* 1997;13:327–331.

Kost RG, Strausee SE. Post-herpetic neuralgia: pathogenesis, treatment, and prevention. *N Engl J Med* 1996;335:32–42.

Nathwani D, MacDonald T, Davey P. Cost-effectiveness of acyclovir for varicella infections in immunocompetent patients: a british perspective. *Infectious Disease Clinical Practice* 1995;4:138–145.

Rowbotham MC, Davis PS, Verkempinck C, et al. Lidocaine patch: double-blind controlled study of a new treatment method for post-herpetic neuralgia. *Pain* 1996;65:39–44.

Watson CPN, Evans RJ, Watt VR, et al. Post-herpetic neuralgia: 208 cases. *Pain* 1998;35:289–297.

Watson CPN, Deck JH, Morshead C, et al. Post-herpetic neuralgia: further post-mortem studies of cases with and without pain. *Pain* 1991;44:105–117.

CHAPTER 34

Peripheral Neuropathies

Anne Miller

Entrapment neuropathies occur as a result of external pressure to peripheral nerves, causing focal damage to the nerve and thereby producing the largely sensory disturbance. Peripheral nerves are most vulnerable to this type of injury at locations in the body where the nerves are superficial and in close apposition to bone, surrounded by large muscles, or pass through fibrous tissue structures. The compression may occur as a result of pressure completely extrinsic to the body, as in the lengthy application of a tourniquet, prolonged contact with a hard surface, or in the wearing of constrictive garments. Muscle hypertrophy as a result of repetitive exercise may compress a peripheral nerve, as can the changes in local anatomy caused by rapid weight loss or weight gain. Masses such as tumors or scar tissue may do the same. Whereas any individual exposed to these conditions may sustain damage to a peripheral nerve, those with specific systemic illnesses that predispose them to generalized polyneuropathies (diabetics, alcohol abusers, patients with renal failure, among others) are at higher risk of developing entrapment neuropathies.

A careful, directed neurological history and examination is essential to the accurate diagnosis of entrapment neuropathy. On questioning, one may elicit a history of a recent drinking binge with a new neurological deficit on awakening. The patient may have had recent surgery and therefore positioning on an operating table. Pregnancy may have produced a new tingling in the anterior thigh or the palm of the hand. As mentioned above, the deficit usually is that of a peripheral sensory disturbance in the cutaneous distribution of the peripheral nerve, often characterized by hypesthesia, dysesthesia, and hyperalgesia. If the entrapped peripheral nerve contains motor fibers at the site of entrapment, muscle wasting, and decreased reflexes may be present as well.

The most common diagnostic dilemma in sorting out these lesions occurs in distinguishing between entrapment of a peripheral nerve, a plexopathy, or a root compression.

Again, a precise sensory examination often clarifies the diagnosis. However, a few tools are available to help delineate the precise location of the entrapment. Radiologic studies may suggest entrapment. Electromyography may confirm the clinical impression of motor involvement by demonstrating denervation or reinnervation potentials in the muscles tested; however, these findings merely confirm the presence of a lesion, but do not necessarily tell us where in the peripheral nerve the lesion resides. Nerve-conduction velocities provide us with the most useful information in locating the site of entrapment. Regional slowing of conduction because of demyelination may be detected, as well as decreased amplitudes of sensory and motor action potentials as a result of damage to axons. Unfortunately, this test, although helpful, is time consuming and uncomfortable for the patient, and one may meet some resistance when ordering this exam.

MEDIAN NEUROPATHY

Although the median nerve may be compressed at any point during its course through the upper extremity, median neuropathy most commonly occurs as a result of compression at the wrist by the flexor retinaculum, hence the term *carpal tunnel syndrome*. The median nerve at the wrist provides cutaneous innervation to the distal palm of the hand and the palmar surfaces of the four digits. In addition, it provides motor innervation of the adductor pollicis brevis and the first and second lumbricals. The characteristic symptoms of palmar paresthesias and weak grip often are worse on waking in the morning and frequently are exacerbated by activities requiring continuous wrist flexion. Occasionally, the pain may radiate proximally to the forearm and elbow. A positive Tinel's sign often is a diagnostic aid in these patients. Thenar-muscle wasting often is a late sign.

Women in their middle years tend to be the major sufferers of carpal tunnel syndrome, although a space-occupying lesion of the carpal tunnel (such as ganglion cysts, callus from fracture) may precipitate the lesion in any individual. As mentioned earlier, systemic diseases such as obesity, pregnancy, renal failure, and diabetes predispose individuals to develop this problem. Although peripheral nerve block at the wrist may provide symptomatic relief (for some time if steroid is included), long-term treatment tends to be surgical decompression if the condition persists beyond the resolution of the inciting factor.

ULNAR NERVE COMPRESSION

The ulnar nerve is most commonly compressed at the elbow, where it passes through the condylar groove and is quite superficial. Positioning during anesthesia and repetitive elbow flexion are the two major culprits in precipitating this neuropathy. The ulnar nerve is vulnerable to stretch injury at the elbow, and this appears to be the mechanism for ulnar palsy secondary to flexion, which elongates the nerve.

Severe ulnar-nerve damage at the elbow produces claw-hand deformity. Lesser degrees of injury produce pain in the elbow, with paresthesias and dysesthesias of the ulnar surface of the palm and the last two digits. Hypothenar wasting may be apparent, and the interossei are involved.

Compression of the ulnar nerve at the wrist, although less common than lesions at the elbow, occurs frequently as a result of repetitive trauma, overuse, or space-occupying lesions of Guyon's canal, through which the nerve passes. Because this distal branch of the nerve contains only sensory fibers, paresthesias of the ulnar surface of the palm and digits are the sole features of this lesion; weakness of the flexor carpi ulnaris and flexor digitorum profundus muscles with the accompanying hypothenar wasting are not observed with distal-nerve compression at the wrist. As with median nerve compression, peripheral-nerve block with steroid may provide symptomatic relief, but often surgery is inevitable if the lesion is felt to be anatomic in nature.

RADIAL NERVE COMPRESSION

The radial nerve is vulnerable to compression injury in the arm as it travels around the humerus, closely apposed to the bone in a spiraling course. Humeral fractures can cause nerve injury, as can improper padding of the dependent arm during anesthesia in the lateral-decubitus position. The syndrome familiarly known as *Saturday night palsy* occurs typically after lengthy compression of the nerve during sleep or with the arm slung over the back of a chair, an event occasionally associated with an inebriated state (hence the name). Characteristic features of this syndrome include wrist drop and ill-defined pain in the radial distribution

When the radial nerve is compressed at the level of the elbow in the radial tunnel as the nerve courses between the superficial and deep heads of the supinator muscle, the patient experiences deep pain in the forearm and difficulty extending the thumb and fingers at the metacarpophalangeal joints. A purely sensory deficit occurs if the radial nerve is compressed at the wrist where injuries commonly occur as a result of distal radius fractures or constriction from encircling objects of the wrist. Paresthesias are described in the radial sensory distribution, on the dorsum of the thumb, and the index finger.

THORACIC-OUTLET SYNDROME

True neurologic thoracic-outlet syndrome (TOS) is a rare entity. In the literature, the term TOS has been used to denote many disorders, including arterial TOS, venous TOS, nonspecific neurologic TOS, and true neurologic TOS, with various permutations and combinations of the above.

True neurologic TOS presents with insidious wasting and weakness of the hand, usually unilateral. Young to middle-aged females seem most at risk for developing this lesion, most often ascribed to a rudimentary cervical rib (actually, an unusually long C7 transverse process). This causes stretch to occur on the C8 and T1 ventral rami on the lower trunk of the brachial plexus. Presenting symptoms are paresthesias on the ulnar surface of the forearm and hand, and neurologic examination usually demonstrates weakness of the ulnar-innervated muscles of the hand. A feature that distinguishes this entity from ulnar neuropathy is that the lesion rarely causes a split in sensory loss of the fourth digit. Often, particularly in advanced cases, all the intrinsic muscles of the hand become wasted and weak; most involved are the thenar muscles, thereby causing the clinician to think of carpal-tunnel syndrome.

MERALGIA PARESTHETICA

Meralgia paresthetica, or entrapment of the lateral-femoral cutaneous nerve of the thigh, is a common malady producing paresthesias and dysesthesias of the anterior and lateral aspects of the thigh. The deficit is purely sensory, as the lateral femoral cutaneous nerve of the thigh has as its origins the posterior divisions of the L2 and L3 nerve roots. Although compression from a pelvic mass (or pregnant uterus) is possible as the nerve emerges from the psoas muscle and travels between the iliacus muscle and its fascial covering, the most common point of compression is where the nerve exits the pelvis deep to the inguinal ligament and medial to the anterior–superior iliac spine. Here, it is exposed to external pressure from tight clothing, a protuberant abdomen overhanging the inguinal ligament, or trauma from contact of the iliac spine with counters, tables, etc.

Meralgia paresthetica may masquerade as lumbar-root compression; a peripheral nerve block at the point where the nerve dives below the inguinal ligament will clarify the etiology of the deficit. Injection of a small (ten to 12 mL) volume of local anesthetic mixed with steroid at the point where the nerve emerges from deep to the inguinal ligament will make the diagnosis, and often will provide prolonged relief from the discomfort. It may be necessary to repeat the block a few times in relatively close succession to ensure results, but often this proves to be therapeutic and the condition requires no further intervention.

PIRIFORMIS SYNDROME

The sciatic nerve is composed of the common peroneal nerve, which arises from the posterior divisions of L4, L5, S1, and S2, and the tibial nerve, which derives from the anterior divisions of L4, L5, S1, S2, and S3. The sciatic nerve courses posteriorly and caudally in the pelvis to exit the pelvis via the sciatic notch. Here, it is bound superiorly by the piriformis muscle and, as it courses between the greater trochanter and the ischial tuberosity, it is covered by the gluteus muscles and hamstrings. These are antigravity muscles, the largest in the body, and hypertrophy or spasm, particularly of the piriformis muscle, can cause compression of the sciatic nerve as it emerges from the pelvis. Pelvic fracture or hip fracture/dislocation also can produce compression injury to the sciatic nerve, as can intramuscular injections delivered erroneously directly into the nerve.

Piriformis syndrome typically produces the symptoms of "sciatica" — aching, occasionally burning pain of the buttock, progressing down the posterior aspect of the thigh and leg. Often, injection of the muscle either with local anesthetic mixed with steroid, or even simply "dry needling" to discharge the hypertonic muscle, may be therapeutic. These maneuvers may need to be repeated a few times in relatively close succession for the patient to derive prolonged benefit. Occasionally, local anesthetic combined with hyaluronidase (lyophilized Wydase, Wyeth-Ayerst Laboratories, Philadelphia, PA, U.S.A.) may effectively lyse scar tissue and provide more lasting results. Although this intervention is becoming less popular with the increasing availability of botulinum toxin, or Botox (Allergan, Inc., Irvine, CA, U.S.A.). Injection of Botox into a muscle results in a semipermanent weakening of the muscle contraction. The effect usually lasts only a few months and may be less effective for some people upon retreatment.

PERONEAL NERVE PALSY

As noted previously, the common peroneal nerve is a branch of the sciatic nerve and derives from the posterior divisions of L4, L5, S1, and S2. It travels with the tibial nerve as the sciatic nerve down the posterior thigh until it reaches the upper portion of the popliteal fossa, where the two separate. At this point, the common peroneal moves laterally to pass superficial to the fibular neck. The common peroneal nerve may be compressed externally against the fibular neck, or injury may occur distal to this point after the common peroneal divides into the deep peroneal and the superficial peroneal nerves. Placing the legs in stirrups during general anesthesia, immobility associated with generalized wasting such as during coma, or prolonged crossing of legs may produce this syndrome. As is the case with all focal peripheral nerve entrapment syndromes, peroneal nerve entrapment is more common in patients with preexisting systemic disease predisposing them to generalized polyneuropathies.

Symptoms of common peroneal-nerve syndrome include weakened dorsiflexors and sensory deficits including dysesthesias and paresthesias over the anterolateral aspect of the leg and the dorsum of the foot.

TARSAL TUNNEL SYNDROME

The tibial nerve, a branch of the sciatic, courses superficially along the medial aspect of the ankle and passes under the flexor retinaculum of the dorsum of the foot. Distal to the flexor retinaculum, the tibial nerve divides into plantar nerves, which supply motor function and sensation to the anterior two thirds of the sole of the foot.

Compression of the distal portion of the tibial nerve as it dips under the flexor retinaculum, or of the plantar nerves just distal to the flexor retinaculum, produce painful dysesthesias and paresthesias of the sole of the foot, as well as weakness of the foot muscles. This injury may occur with tight or poorly fitting shoes or other footwear, and may be compounded by resulting scar tissue formation and chronic compression.

OCCIPITAL NEURALGIA

The dorsal ramus of the second cervical spinal nerve is known as the greater occipital nerve. Compression of this nerve is theoretically possible as it courses up the neck, piercing semispinalis and trapezius muscles or the aponeurosis of the trapezius. It is felt by some that this type of compression may be precipitated by whiplash or hyperextension injury, as a similar constellation of symptoms may be seen following compression of the nerve by leaning the head against the back of a chair for a period of time, etc.

The classic symptoms of occipital neuralgia are unilateral continuous or intermittent paresthesias, or numbness radiating to the vertex of the head in the C2 distribution. Often, the course of the nerve may be tender to palpation, particularly at the base of the occiput. There may be a positive Tinel's sign. Often, a peripheral nerve block with local anesthetic where the nerve pierces the muscles at the base of the skull may be helpful diagnostically, as well as provide temporary relief. Computed tomography or magnetic resonance imaging may be suggestive of external nerve compression, in which case surgical decompression may be a helpful maneuver. Simpler therapies such as wearing a soft cervical collar to support neck muscles may be beneficial. Unfortunately, no electrophysiologic studies have been described as useful in clinching the diagnosis, which remains difficult to make.

SELECTED READINGS

Dellon AL. Management of peripheral nerve problems in the upper and lower extremity using quantitative sensory testing. *Hand Clin* 1999;15: 697–715.

Levin SM. Piriformis syndrome. *Orthopedics* 2000;23:183–184.

Loeser JD, Butler SH, Chapman CR, et al., eds. *Bonica's Management of Pain*, 3rd ed. Philadelphia: Lippincott Williams & Wilkins, 2000.

Magnusson T, Ragnarsson T, Bjornsson A. Occipital nerve release in patients with whiplash trauma and occipital neuralgia. *Headache* 1996; 36:32–36.

Mazurek MT, Shin AY. Upper extremity peripheral nerve anatomy: current concepts and applications. *Clin Orthop* 2001;383:7–20.

McCrory P, Bell S. Nerve entrapment syndromes as a cause of pain in the hip, groin and buttock. *Sports Med* 1999;27:261–274.

Stewart JD. *Focal Peripheral Neuropathies* 3rd ed. Philadelphia: Lippincott Williams & Wilkins, 2000.

Murata Y, Takahashi K, Murakami M, et al. An unusual cause of sciatic pain. *J Bone Joint Surg Br* 2001;83:112–113.

Warfield, C, ed. *Principles and Practice of Pain Management*. New York: McGraw–Hill Inc., 1993.

CHAPTER 35

Diabetic Neuropathies

Dhanalakshmi Koyyalagunta

Diabetes mellitus is the most common cause of peripheral neuropathies. Diabetes first was described in Chronicles II of the Bible when King Asa developed gangrene of the feet. In 1887, Pryce described painful, symmetric polyneuropathies both clinically and pathologically in a diabetic patient. Diabetic neuropathy is the most common complication of both insulin-dependent (type 1) and non–insulin-dependent (type 2) diabetes mellitus. Clinical and electrophysiologic evidence of diabetic peripheral neuropathy is estimated to be about 70% and symptomatic neuropathy probably affects around 10% of the diabetic population at any time. Diabetic neuropathy can affect the sensory, motor, or autonomic systems, or any combinations thereof. Sensory disorders are the most frequently encountered symptoms of diabetic neuropathy, and patients may develop symptoms ranging from pain to loss of sensation.

PATHOPHYSIOLOGY

Diabetes damages nerves in a number of ways. Both small, unmyelinated nerve fibers and large, myelinated fibers can be affected together or separately. An important question concerning the pathology of human diabetic neuropathy is whether the Schwann cell or the axon is the primarily damaged structure. Earlier studies of diabetic patients with established neuropathy demonstrated a mixture of both demyelination and axonal degeneration. More recent studies of diabetic patients without evidence of neuropathy have demonstrated demyelination without axonal loss or atrophy, thus suggesting that demyelination and hence involvement of the Schwann cell is primary. With progression of neuropathy, there is progressive axonal degeneration and loss of myelinated fibers. Nerve damage can be focal, as occurs in ischemic mononeuropathies, or can be diffuse, as occurs in peripheral neuropathies. Although there is increasing evidence that the pathogenesis of diabetic neuropathy is multifactorial, the

prevailing theory implicates persistent hyperglycemia as the primary factor within the metabolic hypothesis. The unused glucose in diabetes is shunted into the polyol pathway and converted to sorbitol and fructose by the enzyme's aldose reductase and sorbitol dehydrogenase. Accumulation of sorbitol and fructose in peripheral nerves, as in other tissues, leads to reduced myoinositol levels and inhibition of sodium-potassium ATPase activity. This leads to sodium retention, edema, myelin swelling, axoglial dysjunction, and nerve degeneration. In addition to the metabolic hypothesis, there also is reasonable evidence to suggest other factors responsible for the neuropathy.

The vascular (ischemic–hypoxic) hypothesis implies the combined effects of several metabolic factors to be responsible for the microvascular damage observed in many tissues in diabetes. Some of these factors include the formation of advanced glycosylation end products (AGE), increased oxygen free-radical activity, and reduced endothelial nitric-oxide activity. Immune mechanisms have been implicated in some patients, especially in those with proximal neuropathy and those with a more marked motor component to their neuropathy. Antibodies directed against motor and sensory nerve structures have been detected by immunofluorescence. It also is thought that growth-factor deficiency may play a role in the pathogenesis of diabetic neuropathy. Nerve growth-factor levels are decreased in patients with diabetic neuropathy, and such levels correlate with the severity of the neuropathy. Insulinlike growth factor (IGF)-I and IGF-II have been implicated in the growth and differentiation of neurons. Insulin deficiency leads to a reduced IGF-I concentration. This has been shown to cause marked impairment in peripheral-nerve regeneration. In the laminin of experimental animals, a glycoprotein promotes neurite extension. Lack of normal expression of the laminin gene may contribute to pathogenesis of diabetic neuropathy.

CLASSIFICATION AND CLINICAL FEATURES

Diabetic Autonomic Neuropathy

Autonomic neuropathy often is associated with diabetic predominantly sensory neuropathy. Although clinical assessment of autonomic neuropathy has been confined largely to cardiovascular and genitourinary systems, involvement of every aspect of the autonomic nervous system can be shown (Table 35.1). The sympathetic and parasympathetic nervous systems are involved to differing degrees; studies of baroreflexes indicate that sympathetic dysfunction occurs earlier in the course of diabetes.

Diabetic Polyneuropathy

Polyneuropathy is the most prevalent form of diabetic neuropathy. However, it frequently is asymptomatic. Clinical features are summarized in Table 35.2. The patient usually complains of numbness, dysesthesia, or pain. Sometimes sensations of burning or cold may be the dominant feature. Symptoms are nearly always bilateral and symmetrical, and they affect the distal extremity before the proximal extremity. The symptoms usually are gradual in onset. Some patients may have extreme sensitivity to touch. An occasional nocturnal problem is the "restless legs" syndrome. This is characterized by an

TABLE 35.1. *Clinical Features of Diabetic Autonomic Neuropathies*

System	Features
Cardiovascular	Diminished beat-to-beat variation
	Orthostatic hypotension
	Resting tachycardia
	Painless myocardial infarction
	Sudden death
	Prolonged QT interval
Genitourinary	Diabetic cystopathy
	Male impotence
	Female sexual dysfunction
Gastrointestinal	Esophageal motor incoordination
	Decreased gastric motility, gastroparesis
	Nocturnal diarrhea
	Constipation
	Fecal incontinence
	Gall-bladder hypocontraction
Ophthalmic	Miosis
	Disturbance of dilation
	Argyll Robertsonlike pupils
Neuroendocrine	Reduced pancreatic polypeptide release
	Reduced somatostatin release
	Reduced motilin and gastric inhibitory peptide release
	Enhanced gastrin release
	Impaired glucose-counter regulation
Miscellaneous	Diminished, excessive, or gustatory sweating

TABLE 35.2. *Clinical Features of the Common Diabetic Peripheral Neuropathies*

Lesion	Site	Features
Polyneuropathy	Distal extremities	Tingling, pain, burning, numbness, symmetric distal sensory loss, diminished deep-tendon reflexes
Mononeuropathy	Cranial nerves 3–7 peripheral	Pain, diplopia, nerve dysfunction
Radiculopathy	Cervical, lumbosacral, thoracic, abdominal	Lancinating pain, root distribution, functional and sensory loss
Amyotrophy	Proximal lower limbs	Pain, weight loss, weakness, muscle wasting, tenderness

uncontrollable urge to move the feet, especially at nighttime, thus disrupting the patient's sleep. The patient may obtain relief by pacing the floor or rubbing the feet. The symptoms usually disappear within a few hours.

The majority of patients with diabetic polyneuropathy (DPN) have a number of characteristic physical findings. Early on, diminished thermal sensation may be the only demonstrable finding, while diminished vibration sense is common at later stages. The distal toes are affected first, followed later by loss of sensation in the feet and lower legs. Severe cases have skin-trophic changes with callous formation. Wasting of the small muscles of the feet may be evident. The deep-tendon reflexes at the ankles usually are diminished or absent. The knee deep-tendon reflexes are diminished at later stages. Patients with severe, painful neuropathy often may experience unpleasant sensitivity to touching the feet. Some patients may develop evidence of neuroarthropathy — Charcot's joint. This is characterized by abnormal displacement of foot bones with disintegration of the foot joints. The acute Charcot's joint often is swollen and warm, with a markedly increased blood flow. In evaluating the painful diabetic foot, it is critical to determine if ischemia is present. In diabetic neuropathy, the foot pulses often may be prominent and bounding. In the ischemic foot, pulses usually are absent, the skin is atrophic and dusky, and the capillary filling time is slow. Ischemic rest pain usually is unilateral and well localized, and gangrene may be evident. In patients complaining of pain in the feet, it also is important to ensure that there are no bone fractures or inflammatory arthritic changes such as gout. Cellulitis also must not be overlooked. Plantar fascitis and bone spurs sometimes may cause confusion. Pain from these conditions usually is induced by walking and relieved by rest, while neuropathic pain may be relieved by walking and only symptomatic at rest.

Diabetic Mononeuropathies

Diabetes can affect a variety of cranial and peripheral nerves. The cranial nerves most frequently involved are the third and sixth, while involvement of the seventh is much more rare. The clinical history of diabetic third-nerve palsy is characteristic. The patient usually complains of relatively sudden onset and unilateral, periorbital pain in association with diplopia. Examination may reveal a severe ophthalmoplegia with displacement of the eye laterally and inferiorly in the case of a third-nerve lesion, and there may be ptosis with characteristic sparing of the pupil. The pain may be severe and may persist for weeks. Spontaneous recovery is usual. The condition often causes alarm, and careful evaluation is needed for such possibilities as a berry aneurysm in the posterior communicating cerebral artery and other mass compressive lesions intracranially. The most commonly affected peripheral nerves are the ulnar, median, femoral, and common peroneal nerves. Ulnar nerve lesions are characterized in advanced cases by severe wasting of the small muscles of the hand, particularly the interossei muscles. Median nerve lesions usually present as carpal tunnel syndrome, with pain radiating to the forearm and to the hand. Common peroneal nerve lesions cause characteristic foot drop and the dominant features are weakness of dorsiflexion and eversion of the foot. There sometimes is sensory blunting on the lateral aspect of the outer leg. Pain is variable and may be elicited by pressure around the common peroneal nerve. Spontaneous recovery to near-full function occurs in many patients.

Diabetic Radiculopathy

Diabetic radiculopathy is one of the most dramatic but poorly understood forms of diabetic neuropathy. It most frequently affects the nerve roots in the thoracolumbar areas. Involvement of the nerve roots to the muscles of the proximal lower limbs has many similarities to and overlaps with diabetic amyotrophy. In an extensive series of studies from the Mayo Clinic, polyradiculopathy was found to affect the chest wall, abdomen, back, anterior thigh, buttock, and foot regions. It may be bilateral and symmetrical or unilateral. The usual history demonstrates relatively sudden onset pain in the chest, abdomen, back, or limbs. Truncal radiculopathy may simulate a variety of thoracic and abdominal problems. Clinical findings are variable. When the chest and thorax are involved, some sensory blunting may be found on the anterior chest or abdomen. Herpes zoster often is suspected, but skin lesions do not develop. Sensory loss may not be demonstrable. It is difficult to demonstrate loss of muscle power in these regions. When radiculopathy affects the lower limbs, there may be segmental reflex loss at the ankle, or, more commonly, at the knees. Sensory loss again usually is not a prominent feature. In contrast to root-compressive lesions caused by degenerative intervertebral disc disease, the straight-leg raising test usually does not elicit pain. The term "neuropathic cachexia" has been employed to describe a group of patients with a syndrome resembling polyradiculopathy of lower limbs. The syndrome has many similarities to diabetic amyotrophy and indeed the condition appears to overlap with this type of neuropathy. Severe pain, depression, weight loss, and impotence are the dominant features. Patients usually require an extensive work-up for underlying malignancy because of weight loss and depression, although usually no malignancy is found. Slow spontaneous recovery appears in most patients over a period of 1 to 2 years.

Diabetic Amyotrophy

Diabetic amyotrophy, which also has been termed diabetic myelopathy, is a characteristic clinical syndrome. Its pathophysiology is obscure. Diagnosis primarily is based on the history and physical findings, as specific laboratory tests do not exist. Patients usually present with a history of severe pain and weakness in the proximal lower limbs, gluteal region, anterior thigh, or, more rarely, the distal extremity. The pain often is asymmetrical — first developing in one limb, gradually improving spontaneously, and subsequently involving the opposite limb. The upper limbs usually are not affected. Weight loss nearly always occurs in these patients and may be profound. The condition does not clearly seem to be related to the magnitude of glucose intolerance and occurs in patients who often have mild diabetes. On examination, the patients usually are depressed. Wasting of the proximal muscles in the lower limbs and gluteal region is common, and certain muscle groups may be tender to palpation. Profound weakness may be demonstrable and usually is asymmetric. A degree of polyneuropathy may be found in the distal extremity, but this does not extend proximally. Proximal sensory loss usually is not demonstrable. Certain cases have been found to have extensor plantar responses. Other features of myelopathy usually are not demonstrable, however. Spontaneous recovery over 1 to 2 years occurs in most patients, although residual disability does occur.

INVESTIGATIONS

It is tempting to order nerve-conduction velocity and other neurophysiological studies in patients with painful diabetic neuropathy. The objective of diagnostic tools is twofold: first, to measure the severity of the DPN, and, second, to quantify changes induced by specific treatment. Nerve-conduction studies: abnormalities of sensory-nerve conduction and amplitude of sensory or motor-nerve action potentials are indicators of neuropathy. Nerve-conduction studies are useful for establishing the anatomic distribution of the neuropathy. The earliest abnormality of DPN is slowed nerve conduction and/or decreased amplitude of the sural-nerve action potential. Nerve-conduction studies usually tend to measure the integrity of large, myelinated fibers, while painful neuropathies may predominantly affect small myelinated or unmyelinated nerves. Paradoxically, patients may have few abnormal physical findings and minimal electrophysiological abnormalities and may still have severe, painful neuropathies. Quantitative sensory testing (QST) is used in clinical trials to assess disease severity and treatment effects on small-nerve fibers. It has been established that QST has a definite role in monitoring patients in clinical trials, although it should be used only as one component of the patient evaluation. Computer-assisted sensory examination intravenous instruments are the most widely used QST instruments.

Skin biopsy. The biopsy of intraepidermal nerve fibers is a recent technique, which facilitates the study of small-fiber neuropathies. Cerebrospinal fluid (CSF) examination may be indicated in patients with polyradiculopathy and amyotrophy where infection or malignancy is being considered. Quite frequently, CSF protein is elevated, however this is not a specific feature and is found in long-standing diabetics. CSF cellular counts usually are normal. *Tabes dorsalis* should, of course, be ruled out in patients with atypical features by appropriate serology. Nerve biopsy rarely is indicated. Muscle biopsy usually is unrevealing in cases of diabetic amyotrophy, but occasionally may be necessary to distinguish polymyositis and other inflammatory conditions of muscle. X-rays of the feet should be obtained when osteomyelitis, bone spurs, Charcot's joints, or bone fractures are suspected. Finally, it is important to rule out conditions that may be confused with neuropathy and to identify by appropriate studies nondiabetic causes of neuropathy, such as alcohol, uremia, malignancy, and vitamin deficiency.

MANAGEMENT

Control of pain constitutes one of the most difficult management issues in diabetic neuropathy. Assessment of pain severity frequently is complicated by the presence of depression, thus making recognition of the underlying depression and its treatment an essential part of patient care. The natural history of most diabetic neuropathies is for pain to gradually remit. However, there are patients in whom symptoms do not remit even after several years. The majority of painful peripheral neuropathies spontaneously resolve on their own, leaving the patient with loss of sensation. It is important to counsel these patients regarding this fact, because it can make the pain easier to tolerate in the short term.

Glycemic Control

Of all the treatments, tight and stable glycemic control is probably the only one that may provide symptomatic relief as well as slow the progression of neuropathy. It should be noted, however, that rapid normalization of blood-glucose levels with insulin has been associated with painful insulin neuritis, and care should be taken when attempting to restore normoglycemia in newly diagnosed diabetic patients.

Analgesics are effective rarely in the treatment of painful diabetic neuropathy, although they may be of some use on a short-term basis for self-limited syndrome, such as painful diabetic third-nerve palsy, or for chronic painful neuropathy associated with musculoskeletal and joint abnormalities. Clinical trials have demonstrated efficacy with ibuprofen (600 mg q.i.d.) and sulindac (200 mg b.i.d.) in relieving neuropathic pain. Nonsteroidal antiinflammatory drugs must be used cautiously in diabetic patients, however, because of the risk of nephrotoxicity. With the use of narcotics, there is the risk of addiction and constipation, which may exacerbate features of autonomic neuropathy. Use of opiates to treat nonmalignant pain remains controversial because of both their questionable efficacy and their effects on the social functioning. Pain management of diabetic neuropathy requires individualized palliative treatment that may include long-term opiates in certain groups of patients.

Tricyclic Antidepressants

Tricyclic antidepressants (TCAs) have long been appreciated as adjuncts in the treatment of neuropathic pain. TCAs are thought to relieve pain by blocking the neuronal reuptake of norepinephrine and serotonin, thereby potentiating the inhibitory effect these neurotransmitters have in nociceptive pathways. Unfortunately, the anticholinergic side effects of tricyclics can interfere with symptomatic treatment. Dry mouth, urinary retention, cardiac arrhythmias, memory loss, and impotence can be major impediments to pain management. Other side effects consist of the predominantly α-adrenergic blocking effects of orthostatic hypotension and the antihistaminergic effects of sedation. Amitriptyline is the most anticholinergic, followed by protriptyline, clomipramine, doxepin, imipramine, nortriptyline, and desipramine.

Serotonin Reuptake Inhibitors

Use of selective serotonin reuptake inhibitors has had mixed reviews. In the literature, paroxetine and citalopram have been shown to relieve pain associated with diabetic neuropathy. Fluoxetine has been shown to decrease symptoms of painful neuropathy only in depressed patients. In one clinical study, sertraline has been shown to be effective in the treatment of diabetic neuropathy.

Anticonvulsants and Antiarrhythmics

Anticonvulsants and antiarrhythmics often are second-line drugs after use of TCAs for neuropathic pain. These agents act by reducing spontaneous discharges from damaged primary small-fiber nociceptors. Dilantin and carbamazepine have been helpful in limited populations with neuropathic pain. Gabapentin has been shown to be effective in relieving pain of diabetic neuropathy. But it does not appear to offer considerable advantage over amitriptyline and is more expensive. Lidocaine provides relief of intractable pain for 3 to 21 days. If successful, therapy may be continued with oral mexiletine, a structural analogue of lidocaine. Clonazepam has been shown to relieve symptoms of restless-leg syndrome. *Capsaicin*, the active "hot" ingredient of peppers, acts mainly on C nociceptors, thereby producing depletion of substance P in C fibers. Marked hyperesthesia with burning, lancinating, dysesthetic pain is typical of C-fiber pain and may respond to capsaicin applied topically three or four times daily. There is initial exacerbation of symptoms followed by relief in 2 to 3 weeks. *Clonidine*: It is thought that there is an element of sympathetic mediation of C-fiber–type pain, which can be overcome with clonidine (or phentolamine). An infusion of phentolamine can be tried, if a positive response is seen, oral or topical clonidine can be used. *Dextromethorphan (DXM)* is an antagonist to the glutamate receptor subtype *N*-methyl-D-aspartate (NMDA). Activation of the NMDA receptor by glutamate and aspartate is believed to play a role in the phenomenon known as "wind-up." Clinical studies provide modest evidence that DXM may be an effective treatment in patients with painful peripheral diabetic neuropathy. *Calcitonin* has shown to be efficacious in treating pain associated with diabetic neuropathy. A recent study demonstrated a significant improvement in peripheral neuropathy following 12 months of treatment with the angiotensin-converting enzyme inhibitor trandolapril. Tramadol has been used in some patients with good results.

Other Measures

Nocturnal doses of pulsed-electrical stimulation may be effective in alleviating subjective, burning, diabetic–neuropathic pain. Application of transcutaneous electrical nerve stimulation to the skin of the lumbar area may be an effective treatment in some patients. Electroacupuncture has been shown to be useful in alleviating pain of diabetic neuropathy. Electrical spinal-cord stimulation offers a new and effective way of relieving chronic diabetic-neuropathic pain and improves exercise tolerance. The technique should be considered in patients with neuropathic pain who do not respond to conventional treatment.

Therapies Aimed at Pathogenetic Mechanisms

Aldose reductase inhibitors reduce the flux of glucose through the polyol pathway, thus inhibiting tissue accumulation of sorbitol and fructose and preventing reduction of redox potentials. Aldose reductase inhibitors now are commercially available in Europe. Gangliosides are sialoglycolipids that are essential components of nerve-cell membranes. Some studies have shown small but statistically significant improvement in motor and sensory conduction in patients treated with gangliosides. A recent multicenter, double-blind, placebo-controlled trial using gamma-linoleic acid showed significant improvement in diabetic neuropathy. Myoinositol supplementation has been shown to improve neuropathy in several studies. *N*-acetyl-L-carnitine has been shown to have therapeutic benefit in animal models of diabetes. In patients with diabetic neuropathy that is associated with signs of antineuronal autoimmunity, intravenous immunoglobulin has been shown to have potential benefit. Lipoic acid, a powerful lipophilic free-radical scavenger that increases glucose entry and improves experimental diabetic neuropathy, has been used extensively for the treatment of painful diabetic neuropathy in Germany. Several trials are underway to study and assess the role of nerve-growth factors in the treatment of diabetic neuropathy.

ACKNOWLEDGEMENT

The author thanks James O'Hare, M.D., for research used in this chapter.

SELECTED READINGS

Archer AG, Roberts VC, Watkins PJ. Blood flow patterns in painful diabetic neuropathy. *Diabetologia* 1984;27:563–567.

Archer AG, Watkins PJ, Thomas PK, et al. The natural history of acute painful neuropathy in *diabetes mellitus. J Neurol Neurosurg Psychiat* 1983;46:491–499.

Bastron JA, Thomas JE. Diabetic polyradiculopathy. Clinical and electromyographic findings. *Mayo Clin Proc* 1981;56:725–732.

Boulton AJM, Armstrong WD, Scarpello JHB, et al. The natural history of painful diabetic neuropathy — a four-year study. *Post Grad Med J* [London]. 1983;59:556–559.

Boulton AJM, Drury J, Clarke B, et al. Continuous subcutaneous insulin infusion in the management of painful diabetic neuropathy. *Diabetes Care* 1982;5:386–390.

Boulton AJM, Malik RA. Prevention and treatment of diabetes and its complications. *Med Clin North Am* 1998;82:909–929.

Boulton AJM, Worth RC, Drury RC, et al. Genetic and metabolic studies in diabetic neuropathy. *Diabetologia* 1984;26:15–19.

Brown MJ, Asbury AK. Diabetic neuropathy. *Ann Neurol* 1984;15:2–12.

Brown MJ, Martin JR, Asbury AK. Painful diabetic neuropathy. A morphometric study. *Arch Neurol* 1976;33:164–171.

Calcutt NA, Dunn JS. Pain: nociceptive and neuropathic mechanisms. *Anesthesiology Clinics of North America* 1997;15:429–444.

Dyck P, Lambert E, O'Brian P. Pain related to peripheral neuropathy related to rate and kind of fiber degeneration. *Neurology* 26:466–471.

Ellenberg M. Diabetic Neuropathy. In: Ellenberg M, Rifkin H Eds. *Diabetes Mellitus: Theory and Practice.* New York: Medical Examination Publication House Co. Inc., 1983;38:777.

Garland H, Taverner D. Diabetic myelopathy. *Br Med J* 1953;1:1406–1408.

Green DA, Brown M, Braunstein SN, et al. Comparison of clinical course and sequential electrophysiological tests in diabetics with symptomatic polyneuropathy and its implications for clinical trial. *Diabetes* 1981;30:139–147.

Green DA, Lattimer SA, Sima AAF. Sorbitol, phosphoinositides and sodium-potassium-ATP-ase in the pathogenesis of diabetic complications. *N Engl J Med* 1986;316:599–606.

Harati Y. Chronic complications of diabetes. *Endocrinol Metab Clin North Am* 1996;25:325–359.

Kaplan WE, Abourizk NN. Diabetic peripheral neuropathies affecting the lower extremity. *J Am Pod Ass* 1981;7:356–363.

Kvinesdol B, Molin J, Froland A, et al. Imipramine treatment of painful diabetic neuropathy. *JAMA* 1984;251:1727–1730.

Lewin IG, O'Brian IAD, Morgan MH, et al. Clinical and neurophysiological studies with the aldose-reductase inhibitor, sorbinil in symptomatic diabetic neuropathy. *Diabetologia* 1984;26:445–448.

O'Brien SP, Schwedler M, Kerstein MD. Peripheral neuropathies in diabetes. *Surg Clin North Am* 1998;78:393–408.

Pain perception in diabetic neuropathy. *Lancet* 1985;1:83–84.

Porte D, Graf RJ, Halter JB, et al. Diabetic neuropathy and plasma glucose control. *Am J Med* 1981;70:195–200.

Turkinton RW. Depression masquerading as diabetic neuropathy. *JAMA* 1980;243:1147–1150.

Vinik AI. Diabetic neuropathy: pathogenesis and therapy. *Am J Med* 1999;107:17S-26S.

Vinik AI. Diagnosis and management of diabetic neuropathy. *Clin Geriatr Med* 1999;15:293–320.

Ward JD. The diabetic leg. *Diabetologia* 1982;22:141–147.

Watkins PJ. Pain and diabetic neuropathy. *Br Med J* 1984;288:168–169.

Young RJ, Clarke BF. Pain relief in diabetic neuropathy: the effectiveness of imipramine and related drugs. *Diabetic Med* 1985;2:363–366.

Young RJ, Ewing DJ, Clarke BF. A controlled trial of sorbinil, an aldose-reductase inhibitor, in chronic painful diabetic neuropathy. *Diabetes* 1983;32:938–942.

CHAPTER 36

Acute Pain Management

Christine Peeters-Asdourian

Since the discovery of opioid receptors in 1978, efforts have been made to improve the delivery of analgesic drugs in a more effective way. Thanks to these advances in basic science on the clinical front, the last two decades have witnessed major strides in postoperative analgesia with the creation of acute-pain services, the increased use of epidural analgesia and the introduction of the concept of patient-controlled analgesia (PCA).

Numerous guidelines have been published about the management of postoperative pain. First the Agency for Health Care Policy and Research (AHCPR) took the lead in educating caregivers as well as the public! The American Pain Society as well as the American Society of Anesthesia then followed suit and now, to be implemented in 2001, the Joint Commission on Accreditation of Healthcare Organizations (JCAHO) has published *Standards for Pain Management in Hospital Settings.*

PAIN AS THE FIFTH VITAL SIGN

The guidelines from JCAHO plan to incorporate pain measurements onto the bedside chart, tracking the patient's temperature, blood pressure, heart rate, and respiratory rate, thus making pain rating the fifth vital sign.

However, a simple numerical assessment of pain on the visual analog scale or verbal rating scale does not differentiate between pain at rest and pain with movement or incident pain, which usually is more challenging to manage.

Also, to effectively adjust the analgesic regiment, one needs to track sedation and other possible adverse effects associated with the administration of analgesics such as nausea/vomiting, respiratory depression, and/or cognitive impairment.

The importance of good postoperative analgesia and its impact on favorable postsurgical outcomes are undeni-

able. Pain in the postoperative period may contribute to adverse outcomes including thromboembolic and pulmonary complications.

POSTOPERATIVE PAIN: THE PROBLEM

A surgical incision cuts through a variety of tissues including nerve endings and activates specific nociceptors (pain receptors) as well as free nerve endings. It is associated with the release of inflammatory mediators such as bradykinin, serotonin, and histamine, which contribute to *peripheral sensitization.* Clinically, this phenomenon is manifested by *hyperalgesia,* which is an amplification of noxious pain signals. These painful signals are transmitted to the dorsal horn of the spinal cord in an amplified fashion and are increased in duration.

The nociceptor information is transmitted to the cord by way of the A-δ (myelinated) fibers and the C (unmyelinated) fibers. When peripheral sensitization occurs, painful information also can be carried by A-α and A-β fibers. This is manifested by *allodynia,* a pain state where non-noxious stimuli are transformed and expressed as painful. Signals entering the central nervous system from the periphery will be increased in amplitude and duration. This is the phenomenon of "wind up" or central sensitization.

Analgesic techniques, to be effective, will need to counteract these activations of nociceptors at the periphery as well as centrally, thus the need for a multimodal or "balanced" analgesia to insure patient comfort, to improve early mobilization and decrease the consequences of the postsurgical stress.

Traditional methods of intermittent on request, intramuscular or subcutaneous administrations of opioids have failed to provide satisfactory analgesia. Failure to adequately relieve postoperative pain contributes not only to postdiscomfort, but also to postoperative morbidity, poor patient outcome and prolonged hospital stay.

Options for pain management in the postoperative period include the following:

1. Systemic analgesics
2. Neuraxial opioids and local anesthetics
3. Regional anesthetic techniques
4. Adjunct treatments like transcutaneous electrical-nerve stimulation (TENS) unit, heat application, self-hypnosis, etc.

SYSTEMIC ANALGESICS

Opioids

Opioids remain the mainstay of postoperative analgesia and have demonstrated their efficacy in the management of severe pain. The main concerns about the use of opioids remain their side effects: nausea, vomiting, ileus, biliary spasms, respiratory depression, and the potential for abuse, although in the immediate postoperative period this is rarely an issue. Opioids can be administered intramuscularly, subcutaneously, or intravenously.

The administration of opioids by intramuscular injections prescribed on an as-needed basis provide fluctuating opioid levels resulting in sedation and other adverse effects when levels are high, and inadequate analgesia when levels are low. A better method of administration of opioids is by way of a microprocessor-controlled infusion pump or PCA.

A preset dose of opioids is delivered to the patient when activating the demand switch, given that a predetermined time has elapsed since the previous dose, this is the "lock-out" time. An upper limit per hour or per 4 hours is predetermined and set in the program as an additional safety device. Numerous studies have demonstrated the safety and opioid-sparing effect of the PCA (Table 36.1).

Patients taking opioids preoperatively will show some tolerance intraoperatively and postoperatively. One can safely assume that patients taking two tablets of combination analgesics such as Percocet (Endo Laboratories, Chadds Ford, PA, U.S.A.) (5-mg oxycodone/tablet) or Vicodin (Knoll Laboratories, Mount Olive, NJ, U.S.A.) (5- or 7-mg hydrocodone) q.i.d. will require 1-mg morphine/hour postoperative to replace their regular opioids.

Nonopioid Analgesics

With opioids alone, intramuscular or intravenous (i.v.), the analgesia may be marginal and side effects intolerable (nausea, vomiting, sedation), thus the need for synergy, choosing drug classes that will overlap for analgesia but not for side effects. Drug classes that fit these requirements are as follows: cyclooxygenase inhibitors, α_2-agonists, nitric-oxide synthetase inhibitors, N-methyl-D-aspartate (NMDA)-receptor blockers, and local anesthetics when delivered by thoracic-epidural catheters. This balanced analgesia or delivery of different classes of analgesics will result in effective pain relief by synergistic or additive effect with reduced incidence of side effects.

Nonsteroidal Antiinflammatory Drugs

Nonsteroidal antiinflammatory drugs (NSAIDs) produce their effect inhibiting the prostaglandin synthesis and release at the level of cyclooxygenase. These drugs have proven efficacy as the sole analgesic agent for management of mild-to-moderate pain in minor surgical procedures.

Ketorolac, the only parenteral NSAID presently available, is a nonspecific inhibitor of both cyclooxygenase isoenzymes (Cox-1 and Cox-2). The Cox-1 isoenzyme is normally found in blood vessels, platelets, the gastrointestinal tract and the kidney. On the other hand the Cox-2 isoenzyme is induced by inflammation in peripheral tissues. The inhibition of the Cox-1 isoenzyme is responsible for the gastric and renal side effects of NSAIDs and for its inhibitory effect on platelet function.

One should be cautious when using NSAIDs in the immediate postoperative period and take into consideration risk factors such as a history of bleeding peptic

TABLE 36.1. *Patient-Controlled-Analgesia–Suggested Dosing*

	PCA dose	Lock-out time	1-h limit	Basal rate[b]
Morphine 1 mg/mL	0.5–3 mg	5–10 min	10–20 min	0.5–2 mg/h
Hydromorphone 0.2 mg/mL	0.1–0.5 mg	5–10 min	1–2 mg	0.1–0.2 mg/h
Fentanyl	25–50 µg	5–10 min	250 µg	25–50 µg/h
Meperidine 10 mg/mL	10–20 mg	5–10 min	100 mg[a]	100–200 mg/h

[a]Toxic metabolite normeperidine may accumulate rapidly, if patient is getting more than 1,000 mg/day.
[b]Basal rates should not be used routinely and can be reserved for nighttime, when indicated.

ulcers, volume depletion (for NSAID-induced acute renal failure) especially in elderly patients or when the risk of hemorrhage is considerable and the surgical site involves the airway. The usual dose of ketorolac is 15 mg i.v. q6 hours for 24 to 48 hours. Cox-2 inhibitors appear to be safer but parenteral forms of these molecules are not yet available.

Analgesic Adjuvants

Other classes of drugs may enhance the effects of opioids or may have independent analgesic effects. Most of these drugs are not available in parenteral forms and usually are reserved for patients not responding to more routine therapies. The addition of an α-2 agonist may be beneficial and opioid sparing. Clonidine, dexmedetomidine, and tizanidine are representative of that class but only clonidine is Food and Drug Administration approved and may contribute to hypotension in the perioperative period.

Antihyperalgesic drugs, which block the effect of the transmitter release, include nitric oxide synthetase inhibitors and NMDA-receptor blockers. There is no available pure nitric-oxide synthetase inhibitor. However, there is some evidence that acetaminophen exerts its action by inhibition of nitric-oxide production. For this reason, acetaminophen administered around the clock in the immediate postoperative period may be very useful. Proparacetamol, the precursor of acetaminophen, is being clinically investigated in a parenteral form. Otherwise, acetaminophen is available orally (pill form and elixir) and rectally. The only concern may be that acetaminophen, because of its antipyretic properties, will mask febrile states in the immediate postoperative period.

Dextromethorphan is the most readily available NMDA blocker, though often in combination with other drugs such as cough suppressants. The clinically useful dose appears to be 30 to 60 mg every 4 to 6 hours. Ketamine in low doses (up to 10 mg/hour i.v.) also may be a useful NMDA blocker for postoperative pain.

NEURAXIAL OPIOIDS AND LOCAL ANESTHETICS

Neuraxial opioids and local anesthetics can be provided by way of epidural or intrathecal route. Of these, epidural catheter infusion is the most commonly used method and recently, a cumulative meta-analysis of various postoperative therapies shows that epidural opioids and epidural local anesthetics with or without opioids decreased the incidence of pulmonary complications as opposed to systemic opioids. Epidural analgesia also is associated with a lower incidence of cardiovascular events and provides a decreased stress response to surgery, earlier ambulation, rapid return of bowel function, shortened hospitalization, reduced costs, and overall, a lower mortality.

Large surveys show that the most effective placement of the epidural catheter for infusion of local anesthetic (bupivacaine or ropivacaine in dilute concentration) with a lipophilic opioid such as fentanyl, is the upper thoracic region (T3) for thoracic surgery, the mid-thoracic region (T6) for upper-abdominal surgery, and the lower-thoracic region (T9) for lower-abdominal surgery (Table 36.2).

The amount of opioids needed by neuraxial route to provide effective analgesia is less than by systemic route, especially when combined with local anesthetics. This is definitely the case with morphine and to a lesser degree with fentanyl and hydromorphone, but systemic side effects of opioids may be less frequent.

When using a combination of local anesthetic and opioids, an infusion technique is required. The advantages of the combination are a synergistic effect with lower opioid doses and overall fewer side effects. However, with an infusion technique there is a risk of local anesthetic toxicity, a risk for catheter migration, potential sympathetic block, and orthostatic hypotension (Table 36.3).

A large recent study shows an incidence of respiratory depression of 0.07%, nausea and vomiting 22%, and pruritus 22%. Another equally large study showed an overall rate of complications of 3% associated with the placement of thoracic-epidural catheters. The complications

TABLE 36.2. *Epidural Catheter Insertion Site*

Cord segment	Target for	Central bony location	Landmark
Upper thoracic cord	Thorocotomy	T_3	Root of scapular spine
Lower thoracic cord	Upper abdominal surgery	T_6	Scapular tip
Lumbosacral cord	Lower abdominal surgery	T_{11-12}	12th tip
	Lower extremity surgery above the knee	L_1-L_2	12th tip
	Perineal surgery	L_{3-4}	Tuffier's line $L_{(4-5)}$
	Lower extremity surgery below the knee	L_{3-4} L_{4-5}	Tuffier's line $L_{(4-5)}$

TABLE 36.3. *Epidural Local Anesthetic and/or Opioid*

Local anesthetic		Opioid
Bupivacaine	0.0625% to 0.125%	Morphine 25–50 mg/mL
Ropivacaine	0.05% to 0.2%	Hydromorphone 3–13 mg/mL
		Fentanyl 1–10 μg/mL
Usual rate, 4–16 mL/h		

included dural perforation (0.7%), unsuccessful catheter placement (1.1%), postoperative radicular type of pain (0.2%) responsive to catheter withdrawal in all cases, and peripheral-nerve lesions (0.6%), 0.3% of which were peroneal nerve palsies probably related to surgical positioning and other transient-peripheral nerve lesion (0.2%).

Coagulopathy and systemic infection associated with bacteremia are definite contraindications to neuraxial techniques.

Anticoagulation is a relative contraindication. The American Society of Regional Anesthesia recently published a concern statement on neuraxial anesthesia and anticoagulation. For postoperative analgesia, the timing of the epidural catheter removal is important as most case reports of epidural hematomas have been documented upon removal of the epidural catheter.

Patients receiving low-dose *warfarin* therapy during epidural analgesia should have their prothrombin time and international normalized ratio (INR) monitored on a daily basis, and checked before catheter removal, if the initial dose of was more than 36 hours before. Initial studies evaluating the safety of epidural analgesia in association with oral anticoagulation utilized low-dose warfarin may require more intensive monitoring of the coagulation status.

Neurologic testing of sensory and motor function should be performed routinely on patients on anticoagulation with epidural analgesia and continue for at least 24 hours after. An INR greater than three should prompt the physician to withhold or reduce warfarin dose in patients with indwelling neuraxial catheters.

The use of *antiplatelet drugs* alone does not create a level of risk that will interfere with the performance of neuraxial blockade. When used in combination with other anticoagulant regimens, there may be an increased chance of hematoma formation.

It is recommended that indwelling catheters be removed prior to initiation of low-molecular-weight heparin thromboprophylaxis. If a continuous technique is selected, the epidural catheter may be left indwelling overnight and removed the following day with the first dose of low-molecular-weight heparin administered 2 hours after the catheter removal.

For any low-molecular-weight heparin prophylaxis regimen, catheter removal should be delayed for at least 10 to 12 hours after a dose of low-molecular-weight heparin.

A single, intrathecal opioid injection can be used either alone or in combination with epidural infusion and other methods for pain control. However, the pain relief achieved with this method usually is not longer than 12 to 18 hours and the need for monitoring for possible respiratory depression is the same as for epidural opioid administration.

With the use of neuraxial opioids, it is paramount to adequately educate the nursing and support staff to the monitoring and possible side effects of the techniques. Policies and protocols need to be in place to insure patients' safety and it has been demonstrated that an organized acute-pain service provided superior postoperative analgesia care compared to standard delivery of analgesics.

For both PCA and epidural analgesia, standard orders for monitoring and for medications such as antiemetics (droperidol, etc.) antipruritus agents (diphenhydramine, etc.) as well as orders for small titrations greatly facilitate the delivery of postoperative care (Figs. 36.1 and 36.2).

Nonpharmacologic methods of pain management and stimulation-induced analgesia can be used in the postoperative period with either acupuncture or transcutaneous electrical-nerve stimulation (TENS). With TENS, a small electrical current presumably stimulates the touch pressure and proprioception fiber (A–B) to release endogenous opiates and close the "gate" of pain transmission at the spinal level. The TENS technique is considered safe but does not reliably provide analgesia in all cases. It is best used for amputations, back surgery, and postcaesarian sections. Sterile electrodes are available to be placed close to surgical sites. TENS is contraindicated in patients with demand pacemakers and may interfere with electrocardiogram monitoring.

Behavioral techniques such as relaxation therapy and hypnosis also have been used successfully in the treatment of preoperative pain but these techniques require preoperative preparation and motivation on the part of the patient to be effective in the immediate postoperative period.

ALLERGIES — NONE KNOWN ☐ IF YES, LIST		

DATE HOUR	ORDER	POSTED	ORDER DATE	TIME	START DATE	
	Patient - Controlled Analgesia (PCA)	BY _____	**LOADING DOSE**			
	Acute Pain Service Order Form		**Rx**			
		TIME:	_____ _____ mg.			
	1. NO OTHER NARCOTICS MAY BE GIVEN		q_____min. PRN for Pain Score≥ 5, and sedation			
	EXCEPT BY ORDER OF THE APS PHYSICIAN.	_____	score ≤ 1, for maximum dose of _____ mg. If pain score remains ≥ 5, despite max. dose, call Acute Pain Service. When pain score is ≤ 5 and sedation score ≤ 1 start PCA and instruct patient in usage.			
	2. Monitoring:		SIGNATURE		MD	PAGE I.D.#
	a. Respiratory rate, pain score (at rest and	POSTED	ORDER DATE	TIME	START DATE	
	with movement) and sedation level		**MORPHINE** (CIRCLE DOSE)			
	q̄ 2h x 8h, then q̄ 4h while the patient	BY _____	PCA dose 0.5mg 1mg 1.5mg 2mg _____mg			
	is on PCA therapy. Please document		Lockout Interval _____ minutes			
	responses in the progress notes.	TIME:	Basal Rate _____ mg(s)/hour			
			1-Hour Maximum Limit _____ mg(s)			
	b. Verbal Analogue Scale (VAS) - Pain Score	_____	SPECIAL ORDERS			
	(0-10) 0 = No Pain 10 = Worst Pain Possible	SIGNATURE			MD	PAGE I.D.#
	c. Sedation Scale:	POSTED	ORDER DATE	TIME	START DATE	
	0 = NONE		**DILAUDID (HYDROMORPHONE)** (CIRCLE DOSE)			
	S = SLEEP (normal sleep, easy to arouse)	BY _____	PCA dose 0.05mg 0.125mg 0.25mg 0.375mg _____mg			
	1 = MILD (occ. sleepy, easy to arouse)		Lockout Interval _____ minutes			
	2 = MODERATE (freq. drowsy, easy to arouse)	TIME:	Basal Rate _____ mg(s)/hour			
	3 = SEVERE (somnolent, difficult to arouse)		1-Hour Maximum Limit _____ mg(s)			
		_____	SPECIAL ORDERS			
	4 = UNRESPONSIVE	SIGNATURE			MD	PAGE I.D.#
	3. Call Acute Pain Service:	POSTED	ORDER DATE	TIME	START DATE	
	a. Sedation level = 3, **OR** RR less than 10/min.		**SUBLIMAZE (FENTANYL)** (CIRCLE DOSE)			
	b. Inadequate analgesia or other	BY _____	PCA dose 12.5mcg 25mcg 37.5mcg 50mcg _____mcg			
	problems related to PCA.		Lockout Interval _____ minutes			
	c. Page Anesthesia **STAT** for sedation	TIME:	Basal Rate _____ mcg(s)/hour			
	level = 3 **AND** RR less than 10/min.		1-Hour Maximum Limit _____ mcg(s)			
		_____	SPECIAL ORDERS			
	d. Page Anesthesia **STAT** if patient is	SIGNATURE			MD	PAGE I.D.#
	UNRESPONSIVE.	POSTED	ORDER DATE	TIME	START DATE	
	4. Thank you.		**DRUG:**			
		BY _____	PCA dose _____ mg(s)			
			Lockout Interval _____ minutes			
		TIME:	Basal Rate _____ mg(s)/hour			
			1-Hour Maximum Limit _____ mg(s)			
		_____	SPECIAL ORDERS			
SIGNATURE MD		SIGNATURE			MD	PAGE I.D.#

FIG. 36.1. Patient-Controlled Analgesia (PCA) Acute Pain Service Order Form. Anesthesia & Nursing Services, Beth Israel Deaconess Medical Center, Boston, MA.

ALLERGIES — NONE KNOWN ☐   IF YES, LIST

DATE
HOUR

1. **NO OTHER NARCOTICS OR SEDATIVES** may be given to patient unless ordered by Acute Pain Service.

2. **Monitoring:**

   A. Keep head of bed ≥30° at all times.

   B. Blood pressure and pulse rate $\overline{15}$ min x 2, then $\overline{30}$ min x 3, then $\overline{4}$ hours for remainder of therapy, **AND** after any dose increase.

   C. Respiratory rate and sedation level *$\overline{30}$ min x 4, then $\overline{2}$ hours for the remainder of therapy, **AND** after any dose increase.

   D. Sensory level and motor function $\overline{2h}$ while awake.

   E. Pain score ** (at rest and with movement) $\overline{2h}$ while awake.

   F. Postural BP/pulse prior to first ambulation.

   G. *Sedation Scale:
   0 = NONE
   S = SLEEP (normal, easy to arouse)
   1 = MILD (occassionally sleepy, easy to arouse)
   2 = MODERATE (frequently drowsy, easy to arouse)
   3 = SEVERE (somnolent, difficult to arouse)
   4 = UNRESPONSIVE

   H. **Verbal Analogue: Scale
   Pain Score (0-10), 0 = No Pain,
   10 = Worst Pain Possible.

3. **Activity**
   Patient must be accompanied at all times during ambulation.

4. **Fluids**
   Patient must have patent IV while epidural catheter is in place. Fluids as ordered by team; or Lactated Ringers solution to keep vein open.

5. **Notify Acute Pain Service for the following:**
   A. SBP < _____ mmHg and/or P < _____ / min.
   B. Postural BP drop = 15 mm Hg and/or HR _____
   C. RR = 9/min.
   D. Sedation level = 3,
   E. Pain score of zero (0/10) at rest **AND** with movement.
   F. Inadequate analgesia or other problems related to the epidural

6. **Page Anesthesia STAT for:**
   A. Sedation level = 3 **AND** RR < 9/min.
   B. If patient is unresponsive.
   C. Numbness above nipples and/or inability to bend knees.
   D. If patient has syncope, circumoral numbness, or tinnitus,

   Stop the infusion and page Anesthesia **STAT**.

7. Infusion started at _____ hours.

8. **Thank you.**

DOSE GIVEN AT

_____ AM, _____ PM

TIME FAXED _____

POSTED BY _____

ORDER CHECKED BY

_____ RN

ORDER DATE	TIME	START DATE	H O U R S	A M
D/C DATE/TIME OR NUMBER OF DOSES				P M

℞

Fentanyl   4mcg/ml
Bupivacaine PF   1mg/ml (0.1%)
Infuse via lumbar/thoracic catheter at
_____ ml/hr

SIGNATURE   PAGE I.D.#
                                    M.D.

ORDER DATE	TIME	START DATE	H O U R S	A M
D/C DATE/TIME OR NUMBER OF DOSES				P M

℞

Fentanyl   4mcg/ml
Bupivacaine PF   0.5mg/ml (0.05%)
Infuse via lumbar/thoracic catheter at
_____ ml/hr

SIGNATURE   PAGE I.D.#
                                    M.D.

ORDER DATE	TIME	START DATE	H O U R S	A M
D/C DATE/TIME OR NUMBER OF DOSES				P M

℞

Fentanyl   2mcg/ml
Bupivacaine PF   1mg/ml (0.1%)
Infuse via lumbar/thoracic catheter at
_____ ml/hr

SIGNATURE   PAGE I.D.#
                                    M.D.

ORDER DATE	TIME	START DATE	H O U R S	A M
D/C DATE/TIME OR NUMBER OF DOSES				P M

℞

Bupivacaine PF   1mg/ml (0.1%)
Infuse via lumbar/thoracic catheter at
_____ ml/hr

SIGNATURE   PAGE I.D.#
                                    M.D.

ORDER DATE	TIME	START DATE	H O U R S	A M
D/C DATE/TIME OR NUMBER OF DOSES				P M

℞

Hydromorphone   0.02mg/ml
Bupivacaine PF   1mg/ml (0.1%)
Infuse via lumbar/thoracic catheter at
_____ ml/hr

SIGNATURE   PAGE I.D.#
                                    M.D.

MC 0540-1

FIG. 36.2. Epidural Analgesia Standard Order Form. Acute Pain Service. Anesthesia & Nursing Services, Beth Israel Deaconess Medical Center, Boston, MA.

ALLERGIES — NONE KNOWN ☐   IF YES, LIST

DATE	
HOUR	

1. **NO OTHER NARCOTICS OR SEDATIVES** may be given to patient unless ordered by Acute Pain Service.

2. **Monitoring:**

   A. Keep head of bed ≥30˚ at all times.

   B. Blood pressure and pulse rate $\overline{15}$ min x 2, then $\overline{30}$ min x 3, then $\overline{4}$ hours for remainder of therapy, **AND** after any dose increase.

   C. Respiratory rate and sedation level *$\overline{30}$ min x 4, then $\overline{2}$ hours for the remainder of therapy, **AND** after any dose increase.

   D. Sensory level and motor function $\overline{2}$h while awake.

   E. Pain score ** (at rest and with movement) $\overline{2}$h while awake.

   F. Postural BP/pulse prior to first ambulation.

   G. *Sedation Scale:
      0 = NONE
      S = SLEEP (normal, easy to arouse)
      1 = MILD (occassionally sleepy, easy to arouse)
      2 = MODERATE (frequently drowsy, easy to arouse)
      3 = SEVERE (somnolent, difficult to arouse)
      4 = UNRESPONSIVE

   H. **Verbal Analogue: Scale
      Pain Score (0-10), 0 = No Pain,
      10 = Worst Pain Possible.

3. **Activity**
   Patient must be accompanied at all times during ambulation.

4. **Fluids**
   Patient must have patent IV while epidural catheter is in place. Fluids as ordered by team; or Lactated Ringers solution to keep vein open.

5. **Notify Acute Pain Service for the following:**
   A. SBP < _____ mmHg and/or P < _____ / min.
   B. Postural BP drop = 15 mm Hg and/or HR _____
   C. RR = 9/min.
   D. Sedation level = 3,
   E. Pain score of zero (0/10) at rest **AND** with movement.
   F. Inadequate analgesia or other problems related to the epidural

6. **Page Anesthesia STAT for:**
   A. Sedation level = 3 **AND** RR < 9/min.
   B. If patient is unresponsive.
   C. Numbness above nipples and/or inability to bend knees.
   D. If patient has syncope, circumoral numbness, or tinnitus,

      Stop the infusion and page Anesthesia **STAT.**

7. Infusion started at _____ hours.

8. **Thank you.**

DOSE GIVEN AT

_____ AM, _____ PM

TIME FAXED _____

POSTED BY _____

ORDER CHECKED BY

_____ RN

ORDER DATE	TIME	START DATE	H O U R S	A M
D/C DATE/TIME OR NUMBER OF DOSES				P M

℞

Special Epidural Solution

Infuse via lumbar/thoracic catheter at _____ ml/hr

SIGNATURE		PAGE I.D.#
	M.D.	

DOSE GIVEN AT

_____ AM, _____ PM

TIME FAXED _____

POSTED BY _____

ORDER CHECKED BY

_____ RN

ORDER DATE	TIME	START DATE	H O U R S	A M
D/C DATE/TIME OR NUMBER OF DOSES				P M

℞

Diphenhydramine

12.5-25mg IV/PO every 6 hours
PRN Itching

SIGNATURE		PAGE I.D.#
	M.D.	

DOSE GIVEN AT

_____ AM, _____ PM

TIME FAXED _____

POSTED BY _____

ORDER CHECKED BY

_____ RN

ORDER DATE	TIME	START DATE	H O U R S	A M
D/C DATE/TIME OR NUMBER OF DOSES				P M

℞

Droperidol

0.625mg IV every 6 hours
PRN Nausea

SIGNATURE		PAGE I.D.#
	M.D.	

DOSE GIVEN AT

_____ AM, _____ PM

TIME FAXED _____

POSTED BY _____

ORDER CHECKED BY

_____ RN

ORDER DATE	TIME	START DATE	H O U R S	A M
D/C DATE/TIME OR NUMBER OF DOSES				P M

℞

SIGNATURE		PAGE I.D.#
	M.D.	

DOSE GIVEN AT

_____ AM, _____ PM

TIME FAXED _____

POSTED BY _____

ORDER CHECKED BY

_____ RN

ORDER DATE	TIME	START DATE	H O U R S	A M
D/C DATE/TIME OR NUMBER OF DOSES				P M

℞

SIGNATURE		PAGE I.D.#
	M.D.	

MC 0540-2

FIG. 36.2. *Continued.*

SELECTED READINGS

Acute Pain Management Guidelines Panel. *Acute Pain Management: Operative or Medical Procedures and Trauma. Clinical Practice Guideline.* AHCPR Pub. No. 92-0032, Rockville, MD: Agency for Health Care Policy and Research, Public Health Service, U.S. Dept. of Health and Human Services, Public Health Service, 1992.

Basbaum AI. Spinal mechanisms of acute and persistent pain. *Reg Anesth Pain Med* 1999;24:59–67.

Ballantyne JC, Carr DB, deFerranti S, et al. The comparative effects of postoperative analgesic therapies on pulmonary outcome: cumulative meta-analysis of randomized, controlled trials. *Anesth Analg* 1998;86:598–612.

Bylon JF, Katz J, Kavanagh BP, et al. Epidural bupivacaine-morphine analgesia versus patient-controlled analgesia following abdominal aortic surgery. *Anesthesiology* 1998;89:585–593.

Grace RF, Power I, Umedaly H, et al. Preoperative dextromethorphan reduces intraoperative but not postoperative morphine requirements after laparotomy. *Anesth Analg* 1998;87:1135–1138.

Katz J, Kavanagh BP, Sandler AN, et al. Preemptive analgesia: clinical evidence of neuroplasticity contributing to postoperative pain. *Anesthesiology* 1992; 77:439–446.

Kohrs R, Durieux ME. Ketamine: teaching an old drug new tricks. *Anesth Analg* 1998;87:1186–1193.

Liu S, Carpenter RL, Neal JM. Epidural anesthesia and analgesia. *Anesthesiology* 1995;76:342–53.

ASA Task Force on Pain Management. Practice guidelines for acute pain management in the perioperative setting. *Anesthesiology* 1995;82:1071–1081.

Steinbrook RA. Epidural analgesia and gastrointestinal motility. *Anesth Analg* 1998;86:837–844.

Woolf CJ. Wind-up and central sensitization are not equivalent. *Pain* 1996; 66:105–108.

Yeager MP, Glass DD, Neff RK, et al. The safety and efficacy of intrathecal opioid analgesia for acute postoperative pain: seven years experience with 5969 surgical patients at Indiana University Hospital. *Anesth Analg* 1999;88:599–604.

CHAPTER 37

Labor Pain

Kimberly A. Cox and Mukesh C. Sarna

Labor is defined as the progressive dilation of the uterine cervix in association with repetitive uterine contractions. Childbirth is defined as the act of bringing forth offspring. When two very dynamic processes are embodied into one uniquely female experience, it is not hard to imagine the complexity of such a process. Besides the neurophysiological aspect of labor, there are psychological, cultural, and societal issues associated with childbirth and its associated pain and, in particular, *relief* of labor pain. Distention of the cervix and contraction of the uterus is painful. It has been well documented that uterine contraction pain can evoke a generalized neuroendocrinal stress response. This chapter will describe the pain pathways involved in labor pain and currently available methods of alleviating pain associated with labor. Particular focus will be made on recent advances in neuraxial blockade. In addition, labor analgesia during the *fourth* stage of labor will be addressed.

LABOR PAIN PATHWAYS

The exact neurophysiologic mechanism of labor pain is unknown. It appears that the pain associated with labor arises primarily from nociceptors in uterine, cervical, and perineal structures. The pain associated with uterine contractions may be partially because of myometrial and cervical ischemia. There is some evidence that compression of the lumbosacral trunk may be the source of "back labor" for some patients. The pain of labor includes both a visceral and a somatic component. The visceral component primarily involves the cervix and the lower-uterine segment but also may involve the body of the uterus and the adenexa.

During the first stage of labor (the interval between the onset of labor and full cervical dilation), bare-nerve terminals of A-δ and C fibers in visceral afferents to the uterus and cervix transmit pain sensation by way of the uterine and cervical plexus to the inferior, middle, and superior hypogastric plexus. These fibers, along with sympathetic fibers, enter the neuraxis at the tenth, 11th, and 12th thoracic and first lumbar-spinal segments (Fig. 37.1). They synapse and make connections with ascending and descending fibers in the dorsal horn particularly in Rexed lamina V (Fig. 37.2).

Bilateral lumbar-sympathetic block will interrupt pain impulses from the uterus, cervix, and upper vagina and will provide analgesia during the first stage of labor. During the second stage of labor (interval between full cervical dilation and delivery of the infant), pain is caused by distension and tearing of the perineum, which causes stimulation of A-δ and C fibers of somatic afferents to the vagina and perineum. These fibers travel through the pudendal nerves and enter the neuraxis at the second, third, and fourth sacral segments. Bilateral pudendal nerve blocks will relieve perineal pain during the second stage of labor. The third stage of labor encompasses the period between the delivery of the infant and delivery of the placenta. This stage may have similar pain pathways to that of the first stage of labor. The fourth stage of labor, a term that we have chosen to coin and define as the recovery period, begins following delivery of the placenta. During this stage, there may be significant perineal pain as the result of vaginal lacerations, episiotomy, lack of pelvic-floor muscular tone, and uterine "shrinkage." The pain associated with the fourth stage of labor often is underappreciated and undertreated. A few studies have shown that a single dose of epidural morphine may lessen pain during this stage of labor.

Peripheral afferents coming from the uterus, cervix, and perineum enter the spinal cord, where they synapse extensively and ascend via the spinothalamic tract to the brain stem and cortex (Fig. 37.3). Within the central nervous system, this information undergoes considerable modulation. The impulses can be inhibited, enhanced, and/or referred.

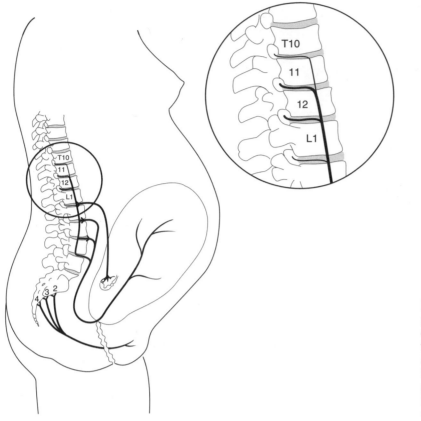

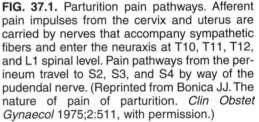

FIG. 37.1. Parturition pain pathways. Afferent pain impulses from the cervix and uterus are carried by nerves that accompany sympathetic fibers and enter the neuraxis at T10, T11, T12, and L1 spinal level. Pain pathways from the perineum travel to S2, S3, and S4 by way of the pudendal nerve. (Reprinted from Bonica JJ. The nature of pain of parturition. *Clin Obstet Gynaecol* 1975;2:511, with permission.)

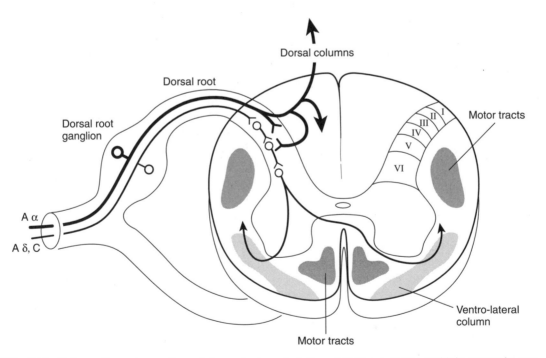

FIG. 37.2. Schematic cross-section of the spinal cord. A-δ and C fibers make multiple synaptic connections in the dorsal horn. Cell bodies in lamina V send axons to the ipsilateral and contralateral ventral column to make up the spinothalamic system. (Reprinted from Bonica JJ. The nature of pain of parturition. *Clin Obstet Gynaecol* 1975;2:511, with permission.)

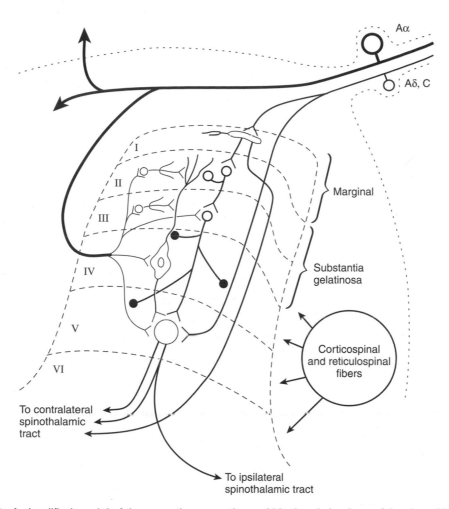

FIG. 37.3. A simplified model of the synaptic connections within the six laminae of the dorsal horn. Pain impulses during parturition are transmitted via A-δ and C fibers to the dorsal horn, where multiple synaptic connections are made. Descending corticospinal and reticulospinal fibers carry impulses that may modulate pain information at the dorsal horn, a possible neurophysiologic mechanism for cortical modification of afferent pain stimuli. (Reprinted from Bonica JJ. The nature of pain of parturition. *Clin Obstet Gynaecol* 1975;2:511, with permission.)

WHY IS PAIN IN LABOR POTENTIALLY "BAD"?

It has been shown that labor can evoke a neuroendocrine reaction. There have been reported prolonged increases in plasma cortisol levels in early labor, increases of both adrenocorticotropin hormone (ACTH) and cortisol during labor and immediately postpartum. There also have been reports of increases of epinephrine, norepinephrine, and β-endorphins throughout labor. Animal studies indicate that both epinephrine and norepinephrine can decrease uterine blood flow and cause fetal asphyxia. Maternal psychological stress can detrimentally affect the fetal cardiovascular system and acid-base status as demonstrated in baboons and monkeys. Anxiety, pain, and labor are forms of stress, which may be harmful to the fetus and counterproductive to the birthing process.

Anesthesia, by alleviating pain, can minimize the effects of stress. Epidural anesthesia prevents increases in both cortisol and 11-hydroxycorticosteroid levels during labor. Epidural anesthesia also attenuates elevations of epinephrine, norepinephrine, and endorphin levels. Presumably, regional anesthesia blocks afferent stimuli to the hypothalamus and thus inhibits the body's response to stress. Some of the responses to the stress of labor and the effects of epidural anesthesia on these responses are presented in Figure 37.4.

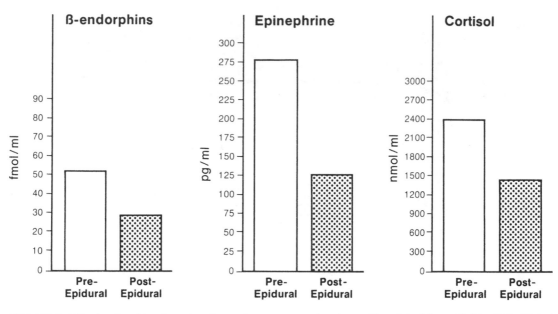

FIG. 37.4. Effects of epidural analgesia on the response to stress (Reprinted from Gabbe SG, Niebyl JR, Simpson JL, eds. *Obstetrics: Normal & Problem Pregnancies*, 3rd ed. New York: Churchill Livingstone, 1996, with permission.).

METHODS OF PAIN RELIEF DURING LABOR

Pain relief in childbirth involves interrupting the pain pathways anywhere from the point of initiation of the painful stimulus to the central perception of pain. Pain relief can be accomplished by (a) blockade of peripheral-pain receptors; (b) peripheral-nerve block; (c) spinal-cord blockade; (d) stimulating endogenous opiate receptors in the central nervous system; (e) altering central responsiveness to pain (i.e., with systemic narcotics); (f) enhancing inhibitory pathways (i.e., through the use of Lamaze technique; (g) other techniques whose mechanisms are not fully known (Tables 37.1 and 37.2).

Central Neuronal Blockade

One of the most common ways to provide pain relief during labor is with systemic narcotics. However, complete analgesia for labor and vaginal birth cannot be achieved in most parturients without also producing severe hypoventilation, obtundation of reflexes, and postural hypotension. In contrast, epidurally administered narcotics in appropriate doses causes less severe side effects and provides better analgesia than systemically administered narcotics. One of the goals of an obstetrical anesthesiologist is to provide the parturient with a very tailored and safe anesthetic. In the past decade, obstetrical anesthesiologists have focused on "analgesia" during labor. Obviously, epidural anesthesia and epidural analgesia are by no means interchangeable. Epidural analgesia for labor should preserve the normal labor and delivery process with the added benefit of preventing the deleterious effects of severe pain. Epidural anesthesia may be extended to the laboring patient when a number of circumstances warrant it. For example, for an operative delivery, instrumental delivery, for repair of vaginal lacerations, episiotomy, or for removal of retained placenta.

Epidural Analgesia

An epidurally administered drug by way of a catheter provides excellent pain relief and the ability to extend

TABLE 37.1. *Regional Anesthetic Techniques for Relief of Labor Pain*

		Area of anesthesia
Central neuronal blockage	Epidural (lumbar or caudal), spinal combined spinal–epidural	T10–S5
Peripheral neuronal blockade/plexus block	Bilateral pudendal nerve block	S2–S4
	Lumbar sympathetic block	T10–L1
	Paracervical block	T10–L1
Infiltration	Local anesthetic to perineal skin tissue	Perineum

TABLE 37.2. *Methods of Pain Relief During Labor*

Method	Proposed mechanism
Systemic narcotics	Stimulate opiate receptors and thus alter central responsiveness to pain
Inhalation analgesia	Diminished reception of responsiveness to pain by a change in membrane properties of brain tissue
Lamaze	Decreasing pain by decreasing anxiety, through prenatal education and relaxation techniques
Hypnosis	Enhancement of descending inhibitory pathways. Altered state of consciousness involving profound relaxation
Acupuncture	Endorphin-mediated mechanism
TENS	Activation of A-δ afferent fibers, which inhibit transmission of impulses in the spinothalamic tract
Sterile-water blocks	Intradermal injection of hypotonic sterile water causes a strong sensory stimulation of the surrounding skin. The analgesia produced by this stimulation may originate in the midbrain or may be referred analgesia
Biofeedback	Relaxation therapy by which one learns to discriminate and control muscle tension

TENS, transcutaneous electrical nerve stimulation

the duration of the block to match the duration of labor. The technique of choice usually is percutaneous placement by the loss of resistance to saline or air, performed at the L2–L3 or L3–L4 interspace. Several drugs have been tried epidurally in the obstetrical population. Local anesthetics and opioids are the ones most commonly used. However, clonidine—a drug of recent interest—is being used epidurally in the obstetric patient.

Local anesthetics work by inhibition of sodium-ion influx across the neuronal-cell membrane. They also alter potassium and calcium-ion conductance across excitable membranes to produce blockade of nerve impulses. Local anesthetics have several advantages when used epidurally. They provided effective, controllable analgesia and are safe for the mother when properly administered and appropriately monitored. Local anesthetics administered epidurally in proper doses have not been shown to cause fetal depression. There are several local anesthetics available for epidural use, each of which has its own particular profile of advantages and side effects (Table 37.3).

Epidural administration of local anesthetics has the potential to cause hypotension. As with spinal anesthesia, the hemodynamic changes are believed to result from venous and arterial dilation induced by sympathetic blockade. In fact, one of the major drawbacks of using local anesthetics alone to obtain adequate analgesia is the risk of inducing maternal hypotension. It has been shown that boluses of local anesthetics decreased the time to achieve maximum block but also increased the incidence of hypotension.

Epidurally administered opioids work by binding to receptors in the dorsal horn of the spinal cord. Binding of opioid receptors causes a modulation of nociceptive impulses transmitted by C and A-δ fibers before they are relayed to the ascending spinothalamic tract. Intraspinal opioids do have a ceiling affect beyond which further dosing increases the incidence of undesirable side effects, most likely because of rostral spread of the medication. Some of the side effects associated with increasing doses of opioids are pruritus, sedation, and respiratory depression. The ceiling effect of intraspinal opioids is overcome by using mixtures of opioids with local anesthetics.

TABLE 37.3. *Local Anesthetic Profiles*

Local anesthetic	Advantage	Side effect/disadvantage
Lidocaine	Dependable analgesia with duration of action about 60 min Relative fast onset	Placental transfer is appreciable
Etidocaine	Intense sensory block	Intense motor block that tends to outlast the sensory block
Prilocaine	Rapid breakdown Low acute toxicity	Phenolic breakdown product that causes significant methemoglobinemia in dose above 600 mg
Mepivacaine	Intermediate duration of action	Long half-life in the neonate
Ropivacaine	Less cardiotoxicity when compared to bupivacaine	Less anesthetic potency than bupivacaine
Bupivacaine	Long duration of action High quality of analgesia with minimal motor block	Slow to produce surgical anesthesia Cardiotoxicity
Chloroprocaine	Fastest-acting local anesthetic Short plasma half-life Extremely safe for mother and infant	Backache with doses greater than 23–25 mL Impairs the subsequent action of epidural bupivicaine, fentanyl, and morphine

TABLE 37.4. *MLAC of Bupivacaine and Fentanyl Concentrations Compared with MLAC of Control*

	MLAC	P	Pa
Bupivacaine	0.069 (0.057–0.080)		
Fentanyl 1 μg mL^{-1}	0.057 (0.047–0.066)	0.14 (–0.003–0.027)	0.52 (–0.008–0.032)
Fentanyl 2 μg mL^{-1}	0.048 (0.037–0.059)	0.008 (0.006–0.036)	0.03 (0.0013–0.041)
Fentanyl 3 μg mL^{-1}	0.031 (0.017–0.045)	<0.0001 (0.022–0.054)	<0.0001 (0.018–0.058)
Fentanyl 4 μg mL^{-1}	0.015 (0.004–0.025)	<0.0001 (0.039–0.069)	<0.001 (0.035–0.073)

MLAC, minimum local analgesic concentration using the method of Dixon and Massey; P, P value (95% confidence interval) using modified *t* tests *vs* MLAC of control.

aP, P value (95% confidence interval) with Bonferroni correction.

Reprinted from Lyons G, Columb M, Hawthorne L, et al. Extradural pain relief in labour: bupivacaine sparing by extradural fentanyl is dose dependent. *Br J Anaesth* 1997;78:493–497, with permission.

When local anesthetics and opioids are combined, their analgesic properties are synergistic. Lyons et al. reported significant dose-dependent reductions in the minimal local anesthetic concentration of bupivacaine with various doses of fentanyl (Table 37.4). It appears that a continuous infusion of dilute local anesthetic plus opioid provides better pain relief and less motor block. During that study, it was noted that epidural infusion of 0.125% bupivacaine beyond a cervical dilation of 8 cm prolonged the second stage of labor and increased the frequency of instrumental delivery in nulliparous women. Recent studies, however, have disputed this finding. Because studies suggest that a continuous infusion of 0.0625% bupivacaine with 0.0002% fentanyl produces analgesia similar to that provided by the infusion of 0.125% bupivacaine alone, it would seem appropriate to use the least amount of local anesthetic and narcotic that will give analgesia. In fact, some centers are using infusions of 0.04% bupivacaine with 1.67-mcg/cc fentanyl at rates of 10 to 15 cc/hour with good results.

Clonidine is a highly lipid-soluble α-2 adrenergic agonist that acts by way of a nonopioid mechanism involving α-2 receptors in the dorsal horn of the spinal cord. When used alone, large doses are necessary to obtain pain relief with hypotension and sedation as a consequence. Clonidine has been shown to prolong the sensory block of local anesthetics and has a synergistic affect with extradural opioids. Most of the studies on extradural clonidine during pregnancy were done on sheep models. In pregnant ewes, it was noted that with epidurally administered clonidine there was a minor decrease in heart rate without changes in maternal or fetal blood pressure, intrauterine pressure, or uterine blood flow. Presently, the optimal dose of neuraxial clonidine with or without local anesthetics and opioids has not been established for labor analgesia.

Spinal Analgesia

Spinal analgesia can be administered through a one-shot technique or through a continuous infusion by way of a microcatheter. The obvious disadvantage of a one-shot spinal is the limited duration of action and thus the potential need for repeated injections. One-shot spinals are very useful in urgent situations and planned uncomplicated cesarean sections. The advantages of spinal anesthesia include speed of onset and reliable nature of the block. Small doses of drugs are administered, thus decreasing the possibility of adverse effects on the mother and fetus. Some of the possible complications and side-effects of intrathecal opioids are inadvertent overdose, pruritus, nausea, vomiting, hypotension, urinary retention, maternal-respiratory depression, postural-puncture headache, and subarachnoid migration of an epidural catheter if a "combined technique" is utilized (see next section). Studies also have shown that persistent maternal hypotension could have effects on the fetal heart-rate pattern often manifested by late decelerations.

The Food and Drug Administration (FDA) has withdrawn the use of spinal microcatheters in United States because of the association with cauda equina syndrome. Thus, the use of continuous intrathecal administration of labor analgesic solutions is restricted to unintentional intrathecal placement of standard epidural catheters.

Combined Spinal–Epidural Analgesia

The possibility of combining the advantages of both the epidural and spinal techniques of anesthesia and analgesia first was described by Brownridge in 1981. This method allows the reliability of the spinal block to be combined with the flexibility of the epidural block. The combined spinal–epidural (CSE) provides speed of onset with optimum operative conditions with the added advantage of having an epidural catheter for extending the duration of the block and providing postoperative analgesia. The procedure usually is done with a needle-through-needle technique. It can be safely done in a patient who is a candidate for epidural analgesia for labor by carefully selecting the correct medication and dosage. It is particularly useful in multiparous women with a rapidly progressing labor. The spinal portion of a CSE usually is achieved by intrathecal administration of a short-acting, lipid-soluble opioid such as fentanyl 10 to 25 μg or sufentanil 5 to 10 μg plus a local anesthetic such as bupivacaine 2.5 mg. This will provide quick comfort to the laboring woman. The epidural catheter is threaded and checked by aspiration for blood and cerebrospinal fluid (CSF); however, the response to a "test dose" of epidural medication cannot be determined at the time of intrathecal block. This is one obvious disadvantage of this otherwise very helpful technique.

Patient-Controlled Epidural Analgesia

Patient-controlled epidural analgesia (PCEA) first was recommended in 1988. Since then, numerous trials using PCEA have been reported. The advantages of PCEA are minimum drug dose, flexibility, and benefits of self-administration. As in most patient-controlled devices, it provides the patient with a sense of self-control and the maintenance of self-esteem, which may be vital for a positive experience in childbirth. Although PCEA has not been universally accepted among obstetrical anesthesiologists, there is evidence that PCEA achieves analgesia of equivalent high quality while allowing for a reduction in bupivacaine utilization, and a lesser requirement for supplementation and interventions.

THE FOURTH STAGE OF LABOR

Stage four of labor may be accompanied by significant perineal pain as a result of vaginal laceration, episiotomy, or postoperatively, following a cesarean delivery. In recent years, there has been increasing number of studies showing that postoperative pain can be substantially reduced by administering morphine epidurally. It has been shown that 2 mg of morphine given epidurally after vaginal delivery provides superior pain relief for perineal discomfort in patients with and without episiotomy. There were also minimal side effects and better overall patient satisfaction when compared to oral analgesics. Patients reported lower pain scores that lasted for at least 1 week. Other studies have shown that the incidence of postepisiotomy pain can be substantially lessened if epidural morphine is given before the onset of pain. It was also noted in several studies that as pain intensity increases, it becomes more difficult to control with low doses of epidural morphine. Therefore, epidural morphine, given before the onset of pain, is much more effective and may prevent the spinal cord from becoming hyperexcitable.

CONCLUSION

Although, in the past, pain was not thought of as being potentially bad in the laboring patient, it is clear now that the body's normal response to pain can have deleterious effects on the mother and fetus. Labor is a very dynamic process with various degrees of pain. Pain relief during labor often is desirable. Choosing the best method of pain relief during labor depends on an understanding of pain pathways, mechanisms of action of the techniques of pain relief, and the physiological consequences of each method.

SELECTED READINGS

Abboud TK, Sarkis F, Blikian A, et al. Effects of epidural anesthesia during labor on maternal plasma beta-endorphin levels. *Anesthesiology* 1983; 59:1–5.
Adamson K, et al. Production of fetal asphyxia in the Rhesus monkey by administration of catecholamines to the mother. *Am J Obstet Gynecol* 1971;109:248.
Ascanio RS, Mahaney G, et al. A Single dose of epidural morphine alleviates postpartum perineal pain for at least one week: 153.
Behar M, Majora F, Olshwang D, et al. Epidural morphine in treatment of pain. *Lancet* 1979;1:527–529.
Berges PU. Regional Anesthesia for Obstetrics. *Clin Anesth* 1969;2: 141–166.
Birnbach D. *Combined Spinal Epidural (CSE) and Other New Techniques for Labor Analgesia.* New York, NY: 242 SOAP 19
Brownridge P. Epidural and subarachnoid analgesia for elective caesarean section (Letter). *Anaesthesia* 1981;36:70.
Buchan PC, Milne MK, Browning MC. The effects of continuous epidural blockade on plasma 11-hydroxycorticosteroid concentration in labor. *J Obstet Gynecol Br Commonw* 1973;80:974–977.
Burns JK. Relationship between blood levels of cortisol and duration of human labor. *J Physiol (Lond)* 1976;254:12P.
Chestnut DH, Owen CL, et al. Continuous infusion epidural analgesia during labor: a randomized, double-blind comparison of 0.0625% bupivacaine/0.0002% fentanyl versus 0.125% bupivacaine. *Anesthesiology* 1988;68:754–759.
Chestnut DH, Vandewalker GE, et al. The influence of continuous epidural bupivacaine analgesia on the second stage of labor and method of delivery in nulliparous women. *Anesthesiology* 1987;66:774–780.
Coombs DW, Saunders RL, et al. Intrathecal morphine tolerance: use of intrathecal clonidine, DADLE and intraventricular morphine. *Anesthesiology* 1985;62:358–363.
D'Angelo R. Gerancher JC, et al. Epidural fentanyl produces labor analgesia by a spinal mechanism. *Anesthesiology* 1998;88:1519–1523.
Eisenach JC, Castro MI, et al. Epidural clonidine analgesia in obstetrics: sheep studies. *Anesthesiology* 1989;70:50–56.
Eisenach JC, Rauch RL, et al. Epidural clonidine analgesia for intractable cancer pain. Phase I. *Anesthesiology* 1989;71:647–652.
Falconer AD, Powles AB. Plasma noradrenaline levels during labour: influence of elective lumbar epidural blockade. *Anesthesia* 1982;37:416–420.
Ferrante FM, Rosinia FA, Gordon C, et al. The role of continuous background infusions in patient-controlled epidural analgesia for labor and delivery. *Anesth Analg* 1994;79:80–84.
Fletcher JE, Thomas TA, Hill RG. Beta-endorphins and parturition. *Lancet* 1980;1:310.
Gabbe SG, Niebyl JR, Simpson JL, eds. *Obstetrics: Normal & Problem Pregnancies*, 3rd ed. New York: Churchill Livingstone, 1996.
Gambling D, Yu P, Cole C, et al. A comparative study of patient-controlled epidural analgesia and continuous infusion epidural analgesia during labour. *Can J Anaesth* 1988;35:249–254.
Goland RS, Wardlaw SL, Stark, RI, et al. Human plasma beta-endorphin during pregnancy, labor and delivery. *J Clin Endocrinol Metab* 1981;52: 74–78.
James EF, McCroy JW. The loading dose in continuous infusion extradural analgesia in obstetrics. *Br J Anaesth* 1991;67:323–325.
Lederman RP, et al. Endogenous plasma epinephrine and norepinephrine in last trimester pregnancy and labor. *Am J Obstet Gynecol* 1997;129:5.
Loeser JD, Butler SH, Chapman CR, et al., eds. *Bonica's The Management of Pain*, 3rd ed. Philadelphia: Lippincott Williams & Wilkins, 2000.
Lyons G, Columb M, Hawthorne L, et al. Extradural pain relief in labour: bupivacaine sparing by extradural fentanyl is dose dependent. *Br J Anaesth* 1997;78:493–497.
Maltau JM, Eielsen OV, Stokke KT. Effect of stress during labor on the concentration of cortisol and estriol in maternal plasma. *Am J Obstet Gynecol* 1979;134:681–684.
Melzack R, Schaffelberg D. Low-back pain during labor. *Am J Obstet Gynecol* 1987;136:901–905.

Moir C. The nature of the pain of labour. *J Obstet Gynaecol (Br)* 1939;46: 409–425.

Murata K, Nagakawa I, Kumeta Y, et al. Intrathecal clonidine suppresses noxiously evoked activity of spinal wide dynamic range neurons in cat. *Anesthesia and Analgesia* 1989;69:185–191.

Nishikawa T, Dohi S. Clinical evaluation of clonidine added to lidocaine solution for epidural anesthesia. *Anesthesiology* 1990;73:853–859.

Niv D, Wolman I, Yashar T, et al. Epidural morphine pretreatment for postepisiotomy pain. *Clin J Pain* 1994;10:319–323.

Reynolds SRM. Innervation of the uterus: functional features. In: Reynolds SRM, ed. *Physiology of the Uterus.* New York: Harper & Brothers, 1949: 477–490.

Roman-Ponce H, Thatcher WW, Caton D, et al. Effects of thermal stress and epinephrine on uterus blood flow in ewes. *J Anim Sci* 1978;46:167–174.

Rosenfeld CR, Barton MD, Meschia G. Effects of epinephrine on distribution of blood flow in the pregnant ewe. *Am J Obstet Gynecol* 1976;124:156–163.

Russell R, Reynold F. Epidural infusion of low-dose bupivacaine and opioid in labour. *Anaesthesia* 1996;51:266–273.

Schnider SM, Levinson G. *Anesthesia for Obstetrics*, 3rd ed. Baltimore: Williams & Williams, 1993:151.

Sullivan AF, Dashwood MR, Dickenson AH, et al. Alpha 2-adrenoceptor modulation of nociception in rat spinal cord: location effects and interactions with morphine. *Eur J Pharmacol* 1987;138:169–177.

Thoren T, Holmstom B, Rawal N, et al. Sequential combined spinal epidural block versus spinal block for cesarean section: effects on maternal hypotension and neurobehavioral function of the newborn. *Anesth Analg* 1994;78:1087–1092.

Tuimala RJ, Kauppila AJ, Haalahti J. Response of Pituitary adrenal axis on partial stress. *Obstet Gynecol* 1975;46:275–278.

Tzeng JL, Wang JJ, et al. Clonidine potentiates lidocaine epidural anesthesia. *Anesthesia and Analgesia* 1989;68:5298.

Unnerstall JR, Kopajtic TA, Kuhar MJ. Distribution of alpha 2 agonist binding sites in the rat and human central nervous system: analysis of some functional, anatomic correlates of the pharmacologic effects of clonidine and related adrenergic agents. *Brain Research* 1984;319:69–101.

Veillette Y, Orhant E, et al. Addition of clonidine decreases lidocaine absorption after epidural injection. *Anesthesiology* 1989;71:A267.

Vercauteren M, Lauwers E, Meert T, et al. Comparison of epidural sufentanil plus clonidine with sufentanil alone for postoperative pain relief. *Anaesthesia* 1990;45:531–534.

CHAPTER 38

Pain of Trauma

Roy J. Braganza

For all the happiness mankind can gain is not in pleasure, but in rest from pain.—John Dryden

Trauma is a common cause of pain, morbidity, and mortality. Trauma is the third leading cause of death behind cardiovascular disease and cancer. In the below-30 age group, it is the leading cause of death. The trauma patient often is faced with significant amounts of pain. Protective effects of acute pain have been postulated. Pain draws attention to the injury, allowing the patient to seek help. Pain may cause immobilization, preventing further injury. Pain also triggers the release of catechols, resulting in an increase in heart rate and blood pressure, which helps preserve blood flow to vital organs during a time of hypovolemia. Besides location and severity of injury, prolonged pain is a contributor of increased morbidity. Frequently, the patient suffering acute pain is inadequately treated. Studies have shown effective pain therapy leads to shortened hospital stay, decreased morbidity and mortality, and increased patient satisfaction. Despite the benefits of analgesia, the trauma patient presents many challenges that sometimes leave the patient undertreated.

Because the initial care of the trauma patient focuses on assessment of the injuries and stabilization of respiratory and circulatory function, trauma algorithms do not address pain the patient may be experiencing. Life-saving procedures like endotracheal intubations, tracheostomies, and chest tubes are procedures often performed without the benefit of pain medications. The hesitancy in treating patients for pain stems from the fact that small amounts of opiate analgesics may compromise a patient's condition, making breathing or hemodynamics worse. Sedation can cloud adequate interpretation of an abdominal or neurological exam. If a head injury is suspected, opiates may not be desirable, as a patient's decompensation may not be detected as early if incorrectly ascribed to the sedating effects of the pain killer. Furthermore, the potential retention of carbon dioxide from opiate-mediated respiratory depression may worsen a rising intracranial pressure.

So what can one do to treat the pain of the trauma patient acutely? It is important to assess the patient's pain for severity and location. Psychosis, dementia, having decreased consciousness secondary to injuries, or being under the influence of drugs or alcohol all are conditions that may prevent a patient from expressing his complaints. In these situations, changes in blood pressure, heart rate, pupil size, sweating, and respiratory rate may help in determining the level of pain and subsequent necessary analgesia.

In the acute setting, collecting a patient's history for other medical conditions, medications, pain history, and psychosocial issues will later impact on the patient's pain management. The trauma patient in the emergency room will benefit from reassurance and from being told what is going on and what to expect, when possible. Acknowledging a patient's pain can lead to immobilization of limbs and better care when moving the patient, thereby decreasing discomfort. Finally, after consultation with the other physicians taking care of the patient, small doses of opiates may be able to be titrated safely without masking future clinical findings.

After the patient has been stabilized, a more detailed history of coexisting diseases will enable a more complete and prudent care plan. For example, there may be more detriment to the patient's cardiovascular system in not treating an overactive sympathetic response in a patient with coronary-artery disease. A patient with aortic stenosis or relative hypovolemia may not tolerate the use of an epidural with local anesthetic blockade of sympathetic fibers. A patient's preexisting hepatic disease or renal failure (chronic or acute from a crush injury) may impact on the metabolism and serum levels of opiates. Patients with pulmonary diseases like asthma or chronic obstructive pulmonary disease may benefit from regional anesthetic techniques, when possible, for surgery or postoperatively.

Patients with seizures or psychiatric disorders often are on medications that interact with the metabolism of sedatives. A higher tolerance to opiates is seen in chronic-pain sufferers or substance abusers. Knowing a patient's history will allow an individualized plan to be formed.

Opiates are the most widespread tool in treating the trauma victim. Regardless of the choice of opiate, it is known that trauma patients are undertreated with pain medications. Besides a concern for hypotension and respiratory depression with opiate use, there are other reasons for treatment inadequacies. Opiate dosing often is written by a physician as a "p.r.n." order for patients who, because of their injuries, may be unable to complain about pain. In addition, there are social stigmas surrounding the use of drugs like morphine and meperidine and the unfounded fear of opiate addiction in the acute-pain setting. Porter reported in 1980 that only four of 12,000 patients became addicted to opiates in the acute-pain setting, a very rare occurrence.

Opiates are the most commonly used drugs for analgesia of trauma pain, and there are a variety of routes for their administration. Oral opiates typically are not desirable. The patient may be at risk for aspiration possibly because of decreased mental status or difficulty swallowing and must be assumed to have a full stomach, necessitating further precautions to minimize the risk of aspiration. Intramuscular (i.m.) and subcutaneous (s.c.) opiates also have gone out of favor because of the discomfort of the needle stick to the patient, the slower and greater variability of onset of pain relief, and less reliable blood-level of drug. The pharmacokinetics of the IM and SC routes are more affected in the trauma patient owning to less predictable blood flow to the more superficial tissues.

Intravenous (i.v.) opiates provide a faster onset and more dependable plasma level than i.m. or s.c. There are a variety of methods for i.v. administration. Patients are commonly put on an i.v. p.r.n dosing of analgesics, which makes the assumption that the patient is able to complain of pain. Alternately, providing analgesics on a scheduled (e.g., every 3 hours) rather than a demand basis enables steadier levels, reducing both patient discomfort and opiate given. Some facilities use a constant infusion of i.v. opiate (e.g., morphine 2 mg/hour) with a p.r.n. regimen as a backup.

Patient-controlled analgesia (PCA) provides yet another method of administering i.v. opiates to the patients able to understand and use the PCA. While first introduced in 1968, PCA efficacy and safety were demonstrated, resulting in a wider use of the device in the 1980s. The benefits of PCA include a decreased lag time until pain relief, less patient anxiety, more stable blood levels of opiate, and an overall decrease in analgesic given. Development of tolerance or addiction is not seen with PCA as patients tapered their own doses in proportion to their healing and diminution of pain.

Though morphine remains the most commonly used drug for PCA, many other opiates have been used as well. Besides the choice of drug, the other variables for PCA are the dose and the lockout interval (minimum time between doses). For morphine, a prescription may be 1 to 2 mg with a lockout of 6 to 8 minutes. A basal rate of 1 to 2 mg/hour also may be added to PCA. PCA dosing should be individualized based on the patient's condition, age, and other medical problems and may have to be altered after instituted based on the patient's response. PCAs have been used in many different types of patients including those with a history of substance abuse and children as young as 7 years old.

Finally, opiates may be administered neuroaxially. Though used less often than the parenteral route, opiates may be given intrathecally or by way of an epidural, allowing analgesia with less sedation. Because the opiate may be given without the concomitant use of local anesthetic, there is no concern about motor or sensory loss. Because of the risk of delayed respiratory depression, patients treated with centrally acting opiates should be monitored for adequacy of respiratory rate and sedation for 18 to 24 hours after the last opiate dose.

While opiates have been given through spinals and epidurals, local anesthetics also have been used for neuroaxial blocks in addition to a variety of other nerve blocks for anesthesia and analgesia. Assuming there are no contraindications like a coagulopathy, sepsis, or patient refusal, regional anesthesia provides an excellent alternative to systemic analgesics for the trauma patient. Lasting analgesia, less sedation, and less hemodynamic fluctuation are some of the benefits of regional anesthesia. The choice of the nerve block depends on the exact location of the body affected, the patient's medical problems, the ability to place the trauma patient in a desired position for the block, and the length of desired anesthesia, always considering the risks of the given block.

A variety of blocks can be used for the upper extremity. Bier blocks, while seldom used for analgesia, can be used for repair of lacerations and fractures of the hand and distal forearm. Application of the Esmarch bandage to the injured limb and the short duration of this block, however, may preclude its use. Brachial-plexus blocks—including interscalene, supraclavicular, infraclavicular, and axillary blocks—also can be performed for the upper extremity. The exact choice of approach to the brachial plexus depends on the location of the injury. One such guideline is the higher up the injury, the higher up the block should be performed. Injuries of the upper arm and shoulder are likely to require an interscalene block. Patchy blocks may be supplemented with individual nerve blocks at the level of the elbow or wrist.

Lower-limb blocks can be utilized instead of an epidural or spinal block. The femoral-nerve block can be performed for mid- to lower-third, femoral-shaft injuries.

With a greater volume of local anesthetic, a "three in one" will include blocking the obturator nerve and lateral femoral-cutaneous nerve, as well as the femoral nerve. This block may be used for injuries of the upper-anterior thigh. The sciatic-nerve block is useful for procedures below the ankle; and for trauma below the knee, a combined femoral and sciatic-nerve block may be chosen. Ankle blocks are popular for surgery on the foot. Epidural or femoral catheters can be kept in place for postoperative analgesia, providing an additional benefit.

The patient with thoracic trauma presents a challenge. Common chest injuries include rib fractures, flail chest, pulmonary contusion with edema, and a pneumothorax with a chest tube. The patient often is able to survive these initial painful injuries, only to be susceptible to hypoventilation, ventilation/perfusion mismatch, atelectasis, pneumonia, and adult respiratory distress syndrome. Appropriate analgesia can aid in decreasing these sequelae. Since 1961, continuous thoracic epidurals have been used for patients with rib fractures eliminating the need for intubation and mechanical ventilation. Appropriate pain management allows effective deep breathing and deeper coughing, and it minimizes splinting. Besides pain relief, thoracic epidurals have been shown to improve lung compliance, increase vital capacity and functional residual capacity, and decrease bronchial resistance. An added benefit of the continuous thoracic epidural is markedly less sedation. If a thoracic epidural cannot be placed, regional alternatives exist. A lumbar epidural dosed with opiate may be used, but it has a slower onset and a risk of delayed respiratory depression. While a lumbar epidural with opiate has the added benefit of ameliorating thoracic, abdominal, and lower extremity pain in the patient with multiple trauma, a thoracic epidural may only help thoracic injuries resulting from the rostral spread of the opiate in the epidural space.

Another choice is the intercostal block, which may be performed over several segments accordingly. While they have shown to be effective, the blocks have to be repeated every 6 to 8 hours to provide adequate comfort; however, a block as long as 16 hours has been reported. Though less effective, alternatives like the interpleural catheter with a continuous infusion and administration of local anesthetic through the chest tube have been used for pain relief.

Many pain centers involve a psychologist, social worker, and physical therapist as part of the care team. The trend of holism extends to alternative medicine, which also may benefit the patient with acute trauma. Acupuncture, guided imagery, and hypnosis have been used to decrease pain and may complement the patient's therapy. Patients want to contribute and take charge more of their care and recovery. Prayer and relaxation techniques allow them to do this while reducing their pain and anxiety. Integration of therapeutic modalities provides synergy that may help limit the patient's disability.

Long after the trauma patient has been declared stable, with wounds healing on the way to recovery, the patient remains at risk for conditions associated with posttraumatic pain. The severity of the injury has no correlation with the severity of the pain syndrome. Though difficult, early diagnosis is important to retard the onset of secondary problems like physical impairment, psychosocial deterioration, and substance dependence.

Myofascial pain is a result of localized areas of hyperirritability. These trigger points begin a variable time after trauma or surgery. The tender spots occurring in the soft tissues may be treated with medications, physical therapy, and injections. Trigger-point injections with 1 cc of lidocaine are used commonly, and stretching and aerobic exercise are thought to help.

Complex regional pain syndrome (CRPS) is a group of disorders consisting of burning pain, hyperalgesia, and allodynia that may or may not have a known preceding traumatic injury proximal to the painful area. Patients with CRPS may start to develop their symptoms either immediately or weeks after the inciting event. CRPS is a progressive disorder with burning, lancinating pain, vasomotor and sudomotor disturbances that can lead to skin and nail changes, and finally contractures with possible disuse of the affected tissue. Early diagnosis and treatment is necessary for improved outcome. Oral administration of α-antagonists like phenoxybenzamine and prazosin has been used. Treatment options include stellate and sympathetic ganglion blocks as well as guanethidine and bretylium intravenously. Many patients benefit from muscle relaxants (such as cyclobenzaprine) or a low-dose tricyclic antidepressant (such as amitriptyline or nortriptyline).

Phantom-limb pain with cramping, shooting, or burning pain may occur in up to 70% of patients who have had an amputation. Melzack characterizes phantom-limb pain as having the following four qualities: (a) pain after healing of the injured tissue (b) trigger zones that may spread to otherwise healthy areas on the ipsilateral or contralateral side of the body (c) it is more likely if there was pain in the extremity before the amputation, and (d) the pain may be abolished on occasion by temporary decreases or increases of somatic input. Sympathetic blocks have been used to rule out CRPS. Pharmacological agents like tricyclic antidepressants, steroids, and anticonvulsants have been used for therapy as well as physical therapy, trigger-point injections, and TENS units.

Myofascial, complex, regional-pain syndrome and phantom-limb pain all are chronic-pain conditions that occur after trauma. While there are many treatment options, long-term opiate use is indicated rarely. For many patients, referral to a pain-management specialist may be indicated.

In summary, physicians are armed with many alternatives to combat pain. A careful history, physical, and evaluation will enable an appropriate therapeutic regimen for the trauma patient.

SELECTED READINGS

Ashburn MA, Fine PG. Persistent pain following trauma. *Mil Med* 1989; 154:86–89.

Dryden J. *The Indian Emperor.* 1665: Act 4. Scene 1.

Loeser JD, Butler SH, Chapman CR, et al., eds. *Bonica's The Management of Pain*, 3rd ed. Philadelphia: Lippincott Williams & Wilkins, 2000.

Ferrante FM, VadeBoncouer TR. *Postoperative Pain Management.* Edinburgh: Churchill Livingstone, 1993.

Porter J. Addiction rare in patients treated with narcotics. *N Engl J Med* 1980;302:123.

Smythe M. Patient controlled analgesia: a review. *Pharmacotherapy* 1992; 12:132–143.

Wall PD, Melzack R. *Textbook of Pain.* Edinburgh: Churchill Livingstone, 1994.

PART IV

Pain Management

Medications

CHAPTER 39

Systemic Analgesics: An Overview

Hilary J. Fausett and Carol A. Warfield

Selecting the most appropriate analgesic for the patient with chronic pain poses a complex challenge to the thoughtful physician, given the staggering array of analgesics, each with specific indications, contraindications, pharmacologic properties, and adverse effects. An appropriate choice depends on multiple factors: the source, character, and location of pain; its duration; the patient's general physical condition; and a complexity of other circumstances associated with the patient's illness. The choice of analgesic for a bedridden patient with a terminal malignancy might be very different, for example, from that which would be prescribe for a healthy patient suffering occasional headaches. Before outlining a reasonable approach to the selection of analgesics, we will discuss the various classes of pain relievers commonly employed. And certainly, this review is not meant as an endorsement for the use of medications instead of non-pharmacologic approaches.

The range of medications available for treating pain syndromes continues to grow. Although opiate medications are commonly considered the "gold standard" of analgesics, it should be remembered that some types of pain, such as neuropathic pain, appear to be unresponsive to opiates. Other types of pain, such as migraine, appear to have a mixed response: some patients need opiates for pain relief while others feel their pain is not affected by the opiate and yet their auxiliary symptoms, such as nausea, get worse.

Pain physicians routinely use nonsteroidal antiinflammatory drugs (NSAIDs) and acetaminophen as analgesics. Many conditions are treated with antidepressants or anticonvulsants, and the use of antiarrhythmic drugs is gaining in popularity. There are a variety of psychotropic drugs that have been shown to be effective in clinical reviews.

OPIOIDS

Since morphine was isolated from opium in 1803, it has maintained its position as the prototype of the opiate analgesics.

The opioids provide analgesia whether given into the spinal cord or into higher centers. The opiates all have other effects. In addition to their "pain relieving" properties, the opiates have a number of other properties: sedation, decreased pain perception, decreased inhibitions, and feelings of apathy and euphoria. Some degree of pain still may be perceived, but it is no longer subjectively disturbing. If the effects of morphine ended there, it would be a very nearly perfect analgesic, but unfortunately, it has several shortcomings. In some patients, the feeling of well-being is replaced by a dysphoric reaction. Recent investigations have suggested that this variant response might be an effect of interactions with endogenous enkephalins and their receptors, which differ in concentration from patient to patient. The opiates also cause lethargy and dulling of consciousness and may induce nausea and vomiting, mediated by way of the medullary-emetic center and the vestibular apparatus. Nausea is much more pronounced with ambulation, thereby often limiting the use of opiates in patients who are not bedridden. The opiates affect the respiratory center in the medulla, causing a dose-related, decreased responsiveness to increasing levels of carbon dioxide and consequent respiratory depression. Orthostatic hypotension often is seen, particularly if the patient is even slightly dehydrated. Thus, opiates should not be withdrawn from patients who become hypotensive until they have had a full trial of vigorous hydration. A decrease in gut, smooth-muscle tone, and motility may be responsible for the constipation that often accompanies the use of opiates, as the gastrointestinal tract is known to have functional opiate receptors; laxatives and enemas should be used when appropriate. Biliary spasm may result from contraction of the sphincter of Oddi, another opiate-receptor–mediated response.

Perhaps the most feared side-effect of the opiates is their tendency to cause physiologic and psychologic dependence. Physiologic dependence is manifested by withdrawal symptoms after abrupt discontinuance of the drug. Psychologic dependence is characterized by intense craving for the substance. There is an additional, apprehensive factor: patients in severe pain may become quite agitated if medication is withheld or if they are merely told their dose is to be lowered, as they anticipate an increase in their discomfort. These patients can be viewed as "pain adverse" although their behavior often mimics that of the person whom is "drug seeking." A cycle eventually may develop in which the patient actually becomes "dependent" on pain as a means of continuing the opiate. This pain behavior is most strikingly observed when drugs are given on a p.r.n. basis. Another important characteristic of the opioids is their propensity to cause tolerance with prolonged use. Patients may require alarmingly large doses, with no side effects. It must be remembered, however, that tolerance may diminish significantly when the inciting pain subsides, and patients then must be observed closely for symptoms of overdose.

All of the opiate analgesics exhibit all of these characteristics to varying degrees. The agonist-antagonist combinations were developed in an attempt to limit the addictive potential and respiratory depression of opiates, but their psychotomimetic potential and propensity to increase cardiac work have limited their use. In any case, it should be remembered that these drugs can precipitate withdrawal when given to replace chronically administered narcotics. These medications do appear to have less addictive potential, and respiratory depression seems to plateau with increasing doses, especially with butorphanol.

Codeine, a direct derivative of opium, has maintained its position as a commonly prescribed analgesic for moderate pain. This is unfortunate, as studies have shown that 10% of the Caucasian population of the United States lacks the enzyme necessary to make codeine into its active form. This means that healthcare practitioners may view these patients as "drug seekers" if they ask for something "stronger" when, in reality, the pain is being inadequately treated. Codeine is well-absorbed orally, and it is believed to have less abuse potential than morphine. This is very likely because of the prominence of the gastrointestinal side effects of nausea, vomiting, and constipation. The patient soon will prefer mild pain to severe constipation.

Oxycodone and hydromorphone are both better analgesics and are better tolerated by patients than codeine. Oxycodone is available in a sustained-relief formula and it is widely used to treat chronic pain, both malignant and nonmalignant. A low dose of OxyContin (Purdue Pharma L.P., Stamford, CT, U.S.A.) may be adequate to help an elderly person with renal insufficiency have enough pain relief from osteoarthritis and compression fractures to be able to perform the activities of daily living required to live independently. OxyContin provides excellent pain relief with minimal side effects and has become a drug of abuse with a very high street value. Propoxyphene has about the same analgesic effectiveness as aspirin and is quite toxic in high doses. The napsylate form has a slower rate of absorption from the stomach, which is particularly helpful in cases of overdose. Its use is not endorsed by most pain specialists, although it continues to be prescribed.

Case Reports

Patient 1

A 91-year-old woman was proud of her independence and her good health. A series of falls, however, had left her with two compression fractures, one at T8 and one at T11. She was unable to move without severe pain and became depressed. A short-acting opiate was prescribed. Oxycodone with acetaminophen provided good but very short-term relief: her pain returned in 3 hours, but because the preparation contained acetaminophen, she was cautioned against using it that frequently. She was started on a very-low dose of sustained-release oxycodone (OxyContin 10 mg) in the morning. Her pain was controlled and her mood improved. She was able to return to caring for herself and baked a batch of her famous oatmeal cookies for the Pain Management staff.

Meperidine, although it has a shorter duration of action than morphine, is similar in its analgesic action. Meperidine usually is used only in its parenteral form, as it is very poorly absorbed in oral form. Its atropinelike effects and incompatibility with monoamine-oxidase inhibitors should be kept in mind. Overuse of meperidine may result in an accumulation of its metabolite, normeperidine. This compound can cause seizures. Because of this risk and the high addiction potential of meperidine, its popularity is waning.

Methadone, which gained popularity as a maintenance drug for narcotic addicts, has been used very successfully in the treatment of severe chronic pain. Its abuse potential is similar to that of morphine, but it produces less sedation, is absorbed very well, and has a duration of action longer than morphine when taken orally. For these reasons, methadone may be the opioid most suited for ambulatory patients with the severe pain of malignancy or conditions that would otherwise require parenteral narcotics. Methadone appears to have N-methyl-D-aspartate antagonistic properties as well, and so may be of benefit in treating neuropathic pain.

Fentanyl is a very potent opiate that is available for intravenous, epidural, and intrathecal use, and it also comes as a transdermal preparation. This fentanyl patch provides 72 hours of slow medication delivery. Although this is a very effective delivery system, care must be used in titrating the dose. If a patient receives too great of a dose and the patch is removed, there may still be some medication that has been absorbed into the dermal-tissue layers that the patient will continue to receive. This delivery system is a very convenient way of providing potent analgesia to patients with severe pain.

Opiates remain the first-line drugs for the treatment of acute, short-term pain. Posttraumatic, postoperative, and acute myocardial pain respond well to parenteral opiates. In these cases, dosage should be increased until adequate analgesia is produced. Inadequate and infrequent medication does not make drug dependence less likely, but serves only to induce intense anxiety in the patient. The choice of drug should be guided by the patient's condition and the physician's experience.

When pain is severe and prognosis is limited, as in terminal malignancy or irreversible sepsis or shock, the physician should not hesitate to resort to parenteral opiates in a bold fashion. When opiates are administered by intravenous drip, the level of narcotization can be monitored in a semiquantitative fashion by observation of the respiratory rate, which will vary inversely with the analgesia obtained, as seen in the following case.

Patient 2

A 62-year-old man with a history of metastatic cancer of the prostate was admitted to the hospital with increasing weakness of the lower extremities. The physical examination was consistent with spinal-cord compression and magnetic resonance imaging revealed a defect at the C5 level. The patient was taken to the operating room for surgical decompression of spinal metastases. The tumor was found to be quite extensive, and despite vigorous surgical excision, the patient's condition deteriorated postoperatively. He experienced increasing pain and weakness of the upper extremities, which progressed to quadriplegia. Intramuscular morphine was unsuccessful in relieving his pain and anxiety, and a closely monitored intravenous morphine drip was started with an infusion pump. The dose was increased rapidly from 2 to 15 mg/hour titrated to reduce the respiratory rate to 10 breaths per minute. This regimen provided excellent analgesia, anxiolysis, and a sense of well-being until the patient's death several days later.

ANTIINFLAMMATORY ANALGESICS

NSAIDs are available over-the-counter and in prescription strength. This category of medications includes aspirin and other drugs that appear to produce analgesia by inhibiting pain-producing substances (e.g., bradykinin) and prostaglandin synthetase, and also the newer Cox-2

inhibitors (see Chapter 41). Newer studies indicate that they also may have an effect on neuronal membranes. This group of drugs characteristically shares analgesic, antipyretic, and antiinflammatory properties of varying degrees. Aspirin is the prototype, but newer agents have been sought in hope of increasing analgesic and antiinflammatory potency, while minimizing side-effects. Unfortunately, most of these agents increase the risk of bleeding by decreasing platelet adhesiveness. Nausea and vomiting, and other troublesome gastric intestinal side-effects, appear to be caused both by direct gastric irritation and by stimulation of central-emetic receptors. The NSAIDs alter prostaglandin production and thus directly affect renal function. These agents usually are avoided in patients with renal insufficiency. Dependence, respiratory depression, and central nervous system depression generally are not associated with these drugs.

Indomethacin first was introduced in 1963 as a potent antiinflammatory, analgesic, and antipyretic medication, but its usefulness has been limited by its gastrointestinal, central nervous system, and hematopoietic toxicity. Abdominal pain, nausea, anorexia, headache, dizziness, and confusion are not rare.

Ibuprofen, although less potent as an antiinflammatory agent, has analgesic potency similar to that of aspirin, but causes less gastrointestinal distress. It has a shorter half-life than some of the other NSAIDs, necessitating more frequent dosing, but still is a very popular drug.

Naproxen boasts both analgesic and antiinflammatory activity comparable with that of aspirin and indomethacin, but with fewer adverse gastrointestinal effects. Naproxen sodium is more rapidly absorbed than naproxen and provides a quicker onset of analgesia.

The COX-2 inhibitors are providing many patients with good pain relief, although the same side effects of gastrointestinal bleeding and renal insufficiency that limit the use of the other NSAIDs also limit their usefulness. Some COX-2 agents provide very good postoperative pain relief, but these agents have not fulfilled the hype (such as being on magazine covers) that accompanied their release.

NSAIDs are particularly useful in the treatment of pain associated with an inflammatory process, such as rheumatoid arthritis, and also have been found to be quite effective in the treatment of dysmenorrhea, perhaps because of their effect on prostaglandin metabolism. Those with more potent analgesic properties may be suitable for treating other types of painful syndromes.

Case Report

A 15-year-old girl was referred to the pain management center with chronic abdominal pain and school avoidance. After several visits she developed a rapport with one of the pain practitioners and confessed that her symptoms were related to her menses. She was started on naproxen twice daily the day before she expected her menstrual cycle to begin. Her pain was well controlled and she returned to school and participation in classroom activities.

Although not a NSAID, acetaminophen is best mentioned here. Acetaminophen remains the most widely used analgesic agent in hospitals and homes. It is available over-the-counter and also as part of prescription preparations of combination therapies. Acetaminophen appears to have synergistic activity with the opiates to provide better pain relief with fewer side effects. Because of the potential for hepatic toxicity, the total daily dose of acetaminophen must be limited. Alcoholics may be at increased risked of developing hepatotoxicity.

PSYCHOTROPIC DRUGS

The relationship between pain and emotion has been demonstrated clearly. Drugs may reduce pain purely by influencing the patient's emotional state, and chronic pain can cause depression and anxiety. Recent investigations into the neurophysiologic basis of pain have linked pain perception to altered levels of certain neurotransmitters, such as serotonin. This chemical imbalance also appears to have an effect on sleep and mood, causing insomnia and depression. The commonly used antidepressants alter the production, utilization, or action of certain neurotransmitters, most notably norepinephrine and serotonin. Aside from their effect on mood, antidepressants have been found to have primary analgesic effects. It has been postulated that their analgesic capabilities stem from their ability to affect multiple receptor types and modulate nerve transmission. A single dose at bedtime for a patient with chronic pain often suffices to provide analgesia and to counteract insomnia as well.

The tricyclic antidepressants (TCAs) remain the most popular of the psychotropic drugs, especially because several new quaternary compounds that may have fewer side-effects have been developed. Because TCAs have a propensity to cause drowsiness, orthostatic hypotension, and anticholinergic effects, such as dry mouth, blurred vision, urinary retention, and increased intraocular pressure, their usefulness may be limited. The choice of antidepressant often depends on the patient's physical and psychologic condition. In our experience, anxious, restless, and sleepless patients often do best with a more serotonergic agent, such as amitriptyline, whereas patients complaining of constant fatigue do better with noradrenergic medications, such as imipramine.

The selective serotonin reuptake inhibitors do not appear to have a direct affect on pain transmission, but may help by improving mood.

Case Reports

Patient 1

A 53-year-old man was referred to the pain management center for evaluation of left-chest pain. He had recently undergone a course of chemotherapy for a lymphoma and subsequently noted a vesicular rash over his left chest and back. He was treated with an antiviral agent and the rash eventually faded, leaving a painful, patchy, white area. Physical examination revealed dysesthesia over the T3 dermatome, along with skin changes consistent with scarring from the episode of zoster. Amitriptyline, 25 mg p.o. at bedtime, was started, and the patient obtained some relief almost immediately, and was able to sleep through the night. The dose was increased to 75 mg and then to 100 mg, and the patient experienced substantial relief of his symptoms.

Other psychotropic drugs useful in the treatment of pain include the antiepileptics. Certain painful syndromes appear to be incited by reverberating cyclic-neuronal stimulation, much like that seen in seizures. Both carbamazepine and phenytoin have proved quite useful in the treatment of trigeminal and many traumatic neuralgias, as in the following case.

Patient 2

A 27-year-old woman was referred to the pain management unit for evaluation of dysesthesia of the scalp. One year earlier, she had been involved in an automobile accident, sustaining lacerations over her left scalp, and had been experiencing increasing feelings of dysesthesia and hyperesthesia over the affected area. The dysesthesia made it very difficult for her to comb her hair, and she stayed at home on windy days because a mere breeze caused severe discomfort. Neurologic examination, electroencephalogram, and computed tomography all were within normal limits. Carbamazepine, 200 mg p.o. b.i.d., was begun, and within 1 week her symptoms had resolved completely.

Some of the new anticonvulsants have gained great popularity. Gabapentin is a membrane-stabilizing agent that does not interfere greatly with the metabolism or protein-binding of other agents. It generally is well-tolerated. Topiramate is used widely for treating diabetic neuropathy, and has a mechanism of action different from the other anticonvulsants: topiramate reduces both the duration of abnormal discharge and the number of discharges with each action potential, as well as enhancing the activity of the inhibitory neurotransmitter γ-aminobutyrate (GABA).

Patient 3

A 57-year-old man was referred to the pain management center with perineal burning following resection of prostate cancer. He was started on desipramine 10 mg p.o. at night and his pain was improved by 50%. He was started on gabapentin 100 mg p.o. at night and the dose was increased every other day until he was taking gabapentin 400 mg p.o. t.i.d. He reported that he was nearly pain-free, except for an occasional "lightening bolt." After over 6 months of pain, with the combination of desipramine 10 mg p.o. b.i.d. and gabapentin 600 mg p.o. t.i.d., he was able to sleep well and return to work and normal daily activities.

The major tranquilizers, including the phenothiazines and butyrophenones, have a place in the treatment of pain because of their antiemetic effects, which often help patients tolerate other analgesics. They cause emotional tranquility by decreasing the alerting effect of the reticular formation. Their propensity for causing extrapyramidal effects and orthostatic hypotension should be kept in mind.

Anxiolytic medications often are prescribed for patients suffering from pain. This is certainly appropriate when the patient's anxiety is contributing significantly to the suffering, but the physician should be mindful of their potential for causing psychologic dependence. The benzodiazepines remain among the most useful anxiolytics, because at low dosages they do not affect cortical function, but exert a calming effect by their action on the limbic system. Of the benzodiazepines currently available, diazepam remains most useful in many musculoskeletal disorders, because it directly decreases tension of striated muscle by a central action. Clonazepam often is used to treat neuropathic pain, as it is an anticonvulsant as well as being a well-tolerated anxiolytic. Barbiturates have very little place in the treatment of pain, because at low dosages they may increase anxiety, restlessness, and pain perception.

Other medications, such as antispasmodics, muscle relaxants, β blockers, and steroids have been used for their analgesic effect, but usually only when appropriate for specific disorders.

Several general principles should be kept in mind with regard to analgesic medication. First, a patient in severe pain should be kept comfortable. All too often, adequate doses of opiates are withheld because of an unwarranted fear of producing dependence. This practice usually serves only to increase the patient's anxiety. It must be remembered that dose requirements vary substantially from patient to patient, especially when tolerance is a factor. With adequate monitoring, one should not hesitate to increase the dose of analgesic as rapidly as appropriate. Good communication with the patient will encourage the diagnosis of other disorders, such as anxiety or depression that then can be treated appropriately, decreasing the likelihood of inappropriate opiate use.

Second, giving analgesics on a timed rather than p.r.n. basis reduces patient anxiety and makes patients less likely to develop pain behavior as a result of being "rewarded" for pain. Evidence also suggests that giving medications on a timed basis decreases tolerance.

Third, choice of drugs should be guided by the requirements of the patient's problem. Severity, character, and expected duration of pain, along with concomitant med-

ical problems, are the relevant factors to consider. Pain should be viewed as a symptom and the underlying diagnosis treated appropriately. The diagnosis of chronic pain should be one of exclusion. Side-effects of each medication always should be borne in mind in formulating a plan for management and follow-up. Medications such as carbamazepine and the NSAIDs may require determination of hematologic values intermittently.

Fourth, the patient should be followed closely to determine when the analgesic need decreases. Patients often are quite fearful of drug withdrawal and may be unable to assess their own pain if they fear that drugs may be withdrawn. Conversely, patients may try to stop medications abruptly and be disappointed that the pain has returned, and that they are not "cured." It is important to provide good education about the nature of chronic pain and about adherence to medical therapy.

Finally, where doubt exists, the physician is well advised to choose analgesics with which he or she is most familiar. This applies especially to the pregnant patient and to those with multiple medical problems, as in the following.

Patient 4

A 57-year-old woman was admitted to the hospital for control of abdominal pain. Three months earlier she began to experience midepigastric pain radiating to the back, and a diagnosis of unresectable cancer of the pancreas was made. She was discharged on oral opiates, but her pain and opiate tolerance continued to increase. She was admitted to the hospital for parenteral-opiate therapy. Morphine sulfate (20 mg q.3.h.) was administered intramuscularly without adequate relief. A neurolytic celiac-plexus block then was performed, resulting in complete pain relief. Subsequently, the patient became quite anxious about withdrawal of her opiate and complained of recurrence of pain whenever a reduction in dosage was mentioned. Equianalgesic doses of oral methadone were substituted for morphine, and a psychiatry consultation was requested. The patient freely discussed with the psychiatrist her fear that the block might not continue to work and that she might die in pain. Discussion with the pain management physician and the clinical nurse specialist helped to alleviate her anxiety. She was assured she would always be treated with whatever medications were needed to control her pain. Over the next 2 weeks, her opiate dose was reduced at a rate of 10% every other day, and by the end of that time she was symptom-free and stopped all medications. She was discharged to home comfortable and happy with the care she had received.

This brief overview is too short to mention adequately all the agents that are used. The next several chapters will deal with some more-specific pharmacologic treatments of pain. For more specific discussions, such as the use of triptans for treating migraines or topical agents for treating postherpetic neuralgia, please refer to the chapter that covers the topic.

SELECTED READINGS

Dallel R, Voisin D. Towards a pain treatment based on the identification of the pain-generating mechanisms? *Eur Neurol* 2001;45:126–132.

Gawel MJ, Worthington I, Maggisano A. A systematic review of the use of triptans in acute migraine. *Can J Neurol Sci* 2001;28:30–41.

Glick SD, Isabelle M, Maisonneuve IM. *New Medications for Drug Abuse (Annals of the New York Academy of Sciences, V. 909)*. New York: New York Academy of Science, 2000.

Goodman LS, Gilman AG, eds. *The Pharmacological Basis of Therapeutics*. New York: MacMillan Publishing Co., 2001.

Hewitt DJ. The use of NMDA-receptor antagonists in the treatment of chronic pain. *Clin J Pain* 2000;16(suppl):S73–S79.

Sawynod J, Cowan A. *Novel Aspects of Pain Management: Opioids and Beyond*. New York: John Wiley & Sons, 1999.

Stein C. *Opioids in Pain Control: Basic and Clinical Aspects*. New York: Cambridge University Press, 1999.

Woolf CJ. Pain. *Neurobiol Dis*. 2000;7:504–510.

CHAPTER 40

Psychotropic Medications

John Sharp

For many years, psychotropic agents have been used and misused, prescribed alone or as adjunctive therapy to narcotics and non-narcotic analgesics for pain control. Their use has stirred controversy over whether they provide increased analgesia or whether reports of pain are fewer as patients are more sedated. Over the past decade, the use of these agents has come under more rigorous scientific scrutiny. While there are many uncertainties about their efficacy in any given clinical encounter, their safety and utility in delivering improved pain control has become more fundamentally accepted. Skillful use of psychotropic drugs — especially as adjunctive agents — often improves analgesia in a wide variety of conditions. A basic understanding of the effects of psychotropic medications can help the physician to include them rationally in the management of pain.

Aside from the narcotic analgesics, many drugs that have an effect on the central nervous system currently are used for pain control. These include antidepressants, neuroleptics ("major tranquilizers"), benzodiazepines ("minor tranquilizers"), psychostimulants, anticonvulsants, cannabinoids, and combinations of these drugs (such as the "Brompton cocktail"). Each pharmacologic class of drugs has specific effects on the central nervous system. Some possess direct-analgesic properties or potentiate narcotic-analgesic activity. However, most work by supplemental means through the activation of additional receptor sites.

ANTIDEPRESSANTS

This is the most studied class of psychotropic agents. Tricyclic antidepressants have a relatively long track record for the treatment of chronic pain. Amitriptyline, desipramine, nortriptyline, and doxepin have been the most studied agents. Many studies have documented the usefulness of antidepressants in certain pain syndromes such as fibromyalgia, postherpetic neuralgia, and dia-

betic-peripheral neuropathy. They inhibit neuronal reuptake of norepinephrine and, to a lesser degree, serotonin in the central nervous system. Further, they seem to potentiate narcotic analgesia and relieve pain associated with depression. Spiegal and coworkers compared the analgesic actions of amitriptyline, morphine, and aspirin in mice. They found that each of the drugs inhibited the animals' writhing dose dependently. Although amitriptyline was less potent than morphine, it was found to be ten times as potent as aspirin. Tricyclics appear to offer enhanced efficacy in the presence of depression but are not limited to use in the depressed patient.

Newer antidepressants also have been shown to primarily increase brain levels of serotonin, a key monamine neurotransmitter. Low levels of brain serotonin have been implicated in both depressive and pain disorders. More research certainly is warranted to better elucidate the analgesic effects of these antidepressants. Current information indicates that they can be useful for treatment of pain from disorders that are not associated with endogenous depression. Fluoxetine and paroxetine have been studied with equivocal results. Newer antidepressants such as venlafaxine and citalopram have been used to treat pain but have not been widely studied for this application. Nonetheless, venlafaxine has gained increasing acceptance owing to its balanced reuptake inhibition of both norepinephrine and serotonin. The hypnotic effects of many antidepressants also have prompted many pain clinics to use them as first-line sleeping medication for patients in pain.

MAJOR TRANQUILIZERS

The use of phenothiazines and butyrophenones to potentiate narcotic analgesia is widespread, but many studies designed to evaluate the narcotic-potentiating properties or analgesic potency have yielded conflicting data. Chlorpromazine has long been used as an analgesic adjuvant, but no well-documented study has satisfactorily proven its analgesic efficacy. Many physicians attribute the appearance of the analgesic effect of phenothiazines to a decrease in the reporting of pain as a result of sedation. Low-dose fluphenazine and haloperidol have gained general acceptability as adjunctive agents for intractable states including chronic headaches, neuropathic disorders, and cancer pain. Further, the butyrophenones have a high affinity for opiate receptors and may be direct-opiate agonists. Finally, the use of phenothiazines and butyrophenones in combination with narcotics often is indicated because of their potent antiemetic effects.

Cancer, antineoplastic chemotherapy, anesthesia, and surgery all are known to cause nausea and vomiting. Indeed, pain alone may produce nausea by delaying gastric emptying, and the narcotics used to treat pain may exacerbate this problem by directly stimulating the chemoreceptor-trigger zone. That problem seems to be more apparent in ambulatory patients, because motion causes vestibular stimulation. Phenothiazines and butyrophenones are powerful antagonists of the nausea produced in the chemoreceptor-trigger zone, probably because of blockade of dopamine receptors. Possible side effects include sedation, hypotension, and extrapyramidal effects. Tardive dyskinesia is a risk of long-term neuroleptic treatment, which is dose- and duration-dependent. Exposure to this risk must be balanced with the apparent benefit to these potentially potentiating agents.

Bourhis and coworkers argued that phenothiazines may have a valid role in chronic-pain therapy; they promote a sense of well-being even though they do not actually alter pain levels. They suggested that "pain infirmity" (the inability to carry out routine activities) and not analgesia was the issue. It must be kept in mind, however, that these agents may contribute to respiratory depression and sedation, especially when used in conjunction with narcotics, and that their use may limit maximal narcotic dosage.

MINOR TRANQUILIZERS

Many of the minor tranquilizers have long been used in conjunction with narcotics for pain relief. Unfortunately, there is little evidence that any of them have analgesic properties or potentiate narcotics. One possible exception is hydroxyzine, which, in addition to its antihistaminic effect, appears to exert analgesic action when given parenterally; it is ineffective when administered orally, presumably because it loses its analgesic capability after hepatic clearance. It can be especially useful in the anxious or nauseated patient. Antihistamines occasionally are useful for anxiety and insomnia in the pain patient.

Anxiolytic medications, such as the benzodiazepines and barbiturates, also have been used in the treatment of pain. It should be remembered, however, that these medications have no primary analgesic effect and serve to allay the anxiety that may contribute significantly to the patient's experience of pain. The benzodiazepines often are useful in this respect, because at low doses, they do not affect cortical function but exert a calming effect by their γ-aminobutyrate (GABA) -ergic action on the limbic system and on the reticular activating system. Some of them, most notably diazepam, also may be useful for treating musculoskeletal pain, as they directly decrease tension in striated muscle through a central action. It should be kept in mind, however, that benzodiazepines, being central nervous system depressants, may ultimately exacerbate the depression so commonly seen in chronic-pain syndromes. Trials of diazepam, clonazepam, lorazepam, and oxazepam have supported their suitability as adjuvant agents.

Barbiturates now have little use in the treatment of pain. At low doses, they may increase anxiety, restlessness, and pain perception. At high doses, they cause excessive sedation and respiratory depression. Their early use in sleep induction has been supplanted by the use of sedating antidepressants.

Alcohol is another drug that has long been used for pain relief, not only by patients who use it because of its common availability, but also by physicians, who may prescribe alcohol as part of a pain "cocktail." Like other drugs of this class, alcohol is an anxiolytic with possible analgesic properties of its own. The misconception, held by many chronic-pain patients, that alcohol readily relieves pain has led to serious problems with abuse and dependency as well as with the overpotentiation of opiates and benzodiazepines.

PSYCHOSTIMULANTS

Perhaps the most common stimulant used in pain treatment today is caffeine. This substance is found in many widely available over-the-counter analgesic preparations. In 1983, Laska and coworkers published a study substantiating the statistically significant efficacy of caffeine as an adjunct of acetaminophen analgesia. The mechanism by which caffeine exerts its analgesic effects is unknown. There are many reports in the literature of caffeine's ability to elevate mood and provide a sense of well-being. It also has been shown to increase alertness, decrease drowsiness, and lessen fatigue. Those effects suggest that caffeine exerts its analgesic properties by way of its elevation of mood, as may occur with the antidepressants.

The analgesic effects of amphetamines also have been long debated. In 1977, Forrest and coworkers reported findings of a double-blind study that demonstrated a twofold greater analgesic effect in postoperative patients given morphine in combination with dextroamphetamine than in patients given morphine alone. The adjunctive use of amphetamines, however, has not gained wide acceptance — possibly because of their sympathomimetic effects on the cardiovascular system and their abuse potential. Nevertheless, in practice, low doses often prove useful to patients by relieving depression, enhancing cognition, and improving the general sense of well-being.

Another stimulant that has been used for more than a century is cocaine. In fact, Coca-Cola originally contained cocaine and was marketed for medicinal purposes, including pain relief. Studies of cocaine have failed to show any analgesic efficacy, however. This drug, too, may induce mood elevation and a sense of well-being that is interpreted as pain relief. It also should be remembered that cocaine has local-anesthetic properties and will provide analgesia when applied topically.

ANTICONVULSANTS

Two anticonvulsants that traditionally have been used for pain relief are phenytoin and carbamazepine. They exert their anticonvulsant action by specifically suppressing spontaneous neuronal firing in the brain, but it has not been established whether they suppress peripheral nociceptive neuronal firing (e.g., in painful neuromas). Their unquestionable efficacy in the treatment of trigeminal neuralgia has prompted their use in many other pain syndromes, especially in peripheral neuralgias and neuropathies such as postherpetic neuralgia that produce pain and hyperesthesia. To date, their usefulness in pain syndromes other than trigeminal neuralgia is anecdotal. Lately, gabapentin has been used in the treatment of postherpetic neuralgia and other neuropathic-pain syndromes. This is a remarkably well-tolerated agent with some mild anxiolytic and mood-stabilizing properties as well.

CANNABINOIDS

Several studies have demonstrated that one of the active ingredients in marijuana has pain-relieving capabilities. In addition, tetrahydrocannabinol seems to increase appetite, combat nausea, and elevate mood. Unfortunately, these effects often are outweighed by many undesirable side effects, such as sedation, hypotension, and bradycardia.

COCKTAILS

Mention must be given to the many pain-relieving "cocktails" that have been used in recent years. These have contained a variety of drugs including narcotics, cocaine, alcohol, amphetamines, and chloroform water. In 1952, the Brompton Hospital published the composition of a pain-relieving elixir that became known as the Brompton cocktail. It contained 15 mg of morphine, 10 mg of cocaine, 2 mL of 90% alcohol, 15 mL of chloroform water, and 4 mL of flavored syrup. Earlier versions used gin and honey in place of the alcohol and syrup. Those combinations have been dismissed as pharmaco-

logic nonsense by some. Melzak, Mount, and Gordon published a double-blind study comparing the analgesic efficacy of morphine alone with a Brompton mixture containing morphine, cocaine, ethyl alcohol, syrup, and chloroform water. Their data showed no statistically significant difference (with respect to pain relief, confusion, nausea, and drowsiness) between the Brompton mixture and orally administered morphine.

Liquid forms of medication undoubtedly are useful in many cases. The physician should be leery, though, of haphazard combinations of drugs in the form of an elixir or cocktail. It also must be kept in mind that the addition of some psychotropic drugs may cause enough sedation and respiratory depression to preclude the use of the higher doses of narcotics that may be necessary to provide adequate pain relief.

Psychotropic drugs do have a role in the treatment of both acute and chronic-pain syndromes. A comprehensive understanding of their classification and action is necessary to take full advantage of them. Further controlled studies are needed to clarify and confirm their specific utility. This is not to suggest that these drugs are not suited for algorithmic inclusion in clinical trials. Their complex effects may be quite desirable and there are many valid indications for their use. The physician must realize, however, that these drugs generally do not have direct analgesic-potentiating properties. Many of them are potent antiemetics, and their concomitant use with narcotics may allow higher narcotic doses when nausea is a limiting factor. Their adjunctive use is often their best use, providing the distressed patient a marginally improved pain regimen and quality of life.

SELECTED READINGS

Beydoun A. Postherpetic neuralgia: role of gabapentin and other treatment modalities. *Epilepsia* 1999;40(suppl 6):S51–S54.

Bourhis A, Boudouresque G, Pellet N, et al. Pain infirmity and psychotropic drugs in oncology. *Pain* 1978;5:263–274.

Breitbart W. Psychotropic adjuvant analgesics for pain in cancer and AIDS. *Psychooncology* 1998;7:333–345.

Cameron LB. Neuropsychotropic drugs as adjuncts in the treatment of cancer pain. *Oncology* 1992;6:65–72.

Forrest NH, Brown BW, Brown CH, et al. Dextroamphetamine with morphine for treatment of post-operative pain. *NEJM* 1977;296:712–715.

Godfrey RG. A guide to the understanding and use of tricyclic antidepressants in the overall management of fibromyalgia and other chronic pain syndromes. *Intern Med* 1996;156:1047–1052.

Gruber AJ, Hudson JI, Pope HG Jr. The management of treatment-resistant depression in disorders on the interface of psychiatry and medicine. *Psychiatr Clin North Am* 1996;19:351–369.

Laska EM, Sunshine A, Zighelboim I, et al. Effect of caffeine on acetaminophen analgesia. *Clin Pharmacol Ther* 1983;33:498–509.

Magni G. The use of antidepressants in the treatment of chronic pain. A review of the current evidence. *Drugs* 1991;42:730–748.

Portenoy RK. Adjuvant analgesic agents. *Hematol Oncol Clin North Am* 1996;10:103–146.

Spiegel K, Kalb R, Pasternak GW. Analgesic activity of tricyclic antidepressants. *Ann Neurol* 1983;13:462–465.

Watson CP. Antidepressant drugs as adjuvant analgesics. *J Pain Symptom Manage* 1994;9:392–405.

CHAPTER 41

Nonsteroidal Antiinflammatory Drugs

Frederic J. Curlin IV

Nonsteroidal antiinflammatory drugs (NSAIDs) are the cornerstone of treatment for mild-to-moderate pain. The use of NSAIDs is one of the foundations of the World Health Organization's (WHO) suggested algorithm for approaching patients with pain. The action of NSAIDs is threefold: analgesic, antiinflammatory, and antipyretic. NSAIDs act to inhibit cyclooxygenase (COX), an enzyme system that catalyzes the formation of inflammatory mediators known as prostaglandins or eicosanoids. COX inhibition decreases prostaglandin formation resulting in circulatory changes including ischemia of visceral organs (kidney, gastric-mucosal lining), and hepatotoxicity. There are at least two different COX enzymes, and current research suggests the possibility of more. COX-1 and COX-2 mediate different effects. The clinically desirous effect of analgesia appears to be mediated by the COX-2 enzyme family, while the side effects so often associated with NSAID usage, such as gastritis, are more dependent on COX-1 activation. Newer, selective COX-2–specific agents have been developed, however, their ultimate clinical role has not yet been defined. There also may be antiplatelet and weak central nervous system effects from these COX-2 agents. There is little difference in clinical efficacy between different agents in most cases. Prescribing choices generally are dictated by side-effect profile, pharmacokinetic characteristics, and prescriber preference. Side effects may be allergic or may be attributable to enzyme inhibition. Pharmacologic treatment and appropriate dose selection can modify these adverse effects.

PHARMACOLOGY

Prostaglandins have widespread metabolic effects including modulation of pain transmission, inflammation, and body temperature. Arachidonic acid, found in the cell membrane, is acted upon by cyclooxygenase enzymes to produce the unstable prostaglandin intermediates PGG2 and PGH2. These are further modified to produce active prostaglandins, as well as other eicosanoids such Thromboxane A2 (TXA2). Leukotrienes (LKT) are potent mediators of inflammation produced by lipoxygenase; it is important to note that LKT3 production is a separate pathway not affected by COX inhibition.

Unopposed LKT3 production may lead to bronchospasm in susceptible patients. Those with the triad of asthma, rhinitis, and nasal polyps appear to be uniquely sensitive to acetyl-salicylic acid and are cautioned to avoid aspirin.

TXA2 is produced from PGH2 in platelets. TXA2 is essential in platelet aggregation. Aspirin irreversibly acetylates platelet COX, resulting in impairment of platelet adhesion. Nonacetylated salicylates such as Trilisate (The Purdue Frederick Company, Norwalk, CT, U.S.A.) do not inhibit platelet aggregation. Other NSAIDs inhibit cyclooxygenase only as long as an effective serum-drug concentration is present.

COX is found in at least two forms. COX-1 has a baseline rate of activity and is found in blood vessels, stomach, and kidney. Prostaglandins may promote vasodilation or vasoconstriction depending on the specific vascular bed and prostaglandin involved. Locally produced prostaglandins increase renal–cortical blood flow and promote diuresis. Prostaglandins are important cytoprotective agents for gastric mucosa by inhibiting gastric acid secretion, increasing mucosal blood flow, and promoting the secretion of gastric mucus.

COX-2 is found in most tissues. Tissue damage, trauma, and inflammation increase COX-2 activity. This results in the production of PGG2 and PGH2, followed then by the products of the inflammatory cascade. Prostaglandins, especially PGEs and PGI2, sensitize pain receptors by lowering the threshold of chemical and mechanical stimulation necessary to produce painful stimuli.

NSAIDs inhibit COX function. This decreases prostaglandin formation, hence less sensitization of peripheral-nerve terminals is seen. The inhibition of prostaglandin generation also decreases the local inflammatory response to injury, resulting in less swelling and less fluid extravasation, which thus decreases the "inflammatory soup" seen after injury. It is possible that NSAIDs have a direct action on the nervous system as well, although this has not yet been proven. They are effective when inflammation has sensitized peripheral receptors to produce pain from usually painless stimuli, such as standing on a sprained ankle. The analgesic effect usually is seen with the first dose but the inflammatory effects may require several days and higher dosage ranges before they become apparent.

Antipyretic actions of NSAIDs are mediated by the central nervous system. Normal body temperature is maintained by the hypothalamus, which regulates the balance between heat production and heat loss. Fever is the result of an elevated hypothalamic set point, controlled by increased PGE2 in hypothalamic tissues. NSAIDs inhibit PGE2 formation and hence suppress this response.

The adverse effects some patients experience from NSAIDs may be an allergic response to the medication or related to the acknowledged result of enzyme inhibition. As noted above, unopposed leukotriene formation may lead to bronchospasm in susceptible patients. Patients with asthma and nasal polyps appear to have increased sensitivity to aspirin.

Platelet inhibition may lead to coagulation abnormalities, with the possibility for clinically significant bleeding with minor trauma or surgical procedures. Pyrazolone derivatives such as phenylbutazone have the rare but significant possibility of producing aplastic anemia, and hence remain third-line agents.

Gastrointestinal (GI) irritation is common, and occult blood frequently is found in the GI tract of patients taking NSAIDs. Dyspepsia, nausea, constipation or diarrhea may be seen. Occult blood may be seen in the stool. There is up to a fivefold increase in gastric ulceration with occasional perforation for which dyspepsia is not predictive. These risks are increased by a history of previous ulceration, concomitant corticosteroid administration, or advanced age.

Hepatic and renal toxicity may occur as well. NSAIDs are hepatically biotransformed and renally eliminated. Acetaminophen overdose may cause fatal hepatic injury. Patients with impaired renal function or perfusion may rely on renally produced prostaglandins to regulate renal-blood flow. Their absence may cause acute renal ischemia or injury after few doses. Alterations in glomerular filtration may result in sodium and water retention as well as hyperkalemia. Long-term, high-dose treatment has been associated with chronic renal failure, marked by interstitial nephritis or "analgesic nephropathy." Patients with low-flow states such as congestive heart failure, intravascular volume depletion, and vascular disease have an increased risk for nephropathy. Other risk factors include collagen-vascular disease and hepatic cirrhosis (which may decrease NSAID clearance).

Central nervous system effects are common, particularly in the elderly. Headache, confusion, depression, vertigo, and sedation all have been observed.

FAMILIES OF NONSTEROIDAL AGENTS

The majority of NSAIDs are organic acids (Table 41.1). If a hypersensitivity reaction is observed, selection of an NSAID from a different family may be advisable.

Salicylates

Aspirin—acetylsalicylic acid (ASA)—is the prototype NSAID. ASA covalently binds COX, inhibiting platelet aggregation and adhesion for the life of the exposed platelets in a dose-dependent fashion. ASA is highly effective against pain and inflammation, however hematologic side effects can be limiting. Patients taking anticoagulants are at increased risk of bleeding. ASA also is used precisely to inhibit hemostasis in patients vulnerable to conditions such as deep-venous thrombosis and coronary-artery disease.

Preeclampsia has been treated with low-dose ASA therapy, by inhibiting TXA2 synthesis. Although there has been no shown benefit to patients treated with ASA, the possibility of modifying or eliminating a disease by altering enzyme production remains intriguing.

Salicylates also have been used in the treatment of inflammatory-bowel disease. They are one of the classic agents and have provided many patients with relief. Overdose of salicylates is notable for a metabolic acidosis with an associated respiratory alkalosis. Fever may be seen with high ASA doses. The administration of ASA to children and adolescents with viral illnesses has been associated with Reye's syndrome, an often-fatal hepatic collapse. For this reason, aspirin use is avoided in anyone under the age of 18.

Choline magnesium trisalicylate has no antiplatelet effects and significantly lower GI side effects.

Indole Derivatives

Indomethacin is used frequently in the treatment of rheumatoid arthritis. Indomethacin also is a tocolytic for women in preterm labor. Intravenous indomethacin has been used in preterm infants to promote closure of a patent ductus arteriosus. It also is uniquely effective against the benign paroxysmal hemicranium syndrome in adult patients. Unfortunately, 33% to 50% of patients experience toxic side effects of indomethacin, including

TABLE 41.1. *NSAID Dosage (Adults)*

Generic name	Trade name (manufacturer)	Dose	Half life	Notes
Aspirin	Many	325–650 mg p.o. q.i.d.	2–20 h	Half life depends on dose
Choline magnesium trisalicylate	Trililisate (Purdue Frederick, Norwalk, CT)	500 mg p.o. t.i.d.	2–20 h	Half life depends on dose
Diclofenac	Voltaren, Cataflam (Novartis, East Hanover, NJ)	50 mg p.o. b.i.d./t.i.d.	2 h	
Etoloidac	Lodine (Wyeth–Ayerst, Philadelphia, PA)	200–400 mg p.o. b.i.d./t.i.d.	7 h	Less renal side effects
Ibuprofen	Motrin, Advil (McNeil Consumer, Fort Washington, PA)	200–800 mg p.o. t.i.d.	2 h	
Indomethacin	Indocin (Merck, West Point, PA)	25–50 mg p.o. t.i.d.	5 h	High side-effect profile
Ketoprofen	Orudis (Wyeth–Ayerst)	50–75 mg p.o. t.i.d.	3 h	
Ketorolac	Toradol (Roche Laboratories, Nutley, NJ)	15–30 mg i.v. q.i.d.	2 h	Only parenteral NSAID; limit to 3-day use esp. in elderly
Namebutone	Relafen (Smith Kline Beecham, Philadelphia, PA)	500–750 mg p.o. q.d./b.i.d.	24 h	Less GI and platelet side effects
Naproxen	Naprosyn (Roche Laboratories)	250–500 mg p.o. b.i.d.	13 h	
Oxaprozin	Daypro (G. D. Searle, Chicago, IL)	1200 mg p.o. q.d.	40 h	
Piroxicam	Feldene (Pfizer, New York, NY)	20 mg p.o. q.d.	50 h	Higher GI side effects
Sulindac	Clinoril (Merck)	150–200 mg p.o. b.i.d.	8 h	Less renal side effects
Tolmetin	Tolectin (Ortho–McNeil Pharmaceutical, Raritan, NJ)	200–600 mg p.o. t.i.d.	3 h	Higher GI side effects

GI, gastrointestinal; NSAID, nonsteroidal antiinflammatory drug.

GI symptoms such as dyspepsia, headache, and, rarely, hematopoietic reactions.

Sulindac (Clinoril, Merck & Co., Inc., West Point, PA, U.S.A.) is administered as an inactive prodrug that is metabolized to the active form. The active metabolite has a 16-hour half-life.

Aryl Acetic Acid Derivatives

Tolmetin is highly protein bound, well absorbed orally, and as effective as indomethacin for providing relief of patients with rheumatoid arthritis, and appears to be better tolerated.

Ketorolac is more potent as an analgesic than as a systemic antiinflammatory. Ketorolac has unique efficacy against mild-to-moderate pain when given intravenously or intramuscularly. Because of the potential for gastropathy or nephropathy, use should be restricted to 48 hours, with caution in the elderly or those whose systemic circulation is in a low-flow state such as congestive heart failure. Although ketorolac has been used safely in selected, carefully monitored patients for longer than 48 hours, such usage currently is not recommended.

Diclofenac is a potent and well-absorbed NSAID, which is useful for the short-term treatment of acute muscle injury as well as other mild-to-moderate pain states. Diclofenac is well-tolerated by most patients, and only 20% of patients report GI symptoms, which usually are so mild that only 2% of uses need to discontinue therapy.

Diclofenac is not recommended for use in children or in pregnant or nursing women.

Propionic Acid Derivatives

These agents share both efficacious and detrimental features. They often are better tolerated than aspirin. Drug selection is best guided by cost and patient tolerance, as there are few significant differences between group members. Ibuprofen is the best known of these agents.

Ibuprofen is available over-the-counter or by physician prescription in higher doses. It is the most widely used antiinflammatory agent. It is used for a variety of pain syndromes. Ibuprofen also is used as an antipyretic and is safe to use in children. Ibuprofen may be used by nursing mothers, as the level of drug in breast milk is felt to be very low. Nevertheless, all nursing women should be advised of the risk of using any medications while nursing. Because of the effects on the developing fetus, it is not safe for pregnant women to use ibuprofen.

Naproxen (Naprosyn, Roche Laboratories Inc., Nutley, NJ, U.S.A.) has a long half-life allowing twice-daily dosing with improved compliance. Naproxen is available over-the-counter and in higher dosages by physician prescription. It is an effective analgesic and antiinflammatory agent. It commonly is prescribed to treat dysmenorrhea as well. The naproxen-suppression test is used as part of the diagnostic work-up for fever of unknown origin. Naproxen also has been used safely in nursing mothers, with the same caveats as for ibuprofen; use in pregnancy is contraindicated.

Piroxicam

The major advantage of piroxicam is its long half-life, which allows single daily dosing. The analgesic and anti-inflammatory properties are not felt to be otherwise superior, and the side-effect profile is similar to other agents.

Fenamates

Mefenamic acid and meclofenamate sodium may be used in the treatment of arthritic and soft-tissue disorders and primary dysmenorrhea. GI toxicity usually is the limiting factor although hemolytic anemia has been seen. These are considered to be third-line agents, based on the hematologic side effects.

Pyrazolone Derivatives

Phenylbutazone is the only agent in use today. Toxicity, including water retention, hypersensitivity reactions, and aplastic anemia, which may be fatal, limit its use to acute-refractory arthritic episodes.

COX-2 Agents

COX-2 is induced as part of the inflammatory cascade in response to injury. COX-2–derived products play a central role in increasing the transmission of pain messages by lowering the threshold for pain receptors to discharge, as well as by contributing to the "inflammatory soup," which maintains the local response to inflammation (Table 41.2). Presumably, a COX-2–selective enzyme inhibitor would block this cascade while not affecting COX-1–derived prostaglandins in gut, kidney, and elsewhere. This would theoretically lead to analgesic action without the gastropathy and nephropathy seen with many NSAIDs, nor the antiplatelet activity also seen.

These agents proved extremely popular with clinicians, with nearly one in three arthritis patients prescribed COX-2 agents by 1999. Recent studies, however, have not borne out this promise. COX-2 agents are no more effective in treating pain than traditional NSAIDs, and they are associated with an equivalent incidence of dyspepsia. A recent study showed a slightly lower incidence of serious GI side effects—0.76% in patients receiving COX-2 agents versus 1.45% in patients receiving traditional NSAIDs. Counterbalanced against this is a roughly twofold increase in thromboembolic cardiovascular events. This finding is not unexpected in view of the absence of platelet inhibition with COX-2 agents. Low-dose aspirin has been used with COX-2 agents; however such use completely negates the beneficial GI side effects of COX-2 agents. The precise clinical role these drugs will play has not been defined yet. Perhaps as newer agents are introduced, the promise of better analgesia with fewer side effects will be met.

Acetaminophen

Acetaminophen is an analgesic and antipyretic agent with little to no antiinflammatory activity. Although it is not an NSAID, it is fitting to discuss acetaminophen here. Acetaminophen may have a direct effect on the nervous system. Acetaminophen lacks the antiplatelet effects of aspirin and is not associated with Reye's syndrome. Overdosage of acetaminophen can be catastrophic and can result in fulminant-hepatic failure. Aggravating factors that increase the likelihood of untoward effects with acetaminophen include preexisting hepatic stress such as severe illness, congestive heart failure or other low-flow states, or concomitant ethanol administration.

The toxic dose of acetaminophen is 150 to 250 mg/kg. Doses over 400 mg/kg usually are fatal. The liver may be vulnerable to acetaminophen toxicity, which can present after as little as 1 to 3 days use of the maximal recommended dose if aggravating factors are present. Toxicity may present in a subacute fashion over 24 to 48 hours. Treatment includes replenishment of hepatic glutathione stores by administration of N-acetyl-cysteine or Mucomyst (AstraZeneca Pharmaceuticals, L.P., Wilmington, DE, U.S.A.).

CLINICAL USE

NSAIDs are ubiquitous in the treatment of mild-to-moderate pain and inflammation, fever, rheumatoid arthritis, osteoarthritis, and simple acute musculoskeletal syndromes. In rheumatic conditions NSAIDs treat symptoms but do not modify disease process, unlike immune suppressant therapy. Osteoarthritis treatment involves a balance between the risks and benefits of the NSAIDs. Although these agents may provide tremendous relief, due to the chronicity of use and the advanced age of many sufferers, long-term therapy with NSAIDs should be undertaken cautiously and under the supervision of a health provider. Systematic randomized studies have

TABLE 41.2. *COX-2 Specific Agents*

Generic name	Trade name (manufacturer)	Dose	Half life	Notes
Celecoxib	Celebrex (G.D. Searle & Co., Chicago, IL)	100–200 mg p.o. b.i.d. or 200 mg p.o. q.d.	10 h	Allergic reaction crossreacts with sulfa
Rofecoxib	Vioxx (Merck & Co., Inc., West Point, PA)	12.5–50 mg p.o. b.i.d.	10 h	

found little significant differences in efficacy between different NSAIDs or dosage regimens. Idiopathic effects of a particular NSAID may be treated by switching to a different class of medications, although there is no compelling evidence favoring one NSAID over another for most painful conditions. Significant differences in toxicity were noted with higher doses of medications. High dose NSAIDs are unlikely to be beneficial for the treatment of pain, and carry the risks of bleeding and hepatorenal toxicity.

GI side effects can be treated with mucoprotective agents. Proton-pump inhibitors and misoprostol have been found to decrease the incidence of upper-GI ulceration. The use of misoprostol, however, has increased rates of diarrhea and abdominal cramping compared with proton-pump inhibitors. Histamine-2 receptor blockers such as cimetidine were found to be inferior to either proton-pump inhibitors or misoprostol in preventing GI complications. Nabumetone, etodolac, and salsalate appear to have lower rates of GI complications than other agents.

Effective pain treatment requires an adequate trial. For pain of malignant origin, 1 week of the maximum recommended dose is adequate while for nonmalignant pain, 2 weeks maximal dose are suggested. Should one NSAID produce inadequate analgesia, switching to an alternate class is recommended. If analgesia is obtained in the face of unacceptable side effects, an alternate agent in that same class may be tried.

SELECTED READINGS

Gotzsche P. NSAIDs *Clinical Evidence 4*. London: BMJ Publishing Group, 2000.

Hawkey CJ. Omeprazole compared with misoprostol for ulcers associated with NSAIDs. *NEJM* 1998;338:727–734.

Insel P. Analgesic-antipyretic and antiinflammatory agents. In: *Pharmacologic Basis of Therapeutics*, 9th ed. New York: McGraw–Hill, 1996: 617–658.

Kaplan-Machis B. The cyclooxygenase inhibitors: safety and effectiveness. *Ann Pharmacother* 1999;33:979–988.

Portenoy RK. Adjuvant analgesic agents. *Hematol Oncol Clin North Am* 1996;10:103–119.

Portenoy RK. Current pharmacotherapy of chronic pain. *J Pain Symptom Manage* 2000;19:S16–S20.

CHAPTER 42

Antidepressants

Eran D. Metzger

Antidepressant medications are among the most commonly prescribed psychotropic drugs used as single or adjuvant agents in the treatment of pain syndromes. This chapter will focus on two classes of antidepressant medications, the tricyclic antidepressants (TCAs) and the selective serotonin reuptake inhibitors (SSRIs).

Reports of improvement of pain syndromes with antidepressant medication use began to emerge shortly after the introduction of these drugs in the late 1950s. Over the ensuing 40 years, dozens of placebo-controlled studies have established TCAs as important components of the armamentarium against a number of pain syndromes. Furthermore, there now are sufficient data to conclude that the TCAs have direct analgesic effects, as opposed to improving pain indirectly by improving mood. Some studies have documented improvement in pain in nondepressed patients, and others have demonstrated pain improvement in depressed, chronic-pain patients with no improvement in mood.

In the past decade, newer antidepressants have overtaken the TCAs in popularity for the treatment of depression, largely because of their improved side-effect profiles and ease of administration. While newer agents such as SSRIs appear to be as effective as the TCAs in the treatment of severe depression, their efficacy in the treatment of pain has not been established.

TRICYCLIC ANTIDEPRESSANTS

The TCAs or "tricyclics" are referred to as such because of their characteristic molecular structure, two benzene rings joined by a seven-member ring, to which is also attached a carbon side chain. The TCAs are further categorized as either secondary or tertiary amine agents, based on the amine group at the end of the carbon side chain.

The mechanism responsible for the antidepressant effect of TCAs is unknown. TCAs act in the central nervous system at brain neurons to block the reuptake of the monoamine neurotransmitters norepinephrine and, in the case of the tertiary amine agents, serotonin from the synaptic cleft. This effect occurs shortly after introduction of the agent and therefore does not explain the clinical experience of response latency—improvement of depressive symptoms only after 3 to 6 weeks of treatment. Other proposed mechanisms that take this response latency into consideration include down-regulation of particular adrenergic receptors and changes in neuronal-gene expression.

The secondary- and tertiary-amine TCAs are considered to be equally efficacious in the treatment of depression, and the choice of agent therefore is often determined by the side-effect profile. The chief sites for the side effects of these agents are the muscarinic, histaminic, and α_1 receptors. As illustrated in Table 42.1, the secondary amines generally have less effect at these receptors. Clinically, patients taking secondary amine TCAs thus may be expected to experience less dry mouth, constipation, and tachycardia (anticholinergic side effects), less sedation (antihistaminergic effects), and less-severe postural hypotension (less α_1 blockade). Clinicians find that starting a patient on a low dose and increasing the dose slowly significantly ameliorates some of these side effects.

Prior to a discussion of specific chronic-pain conditions, certain generalizations may be made about the clinical evidence to date. Dose ranges tend to be significantly lower in pain-treatment studies than in studies of TCAs for depression. While this undoubtedly spares study subjects some of the side effects of these medications, it remains unknown to what extent efficacy is compromised. Response latency in the treatment of pain often is shorter than that seen in the treatment of depression. This is further "circumstantial evidence" that the antipain mechanism of these agents differs from their antidepressant mechanism.

TABLE 42.1. *Side Effect Profiles of Selected Tricyclic Antidepressants*

	Antihistaminergic effect	Anticholinergic effect	α_1 blockade
Tertiary amines			
Amitriptyline	High	High	High
Clomipramine	High	High	High
Doxepin	High	High	Moderate
Imipramine	Moderate	Moderate	High
Secondary amines			
Desipramine	Low	Low	High
Nortriptyline	Low	Low	Low

Adapted from Hyman SE, Arana GN, Rosenbaum JF. *Handbook of Psychiatric Drug Therapy,* 3rd ed. Boston: Little, Brown and Co., 1995:61, with permission.

Chronic-Pain Conditions

Most of the placebo-controlled studies of TCAs for chronic pain have targeted neuropathic-pain syndromes. Animal studies using various models suggest that the TCAs' mode of analgesic action is related to their monoamine neurotransmitter activity and ability to interfere with sensitization of dorsal-horn neurons. As important as the preclinical studies may be, their findings must be applied with caution to the complex nature of the human neuropathic-pain syndrome. As reviewed by Woolf and Mannion, patients who present with neuropathic pain are a heterogeneous group, not only with regard to the origin of the pain syndrome [e.g., diabetes mellitus, trigeminal neuralgia, human immunodeficiency virus (HIV)] but also in terms of pain mechanisms. No single pain mechanism can be associated reliably with any one type of neuropathy, and more than one pain mechanism may be present in a single patient.

Reviews (Magni) and metaanalyses (Philipp and Fickinger) of the placebo-controlled literature have highlighted the difficulty in drawing conclusions from studies with often-significant differences in methodology. In contrast to the findings in depression, there is evidence suggesting that the tertiary-amine TCAs may be more effective than secondary-amine agents. This has prompted speculation that the increased serotonergic activity of the tertiary-amine TCAs may be responsible for their better performance. A study by Max et al. found amitriptyline and desipramine *equally* effective in the treatment of diabetic neuropathy pain, and it is possible that the findings of tertiary-amine superiority are an artifact of their having been studied more. Postherpetic neuralgia also has been treated successfully with amitriptyline. Two additional neuropathic-pain syndromes warrant specific mention. Patients with trigeminal neuralgia have a gratifying response to carbamazepine that, while tricyclic in structure, is not considered a TCA because of its lack of antidepressant properties. Patients with HIV polyneuropathy, in contrast, have shown poor response to TCAs.

Studies of TCAs for the treatment of fibromyalgia have found that agents such as amitriptyline and clomipramine

were more effective than placebo. Results in this difficult-to-treat population are never robust, however, with response rates below 50%. Doses used in these studies generally are below those used for depression, which may contribute to the modest results. Most of the studies did not exclude subjects with depression, and improvement of mood may well have accounted for much of the overall improvement observed. Studies of other rheumatic conditions employing TCAs as either monotherapy or adjuvants are less encouraging. The few placebo-controlled studies have been hampered by insignificant findings as a result of large placebo response. Doses used generally are low and the influence of depression difficult to assess.

Other chronic-pain syndromes for which TCAs have been studied include back pain, cancer pain, and headache. Where doses have approximated those used in the treatment of depression, TCAs have been shown to be effective in treating chronic back pain. In the treatment of cancer pain as a result of tumor growth, cancer therapy, or medical complications, TCAs have been used as adjuvants to narcotic analgesia. Unfortunately, the current literature provides only anecdotal and open-study support for such use. Stronger data support the use of TCAs for headache pain. Amitriptyline is the best-studied drug, and although doses employed in studies are frequently low, positive results have been obtained for both tension and migraine-headache prophylaxis.

Clinical Approach

For the patient who can tolerate the side effects, a trial of a tertiary-amine TCA probably offers the best likelihood of response. A typical starting dose of 50 mg per day can be increased safely every week, however the wide variability in response rates and doses dictates waiting at least 3 weeks before titrating upward. Patients should take these medications in the evening because of their sedating effect. Patients also should be advised about the possibility of constipation; they can minimize discomfort by increasing dietary fiber or using a laxative or stool softener. Dry mouth is an additional consequence of these medications' anticholinergic effects. Because salivary enzymes are protective against dental caries, patients should be advised to minimize sugar and use sugarless hard candy for symptomatic relief. Finally, α_1 blockade can cause lightheadedness or even syncope upon rising. Preventive measures include sitting on the edge of the bed and dangling one's legs for a moment before rising and avoiding dehydration.

A common cause of poor response to a TCA is an inadequate trial. Patients may discontinue the medication because of side effects, either because the starting dose was too high or the dose was increased too rapidly. Clinicians may discontinue the medication before having reached an adequate dose. If a dose of 200 mg of a tertiary-amine TCA has produced no therapeutic effect, a blood level should be checked 12 hours after dosing. Differences in pharmacokinetics as a result of genetics, concomitant medication administration, and aging may result in as much as 50-fold differences in drug levels between patients. If a TCA is to be discontinued, dosage should be decreased slowly to prevent withdrawal side effects such as restlessness and diarrhea.

For patients who are unable to tolerate a medication from the tertiary-amine class, perhaps because of advanced age or medical illness, a secondary-amine TCA may be administered in the same manner as described above. Nortriptyline is considered twice as potent as the other TCAs, so that a typical starting dose is 25 mg and a typical maximum dose is 75 to 100 mg. Nortriptyline is also unique in having a therapeutic window, such that blood levels above the therapeutic range have caused *worsening* of mood symptoms. Desipramine is less predictably sedating than the other TCAs, and some patients find it mildly stimulating.

Patients undergoing a TCA trial of whatever class should receive a screening electrocardiogram (ECG). TCAs have quinidinelike effects on cardiac conduction and should not be used in patients after acute myocardial infarction or in patients with intraventricular conduction delays, sick-sinus syndrome, second-degree heart block, bifascicular heart block, or prolonged QT interval. TCAs should be used with caution in patients with other forms of heart block. ECG should be repeated after each dose increase. These cardiac effects make the TCAs quite lethal in the event of overdose, so that screening for depression, impulsivity, and suicide risk should be included in the pretreatment evaluation. While many patients starting TCAs may experience some transient blurring of near vision, patients at risk for narrow-angle glaucoma should not be prescribed one of these agents.

Older patients represent an increasing proportion of medical practices and warrant special consideration with regard to TCAs. Normal changes of aging include an increase in the proportion of body fat; hence, the volume of distribution of these lipophilic drugs may be increased. Decreased phase I hepatic metabolism, decreased plasma proteins, and increased receptor sensitivity all may contribute to the older patient being exposed to more free drug per dose than younger patients. Some of the side effects to which older patients are particularly prone include constipation, urinary retention, and orthostatic hypotension. Falls among the elderly are a major public-health concern, and increased fall rates have been associated with TCA use. Older patients are more vulnerable to the development of delirium, so that the anticholinergic effects of these medications are particularly unwelcome. The adage in geriatric medicine, "start low and go slow," is thus particularly relevant for the prescription of TCAs.

SELECTIVE SEROTONIN REUPTAKE INHIBITOR ANTIDEPRESSANTS

The approval in this country in 1987 of fluoxetine for use in depression was followed soon thereafter by the approval of sertraline and paroxetine. The more recent additions of fluvoxamine and citalopram complete the list of SSRIs currently available (Table 42.2). These agents prolong the presence of serotonin in the synaptic cleft by blocking its reuptake into presynaptic neurons. Since being introduced, these medications have earned approval for use in additional psychiatric disorders including obsessive-compulsive disorder, panic disorder, bulimia nervosa, and social phobia.

Chronic-Pain Conditions

The few preclinical studies of the SSRIs have yielded conflicting results. On balance, the SSRIs have not compared favorably to the TCAs in animal models of pain. There have been mixed results from three placebo-controlled clinical studies of neuropathic pain, with fluoxetine not significantly better than placebo in the study of diabetic neuropathy by Max et al., but paroxetine and citalopram showing effectiveness in studies by Sindrup et al. As reviewed by Jung et al., similarly mixed findings also have been obtained in the few studies of SSRIs in fibromyalgia and headache.

TABLE 42.2. *Half-lives and Dose Ranges for Some Selective Serotonin Reuptake Inhibitors*

	Half-life (h)	Starting dose (mg)	Maintenance dose (mg)
Citalopram	35	20	20–60
Fluoxetine	96–144	10–20	20–60
Fluvoxamine	16	50	150–300
Paroxetine	21	10–20	20–60
Sertraline	26	25–50	75–200

Clinical Approach

The popularity of the SSRIs in the treatment of psychiatric disorders is the result of their ease of use and safety. Because of their benign side-effect profiles, dose titration of the SSRIs often is unnecessary. Starting and maintenance doses for treatment of depression are provided in Table 42.2. Given the paucity of controlled studies, guidelines for dosages in the treatment of pain do not exist. As with the TCAs, there is considerable response latency, and a trial of the long half-life agent fluoxetine should be given at least 6 weeks before a change is made. Patients who are being withdrawn from high doses of paroxetine should have the medication decreased slowly, as withdrawal symptoms including vertigo, nausea, and diarrhea have been reported.

Paroxetine's anticholinergic effects generally are milder than those seen with any of the TCAs. Side effects related to the serotonergic activity of these drugs include headache, nausea, and diarrhea, and usually are short-lived. Sexual dysfunction including decreased libido and delayed orgasm are reported by up to one third of patients taking SSRIs for mood disorders. This rate is probably not significantly higher than for the TCAs but has gotten more attention because of the popularity of these medications. Because of serotonin's inhibitory effect on dopamine systems in the substantia nigra and striatum, SSRIs may exacerbate the symptoms of Parkinson's disease.

The pharmacokinetic and pharmacodynamic considerations described above for TCA use in the elderly apply to the SSRIs as well. Because older patients are more likely to be taking multiple medications, special attention should be given to the effects of SSRIs on hepatic metabolism. Fluoxetine and paroxetine are potent inhibitors of the cytochrome P_{450} isoenzyme IID_6. Clinically relevant substrates of this isoenzyme include numerous psychiatric medications, β-blockers, and some antiarrhythmics. Fluvoxamine inhibits the cytochrome P_{450} isoenzymes IA_2, IIC_9 and $IIIA_4$ and may inhibit the metabolism of warfarin, theophyline, propanolol, and alprazolam. Caution must be used to avoid toxicity of these substrates when fluoxetine, paroxetine, or fluvoxamine is added to a patient's drug regimen.

SUMMARY

Results from placebo-controlled studies support the use of TCAs for the treatment of diabetic neuropathy and postherpetic neuralgia, fibromyalgia, chronic back pain, and tension or migraine headache. TCAs with combined noradrenergic and serotonergic effects appear to be particularly effective. TCAs have significant side effects and are contraindicated in some patient populations. Studies of the newer SSRIs are emerging but do not yet support the use of these agents as first-line agents for chronic-pain syndromes. These agents deserve further research, which should address issues including appropriate dose range and possible use as adjuvant therapy. In 1994, venlafaxine was approved for use in this country. This novel antidepressant combines the effects of the TCAs and SSRIs without the typical side effects of TCAs and has proven effective in the treatment of depression. Newer antidepressants such as mirtazapine are emerging that target specific serotonin-receptor subtypes. Research into the effects of these newer agents on various forms of chronic pain may shed further light on the role of norepinephrine and serotonin in these clinically challenging syndromes.

SELECTED READINGS

Baldessarini RJ. Drugs and the treatment of psychiatric disorders. In: Gilman AG, Rall TW, Nies AS, et al., eds. *Goodman and Gilman's The Pharmacological Basis of Therapeutics*. 8th ed. Elmsford, NY: Pergamon Press Inc., 1990:404.

Thapa PB, Gideon P, Cost TW, et al. Antidepressants and the risk of falls among nursing home residents. *N Engl J Med* 1998;339:875–882.

Egbunike IG, Chaffee BJ. Antidepressants in the management of chronic pain syndromes. *Pharmacotherapy* 1990;262–270.

Godfrey R. A guide to the understanding and use of tricyclic antidepressants in the overall management of fibromyalgia and other chronic pain syndromes. *Arch Intern Med* 1996;156:1047–1052.

Hyman SE, Arana GW, Rosenbaum JF. *Handbook of Psychiatric Drug Therapy*, 3rd ed. Boston: Little, Brown, and Co., 1995:61.

Jett MF, McGuirk J, Waligora D, et al. The effects of mexiletine, desipramine, and fluoxetine in rat models involving central sensitization. *Pain* 1997;69:161–169.

Jung AC, Staiger T, Sullivan M. The efficacy of selective serotonin reuptake inhibitors for the management of chronic pain. *J Gen Intern Med* 1997; 12:384–389.

Kieburtz K, Simpson D, Yiannoutsos C, et al. A randomized trial of amitriptyline and mexiletine for painful neuropathy in HIV infection. *Neurology* 1998;51:1682–1688.

Magni G. The use of antidepressants in the treatment of chronic pain. A review of the current evidence. *Drugs* 1991;42:730–748.

Max MB, Lynch SA, Muir J, et al. Effects of desipramine, amitriptyline, and fluoxetine on pain in diabetic neuropathy. *N Engl J Med* 1992;326: 1250–1256.

Philipp M, Fickinger M. Psychotropic drugs in the management of chronic pain syndromes. *Pharmacopsychiatry* 1993;26:221–234.

Sindrup SH, Bjerre U, Dejgaard A, et al. The selective serotonin reuptake inhibitor citalopram relieves the symptoms of diabetic neuropathy. *Clin Pharmacol Ther* 1992;52:547–552.

Woolf CJ, Mannion RJ. Neuropathic pain: aetiology, symptoms, mechanisms, and management. *Lancet* 1999;353:1959–1964.

CHAPTER 43

Antiepileptics

Zahid H. Bajwa, Naveed Sami, and Charles C. Ho

Antiepileptics have been used in the treatment of chronic-pain syndromes for more than 50 years. Phenytoin has been extensively used for the treatment of neuropathic pain in the last 50 years. Carbamazepine was the first antiepileptic used and extensively studied specifically for the treatment of trigeminal neuralgia. Since then, a variety of neuropathic syndromes have been treated with antiepileptics including diabetic neuropathy, postherpetic neuralgia, glossopharyngeal neuralgia, postsympathectomy neuralgia, and postthoracotomy-pain syndromes. These medications range from the older antiepileptics like phenytoin, carbamazepine, and valproic acid to newer agents, which include gabapentin, lamotrigine, felbamate, topiramate, vigabatrin, tiagabine, levetiracetam, zonisamide, and oxcarbazepine.

Neuropathic pain is defined as pain resulting from dysfunction of the nervous system in the absence of ongoing tissue damage. This pain is characterized as sharp, shooting, or burning with a sensation that usually is felt in the area of sensory deficit. It usually is worsened by mild stimuli that normally would not produce pain, such as light touch or cool air. Because of the pathology as a result of permanent metabolic, infectious, or mechanical damage to the nerves, this type of pain tends to be chronic causing great discomfort to the patients.

These symptoms have led to various hypotheses about the pathophysiological mechanisms of neuropathic pain with relevance to antiepileptic medications. When the peripheral nerves become damaged, axons grow towards the formerly innervated area directed by an intact connective-tissue sheath. If this sheath also is damaged, then axon extensions grow without any direction and become tangled into a structure called a neuroma. Neuromas can generate ectopic electrical impulses at the regenerating tips in the damaged primary nociceptive afferents at various levels in the nervous system from the dorsal-root ganglia to demyelinated regions of a root or nerve. Because nerves have been damaged, there is a potential disruption in the balance of the excitatory (e.g., glutamate) and inhibitory [e.g., γ-aminobutyric acid (GABA)] neurotransmitters. This disruption leads to hyperexcitability of the neuronal membrane sodium channels and voltage-dependent calcium channels causing rapid ectopic firing.

Although antiepileptics provide at least partial pain relief in a large percentage of patients with a variety of neuropathic-pain syndromes, their use is limited by side effects in a substantial percentage of patients. Additionally, older antiepileptics (phenytoin, carbamazepine, valproic acid) also require monitoring of blood counts and liver function tests as a result of their hematologic and hepatic toxicity, leading to poor compliance. Newer antiepileptics (with the exception of felbamate) generally are not associated with life-threatening side effects and are easier to use.

The individual antiepileptics will be briefly reviewed before discussing general guidelines for their use in pain control.

PHENYTOIN

Phenytoin is an antiepileptic used to control generalized tonic, clonic, and complex partial seizures. For years, it was the most commonly used single antiepileptic for the treatment of a wide variety of pain syndromes. Phenytoin has been reported to be effective in the treatment of diabetic neuropathy, trigeminal neuralgia, neuropathic cancer pain, postherpetic neuralgia, complex regional-pain syndrome (CRPS) types 1 and 2, and postsympathectomy neuralgia. The proposed mechanism of action is reduction of neuronal hyperexcitability by decreasing the activity of the sodium channels thus stabilizing the neural membrane. Phenytoin is available as 30-mg, 50-mg, and 100-mg tablets, also as a liquid 125 mg/5 mL and 50 mg/1 mL solution for injection. The recommended dose for epilepsy in most patients is 300 mg/day.

However, an exact dose needed to achieve adequate analgesia has not been defined. Phenytoin use as a neuropathic analgesic should follow the guidelines for its use for epilepsy. Phenytoin has the added advantage of once-a-day dosing and is relatively inexpensive. However, a narrow therapeutic window and its short- and long-term side effects limit use. Because of its narrow therapeutic window and short-term side effects on the bone marrow and liver, complete blood counts (CBCs), liver function tests (LFTs), and serum-drug levels need to be closely monitored, particularly in the first 6 months. Long-term use can result in cosmetic side effects such as gingival hyperplasia, hirsutism, coarsening of the facial features, and rarely cerebellar atrophy and peripheral neuropathy.

CARBAMAZEPINE

Carbamazepine interestingly has structural similarities to tricyclic antidepressants, making it a particularly desirable drug in chronic-pain syndromes. It has been widely prescribed as the drug of choice for trigeminal neuralgia and is considered the best neuropathic analgesic for lancinating or electriclike pain. Carbamazepine is effective in other neuropathic pain syndromes such as glossopharyngeal neuralgia, diabetic neuropathy, and pain syndromes associated with multiple sclerosis. It also has been used for the treatment of migraine headaches in pediatric populations. Carbamazepine has been shown to enhance antidepressant effects and also is an effective mood stabilizer. Its mechanism of action is similar to that of phenytoin in stabilizing neuronal membranes. Carbamazepine is available as 100 mg, 200 mg, 100 mg XR, 200 mg XR, and 400 mg XR tablets, also as a suspension of 100 mg/5 mL. The initial starting dose of carbamazepine is between 100 and 200 mg/day and can be slowly increased over several weeks as needed to a maximum total dose of 1,200 mg/day. Prior to initiating therapy, a baseline CBC and LFT should be obtained with frequent monitoring thereafter particularly in the first 6 months. Carbamazepine, like phenytoin, has a narrow therapeutic window and requires frequent monitoring of CBC because of its hematological toxicity, which may result in agranulocytosis and aplastic anemia. Other side effects of concern are hypersensitivity reactions manifesting as Stevens–Johnson syndrome with lymphadenopathy and rare cases of liver failure.

VALPROIC ACID

Valproic acid is a broad-spectrum anticonvulsant used to treat various epileptic syndromes. Although valproic acid has been used in the management of chronic pain, it has been mainly indicated in the preventive treatment of migraine, cluster, and tension-type headaches. It has several proposed mechanisms of action including increasing GABA brain concentrations by inhibition of GABA-aminotransferase and succinic semialdehyde dehydrogenase (enzymes involved in the synthesis and degradation of GABA), selectively enhancing postsynaptic GABA responses, direct effect of the drug on neuronal membranes, and reduction of excitatory transmission by aspartate. Valproic acid is available as 250-mg tablets and syrup 250 mg/5 mL. The starting dose of valproic acid usually begins at 250 mg/day and is titrated slowly upwards to a maximum dose of 1,000 to 2,000 mg/day usually in divided doses. Valproic acid, like carbamazepine, also is an effective mood stabilizer. Limitations for the use of valproic acid include drug interactions and drug-related side effects including central nervous system depression, and hepatic and hematological toxicity. Frequent monitoring of these parameters should continue during the first year of therapy and occasionally thereafter.

CLONAZEPAM

This benzodiazepine has been used successfully in providing relief for both chronic-malignant and nonmalignant pain syndromes including headaches, temporomandibular-joint dysfunction, and phantom-limb pain. Its mechanism of action is through enhancing GABA-receptor–mediated chloride channels. Clonazepam is available as 0.5 mg, 1 mg, and 2 mg tablets. The dose of clonazepam initially should be 0.5 mg at bedtime to be slowly increased to 0.5 to 1 mg three times a day. Doses of up to 20 mg/day have been used in epilepsy. One to 6 mg/day generally is successful in treating headache and pain. Clonazepam is particularly effective when used in combination with other neuropathic analgesics and in patients with prominent anxiety disorder and insomnia. The most commonly occurring side effects are drowsiness, dizziness, fatigue, and sedation. Clonazepam, being a benzodiazepine, may produce physical and psychological dependence, therefore abrupt discontinuation is strongly prohibited.

GABAPENTIN

Gabapentin is one of the newer antiepileptic medications that have been approved for adjunctive treatment of partial seizures. In recently published anecdotal reports followed by multicenter, randomized, placebo-controlled studies, this drug was efficacious in the treatment of postherpetic neuralgia, diabetic neuropathy, refractory CRPS type 1, and migraine headaches. Efficacy and safety of gabapentin in treating a variety of chronic pain states has renewed clinicians' interest and enthusiasm in trying new and old antiepileptics in the treatment of chronic pain. The exact mechanism of action for gabapentin is unknown. It is structurally related to the inhibitory neurotransmitter, GABA, and postulated to increase the level of GABA in the nervous system. However, gabapentin does not interact with any of the GABA receptors nor is it converted to GABA and does not affect the metabolism of GABA in the neurons. It does not act at or bind to most receptors tested including N-methyl-D-aspartate (NMDA) and kainate receptors, and does not directly act at the calcium or sodium channels. Gabapentin is available as 100 mg, 300 mg, 400 mg, 600 mg, and 800 mg tablets. Patients generally have reported adequate relief in dosages ranging from 900 to 2,400 mg/day. It generally is well tolerated at even higher dosages, which some patients require for optimal analgesia. The most common adverse effects of gabapentin include somnolence, diarrhea, mood swings, ataxia, fatigue, nausea, and dizziness.

LAMOTRIGINE

Lamotrigine is a novel antiepileptic, which is chemically different from other antiepileptics. There are no published placebo-controlled studies that look at the efficacy of lamotrigine in treating neuropathic pain. However, there have been anecdotal reports, including a large series, of the successful use of lamotrigine in the treatment of refractory trigeminal neuralgia and facial pain. The exact mechanism of action still is unknown. It does not affect NMDA or GABA receptors directly. However, lamotrigine is thought to stabilize neuronal membranes through the inhibition of sodium channels. Lamotrigine is available as 25 mg, 100 mg, 150 mg, and 200 mg tablets. The starting dose is 25 to 50 mg and it should be increased slowly to 100 mg twice a day. Caution is required when lamotrigine is used in a patient on valproic acid because it significantly slows the clearance of lamotrigine. The dose should be cut by at least 50% and should not exceed 150 mg/day. In treating epilepsy, lamotrigine doses range from 200 to 500 mg/day in two divided doses, but there are no defined doses for lamotrigine in the treatment of neuropathic pain. Patients should be warned of dizziness, ataxia, nausea, and vomiting, which are dose-related side effects but rash remains the most common side effect. Patients should be instructed to inform their physician about any rash or hypersensitivity reaction that could result in life-threatening complications such as Stevens–Johnson syndrome and toxic-epidermal necrolysis. Long-term use of lamotrigine can lead to its accumulation and binding to melanin-rich tissues in the body including the eye, resulting in the blurring of vision.

FELBAMATE

Felbamate is the first one of the new antiepileptics approved by the Food and Drug Administration since 1992. It has been successful in controlling partial seizures in adults and Lennox–Gastaut syndrome in children who are unresponsive to other medications. In a neurobiological study in rats, felbamate was found to reduce mechanoallodynia and hyperalgesia as well as heat hyperalgesia. Because of the epileptiform nature of certain neuropathic pain states, it has been reported to be efficacious in controlling pain in trigeminal neuralgia. Felbamate has multiple mechanisms of action including inhibition of NMDA and α-amino-hydroxy-5-methylisoxazole propionate (AMPA)/kainate receptors, potentiating GABA-receptor–mediated chloride channels, and inhibiting spontaneous discharges from the voltage-dependent sodium channels. Felbamate is available as 400 and 600 mg tablets, and 600 mg/5 mL oral suspension. Felbamate provides effective seizure control between 1,200 and 3,600 mg/day in three divided doses. However, felbamate is rarely utilized except for patients who are refractory to all other antiepileptic medications because of its association with aplastic anemia and fulminant hepatic failure. Patients taking felbamate should have frequent monitoring of CBC and LFTs.

TOPIRAMATE

Topiramate is a novel antiepileptic approved as adjuvantive therapy for partial seizures and generalized tonic-clonic seizures. There are no published placebo-controlled trials examining the efficacy of topiramate in neuropathic-pain syndromes. However, it has been anecdotally reported to relieve pain in postthoracotomy-pain syndrome, intercostal neuralgia, headaches, and other neuropathic-pain states. Pharmacological studies postulate at least three mechanisms of action for topiramate: blocking voltage-dependent sodium channels, potentiating the action of inhibitory GABA transmission, and blocking excitatory AMPA/glutamate receptors. It is available as 15 mg, 25 mg, 100 mg, and 200 mg tablets. In the treatment of partial seizures, the usual starting dose of topiramate is 25 to 50 mg/day, which can be increased to 400 mg/day over 8 weeks in two divided doses. However, the exact dose for neuropathic pain is unknown. Side effects may include anorexia and weight loss. Patients taking topiramate for prolonged periods may develop kidney stones as a result of the inhibition of carbonic anhydrase. Further studies are needed to define its role in the treatment of neuropathic pain and currently are underway.

VIGABATRIN

Vigabatrin is a novel antiepileptic reported to be effective in the treatment of complex partial seizures but currently is not marketed in the United States. Its mechanism of action appears to be by increasing GABA levels through the inhibition of GABA metabolism in the nervous system. Therefore, like many of its predecessors that work through similar mechanisms in controlling neuropathic pain, vigabatrin can be postulated to be an effective alternative to other antiepileptics for patients who fail to achieve adequate analgesia. Vigabatrin has been reported to be well tolerated in patients being treated for epilepsy with minimal central nervous system side effects. Unlike the older antiepileptics, vigabatrin is not metabolized through the liver and therefore has minimal drug interactions with other medications. It has been shown to be effective in controlling epilepsy in doses ranging between 1 to 4 g/day. It is available in 500 mg tablets. The role of vigabatrin in pain management has yet to be defined as there are currently no published, randomized, controlled trials reporting its efficacy in neuropathic pain.

TIAGABINE

Tiagabine, another new antiepileptic, has been shown to be effective in the treatment of complex partial seizures. Tiagabine increases the concentration of GABA by inhibiting the uptake catabolism pathways in presynaptic neurons and thus prolonging the effect of this neurotransmitter. It is available in 4 mg, 12 mg, and 16 mg tablets. The adult maintenance doses range between 32 and 56 mg/day in two to four divided doses for the treatment of epilepsy. This could prove to be effective in the treatment of neuropathic pain because of its mechanism of action. There are some anecdotal reports that suggest its effectiveness in the treatment of neuropathic pain and controlled, multicenter trials currently are underway.

OXCARBAZEPINE

Oxcarbazepine is a new antiepileptic, which is chemically similar to carbamazepine and may prove to be a neuropathic analgesic. It is indicated for monotherapy or adjunctive therapy in the treatment of partial seizures. Oxcarbazepine produces a blockade of voltage-sensitive sodium channels resulting in stabilization of hyperexcited neural membranes, inhibition of repetitive neuronal firing, and diminution of propagation of synaptic impulses. It may modulate high-voltage activated calcium channels and increase potassium conductance. It is available as 150 mg, 300 mg, and 600 mg tablets. The starting dose is 150 to 600 mg/day divided into two doses up to 2,400 mg/day. Monitoring of hepatic enzymes or hematologic parameters is not required with oxcarbazepine to the same degree as with carbamazepine. A recent small study demonstrated its efficacy in trigeminal neuralgia. Further controlled studies currently are underway to determine its efficacy and analgesic dose in the treatment of neuropathic pain.

ZONISAMIDE

Zonisamide is used for adjuvant therapy for partial seizures. It is chemically classified as a sulfonamide and is unrelated to other antiepileptic agents. Zonisamide blocks sodium channels and reduces voltage-dependent T-type calcium currents, stabilizing neuronal membranes and suppressing neuronal hypersynchronization. It binds to the GABA/benzodiazepine receptor and facilitates both dopaminergic and serotonergic neurotransmission. It is available in a 100-mg tablet. The starting dose is 100 mg/day and can be increased up to 400 mg/day. Zonisamide is contraindicated in patients with hypersensitivity to sulfonamides. There are no published reports of its efficacy in treating headache and pain at this point but analgesic efficacy trials currently are underway.

LEVETIRACETAM

Levetiracetam is indicated for adjunctive therapy for partial seizures and may be useful for photosensitive epilepsy. Levetiracetam initially was developed as a cognition-enhancing agent for the treatment of Alzheimer's disease. It has no significant affinity for GABA or benzodiazepine receptors. Levetiracetam appears to act via an unknown binding site in the brain. It is available in 250-mg, 500-mg, and 750-mg tablets. The recommended starting dose is 1,000 mg/day divided into two doses, and the maximum recommended dose is 3,000 mg/day. Adverse effects include drowsiness, memory impairment, depression, nausea, and ataxia. There are no published reports of its efficacy in treating headache and pain at this point.

RECOMMENDATIONS

Despite the increase in the number of antiepileptics available, the rule of "old is gold" continues to be applicable in developing a general strategy to treat neuropathic-pain syndromes. Phenytoin, the ìgrandfatherî of the modern-day antiepileptics, should be tried first because of four major reasons: availability in both oral and injectable forms, which could be helpful in providing immediate relief; lower cost; established safety; and relative ease of use.

There are exceptions to using phenytoin as a first-line therapy as in trigeminal neuralgia where carbamazepine has proven to be more successful than the other antiepileptics. However, if any of the above medications are unsuccessful because of either their inability to provide adequate relief or are intolerable because of their individual side effects, other antiepileptics like valproic acid, gabapentin, lamotrigine, tiagabine, clonazepam, and topiramate should be tried. The newer antiepileptics such as vigabatrin, levetiracetam, zonisamide, and oxcarbazepine do not yet have evidence of proven efficacy in the treatment of neuropathic pain.

Gabapentin has the added advantage of being used in combination with other antiepileptics, which have failed as single agents because of absence of drug interactions with other antiepileptics. Among the newer antiepileptics, gabapentin seems to be the most effective and best tolerated, and other than trigeminal neuralgia, probably should be tried first for most other neuropathic-pain states. For classic trigeminal neuralgia, carbamazepine followed by lamotrigine, topiramate, gabapentin, and oxcarbazepine should be tried either alone or in combination. Preliminary data indicate topiramate to be a promising neuropathic analgesic but results of the placebo-controlled, randomized studies are not yet available. Felbamate only should be used as a last resort because of its association with aplastic anemia and fulminant-hepatic failure. An important point to keep in mind is these medications are antiepileptics first rather than true analgesics and are limited by their adverse effects especially when used chronically. Their use for neuropathic pain generally should follow the same dosing and monitoring guidelines used for seizure control although in our experience, many patients benefit from low doses that are considered subtherapeutic in treating epilepsy and may not require monitoring drug levels.

Today, the number of antiepileptics continues to grow along with our knowledge of the mechanisms of neuropathic-pain syndromes. Epidemiological factors such as an increase in the elderly population will force chronic pain as a manifestation of illnesses like diabetic neuropathy and postherpetic neuralgia to become more prevalent. This will open further research and increase our understanding of antiepileptic agents and their use in pain management.

SELECTED READINGS

DeConno F, Ripamonti C, Sbanotto A, et al. The Pharmacological Management of Cancer Pain. *Ann Oncol* 1993;4:187–193.

Gatti G, Bonomi I, Jannuzzi G, et al. The new antiepileptic drugs: pharmacological and clinical aspects. *Curr Pharm Des* 2000;6:839–860.

Jensen N. Accurate diagnosis and drug selection in chronic pain patients. *Postgrad Med J* 1991;67(suppl 2):S2–S8.

Kloke M, Hoffken K, Olbrich H, et al. Antidepressants and anticonvulsants for the treatment of neuropathic pain syndromes in cancer patients. *Onkologie* 1991;14:40–43.

McQuay H, Carroll D, Jadad AR, et al. Anticonvulsant drugs for management of pain: a systematic review. *Br Med J* 1995;311:1047–1052.

Novel applications of AEDS: current research. Express report from the American Academy of Neurology 48th Annual Meeting, 1996.

Sindrup SH, Jensen TS. Efficacy of pharmacological treatments of neuropathic pain: an update and effect related to mechanism of drug action. *Pain* 1999;83:389–400.

CHAPTER 44

Local Anesthetics

José M. Hernández-García

Local anesthetics have made a significant impact in anesthesia and pain management by producing a transient and reversible blockade of impulse transmission in the peripheral, central, and autonomic nervous systems. The first recognition of the potential of local anesthetic effects was by the Incas of Peru, who chewed coca leaves containing cocaine and found the numbing properties in the mouth. In 1860, Niemann first purified cocaine from coca leaves. Koller, however, was the first to describe its use in 1884, and it was initially utilized in ophthalmology. Procaine was synthesized in 1904 and lidocaine, the first amide local anesthetic, in 1943.

MECHANISM OF ACTION

To understand the mechanism of action, it is necessary to explain the transmission of nerve impulses and the structure of the nerve membrane.

The nerve membrane consists of the characteristic bilayer formed by hydrophobic fatty-acid tails in the center and hydrophilic groups on the outside. Throughout the membrane, there are proteins and ion-conducting channels (Fig. 44.1).

The nerve maintains a resting-membrane potential across the membrane as a result of the different permeability to Na^+ and K^+. The process of transmission of the nerve impulse is by changes in the permeability and diffusion of ions. When a nerve impulse reaches the threshold level, there is an influx or increase in the permeability of extracellular Na^+ ions followed by efflux of intracellular K^+ ions, creating an action potential that is transmitted through the nerve. Eventually, there is a return to baseline or resting-membrane potential by the Na^+-K^+ pump.

Local anesthetics bind to Na^+ channels when they are in the inactive or open state. They cross the axonal membrane and block access to the open pore of the channel from the inner side. In this way, they interfere with the ability to undergo the specific changes that result in the altered permeability to Na^+ and in the altered generation and propagation of nerve-membrane electrical impulses, by inhibiting the function of Na^+ channels.

Nerve fibers are classified into three major classes: myelinated somatic nerves or A fibers (which are divided according to decreasing size in α, β, γ, and δ), myelinated preganglionic autonomic nerves, or B fibers and nonmyelinated nerves or C fibers. Different conduction properties characterize myelinated (saltatory conduction from Ranvier nodes to nodes, faster) and nonmyelinated nerves (uniform, continuous spread of electrical depolarization and slower), because of the thickness of Schwann-cell insulation.

Nerve diameter and myelinization play a significant role in the sensitivity and action of local anesthetics. As the nerve impulse travels from node to node, the thicker the nerve fiber, the longer the distance between nodes and the greater the amount of local anesthetic required to block the conduction. Each nerve has a characteristic or critical blocking length proportional to the diameter, and at least three to five nodes of Ranvier must be exposed to the local anesthetic to obtain a blockade in the conduction of the nerve impulse (Fig. 44.2). This phenomenon is

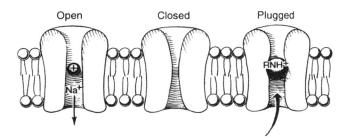

FIG. 44.1. Channel entry. On the left there is an open channel, permeant to sodium ions. The center channel is in the resting, closed configuration. The channel on the right, although in open configuration, is impermeant to sodium ions because it has a local anesthetic cation (RNH^+) bound to the gating receptor site. (Reprinted from DeJong RH. *Local Anesthetics.* St. Louis: Mosby, 1994:49, with permission.)

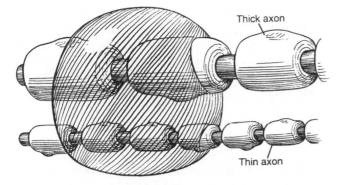

FIG. 44.2. Nodal interval longitudinal blockade. The local anesthetic solution covers three successive nodes of the thin axon but only one of the thick axon. Impulses can skip easily over one and even two inexcitable nodes, enabling conduction along the thick axon to continue uninterrupted. In the thin axon, the conduction is halted. Sufficient volume should be injected to coat at least three consecutive nodes. (Reprinted from DeJong RH. *Local Anesthetics*. St. Louis: Mosby, 1994:68, with permission.)

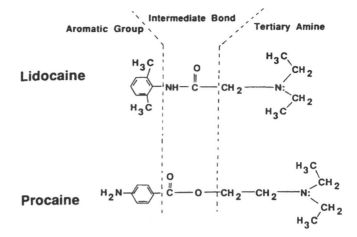

FIG. 44.3. Structures of two local anesthetics, the aminoamide lidocaine and the aminoester procaine. In both drugs, a hydrophobic, aromatic group is joined to a more hydrophilic base, the tertiary amine, by an intermediate bond. (Reprinted from Strichartz GR, Berde CB. Local anesthetics. In: Miller RD, ed. *Anesthesia*, vol. 1. New York: Churchill Livingston, 1994:489, with permission.)

thought to be responsible for the differential blockade of sympathetic, motor, and sensory function in spinal and epidural anesthesia, as well as for the differential blockade by various concentrations of local anesthetics.

STRUCTURE OF LOCAL ANESTHETICS

The basic structure of a local anesthetic consists of a lipophilic aromatic head and a hydrophobic aminoalkyl tail, which are linked by an intermediate chain, which is the base for the classification as esters or amides (Fig. 44.3). The aminoesters are cocaine, procaine, 2-chlorprocaine, tetracaine, and benzocaine. The aminoamides are lidocaine, mepivacaine, prilocaine, bupivacaine, etidocaine, and ropivacaine (Fig. 44.4).

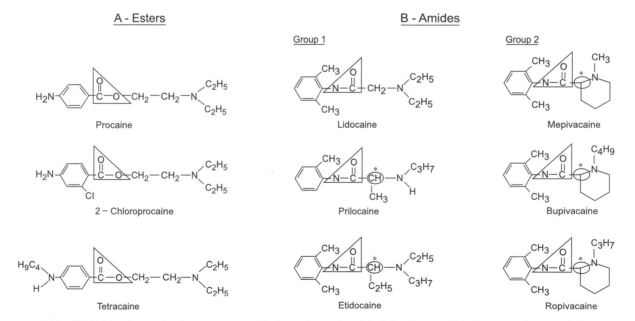

FIG. 44.4. Local anesthetic structures with the ester and amide link shown within the superimposed triangle. When present, the asymmetric carbon is circled, shaded, and marked with an asterisk (*). (Reprinted from DiFazio CA, Woods AM. Pharmacology of local anesthetics. In: Raj PP, ed. *Practical Management of Pain*, 2nd ed. St. Louis: Mosby, 1992.)

TABLE 44.1. *Dissociation Constants*

Local anesthetics	pKa
Benzocaine	3.5
Mepivacaine	7.7
Lidocaine	7.8
Etidocaine	7.9
Prilocaine	7.9
Ropivacaine	8.1
Bupivacaine	8.1
Tetracaine	8.4
Cocaine	8.6
Dibucaine	8.8
Procaine	8.9
Chlorprocaine	9.1
Procainamide	9.3

Local anesthetics are weak bases, lipid soluble, but water insoluble. For this reason, they are marketed in the crystalline-salt form, which is water soluble and more stable in solution. They exist in equilibrium between the uncharged or neutral form and the charged or cationic form. The pKa of the solution and the pH of the medium determine the amount of the neutral and cationic form. The pKa is defined as the pH where 50% of the drug is in the neutral form and the other 50% is in the cationic form (Table 44.1). The pH of the medium is another factor that determines the proportion of the neutral and cationic forms. The pKa is an important determinant of the speed of onset of the local anesthetic. The lower the pKa, the faster the onset. This is because of the higher amount of neutral or base form, which is more lipid soluble and diffuses through the nerve membrane more readily. In the inner space, the base dissociates from the cationic form, which is responsible for binding to the inner pore of the Na^+ channel when it is in the resting or closed state, and producing a change in the configuration that will be impermeable to the Na^+ ions, and therefore produce a blockade in the transmission of the action potential.

PHARMACOLOGICAL CONSIDERATIONS

The properties of local anesthetics are determined by several factors:

Potency

This is related to the lipid solubility. The more lipid soluble, the higher the amount of local anesthetic that crosses the nerve membrane and the more effective the blockade of the nerve impulse.

Protein Binding

There are two plasma proteins that bind to local anesthetics: albumin and α1-acid glycoprotein. Albumin binds a larger amount of drug, although it has less affinity than α1-acid glycoprotein. The higher the amount of local anesthetics bound to plasma proteins, the lesser amount available for blockade. This also is influenced by the pH. In case of acidosis, there is a higher concentration of free drug.

Onset of Action

This is characteristic for each local anesthetic and it depends upon factors such as the dose or concentration used. For example, bupivacaine 0.25% has a slow onset, but this can be increased by using 0.5%. On the other hand, 3% chlorprocaine has a faster onset of action than lidocaine 2%.

Adding bicarbonate to local anesthetics is a common technique used to produce a faster onset of action. This will increase the pH of the solution and therefore the amount of uncharged base form available to cross the neural membrane.

Duration of Action

Chlorprocaine has a short duration. Lidocaine and mepivacaine have an intermediate duration of action, and bupivacaine, ropivacaine, and etidocaine have the longest duration. Duration of action is determined by the amount of drug bound to plasma proteins. Local anesthetics with a high protein-binding capacity have a longer duration of action.

Another important factor is the blood supply to the area of injection. This also will determine the onset of action and toxicity in decreasing order: intercostal, caudal, epidural, brachial plexus, sciatic nerve, and subcutaneous.

Adding vasoconstrictors like phenylephrine, epinephrine, or norepinephrine also will prolong the effect of local anesthetics by decreasing the local absorption of the drug.

Mixtures of Local Anesthetics

The use of combinations of local anesthetics is intended, in most cases, to obtain a blockade with a fast onset of action and a long duration. For this purpose, chlorprocaine and lidocaine have been used with bupivacaine. The result produces a faster onset of action but a shorter duration than bupivacaine alone. This is caused by metabolites of chlorprocaine that interfere with the binding sites for bupivacaine. The effects obtained from mixtures of local anesthetics, therefore, offer little advantage for their clinical use.

METABOLISM AND EXCRETION

Local anesthetics are metabolized according to their chemical structure.

Esters undergo hydrolysis in plasma by the enzyme pseudocholinesterase (or plasma cholinesterase) and the metabolites, such as p-aminobenzoic acid, are excreted in the urine. Patients with abnormal pseudocholinesterase are at increased risk for toxic effects, and the use of esters should be closely evaluated in these cases. Chlorprocaine has the shortest half-life of all local anesthetics and for that reason very little potential for toxicity. Tetracaine, although more potent, is metabolized at a slower rate. Cocaine requires both plasma cholinesterase and liver hydrolysis for elimination.

The aminoamides are metabolized primarily in the liver, but at a rate slower than ester hydrolysis. Their resistance to enzymatic hydrolysis makes them suitable to undergo procedures such autoclaving without loss of potency. Prilocaine has the fastest rate of hepatic degradation, followed by lidocaine.

TOXICITY

Local anesthetics, when used in the appropriate dose and location, should be devoid of side effects. When toxicity does occur, the reactions primarily involve the central nervous system (CNS) and the cardiovascular system.

Central Nervous System

CNS toxicity is most frequently the initial manifestation of overdose in the form of dizziness, circumoral numbness, tinnitus, and blurred vision. In some cases, excitatory symptoms such as agitation, muscular twitching, or tremors precede CNS depression.

Ultimately, convulsions, respiratory depression, and arrest may occur.

The CNS excitatory symptoms may be a result of an initial blockade of inhibitory pathways in the cerebral cortex by local anesthetics, which would increase CNS activity.

The CNS toxic effects are related to the potency and dose of the local anesthetics, bupivacaine being more potent than etidocaine, which is more potent than lidocaine.

Cardiovascular System

Cardiovascular toxicity as in the case of CNS effects may be correlated with the relative potency of local anesthetics, although some animal studies have shown that the dose required to produce cardiovascular effects is three times higher than the dose required for CNS toxicity (Table 44.2).

The first symptoms of cardiac toxicity are dysrhythmias and a fall in blood pressure. This is thought to be because of the inhibition of the Na^+ channels in the cardiac membrane by local anesthetics such bupivacaine and to the negative inotropic action, resulting in a decrease in cardiac output and stroke volume, rather than peripheral vasodilatation.

The cardiovascular toxicity involves a direct effect on the myocardium, vascular tissue, and the central innervation of the heart. If the dose of local anesthetic is excessive, an irreversible cardiac arrest and circulatory collapse may result, making resuscitation prolonged and difficult.

Enhanced cardiac toxicity also may be a result of changes in the acid-base status. Hypercarbia, acidosis, and hypoxia decrease the threshold of local anesthetics to produce cardiodepressant effects and convulsive activity.

Ropivacaine has been shown in clinical studies to be almost equipotent to bupivacaine, although less cardiotoxic, and in dog studies, resuscitation was more effective in cases of ropivacaine toxicity.

Allergies

Allergic reactions to local anesthetics are very rare, but when they occur, are related to the ester group or because of the allergenic properties of the p-aminobenzoic–acid metabolite.

TABLE 44.2. *Comparable Safe Doses of Local Anesthetics (mg/kg)[a]*

Drugs	Peripheral blocks	Plain	With epinephrine 1:200,000	Intercostal blocks with epinephrine 1:200,000
2-Chloroprocaine	–	20	25	–
Procaine	–	14	18	–
Lidocaine	2	7	9	6
Mepivacaine	20	7	9	6
Bupivacaine	5	2	2	2
Tetracaine	–	2	2	–

[a]Estimated to produce peak plasma levels that are less than half the plasma levels at which seizures could occur.

From DiFazio CA, Woods AM. Pharmacology of local anesthetics. In: Raj PP, ed. *Practical Management of Pain,* 2nd ed. St. Louis: Mosby, 1992, with permission.

Allergy to amide local anesthetics is extremely rare. In these cases, it is more frequently from the preservative methylparaben.

Tissue Toxicity

Effects on skeletal muscle have been described with almost all local anesthetics, although the more potent, bupivacaine and etidocaine, seem to cause a greater degree of localized skeletal-muscle damage than the less potent. These changes are reversible and complete regeneration occurs within 2 weeks after the injection.

Chlorprocaine has been described as responsible for some severe cases of neurotoxicity, particularly with the use of a large volume injected in the subarachnoid space, causing neurological deficits. Studies have suggested that the combination of low pH and sodium bisulphite, as a preservative, is responsible for this effect. For that reason, chlorprocaine is marketed now without sodium bisulfite, which has been replaced by EDTA, although some cases of low-back pain have been blamed on the use of this latter combination. Lidocaine, in high concentrations such as 5%, also has been involved in cases of cauda equina syndrome when used through very small 25-gauge catheters, for continuous spinal anesthesia. This has been explained by the overexposure and pooling of the local anesthetic in the distal portions of the cord, and for that reason, the catheter was withdrawn by the Food and Drug Administration.

SELECTED READINGS

Covino BG, Wildsmith JAW. Clinical pharmacology of local anesthetics. In: Cousins MJ, Bridenbaugh PO, eds. *Neural Blockade*. Philadelphia: Lippincott–Raven Publishers, 1998:97–128.

DeJong RH. *Local Anesthetics*. St. Louis: Mosby, 1994.

Strichartz GR, Berde CB. Local anesthetics. In: Miller RD, ed. *Anesthesia*, vol. 1. New York: Churchill Livingston, 1994:489.

Williams MJ. Local anesthetics. In: Raj PP, ed. *Pain Medicine*. St. Louis: Mosby, 1996:162.

CHAPTER 45

Opioids

Michael L. Tran

Since the discovery of opium from the juice of the poppy plant in ancient times, a proliferation of experimental and clinical experience has been established in the area of opioid analgesic. Despite this enormous body of knowledge, surveys of acute- and chronic-pain management have shown unrelieved moderate to severe pain in 25% to 75% of patients. Opioids provide a powerful and flexible tool to manage this pain, which often is associated with medical illnesses. This chapter will involve an overview of opioid pharmacology, individual drugs commonly utilized clinically, and common guidelines for clinical applications.

MECHANISM AND CHARACTERIZATION

The term *narcotic* was derived from the Greek word meaning "stupor." It is used more in a legal context to refer to a variety of abused substances and is not useful in a pharmacological context. Although the term narcotic has been used to generalize opioids, the negative connotations belie the critical role opioids have as versatile and principle analgesics for the management of pain. Opiates are drugs derived from opium and include well-known derivatives such as morphine, codeine, and thebaine. Opioids refer to drugs with morphinelike activity and can be naturally occurring, semisynthetic, or synthetically derived.

Opium contains 20 isolated alkaloids including morphine, codeine, and papaverine. The alkaloids fall into two types, the phenanthrenes (morphine and codeine) and the benzylisoquinoline (papaverine). Modification of some of these alkaloids, specifically morphine and thebaine, give rise to the semisynthetic derivatives including hydromorphone, oxycodone, oxymorphone, and heroin.

Opioid effects are mediated by specific receptors located on cell membranes. These receptors have been identified both pre- and postsynaptically in the central nervous system. As many as five receptors have been identified and have been labeled as mu (μ), kappa (κ), delta (δ), epsilon (ε), and sigma (σ) receptors. The interaction of the agonist opioid with these various receptors results in observable histological changes.

The basic effect of opioids is that of neuronal inhibition either by blocking the release of neurotransmitters or by hyperpolarization of the cell by causing changes in calcium and potassium-ion channels. This physiological reaction is mediated by a second messenger system that uses a G protein.

There are three classification schemes to characterize opioids. The simplest approach is to describe the drug as either weak or strong. Another classification divides the drugs into naturally occurring, semisynthetic, and synthetic compounds based on the chemical derivation. The final categorization method divides the opioids into four categories of agonists, partial agonists, agonist-antagonists and antagonists. This chapter will focus discussion of opioids using this final categorization method.

COMMONLY USED OPIOIDS

Agonist Drugs

Naturally Occurring Opioids

Morphine is the prototypical opioid to which all other analgesics are compared in determining their relative analgesia potency. Its oral bioavailability ranges from 35% to 75%. It undergoes glucuronidation producing morphine-3-glucuronide (M3G) and morphine-6-glucuronide (M6G) in a 2:1 ratio. M6G binds with a higher affinity to the μ receptor. Once inside the central nervous system (CNS), the M6G metabolite is 100 times more potent than morphine, while M3G is inactive or may reproduce hyperalgesia and antagonize M6G. In patients with renal failure, morphine metabolites accumulate resulting in a more prolonged effect and often obtundation and respiratory depression. Relative potency of intramuscular morphine to oral morphine on repeated administration is 1:2 or 1:3. Slow-release formulations of morphine can be administered on an 8-hourly (Oramorph SR, Roxane Laboratories, Inc., Columbus, OH, U.S.A.), 12-hourly (MS Contin, Purdue Frederick Company, Norwalk, CT, U.S.A.), or 24-hourly (Kadian, Zeneca Pharmaceuticals, London, U.K.) basis. These formulations use either hydrophobic or hydrophilic matrices to allow a graded release of the drug as the pill passes through the gastrointestinal tract.

Codeine is considered a weak opioid, commonly used for mild-to-moderate pain. It is a prodrug and is metabolized into a series of metabolites including morphine to produce effect. It has a high oral-to-parenteral ratio (2:1). Codeine can be used in combination with aspirin or acetaminophen. Doses greater than 200 mg orally are associated with significant side effects of nausea and vomiting.

Semisynthetic Opioids

Heroin is semisynthesized from diacetylating morphine. Heroin is a prodrug that is lipid-soluble and rapidly metabolized to 6-acetylmorphine and morphine from which it produces its analgesic effects. Following oral administration of heroin, only morphine can be measured in a patient's blood. It has been demonstrated that by oral route, heroin and morphine are nearly equipotent. A series of studies suggests intramuscular injection is twice as potent as oral morphine, with a faster onset but shorter duration. Because of its great potential for abuse, heroin is not currently legalized in the United States.

Hydromorphone was derived from morphine in the 1920s; it is more soluble than morphine and available in a concentrated dosage form at 10 mg/mL with bioavailability about 30% to 40%. It has a short half-life of 1.5 to 2 hours and is not known to have active metabolites, thus it is useful treatment for the elderly and renal-failure patients.

Oxycodone is a morphine congener with good bioavailability by the oral route. It is commonly used alone or in combination with aspirin or acetaminophen. Relative potency studies show that 15 mg intramuscularly is approximately equal to 10 mg of parenteral morphine. Its half-life is about 2 to 3 hours and is excreted by way of the kidneys. Fixed-dose oxycodone combinations should not be used chronically in large doses for more severe pain because of risk of dose-related toxicity from the nonopioid components.

Synthetic Opioids

Propoxyphene is considered a weak opioid useful for managing mild pain. Its analgesic strength is about one half to two thirds that of codeine. Its oral bioavailability is about 30% to 70% and is demethylated to norpro-

poxyphene. Propoxyphene's half-life is 3 to 4 hours, while that of norpropoxyphene is 23 hours. Propoxyphene causes depression of the cardiac-conduction systems, similar to that produced by lidocaine. Propoxyphene also poses a significant risk for convulsions, CNS depression, and respiratory depression as a result of norpropoxyphene's long half-life contributing to cases of overdose. Naloxone can antagonize these effects.

Methadone is a racemic mixture of which its pharmacological activity comes mostly from the L-isomer. Its analgesic potency is comparable to morphine, and its oral-to-parenteral ratio is 1:2, with a bioavailability greater than 85%. Its plasma half-life ranges from 13 to 50 hours, while duration of analgesia is only 4 to 8 hours. Therefore, repeated doses may lead to drug accumulation. It is a useful second-line drug alternative to morphine, but sophistication of titration is required in its use. Methadone is the main drug of maintenance for the treatment of opioid addiction.

Meperidine is a synthetic opioid analgesic with anticholinergic properties. It is more lipophilic than morphine and produces faster onset and shorter duration of analgesia. It has a bioavailability of 40% to 60%. Repetitive dosing greater than 250 mg/day can lead to accumulation of its toxic metabolite, normeperidine, resulting in CNS hyperexcitability commonly in patients with renal disease. Normeperidine is twice as potent as a convulsant and half as analgesic compared to its parent compound. Naloxone does not reverse meperidine-induced seizure.

Fentanyl is a highly lipophilic opioid agonist with a shorter duration of action than morphine. Its relative potency, as compared to that of morphine, varies between 1:20 to 1:30 in nontolerant, acute patient. It is commonly used to manage acute intra- and postoperative pain. Routes of administration include intravenous, epidural, intrathecal, transmucosal, and transdermal. It is metabolized by the liver into norfentanyl and other inactive metabolites.

Tramadol is a synthetic analogue of codeine, which has very mild agonist effects on the μ receptor (about 1/6000 that of morphine) in addition to inhibitory actions on monoamine reuptake of norepinephrine and serotonin. Tramadol has been associated with seizure, especially when given with antidepressants, particularly those that stimulate norepinephrine such as desipramine and imipramine. It is a very useful intermediate-acting analgesic (6 to 8 hours). Tramadol's elimination half-life is 6.3 hours and it is poorly bound to plasma protein (20%). Tramadol is well tolerated in patients with hypertension, congestive heart failure, or renal insufficiency.

Agonist–Antagonists/Partial Agonist

The mixed agonist–antagonist analgesics include butorphanol, pentazocine, and nalbuphine and are less efficacious than pure agonists, but they cause less respiratory depression and have lower potential for abuse. With this class of opioids there tends to be a ceiling effect to both analgesia and respiratory suppression. They produce analgesia in the nontolerant patients but may precipitate withdrawal in patients who are physically dependent on pure agonists, and are associated with a higher incidence of psychotomimetic effects.

Nalbuphine acts primarily as an agonist at the κ receptor and inhibits the μ receptor. It has an interesting profile where it can reverse respiratory depression while not reversing analgesia. It is equal to morphine in potency and onset. The higher potency and less-pronounced psychotomimetic effects of nalbuphine make it the most useful of this class of drug.

Butorphanol has a similar mechanism to nalbuphine. It is about five times more potent than morphine, and is available in a nasal spray to treat intermittent migraines.

Pentazocine is a partial agonist that binds μ, κ, and δ receptors. Its slow dissociation from the receptors is thought to contribute to its long duration of action and account for naloxone's reduced ability to reverse its effects. It has been used in place of methadone for long-term management of heroin addicts.

Antagonists

This class of opioids has the ability to competitively displace an opioid agonist from its respective receptor. Naloxone and naltrexone are two opioid antagonists. They have a high affinity for μ receptors but also interact with δ and κ receptors at higher doses.

Naloxone is often used to reverse the respiratory depression caused by opioid overdose, at doses of 1 to 5 μg/kg in aliquots of 0.04 mg. Titration of intravenous naloxone often is used to reverse unwanted side effects of pruritus, urinary retention, nausea, and vomiting without significantly affecting analgesia. It is a short-acting medication (30 to 45 minutes), supplemental or intravenous infusion (5 μg/kg/hour) may be needed in patients with long-acting opioid overdose. Rapid intravenous injection may cause nausea and vomiting and cardiovascular stimulation (tachycardia, pulmonary edema, hypertension, dysrhythmia, ventricular fibrillation). This has been attributed to an increase in sympathetic nervous system activity.

Naltrexone acts mainly at the μ receptor. It is active after oral administration and prolongs effect up to 24 hours.

OPIOID PROPERTIES AND SIDE EFFECTS

Side effects of opioids are related to multiple variables including dose dependency; the agent; its half-life; route and speed of administration; and patient factors such as genetic variability, drug interaction, levels of pain, concurrent medical illness, and emotional condition.

Neuromuscular

Opioids reduce cerebrometabolic oxygen consumption, slow electroencephalogram, can cause myoclonus and muscle rigidity, and may cause seizure should they accumulate in the body (e.g., normeperidine, norpropoxyphene, dextromethorphan, tramadol).

Endocrine

Opioids can cause a decrease in levels of testosterone; an increase in levels of prolactin; a decrease in sexual libido; and syndrome of inappropriate diuresis hormone.

Cardiovascular

Opioids produce peripheral vasodilation. Hence, morphine unloads the heart in acute pulmonary edema, but can cause orthostatic hypotension, or bradycardia by increase vagal tone, or can accelerate heart rate notably with meperidine.

Pulmonary

Opioids have a direct effect on the medulla causing depression in cough reflex and respiration. Opioids can have a greater effect on ribcage breathing than diaphragmatic excursion. Therefore, patients with chronic-obstructive pulmonary disease, obesity, or recent abdominal surgery are at the greatest risk for respiratory depression. Also at risk for pulmonary depression are neonates and the elderly who are more sensitive to opioids.

Gastrointestinal

Opioids have a strong effect on the gastrointestinal submucosal plexus, leading to decreased levels of HCl, pancreatic and biliary secretions, and peristalsis. In addition, opioids can increase segmental contractions resulting in nausea, vomiting, reflux, and constipation. Opioids may or may not increase pressure in the sphincter of Oddi.

Gynecological

Opioids relax uterus tone and prolong labor and may well cross the placenta.

Immunological

Opioids reduce immunological responses.

Kidneys

Opioids have no significant effects on kidneys and are generally metabolized by the liver. However, in cases of renal failure, accumulation of problematic metabolites like M6G, norpropoxyphene, and normeperidine may occur. Methadone does not have problematic metabolites but also will accumulate. Hydromorphone, oxycodone, and fentanyl do not have problematic metabolites.

OPIOID-DEPENDENT PATIENTS

The use of opioids as a proper vehicle for pain relief often is followed with concerns about its addictive properties. Studies have shown that there are two forms of dependence that can occur for patients treated with opioids.

Physical dependence represents a physiological response to the effects of chronic opioid use. It describes the phenomenon of withdrawal when an opioid is abruptly discontinued or if an opioid antagonist is administered. Withdrawal syndrome manifested by symptoms of increased sympathetic hyperactivity. It can be prevented by slowly tapering the dose of the opioid or can be reversed by reinstituting the drug in doses of 25% to 40% of previous dose.

Psychological dependence is another term for addiction. It is a psychological and behavioral syndrome characterized by a continued craving for an opioid, which is manifested as compulsive drug-seeking behavior. Anyone who is addicted to opioids is likely to be physically dependent, however, it is possible to be physically dependent without being addicted.

CLINICAL APPLICATION OF OPIOID ANALGESICS

Despite the enormous amount of data available on the pharmacology of opioids, providing a patient with effective analgesia and a precise dosing schedule for a specific pain problem often is difficult and time consuming. This is in part because of the subjectiveness of pain and the difficulties in measuring it; the individual variations in drug requirement; the limited knowledge of the pharmacodynamic relationship of the analgesia; and the side effects of these drugs. Therefore, the following several steps should be considered before prescribing analgesics for an individual patient.

1. Detailed history on effects of the opioids previously used, side effects experienced, long-term usage, and tolerance.
2. Careful physical examination to determine the cause of the painful symptomatology.
3. After the diagnosis is established and the mechanism of pain determined, other factors should be considered prior to a therapeutic plan. Factors that should be accounted for include patient age, physical, nutritional, and mental status; renal and hepatic function; ability to follow instructions; and family support.

By taking into account all of the above factors; an effective analgesic regimen can be formulated. In short, one must use the most effective drug or combination of drugs for a specific pain state that will produce the least serious or distressful side effects.

CONCLUSION

As the understanding of the pharmacological aspects and clinical experience of opioids become more widespread in the medical communities, medical professionals have become more accepting of the use of opioids for the treatment of pain in both acute and chronic settings. The variety of opium derivatives, from naturally occurring to synthetic, allows the medical personnel the flexibility to cater a treatment regimen that takes into account the myriad of medical complexity, types of pain, and potential side effects affecting their patients. Ongoing and future research and advances in the clinical use of opioid drugs together with parallel growth in the understanding of opioid mechanisms hopefully will counteract under treatment of pain and opiophobia.

SELECTED READINGS

Arner S, Myerson BA. Lack of analgesic effect of opioids on neuropathic and idiopathic forms of pain. *Pain* 1988;33:11–23.

Beaver WT. Combination analgesics. *Am J Med* 1984;77:38–53.

Covino BG. Comparative efficacy of post-operative pain control techniques. In: Stanley, TH, Ashburn MA, Fine PG, eds. *Anesthesiology in Pain Management*. Dordrecht, the Netherlands: Kluwer Academic, 1991: 249–256.

Foley KM. The practical use of narcotic analgesics. *Med Clin North Am* 1982;66:1091–1104.

Foley KM. Clinical tolerance to opioids. In: Basbaum AI, Besson JM, eds. *Towards a New Pharmacotherapy of Pain*. Bahlem Konferenzen. Chichester, Great Britain: Wiley, 1991:181–204.

Gibson TP, Giacomini JC, Gibson TP, et al. Propoxyphene and norpropoxyphene plasma concentrations in the anephric patient. *Clin Pharmacol Ther* 1980;27:665–670.

Intrurrisi CE. Effects of other drugs and pathologic states on opioid disposition and response. In: Benedetti C, Giron G, Chapman CR, eds. *Advances in Pain Research and Therapy*, vol. 14. New York: Raven, 1990:171–181.

Intrurrisi CE, Colburn WA. Pharmacokinetics of methadone. In: Foley KM, Inturrisi CE, eds. *Opioid Analgesics in the Management of Clinical Pain*. New York: Raven, 1986:191–199.

Knapp RJ, Malatynska E, Fang L, et al. Identification of a human delta opioid receptor: cloning and expression. *Life Sci* 1994;54:463–469.

Mansson E, Bare L, Yang D. Isolation of a human kappa opioid receptor cDNA from placenta. *Biochem Biophys Res Commun* 1994;202: 1431–1437.

Osborne RJ, Joel S, Trew D, et al. Morphine and metabolite behavior and different routes of morphine administration; demonstration of the active metabolite morphine-6-glucoronide. *Clin Pharmacol Ther* 1990;47: 12–19.

Pick CG, Roques B, Gacel G, et al. Supraspinal $\mu2$ receptors mediate spinal/supraspinal morphine synergy. *Eur J Pharmacol* 1992;220: 275–277.

Portenoy RK. Chronic opioid therapy in nonmalignant pain. *J Pain Symptom Manage* 1990;5:S46–S62.

Portenoy RK, Foley KM, Stulman J, et al. Plasma morphine and morphine-6-glucuronide during chronic morphine therapy for cancer pain: plasma profiles, steady-state concentrations and the consequences of renal failure. *Pain* 1991;47:13–19.

Portenoy RK, Southam MA, Gupta SK, et al. Transdermal fentanyl for cancer pain. *Anesthesiology* 1993;78:36–43.

Portenoy RK, Thaler HT, Inturrisi CE, et al. The metabolite morphine-6-glucoronide contributes to the analgesia produced by morphine infusion in patients with pain and normal renal function. *Clin Pharmacol Ther* 1992;51:422–431.

Porter J, Jick H. Addiction rare in patients treated with narcotics. *N Engl J Med* 1980;302:123.

Raynor K, Kong H, Chen Y, et al. Pharmacological characterization of the cloned kappa-, delta- and mu-opioid receptors. *Mol Pharmacol* 1994;45:330–334.

Rossi G, Pasternak GW, Bodnar RJ. Synergistic brainstem interactions for morphine analgesia. *Brain Res* 1993;624:171–180.

Sawe J, Svensson JO, Odar-Cederlof I. Kinetics of morphine in patients with renal failure. *Lancet* 1985;2:211.

Sawynok J. The therapeutic use of heroin: a review of the pharmacological literature. *Can J Physiol Pharmacol* 1986;64:1–6.

Shepherd K. Review of a controlled-release morphine preparation. In: Foley KM, Bonica JJ, Ventafridda V, eds. *Advances in Pain Research and Therapy*, vol. 16. Second International Congress on Cancer Pain. New York: Raven, 1990:191–202.

Smith MT, Watt JA, Cramond T. Morphine-3-glucuronide — a potent antagonist of morphine analgesia. *Life Sci* 1990;47:579–585.

Wallenstein SL, Kaiko RF, Rogers AG, et al. Crossover trials in clinical analgesic assays: studies of buprenorphine and morphine. *Pharmacotherapy* 1986;6:228–235.

CHAPTER 46

Patient-Controlled Analgesia

Kimberly A. Cox and Hilary J. Fausett

Patient-activated systems for pain control have been described for over 20 years. The initial device was a machine that dispensed intravenous analgesics on demand. The "dropmaster" was a bulky device that consisted of two units, a larger control unit and a smaller unit, which delivered the drug. This smaller unit housed a maintenance-infusion bottle and an analgesic-infusion bottle connected by tubing that passed through a solenoid valve to control the infusion stream. The larger unit housed the following controls: (a) a totalizer, which is now referred to as the drug dose; (b) a refractory-period timer, now known as a lockout-interval; (c) an autodrug changer, which allowed as many as four different drugs in sequence to be dispensed; and (d) a recorder, which registered the drug currently in use. In designing this device, special safety functions were built into the system, which are still used today. The first of these safety devices is that a drug will be dispensed only when requested by a patient. The other safety devices include a solenoid valve (which controls the flow of medication into the intravenous line) that closes in the event of a power failure, a set refractory period, and a set total dose. The ultimate safety factor built into the system was the volume of drug available to enter the system. Only a certain amount of drug was allowed in the system at any given time.

Today, there are several patient-controlled analgesic (PCA) pumps available with different features (Table 46.1). Refinements of this system now permit administration of continuous background infusion superimposed on patient-controlled boluses. These new devices also allow the system to record a profile of a drug administration, including number of requests the patient made for a dose of medication, the requests that did not result in drug delivery, and total amount of the agent that were administered per unit time.

There are several opioids available for PCA use. When choosing a drug for PCA administration, the ideal drug would be highly efficacious, have a rapid onset of action, and a moderate duration of effect. The ideal drug should not accumulate or change pharmacokinetic properties with repeated administrations and should have a large therapeutic window.

Morphine, the drug most widely prescribed by this route, is far from ideal. However, one must keep in mind there is no ideal opioid and all opioid agonists have side effects. Patients who use morphine by way of the PCA pump tend to reach a level of comfort, however, that usually is in balance between acceptable pain and minimal side effects.

With PCA, a patient can maintain a plasma concentration of opioid close to the minimum effective analgesic concentration that approximates the concentration at the receptor site. The most effective protocol for the use of PCA for acute pain is to begin with an intravenous (IV) bolus of morphine, for example, starting with 4 mg for a 70-kg awake adult and then slowly titrate enough IV morphine to have the patient comfortable within 20 to 30 minutes. Patients must be monitored carefully and observed for any signs of drug accumulation and toxicity. Often, this initial loading is done in a recovery-room setting. Once the patient is comfortable, the parameters of the PCA pump are set to deliver a 1- to 2-mg bolus of morphine (depending on the patient's age and surgical procedure) with each request and a lockout period of 6 to 15 minutes. The lockout period prevents redosing before the drug has time to take effect, and thus minimizes the risk of opiate overdose. Table 46.2 represents guidelines regarding bolus doses, lockout intervals, and continuous infusion for various parenteral analgesics when using a PCA system.

Some problems encountered with PCA therapy are primarily the result of operator or mechanical errors. Because patients titrate their own therapy, they must be capable of understanding the concept of the device, be able to activate the device, and be willing to participate in their own treatment plan. It is incumbent upon the physi-

TABLE 46.1. *Patient-Controlled Analgesia Pumps*

Feature	Model						
	Pharmacia-Deltec	Prominject	Harvard PCA 4000	Abbott Lifecare PCA Infusor	ODAC	Cardiff Palliator	Palliator MS 402
Incremental dose[a]	Variable in mg	Variable in units of mass (e.g., mg, μg)	Variable in mL	Variable in mL	Variable in mL	Variable in mL	Variable in mg
Background infusion mode available	Yes	Yes	No	Yes	Yes	No	Yes
Concentration setting	Six preset concentrations	Variable in units of mass/L	No	No; prepacked drugs in special syringes used	Yes; results in printer output in mg	Set as dilution from 1–400 μL/mg	Variable from 1–99 mg/mL
Lockout time[a]	Variable from 5–199 min	Variable from 5–999 min	Variable from 3–60 min	Variable from 5–99 min	Variable from 1–99 min	Variable from 1–99 min	Variable from 1–30 min
Infusion rate or infusion time	1 min/bolus	1 min for bolus dose, 1 h for optional follow-up infusion	Bolus dose 2.5 mL/min	Fixed, 4 mL/min	Background variable in mL/min 0.01–0.99	Variable from 1–99 mL/h	Variable from 3–15 min
Cumulative dose display	Yes	Yes	Yes	Yes	On printer	Yes	Yes
Patient demand signal	Single press	Two presses/1 sec	Single press	Single press	Two presses/1 sec	Two presses/1 sec	Two presses/2 sec
Printer	No	Yes	Yes	Interface	Yes	No	Interface
Battery power	Yes	Yes	Yes	Yes	Yes	No	Yes
Manufacturer	Pharmacia-Deltec	Pharmacia AB, Sweden	C.R. Bard, Inc., United States	Abbott Laboratories, United States	Janssen Scientific, Belgium	Graseby Medical Ltd., U.K.	Graseby Medical Ltd., U.K.

[a]A combination of *dose* setting and *lockout time* setting gives a maximum *dose*/hour for all machines, but this is not a preset feature.

Adapted from Lammer P, Bullingham RES, Jacobs OLR. The PRODAC demand analgesia computer. In: Harmer M, Rosen M, Vickers MD, eds. *Patient-Controlled Analgesia*. Oxford: Blackwell Scientific Publications, 1986:106–107.

TABLE 46.2. *Guidelines Regarding the Bolus Doses, Lockout Intervals, and Continuous Infusions for Various Parenteral Analgesics When Using a PCA System*

Drug	Bolus Dose (mg)	Lockout Interval (min)	Continuous Infusion (mg/h^{-1})
Agonists			
Fentanyl citrate	0.015–0.05	3–10	0.02–0.1
Hydromorphone hydrochloride	0.10–0.5	5–15	0.2–0.5
Meperidine hydrochloride	5–15	5–15	5–40
Methadone hydrochloride	0.50–3.0	10–20	—
Morphine sulfate	0.50–3.0[a]	5–20	1–10
Oxymorphone hydrochloride	0.20–0.8	5–15	0.1–1
Sufentanil citrate	0.003–0.015	3–10	0.004–0.03
Agonist–Antagonists			
Buprenorphine hydrochloride	0.03–0.2	10–20	—
Nalbupine hydrochloride	1–5	5–15	1–8
Pentazocine hydrochloride	5–30	5–15	6–40

[a]For pediatric dosing, see Lubenow TR, McCarthy RJ, Ivankovich AD. Management of acute postoperative pain. In: Barash PG, Cullen BF, Stoelting RK, eds. *Clinical Anesthesia, 2nd ed.* Philadelphia: J.B. Lippincott, 1992:1547–1577, from which this table is reproduced with permission.

cian to ensure the patient has been appropriately educated about the device and oriented to its proper usage. This usually can be accomplished in the recovery room by a properly trained recovery-room nurse.

There has not been much literature generated on the incidence of respiratory depression and/or respiratory arrest in patients on PCA. Many of the case reports concerning untoward outcomes of patients using a PCA were in association with adverse drug interactions, continuous narcotic infusion, nurse and or physician-controlled analgesia, and inappropriate use of PCA by patients.

PCA addressed the problem of inadequate analgesia being given to hospitalized patients. It gives the patient a sense of control over their pain and alleviates much of the fear of future pain. Compared with traditional methods of on-demand analgesic delivery, PCA has been shown to provide superior analgesia with less total drug use, less sedation, fewer nocturnal sleep disturbances, and more rapid return to physical activity.

In delivering analgesia in a very cost-conscious medical system, obtaining pumps for PCA does imply an initial capital investment by the hospital. This cost is offset by the time saved by nursing personnel, who do not have to administer drugs on a routine basis. Effective analgesia is an important factor in preventing postoperative complications and thus helps in decreasing time and cost of hospitalization. Also, patient satisfaction is an invaluable advertisement for a hospital's service.

The use of PCA currently is accepted in most hospitals as an excellent way to control acute pain postoperatively. PCA also is suitable for oncology patients and patients with chronic pain with acute exacerbation such as pancreatitis, and so its usage need not be confined to postoperative patients. PCA is a wonderful tool with rapidly expanding possibilities.

SELECTED READINGS

Barash PG, Cullen BF, Stoelting RK. *Clinical Anesthesia*, 4th ed. Philadelphia: Lippincott Williams & Wilkins, 2000.

Egbert AM, Parks LH, Short LM, et al. Randomized trial of postoperative PCA vs intramuscular narcotics in frail men. *Arch Intern Med* 1990;150:1897–1903.

Forrest WH, Smethurst PW, Kienitz ME, et al. Self administration of intravenous analgesics. *Anesthesiology* 1970;33:363–365.

Sechzer PH. Objective measurement of pain. *Anesthesiology* 1968;29:209.

Tamsen A, Hartvig P, Fagerlund C, et al. Patient controlled analgesic therapy, part one: pharmacokinetics of pethidine in the perioperative periods. *Clin Pharmacokinet* 1982;7:149–163.

White PF. Mishaps with PCA. *Anesthesiology* 1987;66:81–83.

Injection Therapies

CHAPTER 47

Trigger-Point Injections

Eric M. Emont and Hilary J. Fausett

Trigger-point injections are commonly used to treat the painful, taut, knots and bands of myofascial-pain syndromes. A patient who has pain in a particular area first must be carefully examined and diagnosed. Myofascial-pain syndromes may be confused with other regional-pain syndromes, such as bursitis, tendonitis, or nerve-root irritation. Both chronic abdominal pain and chronic pelvic pain may on occasion be secondary to myofascial dysfunction.

There is certainly a tremendous amount of overlap between the presentation of patients with fibromyalgia and with myofascial-pain syndromes. The two entities usually are separated by the history of auxiliary symptoms seen with fibromyalgia and the absence of definitive trigger points on physical examination. Patients with fibromyalgia are much more likely to have "tender points" as opposed to distinct trigger points.

If a patient has symptoms consistent with a myofascial-pain syndrome, the examiner should carefully palpate the area of the patient's pain. The involved muscle is likely to be a taut, tender band that runs parallel to the direction of the muscle. Within this band are discrete, localized areas of tenderness that often are hard or nodular. Placing the muscle under slight tension, with a gentle stretch, often helps to isolate the trigger point. The area should be palpated gently with the fingertips. Some practitioners prefer a gentle circular motion, while others think that stroking the muscle in the direction of the muscle fibers, or perpendicular to them, is the quickest way to determine the presence of any nodules. These are the "trigger points." Trigger points often are located within the mid-depth of the muscle body, but can occur anywhere, even near bony-insertion sites. Pressure with palpation of these nodules should reproduce the patient's pain. Often, palpation of a trigger point will create a radiating band of dysesthesia, or altered sensation. Patients may describe burning, shooting, or numbness. A contraction of the muscle in response to palpation of the trigger point is called a "twitch response" if the same muscle is involved or a "jump sign" if a region distinct to the muscle is involved.

Trigger points are classified further as active or latent and primary or secondary. An active trigger point causes the patient pain without any palpation of the area, whereas a latent trigger point is found on examination, and only when palpated does the patient get the feeling of pain. Primary trigger points are the nidus of the pain syndrome and secondary trigger points develop from another pain syndrome or abnormality (such as an antalgic gait). Treating any instigating or contributing factors is the most important intervention in providing pain relief from trigger points. Thus, if a patient has a gait disturbance, treating the problem appropriately should result in resolution of the secondary trigger-point abnormality.

CASE REPORT

A 22-year-old college student presented to the pain management center with pain in the neck that radiated to the right arm, wrist, and lateral two fingers. She played intramural basketball and was worried that she had injured herself during aggressive play. She reported being in the middle of midterm examinations and had several papers she was in the middle of writing, but now found herself unable to type. Physical examination revealed a muscular young woman with taut and tender muscle bands along her neck, shoulder, and upper back. Pressure on a tender nodule along her scapula reproduced her pain and the burning sensation she had. Further questioning revealed that she had been typing on a laptop computer while sitting on a bed. She was given instructions in proper body mechanics and advised to find a full-sized keyboard, if typing had to remain an activity for her.

She returned 3 weeks later with significant improvement in symptoms, but the trigger point remained. The risks and benefits of injecting the trigger point then were discussed with her.

The pathophysiology of trigger points remains controversial, as testing is difficult to do. Imaging studies and laboratory analysis is within normal limits. Muscle biopsies have not proved diagnostic. There are some reports of electromyographic (EMG) studies revealing a "silent center" to the trigger point that then becomes active with manipulation, but this is controversial and the significance of this finding is unclear.

The generation of trigger points appears to be multifactorial. Overuse and tiring of the muscle and subsequent build up of the toxic byproducts of metabolism may play a role. The release of sensitizing substances from these locally ischemic areas may contribute to the generation of radiating pain. It is possible that the muscle spasm may directly affect a nerve causing impingement, or that the algogenic substances released activate nerve transmission.

The hallmark of treating any myofascial-pain syndrome is to identify any instigating or aggravating factors. Because body positioning, posture, type of physical activity, and stress all play a role in the generation and maintenance of trigger points, all of these factors must be addressed. Some patients may develop trigger points following trauma such as a motor vehicle accident. For these patients as well, the first approach should be the most holistic and noninvasive.

The goal of therapy is to restore the abnormal muscle area to normal-muscle conditions. If physical therapy, massage, stretching, and proper muscle conditioning is not sufficient, the patient may need a trigger-point injection. There are several methods described for injection of a trigger point, and each method has its proponents. The first area of controversy is whether the chosen needle should be small (25 or 30 gauge) to avoid causing further trauma to the muscle, or whether a larger needle (20 or 22 gauge) should be used to "disrupt" the nodule and promote more normal healing. Because there is no consensus as to the pathogenesis of trigger points, there is no agreement on their management.

Whether substances should be injected or whether it is the mechanical aspect of entering the trigger point with the needle that has the therapeutic effect is not clear. This latter technique is called "dry needling" and has many strong proponents, especially amongst homeopathic practitioners. The classic trigger-point injection, however, refers to the injection of local anesthetic into the tender nodule under sterile conditions. Some practitioners add steroid to the local anesthetic to provide some antiinflammatory activity. There is no evidence that the addition of small amounts of steroid makes any difference in the resolution of symptoms, and the complications of intramuscular steroid injection include localized irritation and muscle atrophy as well as systemic effects such as decreased plasma-cortisol levels and increased blood-glucose levels.

TECHNIQUE

With the patient sitting or lying in a comfortable position, the taut muscle band is palpated gently (Fig. 47.1). The nodule of the trigger point is identified and isolated by carefully holding the skin and segment of underlying muscle between the thumb and forefinger (Fig. 47.2). The area is wiped clean with an alcohol wipe or other antiseptic. A 25-gauge needle is advanced until the "twitch response" is seen (Fig. 47.3). The patient may report that the referred pain has been evoked or the practitioner may notice the "jump sign." A small amount of local anesthetic then is injected (perhaps 1 to 2 mL of a mixture of lidocaine 1% and bupivacaine 0.25%). Some advocates suggest following this with a small "fan block" to the area to ensure good spread to the taut muscle. The muscle then is stretched gently to promote distribution of the local anesthetic and, perhaps, increase blood flow to the area.

Patients usually report near-immediate pain relief. During this therapeutic window of analgesia, it is important that the patient practice good body mechanics and initiate gentle stretching exercises.

Case Reports

Patient 1

A 56-year-old college professor was referred to the pain management center with pain in her lower back that

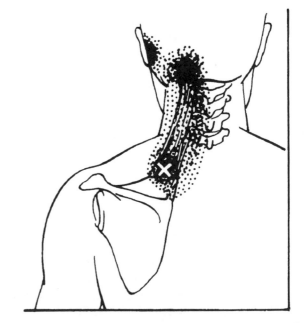

FIG. 47.1. The patient's area of pain should be identified. This illustration shows the trigger point of the levator scapulae muscle and the distribution of the patient's pain. The symptoms can be reproduced by palpation (Reprinted from Loeser JD, Butler SH, Chapman CR, et al., eds. *Bonica's Management of Pain*, 3rd ed. Philadelphia: Lippincott Williams & Wilkins, 2001, with permission.)

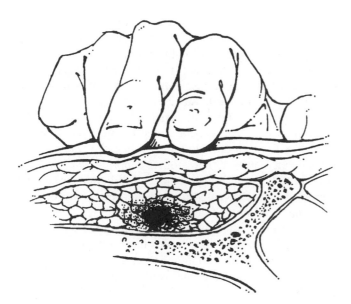

FIG. 47.2. The trigger point is palpated carefully with the fingertips and then isolated by firmly grasping the tense muscle band to hold the trigger point stationary (Reprinted from Loeser JD, Butler SH, Chapman CR, et al., eds. *Bonica's Management of Pain*, 3rd ed. Philadelphia: Lippincott Williams & Wilkins, 2001, with permission.)

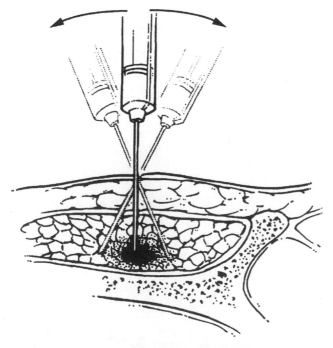

FIG. 47.3. After cleaning the skin with an antiseptic alcohol solution, a fine, 25-gauge needle is advanced into the trigger point. A total of 1.5 mL of local anesthetic (an equal part mixture of 1.0% lidocaine and 0.25% bupivacaine) is injected into the trigger point directly and then "fanned" to the local area. The muscle then is stretched gently (Reprinted from Loeser JD, Butler SH, Chapman CR, et al., eds. *Bonica's Management of Pain*, 3rd ed. Philadelphia: Lippincott Williams & Wilkins, 2001, with permission.)

radiated to her left leg. She also had midback pain that radiated to her left scapula. Physical examination revealed multiple taut muscle bands and several discrete trigger points. Review of her work environment revealed that she was using a computer that was positioned on a credenza and not a desk, because of inadequate office space during a campus-remodeling project. Her employer did not offer any type of ergonomic work-place assessment. Alter carefully educating her and providing her with a referral for physical therapy, the risks and benefits of trigger-point injections were discussed. In the sitting position, her left lower back and left middle back were palpated carefully and the trigger points were marked. Each was individually isolated and held firmly while prepped with alcohol for antisepsis. A new, 25-gauge needle was injected into each trigger point and 1.0 mL of an equal part mixture of lidocaine 1% and bupivacaine 0.25% was injected into each trigger point sequentially until all five trigger points were anesthetized adequately. She reported 50% pain relief that day. She returned weekly for four further treatments. At this point, the remodeling project was complete and she was able to use a normal desk. Her pain was over 75% improved and she saw no further need to continue with injections while she was continuing with physical therapy and an exercise program.

The technique of "dry needling" or using a large-gauge needle to disrupt the trigger point varies somewhat from the technique described above. Once the patient is positioned and comfortable, the trigger point is identified by palpation. The trigger point is injected with 0.5 to 1.0 mL of lidocaine, 1.0%. Once the trigger point is anesthetized, a 20-gauge needle is rapidly advanced in and out of the trigger point several times. The theory is to "break up" the ischemic nodule and improve regional blood flow. Patients will report an increase in their pain for a few days and may experience some localized bruising and perhaps tenderness. Once the area starts to heal, however, the pain should be diminished and the patient should be much improved.

Patient 2

A 29-year-old intensive-care nurse and mother of twin girls complained to her husband, a pain management fellow, of pain in her right upper back and scapula that limited her ability to move her right arm. Her husband diagnosed her with a myofascial pain syndrome and performed three trigger-point injections using a 25-gauge needle and injecting each site with 1.5 mL of 1.0% lidocaine followed by gentle stretching. She reported a decrease in the pain in her shoulder, but felt a new sensation of pain with inspiration. The next day she saw her primary-care physician who ordered a chest x-ray. The radiograph revealed a small apical pneumothorax that did not require any further intervention.

The contraindications to trigger-point injections include infection or other lesion at the site, a coagulopathy, and sepsis (any infection is a contraindication for the use of steroids). The risks of doing trigger-point injections include failure to reveal pain and potential to evoke pain; bleeding; infection; nerve injury; and pneumothorax.

Botulinum toxin is used to treat the muscle spasm of torticollis and blepharospasm. Botulinum toxin A is derived from a culture of *Clostridium botulinum*. The toxin works by irreversibly binding to presynaptic, cholinergic nerve terminals and thus prevents the release of acetylcholine, which should result in sustained muscle relaxation. The nerve endings are a dynamic environment and the blocked receptors eventually are replenished and with reinnervation of the nerve terminal, muscle activity returns to normal. The onset of the effect of the botulinum toxin (Botox, Allergan, Inc., Irvine, CA, U.S.A.) is within 3 to 7 days. The effect lasts a few months, with near-complete return to baseline function by 12 weeks. Repeated injections may lose their effectiveness, as the patient may develop antibodies to the preparation. The use of Botox to treat myofascial-pain syndromes is new and controversial. The other modalities available to treat trigger points should all be tried before proceeding with a Botox injection.

Patient 3

A 41-year-old woman reported 5 years of pain in the left buttocks that radiated to the upper thigh. She had been diagnosed with a myofascial-pain syndrome. She had had multiple trigger-point injections with temporary relief and she continued to do the daily stretching and exercise routine she was taught in physical therapy. Three trigger points were injected in her left lower back with a mixture of Botox 10 mouse units per 1 mL of bupivacaine 0.25%. A total of 4 mL was used for the three sites. She left the pain management center smiling with joy and being pain-free. The patient called the next day to complain that the shot did "nothing." When she was called 1 week later, however, her mother reported that she had gone out shopping and had never felt better. Follow-up visit at 4 weeks revealed mild tenderness along the left lower back but no distinct trigger points.

Trigger-point injections may provide good but temporary relief of pain. Trigger-point injections must be part of a multidisciplinary approach to therapy that likely will include lifestyle changes and well as injections, and perhaps medications.

SELECTED READINGS

Abram SE, Haddox JD. *The Pain Clinic Manual*. Philadelphia: Lippincott, Williams & Wilkins, 2000:167–176.

Newman LD. Myofascial pain syndrome: a comprehensive review. *Clin J Pain* 1998;4:74–85.

Porta M. A comparative trial of botulinum toxin type A and methylprednisolone for the treatment of myofascial pain syndrome and pain from chronic muscle spasm. *Pain* 2000;85:101–105.

Simons DG, Travell JG, Simons LS. *Travell & Simons' Myofascial Pain and Dysfunction: The Trigger Point Manual: Upper Half of Body*. Philadelphia: Lippincott, Williams & Wilkins, 1998.

Travell J, Simons DG. *Myofascial Pain and Dysfunction: The Trigger Point Manual: The Lower Extremities*. Philadelphia: Lippincott, Williams & Wilkins, 1991.

CHAPTER 48

Epidural-Steroid Injections

Charles C. Ho and Zahid H. Bajwa

Steroids can be delivered epidurally by way of a cervical, thoracic, lumbar, caudal, sacral, and transforaminal nerve-root blocks. Epidural steroids are most commonly used for the treatment of lumbosacral radiculopathy and spinal stenosis but have been used for other types and locations of spinal pain. The use of corticosteroids to treat pain caused by inflammation is not a new concept. In the 1920s, Hench first began to use systemic steroids successfully to treat painful arthritis. At about the same time, European physicians began injecting various substances, both intrathecally and epidurally, in an attempt to treat low-back pain. In 1952, the first recorded use of epidural-steroid injections by Robechhi and Capra was a peri-radicular injection of hydrocortisone into the first sacral root. In 1960, Goebert reported successful treatment of sciatica with epidural injection of procaine and hydrocortisone by way of the caudal approach. Since that time, many investigators and clinicians have treated back and radicular pain with intraspinal (epidural or subarachnoid) steroids with varying results. Through decades of clinical experience, the indications and techniques for epidural-steroid injection have been quite well defined, and as a result this therapy now is commonly used to treat spinal stenosis, cervical, thoracic, and lumbosacral radiculopathies.

INDICATIONS

Much of the failure of the early trials of intraspinal steroid therapy may have resulted from inappropriate patient selection. In the early years, the technique was enthusiastically performed on patients with all types of back pain, including muscle strain, fractures, and referred pain. Today it is widely accepted that epidural steroids are most effective for the treatment of spinal-radicular pain.

Radicular pain has characteristic qualities of burning, shooting, or lancinating pain that travels along a dermatomal distribution. There may be motor, reflex, or sen-

sory deficits as a result of spinal-nerve root irritation or compression. The straight-leg raise test is useful in reproducing the symptoms of lumbar radiculopathy. The patient is supine with the knee fully extended and the examiner raises each leg up to approximately 70 degrees. The test is considered positive if there is reproduction of pain radiating below the knee. Pain may be worsened by ankle dorsiflexion or other maneuvers causing traction of the irritated nerve root. Cervical radiculopathy presents as pain radiating into the arm or hand. Patients may have complaint of weakness, numbness, and tingling along the distribution of the cervical roots. Maneuvers to reproduce pain include forced full flexion of the neck and Spurling's maneuver, which is extension and lateral deviation of the neck towards the symptomatic side.

In 1934, Mixter and Barr demonstrated a relationship between intervertebral disc protrusion and radicular pain. They believed that the radiculopathy was caused by the mechanical compression of the nerve roots by the disc. However, mechanical compression alone is not enough to cause symptoms, as there are asymptomatic patients with nerve-root compression secondary to herniated discs. In 1951, Lindahl and Rexed attributed sciatica to a persistent inflammatory irritation of nerve roots, secondary to mechanical compression by herniated disc material or bony contact. The role of inflammation in back pain is supported by the observation during lumbar laminectomy under local anesthesia that inflamed spinal nerves adjacent to a prolapsed disc are very sensitive to minor manipulations, whereas uninflamed nerves can be manipulated with very little discomfort. Because corticosteroids suppress both the early (e.g., edema, capillary dilation) and late (e.g., fibroblast proliferation) manifestations of the inflammatory response, it seemed logical that direct application of those agents into the epidural space, where root compression most commonly occurs, would be of benefit. The theoretical advantages of epidural-steroid injections over systemic steroids include deposition of the drug into the affected area and less systemic side effects from lower blood levels of steroid.

MECHANISM OF EFFECT

The effectiveness of epidural steroids is thought to be the result of reduction of nerve-root swelling and inflammation. Improvement in clinical symptoms has been shown to coincide with improvement of nerve-root edema in the presence of herniated disc. Steroids induce the biosynthesis of a phospholipase A-2 inhibitor. This acts to decrease inflammation by inhibiting the action of phospholipase A-2, which is an enzyme that liberates arachidonic acid from cell membranes. Arachidonic acid is needed for the production of prostaglandins and leukotrienes.

There are other proposed reasons for the effectiveness of epidural steroids in pain relief. Corticosteroids may have a membrane-stabilizing effect by inhibiting discharge from irritated nerve roots. They were found to inhibit ectopic discharge from experimentally created neuromas. Steroids have been found to block transmission of nociceptive C-fiber input by a direct membrane action. Neuraxial steroids may inhibit central sensitization of the dorsal-horn neurons by blocking prostaglandin production. Increased irritation of the dorsal-horn neurons is mediated partly by production of prostaglandins.

PATHOLOGY

Radiculopathy is caused by irritation of the spinal-nerve roots. Intervertebral disc degeneration may cause mechanical compression with subsequent inflammation of the nerve roots. This can be caused by disc herniation or narrowing of the disc space impinging upon the spinal nerve roots as it exits through the intervertebral foramen. Studies by Marshall and Trethwie documented histological evidence of inflammation in the spinal nerve roots of patients undergoing operations for herniated discs. Spondylolisthesis, spondylolysis, and osteophytes are other causes of mechanical-root compression.

Within the intervertebral disc, there is a high concentration of phospholipase A-2. A small leak of phospholipase A-2 can cause an intense inflammatory reaction in the surrounding neural tissue. Its concentration was 20 to 10,000 that of normal tissue when samples were obtained from disk surgery patients. McCarron et al. showed that autologous-nucleus pulposus material in the epidural space caused inflammation in the epidural spaces of dogs. They were found to have biochemical and histological evidence of intense inflammation on gross inspection and microscopic analysis of the spinal cord, dural sac, and nerve roots after daily injections of autologous-nucleus pulposus for 5 days. They were compared to control animals that had saline injections.

CONTRAINDICATIONS

Epidural steroid injection in properly trained hands is considered a safe procedure. Its absolute contraindications include patient refusal and bleeding diathesis. The passage of the epidural needle may puncture an epidural vein resulting in an epidural hematoma. An epidural hematoma can lead to compression, ischemia, or infarction of the spinal cord or nerve roots. It is relatively contraindicated in severe hypovolemia and the presence of infections such as local infection at the site of puncture or septicemia. A profound hypotension may develop with use of local anesthetics causing a sympathectomy. There is a greater risk of developing an epidural abscess in infectious states and in diabetics. Steroids should be used carefully in patients susceptible to fluid retention and congestive heart failure.

There are certain red flags in the physical examination that should prompt further inquiry into the source of pain. A history of trauma may increase the suspicion for fractures. Symptoms of systemic illness such as fever, chills, malaise, and weight loss could signal infection or neoplasm. Recent-onset bowel or bladder dysfunction should be considered spinal-cord compression or cauda equina syndrome until proven otherwise.

ROUTE OF ADMINISTRATION

For many years, there was considerable controversy over whether the injections should be performed in the epidural space or intrathecally. In 1972, Winnie published a study concluding that the procedure was equally effective either way, but the epidural route is preferable for several reasons. Because root compression in discogenic disease occurs most commonly in the epidural space, that seems a logical place for delivery of the corticosteroid. In addition, the epidural route substantially reduces the risk of spinal headache. On the other hand, intrathecal injections may induce more severe postinjection pain, and the vehicle may cause neural damage intrathecally in some circumstances although it is rarely a clinical problem. Some of the preservatives in commercially available steroids such as polyethylene glycol have been shown to be neurotoxic in animal studies. Some clinicians feel that the intrathecal route for steroid injection is indicated in cases of adhesive arachnoiditis, but that remains controversial. The inhibitory effect of intrathecal steroids on the development of reticulin network and cellular elements of arachnoidal adhesions may explain its effectiveness in treating arachnoiditis.

Epidural Administration

The epidural route generally is preferred over the intrathecal route. Epidural-steroid injection should be performed by a skilled specialist who can reliably identify the epidural space even in patients with unusual anatomy, such as that often seen after laminectomy. Another technical requirement is that the injection be given at the level of the affected nerve roots. For example, an epidural-steroid injection should be administered at the L5–S1 interspace in a patient with clinical signs of an L5–S1 disc herniation. The epidural space can be entered through the caudal, sacral, lumbar, thoracic, cervical, and transforaminal routes.

The epidural space is a potential space between the ligamentum flavum and the dura mater. The space exists from the foramen magnum superiorly and extends down to the sacral hiatus inferiorly. The anterior boundary is the posterior longitudinal ligament and the lateral boundaries are the periosteum of the pedicles of the vertebrae and the intervertebral foramina. The structures encountered from the skin in a midline approach are the supraspinous ligament, interspinous ligament, ligamentum flavum, and epidural space. Contents of the epidural space include epidural fat, lymphatics, veins, and arteries. It is possible to inadvertently inject intravascularly or cause spinal-cord ischemia if a spinal artery is traumatized.

The patient may be positioned in the lateral decubitus position with the painful side down to promote contact of the steroid with the affected nerve roots or sitting position, which allows easier location of the midline. After the patient is positioned, the area is prepped and draped. Using sterile technique, the skin and subcutaneous tissues of the appropriate interspace are infiltrated with local anesthetic. The epidural space is entered by three common approaches: midline, paramedian, and caudal. In the midline approach, the needle is placed between the spinous processes. In the paramedian approach, the needle is placed between the lamina avoiding the supraspinous and interspinous ligaments. The needle is placed through the sacral hiatus for the caudal approach. Because the pressure within the epidural space is subatmospheric, a loss of resistance to the air or saline in the attached syringe confirms positioning of the needle in the epidural space. For cervical epidural–steroid injections, the hanging-drop method is commonly utilized. The hanging-drop method uses a drop of fluid on the hub of the needle. When the epidural space is entered, the hanging drop is sucked into the hub. Methylprednisolone acetate (80 to 120 mg) or triamcinolone diacetate (50 to 120 mg) in 5 to 10 mL of local anesthetic or saline is slowly injected. The local anesthetic not only provides analgesia, but the sensory or sympathetic blockade it produces confirms that the needle has been positioned properly.

CHOICE OF INJECTATE

Methylprednisolone acetate and triamcinolone diacetate are the two most commonly used deposteroids for epidural-steroid injections. The amounts range from 50 to 120 mg for triamcinolone to 80 to 120 mg for methyl-

prednisolone. Abram suggests 50 mg of triamcinolone or 80 mg of methylprednisolone for lumbosacral radiculopathy. In 1980, Knight and Burnell recommended that doses of not more than 3 mg/kg methylprednisolone should be given because of risks of systemic side effects. There are published reports of the use of hydrocortisone 25 to 125 mg and prednisone 10 to 50 mg epidurally, however water-soluble preparations of steroids are not commonly used any longer. Oppelt and Rall showed that water-soluble preparations of steroids could cause seizures when injected intrathecally.

The results are comparable for use of either local anesthetic or saline as diluents. The use of local anesthetic can be as a test dose for inadvertent intrathecal injection, reduction of pain for the patient, and as a marker that the steroids are at the correct level. The disadvantages of using local anesthetic include the need for longer monitoring of vital signs, risk of sympathectomy, hypotension, and weakness. In the past, large volumes (average of 72 mL) of normal saline have been recommended to break the fibrous adhesions between the dural sheaths of the nerve roots and the foramina or to displace nerve roots from contact with the herniated disc. Large volumes were found to be painful and resulted in headache and dizziness in some patients. A volume of 6 to 12 mL should provide adequate spread of the deposteroid. The epidural injection of 6 mL of radiopaque dye through the L4–L5 interspace have been shown to spread from L1 down to S5 by Harley.

There may be epidural fibrosis in some patients preventing the steroids from reaching the affected nerve root. Hyaluronidase and hypertonic saline (10% NaCl) may be used to break up the scar tissue. The Racz catheter and epiduroscopy can be used to guide the steroids to the affected area. The Racz Tun-L-Kath is a radiographically visible catheter that can be used to direct injections and break up adhesions. Epiduroscopy provides direct visualization of the epidural space.

Patients may experience onset of pain relief 12 to 24 hours after the administration of epidural steroid, but relief commonly occurs 3 days to 1 week later. Patients are reevaluated 2 to 4 weeks after the injection. At that time, a repeat injection is given if the symptoms improve but reach a plateau or improve temporarily and then recur. The injection is not repeated if the patient reports sustained, satisfactory improvement in symptoms. Lack of response may be from improper placement of the steroid. Most studies reported improvement with one epidural-steroid injection. However, some centers advocate three injections routinely in each patient. The injections may be given up to three times in a 6-month period.

COMPLICATIONS

Serious complications of epidural-steroid injection are rare. Immediate complications include hypotension from sympathetic blockade and problems such as high spinal or intravascular injection secondary to improper needle placement. Nerve-root injury is rare. Patients often may experience discomfort at the injection site or intensification of their pretreatment symptoms for the first 24 to 48 hours; these are presumably related to the minimal tissue trauma inherent in needle placement. Spinal headache consequent to inadvertent puncture of the dura occurs uncommonly in less than 1% of cases. Introduction of air into the subarachnoid space can cause severe headaches distinct from spinal headaches. The epidural space may be missed entirely because of incorrect needle placement. Radiographic studies by Johnson, Schellhas, and Pollei have shown failure to enter the epidural space in up to 30% of injections.

Epidural hematoma, intraocular hemorrhage, and central nervous system infections are serious but extremely rare complications of epidural injection. Intraocular hemorrhages are thought to be from acutely increased cerebrospinal-fluid pressure from compression of the subarachnoid space by the epidural injection. Aseptic meningitis, bacterial meningitis, and epidural abscess have been reported after epidural-steroid injection. Because of the scarcity of reports of such adverse side effects, the advantages of that modality seem to significantly outweigh the disadvantages.

Steroids given by way of the epidural approach are absorbed systemically (as demonstrated by Gorski and coworkers) and can be detected for several weeks after the injection (as demonstrated by Burn and Langdon). Suppression of plasma corticosteroid concentration can be found up to 3 weeks after injection. Side effects from systemic steroids can include fluid retention, hypertension, weight gain, congestive heart failure, elevated serum glucose, and cushingoid appearance. For many years, it was feared that corticosteroids might have a detrimental effect on the neural tissue contained in the epidural space. In 1980, Delaney and coworkers reported that no histological changes in neural tissue were seen after epidural triamcinolone injection in cats. Commercial preparations of steroids contain polyethylene glycol, which has been shown to be neurotoxic. Dilution of the steroid can serve to decrease the concentration of polyethylene glycol.

EFFECTIVENESS

Epidural steroids have been shown to decrease pain, speed return of function, and improve objective-neurologic signs. The procedure can be performed on an outpatient basis, has considerably fewer short- and long-term side-effects compared to surgery, and avoids the addictive potential of long-term use of narcotics. In addition, epidural administration requires a very low dose of steroid, compared with the suggested systemic doses needed to attain antiinflammatory levels intraspinally. In 1975, Green reported the efficacy of systemic steroids in the management of pain caused by lumbar-disc herniation. His patients were given a week-long tapering course, starting at 64 mg/day of intramuscular dexamethasone. The first dose alone was about four times the single dose of steroid given by way of epidural injection. Even with the enormous systemic doses, the relief attained diminished as the drug was tapered.

In 1973, Dilke and coworkers performed a double-blind, controlled, randomized, prospective study of 100 patients. The 50 patients in the treatment group underwent epidural-steroid injection. Those in the control group received only a superficial stick in the back. In the untreated group, 60% of the patients were able to resume work 3 months after injection, compared with 92% of the treated patients. Fourteen percent of the control group and 53% of the treatment group experienced subjective pain relief 3 months after injection. Eighteen percent of the control patients and 48% of the treated patients did not require analgesics 3 months after injection. In a similar study, Brevik and coworkers reported pain relief, objective neurologic improvement, and return to work in 63% of patients treated with a steroid/bupivacaine combination, compared with 25% of patients treated with bupivacaine alone. Arnhoff and coworkers also reported continued improved activity levels and lowered medication use in 151 patients 2 years after epidural-steroid treatment.

In general, epidural-steroid injection seems to be most effective in patients with acute (less than 3-months' duration) rather than chronic pain. Seventy percent to 80% of patients with acute pain may experience improvement, compared with only 40% to 50% of those with chronic pain. A history of previous back surgery seems to be another predictor of outcome; only about 30% to 40% of postsurgical patients improve after epidural-steroid injection. It has been postulated that adhesions and other surgery-related changes may prevent the steroid from reaching the inflamed neural tissue. Success rates also may vary depending on the accuracy of the diagnosis and the technical expertise of the physician; problems in those areas may have accounted for some of the initial disappointing outcomes.

There are a number of factors that may influence the success of epidural-steroid injections. Abram found that success decreased when the patient was injured at work, was out of work because of back pain, was receiving compensation, was involved in legal action, had previous surgery, had a long duration of pain and high pain ratings, or frequently used analgesics. Jamison et al. found that four factors predicted poor outcome at 2 weeks after injections: a greater number of previous treatments, more medications being taken for pain, pain not necessarily increased by activity, and pain increased by coughing. Factors that predicted no benefit 1 year after injection include pain not interfering with activity, unemployment because of pain, normal straight-leg raise test prior to treatment, and pain not being decreased by medication. Sandrock and Warfield felt that there were five factors that influenced the outcome of epidural-steroid injections: accuracy of the diagnosis of nerve root inflammation, duration of symptoms, history of previous surgery, age of the patient, and location of the injection in relation to the pathology.

CONCLUSION

Sciatica and other forms of radiculopathy are very common, often disabling ailments. A multitude of treatments have been proposed, including chiropractic manipulations, potent analgesics and other pharmacologic therapy, and surgery. Epidural-steroid injection has proved to be a safe, quick, and effective mode of therapy, with few risks and many benefits. Relief of the pain may be from resolution of inflammation in spinal-nerve roots, blockage of C-fiber transmission, inhibition of ectopic discharge, or inhibition of central sensitization of the dorsal horn.

The efficacy of epidural steroids has not yet been proven by randomized, controlled trial. Even a widespread treatment such as lumbar-epidural steroid injections is still controversial. The current studies available have flaws in methodology, power, and control. Patient selection, number of injections, volume to be used, and composition of the injectate still remain undefined.

Currently, many different indications for the use of epidural steroids are being explored. Epidural steroids are being used to treat symptoms of spinal stenosis. Its use for pain relief in postherpetic neuralgia is under investigation. The use of steroids with lumbar discectomy to aid in residual radicular pain relief has been found to have some benefit. The efficacy of epidural steroids for these indications is under investigation.

SELECTED READINGS

Abram SE. Treatment of lumbosacral radiculopathy with epidural steroids. *Anesthesiology* 1999;91:1937–1941.

Abram SE, O'Connor TC. Complications associated with epidural steroid injections. *Reg Anesth* 1996;21:149–162.

Arnhoff FN, Triplet HB, Pokorney B. Follow-up status of patients treated with nerve blocks for low back pain. *Anesthesiology* 1977;46:170–178.

Benzon HT. Epidural steroid injections for low back pain and lumbosacral radiculopathy. *Pain* 1986;24:277–295.

Bernat J. Intraspinal steroid therapy. *Neurology* 1981;31:168–171.

Brevik H, Hesla P, Molnar I, et al. Treatment of chronic low back pain and sciatica. In: Bonica J, ed. *Advances in Pain Research and Therapy*, vol 1. New York: Raven Press, 1976.

Brown FW. Management of discogenic pain using epidural and intrathecal steroids. *Clin Orthop* 1972;129:72–78.

Burn JM, Langdon L. Duration of action of epidural methyl-prednisolone. *Am J Phys Med* 1974;53:29–34.

Cuckler JM, Bernini PA, Wiesel SW, et al. The use of epidural steroids in the treatment of lumbar radicular pain: A prospective, randomized, double-blind study. *J Bone Joint Surg Am* 1985;67:63–66.

Delaney T, Rowlingson FC, Carron H, et al. Epidural steroid effects on nerve and meninges. *Anesth Analg* 1980;59:610–614.

Dilke TF, Burry HC, Grahame R. Extradural corticosteroid injection in the management of lumbar nerve root compression. *Br Med J* 1973;2:635–637.

Goebert HW, Jallo SJ, Gardner WJ, et al. Sciatica: treatment with epidural injections of procaine and hydrocortisone. *Cleve Clin Q* 1960;27:191–197.

Gorski DW, Rao TK, Glessor SN, et al. Epidural triamcinolone and adrenal responses to stress. *Anesthesiology* 1981;55:A147.

Green LN. Dexamethasone in the management of symptoms due to herniated lumbar disc. *J Neurol Neurosurg Psych* 1975;38:1211–1217.

Harley C. Extradural corticosteroid infiltration. A follow-up study of 50 cases. *Ann Phys Med* 1967;9:22–28.

Hench PS, et al. The effect of a hormone of the adrenal cortex and of pituitary adrenocorticotropic hormone on rheumatoid arthritis. *Mayo Clinic Proc* 1949;24:181–197.

Hopwood MB, Manning DC. Lumbar epidural steroid injections: is a clinical trial necessary or appropriate? *Reg Anesth Pain Med* 1999;24:5–7.

Johnson BA, Schellhas KP, Pollei SR. Epidurography and therapeutic epidural injections: technical considerations and experience with 5334 cases. *AJNR Am J Neuroradiol* 1999;20:697–705.

Kepes ER, Duncalf D. Treatment of backache with spinal injections of local anesthetics, spinal and systemic steroids. A review. *Pain* 1985;22:33–47.

Lindahl O, Rexed B. Histological changes in the spinal nerve roots of operated cases of sciatica. *Acta Orthop Scand* 1951;20:215–225.

Murphy RW. Nerve roots and spinal nerves in degenerative disk disease. *Clin Orthop* 1977;129:46–60.

Oppelt WW, Rall CP. Production of convulsions in the dog with intrathecal corticosteroids. *Neurology* 1961;2:925–927.

Robecchi A, Capra R. L'idrocortisone (composto F): prime esperienze cliniche in campo reumatologico. *Min Med* 1952;98:1259.

Sehgal AD, Gardner WJ, Dohn DF. Pantopaque "arachnoiditis." *Cleve Clin Q* 1962;29:177.

Sehgal AD, Tweed DC, Foote MK. Laboratory studies after intrathecal corticosteroids. *Arch Neurol* 1963;9:74.

Stanton-Hicks M, Boas R. *Chronic Low Back Pain*. New York: Raven Press, 1982:193–198.

Warfield CA. The use of epidural steroids in the treatment of lumbar radicular pain. A prospective, randomized, double-blind study (letter). *J Bone Joint Surg Am* 1985;67-A:980–981.

Winnie AP, Hartman JT, Meyers HL, et al. Pain clinic II: intradural and extradural corticosteroids for sciatica. *Anesth Analg* 1972;51:990–999.

Wood KM, Arguelles J, Norenberg MD. Degenerative lesions in rat sciatic nerves after local injection of methylprednisolone in sterile aqueous solution. *Reg Anesth* 1980;5:13–15.

CHAPTER 49

Epiduroscopy

Sanjay Gupta

"Epiduroscopy," as the name indicates, is the direct visualization of the epidural space with the help of a fiberoptic device called an "epiduroscope." It provides a unique opportunity to observe a three-dimensional, color view of the epidural anatomy. The technique is relatively new and is slowly evolving and can be a valuable tool for diagnosis and treatment of epidural-space pathology.

HISTORICAL PERSPECTIVE

For a long time, researchers have been trying to find methods to access epidural and spinal space in a minimally invasive manner for diagnostic and therapeutic interventions. Unavailability of fine-caliber, fiberoptic scopes made it almost impossible to achieve that goal in a clinically useful manner until a few years ago. It is interesting to note the evolutionary steps in the development of the epiduroscope, which is now available.

In 1931, Michael Burman, an orthopedic surgeon from New York, removed 11 vertebral columns from cadavers and examined them with arthroscopic equipment. Burman concluded that myeloscopy was limited by the available technology, but with higher-quality instrumentation, the ability to visualize the contents of the spinal canal might be useful in establishing a diagnosis of a tumor or inflammation.

In 1936, Elias Stern from Columbia University's Department of Anatomy was among the first to describe a spinescope. The instrument was never used clinically, but Stern did envision its use for the direct observation of the posterior roots for rhizotomies in patients with intractable pain and sectioning of these roots for treatment of spastic conditions. He also felt that with technologic improvements, epiduroscopy procedures could eliminate the need for extensive, exploratory laminotomies.

In 1942, Pool published a summary of his experience with 400 patients in the journal, *Surgery*. He noted that the myeloscope could help in establishing or confirming a diagnosis, thus avoiding extensive explorations. He was able to identify neuritis, herniated nucleus pulposus, hypertrophied ligamentum flavum, primary and metastatic neoplasms, varicose vessels, and arachnoid adhesions. Surprisingly, no further reports of this technique are found in the literature until 1967. This is perhaps because of the widespread acceptance and ease of performance of myelography, coupled with the inability to record the images with the then-available epiduroscopes.

In the late 1960s and early 1970s, Ooi et al., without knowledge of the American experience, developed an endoscope for intradural and extradural examinations. With the advent of fiberoptic light-source technology in the 1970s, the device was miniaturized enough to be inserted between lumbar-spinous processes in the same manner as a percutaneous lumbar puncture. Ooi and his colleagues performed 208 myeloscopies using various types of equipment. A flexible myeloscope was theorized to have many advantages, but another decade passed before the advent of such a micromyeloscope.

Blomberg of Sweden was the next to describe a method of epiduroscopy and spinaloscopy in 1985. In 1989, Blomberg and Olsson performed ten epiduroscopies on patients scheduled for partial laminectomies for herniated lumbar discs. They determined that the epidural space was indeed only a potential space that remained open for brief periods of time when fluid or air was injected. Blomberg and Olsson also confirmed the presence of a dorsomedian connective-tissue band that divided the epidural space into compartments.

In the late 1980s and early 1990s, the introduction of video chips made it possible to have simultaneous video images while recording all aspects of a surgical procedure. This new technology enabled Shimoji and colleagues to publish their experience using small (0.5 to 1.4 mm), flexible, fiberoptic scopes in 1991. Ten patients with intractable spinal-pain syndromes had flexible, fiberoptic myeloscopes placed into either the subarachnoid space, epidural space, or both, by way of a lumbar paramedian approach through a Tuohy needle. The epidural space, however, could only be visualized after withdrawal of the fiberoptic myeloscope from the subarachnoid position. The authors attributed this to the leak of cerebrospinal fluid into the potential epidural space, which decreased the adhesiveness of the tissues and allowed the lens to achieve its focal length. The fiberoptic scopes could be advanced up to the cisterna magna.

In 1991, Saberski and Kitahata began evaluations of several fiberoptic systems for use in clinical epiduroscopy. The technology had markedly improved, but an appropriate indication for epiduroscopy was not clear. As a diagnostic tool, the uncertainty remained as to whether this technique could provide an advantage over readily available imaging procedures that were noninvasive (e.g., computed tomography scan, magnetic resonance imaging [MRI]). In addition, a number of technological shortcomings needed to be overcome before seriously considering clinical use of these devices. First, the fiberoptic catheters only allowed visualization of tissues that were immediately in front of the lens (i.e., when a 2-mm focal length was maintained). However, this focal distance was difficult to achieve in a potential space like the epidural space. Second, the placement of the device into the epidural space was difficult, even when guided by fluoroscopy. Third, the fiberoptic catheters did not incorporate separate channels that would allow tissue sampling or delivery of medication to the site being investigated. Their work helped in developing the current fiberoptic scope that has a working lumen, has a lens with a short focal length, and incorporates normal saline-flushing channel to prevent tissues or blood from occluding the fiberoptic lens.

SPINAL ENDOSCOPE

The currently available epiduroscope is a flexible, steerable 0.9-mm diameter fiberoptic scope (Fig. 49.1). It provides a 70-degree field of view and has high-resolution optics of around a 10,000-pixel image-fiber bundle. The scope is passed by way of a catheter, which has two, 1-mm lumens. One lumen is used for the spinal endoscope and the other is used for normal saline infusion. The catheter can be maneuvered with two knobs on the proximal ends.

The entry kit is like any other Seldinger-technique kit with a guide wire and a Touhey needle. The scope can be connected directly to a television monitor and the images can be visualized during the procedure. These images also can be recorded or printed using the epiduroscopy apparatus (Fig. 49.2).

INDICATIONS FOR SPINAL ENDOSCOPY

Epiduroscopy is a relatively new procedure and its indications are expanding as the technology and the experience improves. Epiduroscopy at present has both diagnostic and therapeutic indications.

Patients whose MRIs are not able to delineate the cause of pain can be better assessed with the use of epiduroscopy. MRI gives only black-and-white images, and many times in MRI a herniated disc can be a normal finding without any clinical symptoms. With epiduroscopy, three-dimensional color views can show if there is an associated inflammation with the disc herniation and thus can localize the nociceptive source. In addition, because epidural space usually is in a collapsed state, fibrous layers around the nerve roots may not show up that well and thus can be missed with MRI. However, during epiduroscopy, normal saline is used to expand the space and thus, those fibrous layers can be better visualized. Further, possible diagnostic indications for epiduroscopy include diagnosis of arachnoiditis and small, metastatic tumors.

The therapeutic indications at present are lysis of fibrous adhesions using hydrostatic pressure as well as selective injection of steroid around inflamed nerve roots and fibrous tissue. It also possibly can be used for

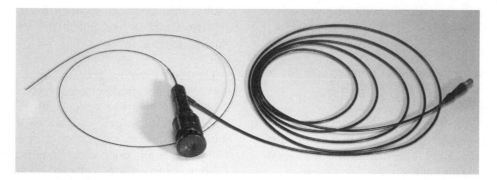

FIG. 49.1. Flexible fiberoptic endoscope. Photo courtesy of Visionary BioMedical, Inc. (*www.myelotec.com*)

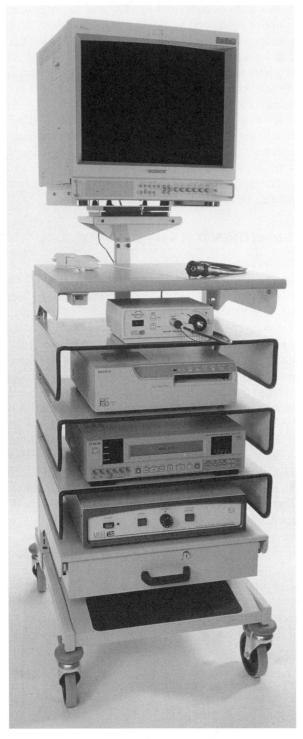

FIG. 49.2. Epiduroscopy apparatus. Photo courtesy of Visionary BioMedical, Inc. (*www.myelotec.com*)

drainage of small epidural abscess and diagnostic biopsies in the epidural tumors. The therapeutic indications will expand further with improvement in technology.

In the pain-management algorithm, patients that have little or no pain relief with epidural-steroid injections may be considered for epiduroscopy. A filling defect seen on an epidurogram correlating to the area of the suspected pain generator may need further confirmatory workup with epiduroscopy. Patients who have failed back-surgery syndrome (FBSS) with a strong radicular component may be evaluated further by epiduroscopy to localize the nociceptive source better.

We had a patient with unilateral leg radicular pain in which MRI did not revel any specific finding. However, an epidurogram showed a filling defect on the affected epidural side. Epiduroscopy further revealed a fibrous strand, which was successfully lysed. The patient remained symptom-free until her 1-year follow-up visit.

CONTRAINDICATIONS

Contraindications are similar to any invasive procedures to epidural space like epidural-steroid injections. Mostly, they are related to coagulation disorders. The main contraindications are coagulopathy, pregnancy, renal insufficiency, chronic-liver dysfunction, a history of adverse reaction to local anesthetics, any local back infections or generalized sepsis, and patients unable to understand informed consent protocol.

EPIDUROSCOPY PROCEDURE

Spinal endoscopy is performed by accessing the caudal canal through the sacral hiatus, a site remote to pathology allowing for a multilevel examination of the spinal canal. The caudal approach to the epidural space offers an advantage over the paramedian-lumbar approach. This approach permits direct access to the epidural space, as opposed to approximate 45-degree bend required to introduce a catheter into the lumbar-epidural space when using the paramedian approach. It is important to note that sacral hiatus is absent in some patients (up to 20%). In those patients, the epiduroscopy procedure cannot be performed with present technology.

Unlike an open surgical procedure where muscle, ligaments, and bone are disturbed, spinal endoscopy is a "gentle" procedure and basically eliminates these potential complications of surgery. Patients are kept preferably awake with conscious sedation for this procedure to be able to diagnose any potential complication. Usually, patients tolerate this procedure well with minimal sedation.

The caudal canal is accessed by way of the sacral hiatus using a modified Seldinger technique and placing an 8-FR introducer. The patients usually are placed in a prone position. To get better access to the sacral hiatus, some practitioners suggest mild inversion of both feet. The procedure is done under fluoroscopy guidance. The 2.7-mm, video-guided catheter containing the epiduroscope is passed through the introducer into the epidural space. Normal saline is used to expand the epidural space and to wash away any debris and blood. The actual amount of normal saline injected varies but up to a liter of normal saline has been safely injected. Epidural space is not usually a tightly contained space, and thus saline leaves the space or is absorbed fairly rapidly. However, caution must be taken and any signs of increased epidural-pressurelike headache, vision changes, etc., should be carefully watched.

Normal saline also is used for breaking any small, fibrous strands around the nerve root. Once the inflamed nerve root is identified, steroids can be selectively injected in that area. Although this is an outpatient procedure, patients should be watched for 1 to 2 hours before being sent home.

COMPLICATIONS

Local complications include bleeding and infection like other invasive procedures. Care should be taken not to puncture dura and entry into intrathecal space should be avoided as that may possibly lead to postdural puncture headache and nerve damage.

Increased epidural pressure and possible air embolisms may lead to headache, transient blindness, nausea, and vomiting, so any signs of increased epidural pressure should be watched carefully.

We currently are working on developing methods of continually monitoring the epidural pressure during the procedure as well as determining the relation between the infusate volume and pressure with the epidural pressure.

FUTURE DIRECTIONS

Epiduroscopy is a procedure that has been practiced only for last few years. In the future, it will likely play an increasing role in diagnosing epidural pathologies including nerve-root inflammations, vascular abnormalities, arachnoiditis, fibrous bands, tumors etc.

It is very likely that further instrumentation including laser will be possible through endoscope to break small adhesions, take biopsies, and drain small epidural abscesses. Work is underway to make it a safer procedure with the help of continuous epidural-pressure measurements and other modifications.

SELECTED READINGS

Blomberg RG. A method for epiduroscopy and spinaloscopy: presentation of preliminary results. *Acta Anaesthesiol Scand* 1985;29:113–116.

Blomberg RG, Olsson, SS. The lumbar epidural space in patients examined with epiduroscopy. *Anesth Analg* 1989;68:157–160.

Blomberg RG. Technical advantages of the paramedian approach for lumbar epidural puncture and catheter introduction. A study using epiduroscopy in autopsy subjects. *Anaesthesia* 1988;43:837–843.

Burman MS. Myeloscopy or the direct visualization of the spinal cord. *J Bone Joint Surg* 1931;13:695–696.

Ooi Y, Morisaki N. Intrathecal lumbar endoscope. *Clin Orthopedic Surgery (Japan)* 1969;4:295–297.

Ooi Y, Satoh Y, Morisaki N. Myeloscopy. *Igakuno Ayumi (Japan)* 1972;81: 209–212.

Ooi Y, Satoh Y, Morisaki N. Myeloscopy. *Int Orthop* 1977;1:107–111.

Ooi Y, Satoh Y, Morisaki N. Myeloscopy. *Orthop Surg (Japan)* 1973;24: 181–186.

Ooi Y, Satoh Y, Morisaki N. Myeloscopy: possibility of observing lumbar intrathecal space by use of an endoscope. *Endoscopy* 1973;5:91–96.

Ooi Y, Satoh Y, Morisaki N. Myeloscopy: a preliminary report. *J Japan Orthop Assoc* 1973;47:619–627.

Ooi Y, Satoh Y, Hirose K, et al. Myeloscopy. *Acta Orthop Belg* 1978;44: 881–894.

Ooi Y, Satoh Y, Inoue K, et al. Myeloscopy, with special reference to blood flow changes in the cauda equina during Lasegue's test. *Int Orthop* 1981; 4:307–311.

Pool JL. Direct visualization of dorsal nerve roots of the cauda equina by means of a myeloscope. *Arch Neurol Psychiatry* 1938;39:1308–1312.

Pool JL. Myeloscopy: diagnostic inspection of the cauda equina by means of an endoscope. *Bull Neurol Inst NY* 1938;7:178–189.

Pool JL. Myeloscopy: intraspinal endoscopy. *Surgery* 1942;11:169–182.

Saberski LR, Brull SJ. Spinal and epidural endoscopy: a historical review. *Yale J Biol Med* 1995;68:7–15.

Satoh Y, Hirose K, Ooi Y, et al. *Myeloscopy in the Diagnosis of Low Back Pain Syndrome.* The Third Congress of International Rehabilitation Medicine Assoc. Basel Switzerland, July 2–9, 1978.

Shimoji K, Fujioka H, Onodera M, et al. Observation of spinal canal and cisternae with the newly developed small-diameter, flexible fiberscopes. *Anesthesiology* 1991;75:341–344.

Stern EL. The spinescope: a new instrument for visualizing the spinal canal and its contents. *Medical Record (NY)* 1936;143:31–32.

CHAPTER 50

Facet Injections

Alicja Soczewko Steiner and Dan P. Gray

Lumbar and cervical spine pain is very common. In most industrialized countries, the lifetime prevalence of back pain is greater than 60% with the annual incidence of at least 5%. Lumbar-facet syndrome has been considered to be a significant source of low-back pain. The prevalence of cervical pain approaches that of the lumbar spine. Thoracic-facet syndrome is a less established cause of pain.

ANATOMIC CONSIDERATIONS

The spine is made up of seven cervical, 12 thoracic, and five lumbar vertebrae. They articulate anteriorly through the discs and posteriorly through two synovial facet joints. Anterior to the ligamentum flavum covering the facet joint is a variable amount of vascularized adipose tissue. This tissue is contained in the epidural space, which is in direct contact with the nerve-root dural sleeve. Enlarged and osteophytic facet joints can contribute to significant narrowing of the neuroforaminal opening and can cause radicular symptoms. There is less agreement on whether the facet joints themselves are pain provocateurs or if alterations in facet-joint anatomy are the benign manifestation of weight-bearing function of these joints.

The space enclosed by the articular cartilage and synovium contains synovial fluid. Computed tomography, magnetic resonance imaging, and intraarticular contrast medium can demonstrate the anatomy of the facet joint. The joint space itself is small. The volume of injectate that can be accommodated by the facet joints varies for different levels as follows: cervical 0.5 mL to 1.0 mL; thoracic 0.4 mL to 0.6 mL; and lumbar 1.0 mL to 2.0 mL.

In the upper lumbar spine, approximately 80% of the facet joints are curved and 20% are flat. This situation is reversed in the lower lumbar spine. The upper lumbar facets are more oriented in the sagittal plane, and by the

L5/Sl level they have rotated more obliquely. The thoracic-facet joints are almost parallel to the coronal plane.

The anatomy of the cervical facets is significantly different from the lumbar facets. The atlantooccipital and atlantoaxial joints are the occiptial-C1 and Cl–C2 facet joints. Their structure, function, and innervation are unique. All of the cervical-facet joints from C2–C3 to C7–Tl are angled 110 degrees from the midline posterior-sagittal plain, which makes their orientation similar to the thoracic facets. The cervical facets play a larger role physically in the spinal-articular tripod structure and are commonly described as the superior and inferior ends of articular pillars. The vertebral artery, which passes through the transverse foramen of the transverse processes of the Cl to C6 vertebra, is a landmark of the cervical spine.

The function of the facet joints appears to be to protect the spine from excessive mobility and to distribute axial loading over a broad area. The orientation and shape of the facets are specifically designed to the stresses and movements expected at each spinal level.

NEUROANATOMY OF THE FACET JOINTS

The poor localization of facet-joint pain is explained by profuse overlapping of sensory innervation. The medial branch supplies the lower facet at its own level as well as the upper part of the joint below. Therefore, each of the facet joints receives innervation from a medial-branch nerve of two posterior primary rami. These nerves also branched out to paraspinal muscles, ligaments, and periosteum with significant dermatomal-sensory overlapping.

In the lumbar region, the medial branch lies in a groove on the base of the superior-articular facet and passes between the mammillary and accessory processes. The medial-branch nerve then runs posteriorly and inferiorly, first sending fibers to innervate the adjacent joint capsule, before sending fibers to the next lower level. The course of the L5 medial branch is different as the transverse process is replaced by the ala of the sacrum. The lumbosacral facet probably has additional innervation from the S1 nerve root.

There is evidence that there is multilevel innervation of the lumbar-facet joints, which includes not only the posterior primary rami, but also the sympathetic and parasympathetic ganglia. The sympathetic fibers have been reported to regulate the activity of sensory neurons, and may contribute to low-back pain.

Thoracic facets have similar innervation to the lumbar spine. Below the T3 level, this pattern is consistent, but the C7 and C8 nerves may travel caudally as far as the T2 and T3 levels.

The exceptions to this description occurred at the midthoracic level where the nerve does not even reliably make bony contact with the superolateral corner of the transverse process. The T11 branch also has different anatomy and runs across the lateral surface of the root of the relatively smaller T12 transverse process. At the T12 level, the medial branch localization is analogous to the lumbar spine.

The cervical-medial branches mainly supply the facet joints with minimal innervation of the following posterior neck muscles: multifidus, interspinalis, semispinalis cervicis, and semispinalis capitis. The C3 dorsal branch is the only cervical-dorsal ramus below C2 that has a cutaneous distribution. Therefore, if neck pain or headache is from cervical-facet disease, cervical-facet joint blocks may relieve it.

The upper-cervical synovial joints, atlantooccipital joints, and atlantoaxial joints are innervated by cervical-ventral rami. Some practitioners advocate direct injection of these upper joints, as attempting to block the innervating branches is likely impossible. The C2–C3 facet joint is innervated mainly by the third occipital nerve and sometimes by the C2 dorsal rami (the greater occipital nerve). There are eight cervical nerves and seven cervical vertebrae. The first seven cervical-nerve roots exit the spine above the vertebral body and they are numbered after the body. The C3–C4 to C7–T1 facet joints are supplied by the medial branches at the same level as the joint and from the segmental level above. These nerves take off from the cervical posterior primary rami and wrap around the waists of the articular pillars.

PATHOGENESIS OF THE FACET SYNDROME

Neurophysiologic studies have shown that the medial-branch nerves transmit nociceptive and proprioceptive signals from the facet joints. Activation of these nerves may be triggered by inflammatory and mechanical factors.

Chronic inflammation with consecutive joint hypertrophy, degeneration, and osteophyte formation may attribute to neural foraminal narrowing and compression of the nerve roots. On occasion, this causes referred pain to the extremities as well abnormal joint stress with possible subluxation and muscle spasm (Fig. 50.1).

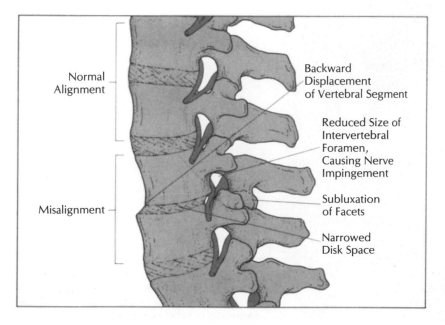

Normal Alignment

Misalignment

Backward Displacement of Vertebral Segment

Reduced Size of Intervertebral Foramen, Causing Nerve Impingement

Subluxation of Facets

Narrowed Disk Space

FIG. 50.1. Disc-space narrowing produces derangement of the mechanics of the spine, with consequent subluxation of the facet joints. Sequelae include nerve impingement, backward displacement of vertebral segment, and restriction of vertebral rotation all of which add up to pain.

INDICATIONS AND CONTRINDICATIONS FOR FACET BLOCKING

The clinical picture of facet-joint syndrome is controversial, as clinicians from different disciplines have varied diagnosis criteria. The diagnosis of facet syndrome often is a "diagnosis of exclusion" based on careful physical examination, medical history, and lack of alternative explanation. The diagnosis is confirmed by reproduction of symptomatic pain during facet injections.

The traditional definition of facet syndrome includes features that are no longer considered strictly diagnostic of pure facet pathology. Pain in the low-back location with occasional radiation to the buttock, groin, hip, and lower extremities usually above knee level (unilateral or bilateral) was considered the classic presentation, but it now is held that radiating pain that ends above the knee may be from nerve-root irritation. Paralumbar tenderness with or without muscle spasm may be from facet syndrome or from a myofascial-pain syndrome. Pain that is dull, deep, and difficult to describe in character may result from a variety of causes. A lack of neurological deficits is not enough to determine that the facet joints are the reason for the pain.

Pain with an onset associated with twisting, bending, or rotation and an elevation of the pain by lateral bending, extension, sitting, and forward flexion in the standing position is considered classic for facet syndrome. It is commonly held that the pain will show improvement by walking, or at least not be made worse by it. There should not be aggravation of pain with Valsalva maneuver. There often is evidence of degenerative changes on radiological studies.

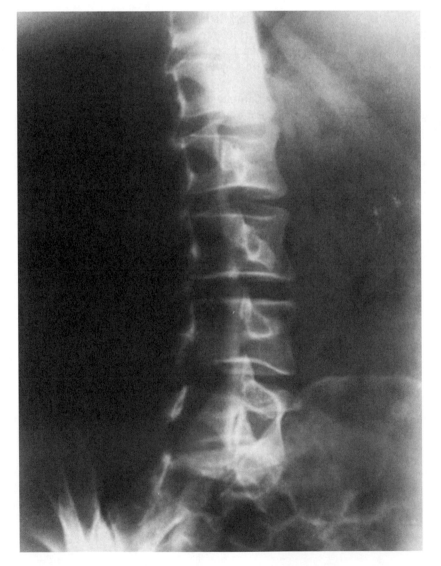

FIG. 50.2. Oblique x-ray of spine shows degenerative changes at L5–S1 facet. Radiographic finding is, however, not specifically diagnostic of facet syndrome.

The thoracic-pain syndrome is considered similar to lumbar-pain syndrome, but there are limited data on this subject. Few studies have been published, and there is primarily anecdotal literature supporting the theories.

Patients with cervicalgia can be divided on the basis of the initiating factors. Patients without history of trauma may have degenerative disease as a primary diagnosis. People with prior trauma may have whiplash syndrome and possible cervicogenic headaches. Pathophysiology of this syndrome is likely from facet-joint sprains with muscle and ligament involvement, as well as occasional periosteal tearing. There may be nerve-root irritation and muscle spasm resulting in the classic distribution of pain.

Radiographic facet-joint changes are common and nonspecific in adults (Fig. 50.2). Routine lumbar radiographs can be normal or can reveal facet degeneration with or without changes in the discs. Arthrography is an additional study, which rarely is performed as the imaging techniques of magnetic resonance imaging (MRI) and computed tomography (CT) have been refined, and CT and MRI examination do not provide specific information about the joints, but provide great information about the surrounding structures. Some studies, however, have suggested that CT and single-photon emission computed topography (SPECT) has some value as a tool to assess clinically significant facet-joint disease. Nevertheless, it seems that a radiographically normal joint is unlikely to be a significant pain generator except in whiplash syndrome.

The clinical criteria for making the diagnosis of facet syndrome are nonspecific, therefore interventional procedures should be offered to patients without neurological deficits or another cause for pain who exhausted conservative treatment measures (analgesics, bed rest, physical therapy). Interventional techniques often are suggested, with the first procedure being the intraarticular or periarticular injections of local anesthetics and steroids.

Diagnostic medial-branch nerve blocks often are used to confirm the diagnosis before trying neuroablative techniques to provide more long-lasting relief. Facet-joint denervation with radiofrequency lesioning or cryotherapy is performed more frequently now than blocks with neurolytic agents. Studies suggest that patients will receive an average of 250 days of pain relief following facet-joint denervation. Some patients will get much longer-lasting relief, while other patients get very little improvement.

Surgical spinal fusion with stabilization of facet joints occasionally is necessary. Only a surgeon can make the determination that surgery is indicated.

In the thoracic and cervical spine, the joints to be injected should be selected based upon the clinical evaluation in conjunction with radiological abnormalities analogous to those described for the lumbar spine.

There are no absolute contraindications to facet injection other than those for any regional block including coagulopathies and systemic or local infection at the site of injection.

FACET BLOCKING TECHNIQUES

Lumbar Facet Block

This procedure is performed with the patient in the prone position. The injection is performed under sterile conditions with continuous vital-sign monitoring. The oblique fluoroscopy view reveals a typical facet-joint picture reminding one of a "scottie dog." This configuration shows the back of the head formed by the inferior articular process and the front feet created by the vertebra below. Local anesthetic is injected where an imaginary line from the center of intensifier intersects the skin on the way towards the facet joint. Either a 20- or 22-gauge, 10-cm spinal needle or a thin probe designed for neuroablation is advanced to the desired position under fluoroscopic guidance (Figs. 50.3 and 50.4). Small amounts of radiological dye (0.25 to 0.5 mL) can be injected to visualize needle-tip placement prior to installment of 1.0 to 1.5 mL of injectate (i.e., 2% to 4% lidocaine with 20 mg triamcinolone or methylprednisolone). The feel of the needle walking off the bone into the joint also can confirm position. Many clinicians ask the patient if entry into the joint recreates their pain. This is known as a pain-provocation test.

Medial-branch blocks are performed using a similar technique, but final needle placement is different. The medial branch is blocked at the junction of the dorsal surface of the transverse process and vertebral body, just caudal to the most medial end of the superior edge of the transverse process. At the lumbosacral level, the posterior primary ramus of L5 is blocked in the groove between the ala of the sacrum and the superior articular process of the sacrum. Blocking a single joint requires that the two medial-branch nerves be injected. At the L5–S1 level, the S1 nerve also should be blocked. It is located cephalad to the S1 posterior opening in a line between the S1 opening and the L5–S1 facet joint. To make a precise injection, the use of a small volume of local anesthetic (0.5 to 1.0 mL) is mandatory.

For therapeutic purposes, a less specific periarticular injection can be done with a larger volume of injectate.

Thoracic-Facet Block

There have been very limited research regarding thoracic-facet denervation and, at this time, the only recommended injections are either intraarticular or periarticular. This procedure is conducted in the prone position using the ribs as a main landmark. The steep angle of the

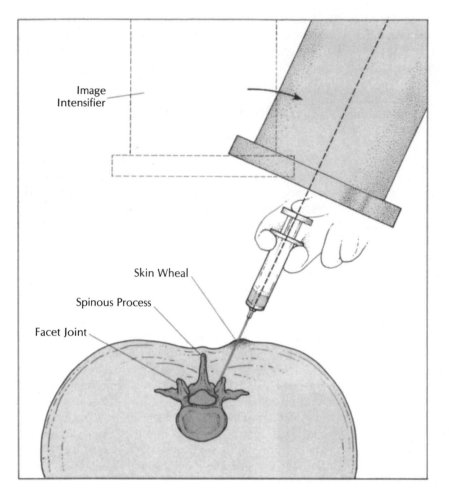

Image
Intensifier

Skin Wheal

Spinous Process

Facet Joint

FIG. 50.3. The only way to make a definitive diagnosis of facet syndrome is by injection of local anesthetic into the facet joint or its nerve supply. Relief of pain confirms the diagnosis. The procedure also may be therapeutic for patients who fail to respond to conservative treatment. The needle can be positioned accurately within the facet joint under fluoroscopic guidance.

joints requires that the skin entry point should overlay the distal pedicle located one or two segments caudally.

Cervical-Facet Block

Blockade of C3–C7 medial branch blocks is done in the lateral position with the side to be blocked superiorly. A 22- or 25-gauge spinal needle is inserted using a posterolateral approach. The target point is the periosteum at the center of the projection of the articular pillar as seen on the lateral fluoroscopic image. After negative aspiration for blood or cerebrospinal fluid, 0.5 mL of local anesthetic is injected. The medial branch of the C8 nerve crosses the T1 transverse process and runs medially onto the lamina of T1 where it should be blocked.

An intraarticular blockade of cervical facets C3 through C7 also can be performed. A 22- or 25-gauge, 10-cm spinal needle should be inserted one to two levels below the joint to be blocked and advanced upward and forward into the joint. A maximum total of 1.0 mL of injectate (including the dye) should be administered to avoid facet-joint rupture.

Blockade of the C2–C3 facet joint requires location of the third occipital nerve. The target points are located along a vertical line bisecting the articular pillar of C3. Injections should be made immediately above the subchondral plate of the C2 inferior-articular process and below the subchondral plate of the C3 superior-articular process as well as at a point between these two. At each of these three sites, 0.5 mL of local anesthetic is injected.

The atlantoaxial joint can be blocked by way of a posterolateral approach in the lateral decubitus position. The head should be slightly flexed and rotated 45 degrees toward the table. The lateral half of the posterior capsule is a final target for a 25-gauge needle. The mastoid process, the occipital prominence, and located between them, the occipital brim are bony landmarks. With oblique imaging, the C-arm and skull/neck are moved until the occipital brim is located over the superior, posterior, and lateral aspect of the joint (the destination point). This procedure is complex. The needle is advanced along this path slowly, confirming its position regularly using a posteroanterior open mouth, lateral and oblique views. Up to 0.5 mL of dye can be used to document the proper needle placement. Aspiration for blood or cerebrospinal fluid should precede the administration of dye and medication (total volume, 1 mL).

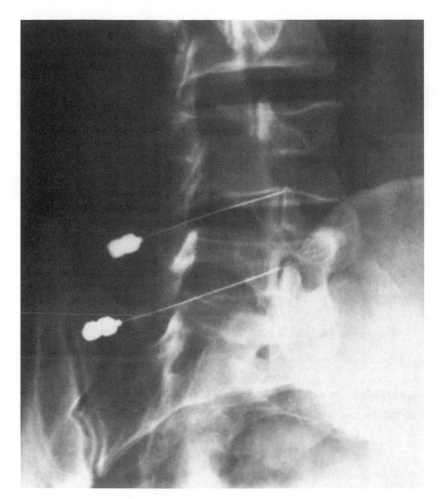

FIG. 50.4. Oblique x-ray shows well-positioned needles within the L4–L5 and L5–S1 facet joints. Facet block with 20 to 40 mg of triamcinolone acetate or methylprednisolone acetate is successful in relieving pain, in many cases.

NEUROABLATION OF THE FACET JOINTS

Facet denervation is performed on the medial-branch nerves with cryotherapy or, more popularly, radiofrequency lesioning using the same technique to locate the nerves as for the medial branch blocks. Previous diagnostic blocks determine which facets will be denervated. A single lumbar-facet denervation requires that two nerves be treated, and three in the case of the L5–Sl facet joint. Two nerves also are denervated for each of the cervical facets, C3–C4 to C7–T1. The technique of denervation of these cervical facets is slightly different. The C2–C3 facet joint requires three-point lesioning as per the technique described above. Because denervation obviously is a destructive procedure and carries a small risk of deafferentation pain and neurological deficits, there must be clear indications that this procedure is needed. The current criteria for facet denervation are not uniform, and so far the best proposal is for clear pain relief after two diagnostic blocks.

Thoracic-medial branch denervation is not recommended because of the lack of a reliable technique for medial-branch blocks at this part of the spine.

ADVERSE EFFECTS

Complications secondary to interventions on the facet joints are rare and usually transient. They include both a failure to relieve pain and the potential of exacerbation of the pain symptoms. Incorrect needle placement or excessive spread of local anesthetic may result in spinal or epidural anesthesia with or without motor and sensory blocks. Injection of material into the intrathecal space may result in chemical meningitis. Whenever a needle is inserted into the back, there is a risk of paraspinal infection and abscess formation. Inadvertent puncture of the vertebral artery may manifest as possible local anesthetic toxicity, with seizure or cardiac arrhythmias. Transient ataxia and unsteadiness as a result of partial blockade of the third occipital nerve and proprioceptive afferents has been reported. Neuroablative procedures may be complicated by persistent motor or sensory deficits.

EFFICACY OF FACET JOINT BLOCKS

The success rate associated with facet-joint injections and neuroablation has varied widely and has been cited as between 16% and 83%. Results have been based mainly on poorly designed studies, which were neither randomized nor controlled trials. Therefore, correct clinical diagnosis and careful patient selection is essential for a good outcome. Other etiology of low-back pain, such as neoplasm, myofascial pain, degenerative-disc disease, infection, and spondylolysis must be excluded.

CONCLUSIONS

In the assessment of patients with spine pain, it is essential to rule out serious pathology that requires surgical evaluation. Facet syndrome still remains a diagnosis of exclusion that cannot be definitively confirmed by any specific laboratory, radiological, or clinical findings. Conservative management should always be offered before scheduling interventional procedures. The patient who has a clinical picture of facet pain, who has been properly examined and screened for other causes of spine pain, and in whom radiological evidence of facet abnormalities correlates with the pain distribution, usually respond to facet injections.

The success rate of facet blockade is reduced significantly in patients with a history of spine surgery, especially fusion. Many clinicians advocate the trial of facet-joint injections in patients with axial back pain, as some of these patients may benefit; and for those who have exhausted most therapies, these injections may provide some relief.

The selection of surgical candidates for spinal fusion based on positive facet diagnostic blocks should be done with the knowledge of their diagnostic limitations. And few surgeons today use the results of facet blockade to aid in their decision-making process. These procedures require further extensive studies and well-designed research.

SELECTED READINGS

Bogduk N. The innervation of the lumbar spine. *Spine* 1983;8:286–293.

Bogduk N, Marsland A. The cervical zygopophysial joints as a source of the neck pain. *Spine* 1988;13:610–617.

Chua WH, Bogduk N. The surgical anatomy of thoracic facet denervation. *Acia Neurochim* 1995;136:140–144.

Cousins MJ, Bridenbaugh PO. In: *Neural Blockade in Clinical Anesthesia and Management of Pain*. 3rd ed. Philadelphia: Lippincott–Raven Publishers, 1998.

Deyo RA, Rainville J, Kent DL. What can the history and physical examination tell us about low back pain? *JAMA* 1992;268:760–765.

Falco FJ. Lumbar spine injection procedures in the management of low back pain. *Occup Med* 1998;13:121–149.

Jerosch J, Castro WH, Liljenqvist U. Percutaneous facet coagulation: indication, technique, results, and complications. *Neurosurg Clin North Am* 1996;7:119–134.

Manchikanti L. Facet joint pain and the role of neural blockade in its management. *Curr Rev Pain* 1999;3:348–358.

Nelemans PJ, deBie RA, DeVelt HC, et al. Injection therapy for subacute and chronic benign low back pain. *Spine* 2001;26:501–515.

CHAPTER 51

Nerve Blocks: An Overview

Hilary J. Fausett and Carol A. Warfield

One of the main reasons a patient is referred to a pain management specialist is for a "nerve block." Local anesthetic blockade of neurotransmission is commonly used by anesthesiologists or surgeons to facilitate surgical procedures. Nerve blocks also are performed for diagnostic and therapeutic purposes.

Diagnostic and surgical nerve blocks are performed with the use of local anesthetics to block nerve transmission for a few hours. These are considered to be temporary blocks and provide temporary pain relief. The nerve, nerve plexus, or nerve ganglion to be blocked is selected on the basis of providing the best anatomic coverage in the least invasive way possible. The risk of the procedure is discussed with the patient ahead of time, and the patient usually is awake or very mildly sedated to reduce anxiety prior to proceeding. In pediatric patients, nerve blocks are occasionally performed following profound sedation or even general anesthesia.

Therapeutic nerve blocks are performed with a mixture of local anesthetic and steroid or a neurolytic substance. The steroid may reduce inflammation and also may decrease aberrant firing of injured nerves. Neurolytic blocks result in the destruction of the nerve, plexus, or ganglion for a variable amount of time. Although the blocks are in theory permanent, there usually is some regrowth of nerve fibers that may result in neuropathic pain. It is for this reason that neurolytic procedures usually are reserved for patients with terminal conditions. The neurolytic, pharmacologic blocks are not the only option. Neurolysis may be done with radiofrequency denervation or with cryoanalgesic ablation. Most pain management specialists are very rigorous in the selection criteria for a neurolytic procedure.

The risk of any nerve block includes causing permanent or temporary injury to the nerve. Because nerve injury may result in a paraesthesia, dysesthesia, or long-lasting anesthesia, this must be discussed with the patient ahead of time. There is a risk of bleeding. To minimize this risk, all patients should be screen for a history of bleeding problems. Patients on antiplatelet medications [such as aspirin or a nonsteroidal antiinflammatory drug (NSAID)] or anticoagulation medication (such as heparin or warfarin) will require additional preparation to minimize the risk of bleeding. There also is a risk of infection. Active infection, infection at the entry site for the nerve block, or bacteremia usually is considered a contraindication for an invasive procedure. Nerve blocks are performed under sterile conditions to avoid introduction of a contaminant.

DIAGNOSTIC NERVE BLOCK

The theory used behind diagnostic-nerve blockade is that by relieving pain by blocking one particular area or one particular type of nerve fiber, a diagnosis can be offered to the patient.

Either an anatomic or a pharmacologic approach may be used. In the anatomic approach, sympathetic- and somatic-nerve blocks are performed sequentially, and relief of pain by selective blockade of either system may aid the physician in determining which nerve system is responsible for the pain syndrome. Alternatively, an anatomic approach in which a block is performed at various points along the course of a nerve may aid in determining where along the neural pathway the pain-producing pathology is located.

The pharmacologic approach to diagnostic neuroblockade takes advantage of the fact that local anesthetics block sympathetic and somatic nerves at different concentrations. Generally, a higher concentration of local anesthetic is required for somatic and motor blockade. Therefore, blockade of a nerve with a low concentration of local anesthetic, which spares sensation but abolishes pain, may point to a sympathetic etiology of the pain.

Unfortunately, the theories used in the application of these differential nerve blocks for the diagnosis of pain may be too simplistic, as they may not take into account alternate pathways of neurotransmission or ephaptic transmission. Nonetheless, sequential differential blockade of nerves with local anesthetic may be a useful technique when other techniques fail to elucidate the etiology of a painful syndrome.

For instance, if a patient has multiple small-disc bulges but the pain felt can be relieved by blocking one specific nerve root (by performing a selective nerve-root block), then the pathology of that particular nerve root is diagnosed as the cause of the patient's pain. Although this makes sense in theory, in practice it is more difficult to make such a simplistic conclusion. First, local anesthetic, no matter how small in amount, may spread. Thus another nerve root may get some of the effects of the block. Second, there is always a "placebo effect" whenever an invasive procedure is done. Thus, unless a block is repeated or done in a "blinded" fashion or with a saline injection, there is a risk that the patient's desire for pain relief may lead him to believe the block helpful. The use of "placebo" nerve blocks with saline to distinguish between an organic and a psychogenic cause of pain is unreasonable because 30% to 40% of patients with an organic cause of pain may be true placebo responders. Third, patients may get relief if the nerve is blocked in a different location, much more distal to the central-putative cause of injury. This has been demonstrated by performing blocks with only subcutaneous injection, nerve-root injection, and sciatic-nerve injection either proximal or distal.

In one study, false-positive results were common, and the authors concluded that the specificity of diagnostic blockade is low. Upon statistical analysis of clinical and technical prognostic factors in this study, the only association with pain relief by any block was the effects of other blocks. There were no associations between the results of blocks and clinical findings (history, physical examination, diagnostic imaging) in these patients, chosen for their homogeneous clinical presentation and absence of functional signs. The authors then conclude that these results indicate a limited role for uncontrolled local anesthetic blocks in the diagnostic evaluation of sciatica and referred-pain syndromes in general. Negative blocks or a pattern of responses may have some predictive value, but isolated, positive blocks are nonspecific.

Case Report

Patient 1

A 51-year-old woman came to the pain management center because of left buttock, thigh, and calf pain of 12 years' duration that had gradually worsened over the past 3 years. Her pain was sharp and intermittent at first but had settled into a continuous burning ache that was greatly exacerbated when she sat on a hard surface or when she walked, but was relieved with recumbency. The pain always radiated from a well-defined point over the sciatic notch, down the thigh, and through the back of the leg to the great toe.

Myelography and computed tomography of the lower-lumbar region revealed no spinal or soft-tissue abnormalities, but electromyography showed changes consistent with denervation of L5 and S1 motor fibers. Weakness of all muscle groups of the left toe (especially the toe extensors) was noted on physical examination; Babinski reflexes were bilaterally positive. Examination of the lower back was negative, but palpation of the left-sciatic notch produced pain in a sciatic distribution. Straight-leg raising caused pain at 60 degrees on the left. Sensory examination revealed diminished vibration and position sense over both legs and diminished pin-prick sensation over the left buttock.

Because the clinical and laboratory findings pointed to a sciatic lesion of nonspinal origin, a sciatic-nerve block was performed at the level of the sciatic notch with 10 mL of 1% lidocaine. It produced relief of both the buttock and leg pains. To more closely pinpoint the cause of pain, a sciatic-nerve block was performed on the left at a point 20 cm below the sciatic notch. This block, however, did not relieve the patient's symptoms, and the lesion thus was definitively localized to the proximal 20 cm of the extrapelvic portion of the sciatic nerve.

The patient was taken to the operating room where the sciatic notch was explored under general anesthesia. The nerve was found to be compressed at the greater-sciatic foramen by a hypertrophied piriformis muscle, and the muscle was lysed. After lysis, the muscle retracted 5 cm into the pelvis. The sciatic trunk was followed 20 cm distally; no other pathology was found, and the operation was completed. Several years after the surgery, the patient remained pain-free.

Diagnostic blocks sometimes are performed to help differentiate between sympathetically maintained pain and somatic pain. Here, the physiologic effects of local anesthetic on nerve transmission are used for diagnostic purposes. Thinner nerve fibers and unmyelinated fibers are more vulnerable to local anesthetic blockade than are thicker fibers and myelinated fibers. Thus, the C fibers that transduce pain and temperature are blocked first, as they are thinner than the A fibers that transduce touch or the myelinated fibers that control motor activity. Because the autonomic fibers of the sympathetic nervous system are blocked first, it has long been taught that relief of pain with preservation of cold perception is diagnostic of sympathetically maintained pain. In practice, few clinicians are able to achieve such delicacy of nerve block to be able to reliably make such a diagnosis.

Another way to diagnose sympathetically maintained pain is by a block of a sympathetic ganglion. This is discussed in detail in Chapter 27 and so will be mentioned only briefly here. If a patient has pain that resolved upon local anesthetic blockade of a sympathetic ganglion, it commonly is held that the patient has a component of sympathetically maintained pain. More current experience suggests, however, that there may be spread of the local anesthetic to somatic fibers, which makes the diagnosis harder to make. Nevertheless, these blocks remain useful tools for treating patients with chronic nonmalignant pain and for many patients with cancer pain as well.

Patient 2

A 51-year-old woman was referred to the pain management center after undergoing surgery for a Colles fracture of the left wrist. A month after the surgery she still had pain in her left hand; it was so severe, despite treatment with oxycodone, that she was unable to participate in physical therapy. Not only was active movement of the hand painful, she would not permit anyone to touch her hand for passive range of motion exercises because of the hyperesthetic quality of her pain.

On physical examination, the hand was swollen, pale, and 3°F colder than the contralateral hand. The hand was diffusely hypersensitive to touch, but otherwise there were no sensory changes. The diagnosis of complex regional pain syndrome (CRPS) with sympathetically maintained pain seemed likely, and a left-stellate ganglion block was performed with 10 mL of 0.25% bupivacaine. That conferred complete and dramatic relief of her pain for approximately 4 days. At that time, a repeat stellate-ganglion block was performed, which provided her with complete pain relief; she remained pain-free several years later.

The blockade of a vicious circle of aberrant nociceptive transmission often has been evoked as an explanation for the long-term relief of pain that may be induced by local injections around a cut or damaged nerve. Furthermore, much has been written about the effects of lowdose, systemic lidocaine infusions providing long-lasting relief of neuropathic pain. This makes it difficult to assume that the direct block of a particular ganglion is necessary for proper treatment and long-term relief.

THERAPEUTIC NERVE BLOCKS

Nerve blocks with local anesthetic in combination with corticosteroids may be useful for treating entrapment neuropathies, such as meralgia paresthetica and carpaltunnel syndrome. Intermittent epidural blocks with local anesthetic in combination with corticosteroids also are commonly used to treat radiculopathy and sciatica.

When corticosteroids accompany the local anesthetic, protracted relief of pain may be attributed to the longterm antiinflammatory effects of the corticosteroids. That may, at least in part, account for the success of these techniques in the treatment of entrapment neuropathies and sciatica. However, even when corticosteroids are not used, intermittent blocks with local anesthetics alone may provide relief that significantly outlasts the expected duration of analgesia from a single injection. That is particularly true in cases of CRPS (see Case Report, Patient 2, above) and certain neuralgias in which pain relief may last months and even years after a course of injections (from one to several blocks over weeks or months).

The mechanism or mechanisms that account for such prolonged analgesia are still unclear. Several theories have been proposed: the disruption of a reverberating cycle of nociceptive nerve transmission; increases in tissue blood flow, muscle relaxation, and restoration of function; and mobility while the local anesthetic provides analgesia. Whatever the mechanism of action, it is well documented that a single block or a series of injections with local anesthetic alone may provide long-term or even permanent relief from disorders such as CRPS.

Another indication for therapeutic nerve blocks is for the facilitation of other procedures, such as physical therapy. For example, intercostal nerve blocks may facilitate chest physical therapy as prophylaxis against respiratory complications in a patient with fractured ribs. Suprascapular nerve blocks may allow manipulation and physical therapy for a frozen shoulder. Epidural analgesia can be useful in allowing passive range-ofmotion exercises in a patient with reflex-sympathetic dystrophy of the leg. A variety of blocks also may be used to relieve muscle spasm or break a cycle of pain and spasm.

Another indication for the use of local-anesthetic blocks is to provide continuous analgesia for patients with severe pain that is not relieved by conventional methods. For example, a terminally ill cancer patient may benefit from continuous infusion of local anesthetic into the epidural space to relieve pain in the lower abdomen or legs. Catheters can be placed for continuous brachialplexus blockade or along distal nerves, like the femoral nerve, for long-lasting pain relief following certain surgical procedures.

When temporary (local anesthetic) blocks fail to provide pain relief of sufficiently long duration, a more permanent type of neural blockade may be sought. However, several misconceptions about the use of so-called permanent nerve blocks must be dispelled. First, no nerve blocks are truly permanent. Most neurolytic blocks will last from days to months, after which time the pain will recur and the block must be repeated. That may be appropriate for a patient with a short life expectancy but may not be appropriate in a patient with benign disease. Because with the risk of nerve regrowth comes the possibility of neuroma formation or neuropathic pain and the repeat block may not be successful, most pain specialists do not perform neurolytic blocks on persons with long life expectancies.

Second, it is not appropriate to perform multiple nerve blocks in patients with diffuse disease, such as multiple bony metastases. Third, neurolytic procedures are most appropriately performed on pure sensory nerves. Although some neurolytic substances preferentially block the pain fibers rather than the motor fibers, blockade of a mixed motor-sensory nerve has the potential for causing motor impairment. Finally, many neurolytic substances may cause skin or mucosal sloughing if injected superficially; these procedures are most appropriate for deep and well-localized structures.

Despite those shortcomings, neurolytic blocks may be appropriate in some circumstances. In any case, it always is appropriate to perform an injection with a local anesthetic before undertaking a neurolytic procedure. This not only gives the patient a chance to "preview" the degree of pain relief and numbness that may be experienced, but also gives the clinician a chance to observe the patient for untoward effects, such as the postural hypotension that may occur after sympathetic blockade.

For all of the reasons outlined above, the celiac plexus is well suited to neurolytic blockade. Because the celiac plexus is composed of a network of the sympathetic and parasympathetic efferent and afferent fibers of most of the upper-abdominal viscera, alcohol block of this structure can be especially useful for patients with painful intraabdominal malignancies, such as cancer of the pancreas.

Case Report

Patient 3

A 74-year-old man was referred to the pain management center with a diagnosis of cancer of the pancreas. Surgical exploration revealed the tumor was inoperable and the patient did well postoperatively, but over the next several weeks he began to experience increasingly severe midepigastric pain that radiated to the back. He was treated with oral opiates in escalating doses, but his pain persisted.

Under fluoroscopic control, a needle was guided to the anterolateral aspect of the body of the first lumbar vertebra, and a celiac-plexus block was performed bilaterally with 15 mL of 1% lidocaine on each side (Fig. 51.1). That provided him with excellent relief of pain, and observation in the recovery room revealed no postural changes in blood pressure. The block therefore was repeated with 15 mL of 95% alcohol on each side, and his pain relief persisted until his death 4 months later.

Historically, many substances, such as oil, hypertonic and hypotonic saline, alcohol, phenol, and chlorocresol have been used to provide chemical destruction of nerves (Table 51.1). Currently, the most commonly used chemical-neurolytic agents are alcohol and phenol. Either may

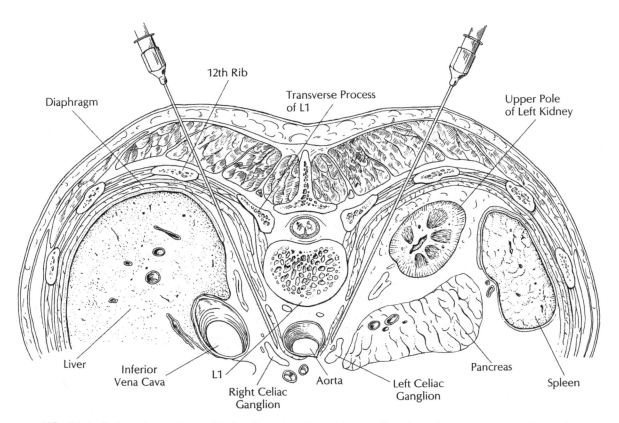

FIG. 51.1. Celiac-plexus block. Under fluoroscopic guidance, the posterior approach to the celiac plexus was used for the cancer patient described. Once the needle placement is confirmed, radiopaque dye can be used to visualize the spread of the solution. If local anesthetic blockade provides symptomatic relief, the block can be repeated with a neurolytic agent for longer-lasting relief.

TABLE 51.1. *Agents Used for Neurolytic Blockade*

Agent	Advantages	Disadvantages
Alcohol (50–100%)	Hypobaric	Neuritis; Solution may spread beyond target; May cause superficial sloughing at injection site
Phenol (6–12% in saline, glycerine or contrast)	Hyperbaric	Less profound block and shorter duration than alcohol; Neuritis; Solution may spread beyond target; May cause superficial sloughing at injection site
Cryoprobe	Reversible small area of destruction. Rare neuritis	Very accurate probe placement required; Large probe needed (12–18 gauge)
Radiofrequency	Small area of destruction	Neuritis can occur; Very accurate probe placement required; Large probe often needed

produce a neuritis, which usually resolves spontaneously, but may cause persistent dysesthetic, hyperpathic burning pain (possibly because of only partial nerve destruction). Although phenol is less likely to produce a neuritis, the block it produces often is less profound and of shorter duration than that achieved with alcohol.

More recently, long-lasting neural blockade has been produced with the use of extreme cold or heat. Cryoanalgesia has the added advantage of producing a completely reversible block that lasts for several weeks (Fig. 51.2). A 12- to 14-gauge cryoprobe must be placed very close to the nerve, and the temperature at the tip is lowered to 20°C for between 60 and 120 seconds, often in several cycles. Because of the size of the probe, there are some technical difficulties in getting the probe to reach deeper structures safely. Also, care must be taken to defrost the tip before removing the probe to minimize tissue damage. Animal studies reveal severe nerve destruction from

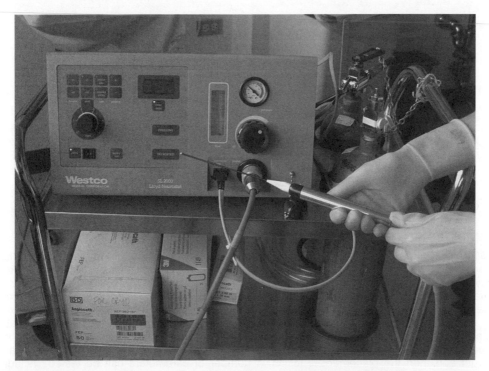

FIG. 51.2. The use of a cryoprobe is reported to block peripheral-nerve function. This procedure has been advocated for the treatment of neuralgia and chronic, intractable, peripheral-nerve lesions. A cryoprobe (must be used with a cooling gas, such as liquid nitrogen, nitrous oxide, or other such compressed gas) produces an ice ball. Within the needle probe, very small, hollow tubes allow the passage of the chosen gas. As the gas expands within the probe, heat is absorbed from the surrounding area, and the temperature rapidly drops. The ice crystals cause tissue changes that block peripheral-nerve function, resulting in an analgesic effect. Because the injured axons regenerate, the analgesia is not permanent. The median duration of pain relief is from 2 weeks to 5 months and can be of benefit in several postoperative circumstances. Cryoanalgesia therapy is most appropriate for painful conditions originating from small, well-localized lesions of peripheral nerves, for sample, neuromas and entrapment neuropathies.

cryoanalgesia and the creation of neuropathic-pain syndromes. In human applications, this syndrome of neuropathic pain does not seem to occur. It is possible that the cryoprobe is merely disrupting nerve transmission without full destruction of the axonal sheath, thereby disrupting the pain signal but not irreversibly damaging the nerve,

Like the cryoprobe, radiofrequency denervation requires very accurate probe placement, as the area of destruction is quite small (Fig. 51.3). The size of the radiofrequency probe varies from and may be as small as 22 gauge or as large as 14 gauge, and the area of destruction is a function of the probe size. The small area of destruction produced with both cryoanalgesia and radiofrequency analgesia precludes the potential side effects that may occur when alcohol or phenol spread beyond the target area and cause block of nearby structures.

The so-called alcohol-spinal block is a technique that was used considerably more widely before the introduction of intraspinal opiates. To perform the technique, a lumbar puncture is made with the patient positioned in a 45-degree lateral tilt with the painful side up (Fig. 51.4) Since alcohol is less dense than cerebrospinal fluid, a small amount of alcohol injected in that position would float upward and bathe only the posterior-sensory roots, leaving the anterior motor roots intact. A potential for motor block does exist, however, especially if the block needs to be performed bilaterally. For that reason, this technique should be performed only by skilled physicians.

Nerve blocks have a definite role in the treatment of painful conditions. In some cases, a single injection or series of injections with local anesthetic alone can provide excellent relief of pain and avoid the long-term use of analgesic medications. These techniques are not without risk, and even temporary blocks carry the risk of local anesthetic toxicity, infection, hematoma, and other, more serious side effects, depending on the location. Side effects and complications, however, are rare. On the other hand, neurolytic techniques require considerably more caution. Careful patient selection and patient preparation are mandatory;

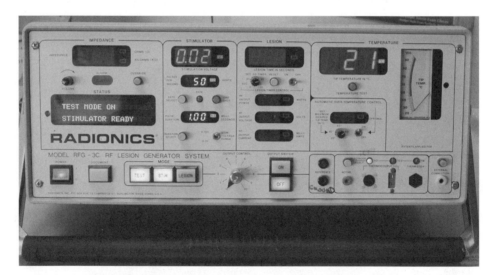

FIG. 51.3. Percutaneous radiofrequency neurotomy is an ablative procedure during which radiowave-induced heat is used to create a lesion in a sensory nerve, thus interrupting the nerve impulse. Radiofrequency lesion generators are used to produce discrete lesions in tissue using small precision-made radiofrequency probes. Radiofrequency lesioning has been used to disrupt nerve transmission for a number of painful conditions, including trigeminal neuralgia (destruction of part of the trigeminal ganglion), complex regional pain syndrome (sympathetic denervation), and facet syndrome (targeting the small somatic nerves that innervate the facet joints). To create the lesion in the desired area, a cannula is placed under sterile conditions near the target. A small needle with an uninsulated tip is passed to the target and then the placement is tested. A number of parameters can be tested, including the response to sensory stimulation or motor-fiber stimulation. Once position is confirmed, the pain clinician starts the lesioning protocol. With the onset of current flow, the temperature at the electrode-tissue interface increases for a period of 40 to 90 seconds. This temperature increases until the energy applied by way of the ablation catheter equals that lost through conduction and convection of heat away from the site. Once this steady-state temperature gradient has been achieved, there is no further lesion expansion. Thus, the total delivered energy can be calculated to be the product of power and duration. The high frequency, alternating current flows from the uninsulated tip of an electrode into the tissue, producing ionic agitation in the tissue about the electrode tip as the ions attempt to follow the changes in direction of the alternating current. This agitation drives water from the cells, leading to desiccation and coagulative necrosis. It also is important to clarify that in frictional heating, it is the tissue about the electrode, rather than the electrode itself, that is the primary source of heat.

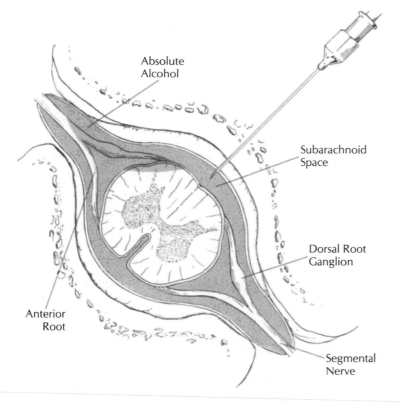

FIG. 51.4. Intrathecal alcohol block. Under fluoroscopic guidance to assure proper needle placement, the intrathecal space is accessed. The patient should be in a semirecumbent position of 45 degrees, with the painful side up. Although the alcohol solution is hypobaric, there is the possibility that motor blockade will occur.

selected use of these techniques can be very effective when conventional modes of pain therapy have failed.

SELECTED READING

Chelly JE. *Peripheral Nerve Blocks: A Color Atlas*. Philadelphia: Lippincott Williams & Wilkins, 1999.

Cousins MJ, Bridenbaugh P. *Neural Blockade in Clinical Anesthesia and Management of Pain*. Philadelphia: Lippincott Williams & Wilkins, 1998.

North RB, Kidd DH, Zahurak M, et al. Specificity of diagnostic nerve blocks: a prospective, randomized study of sciatica due to lumbosacral spine disease. *Pain* 1996;65:77–85.

Waldman SD, Winnie AP. *Interventional Pain Management*. London: WB Saunders Co., 1996.

CHAPTER 52

Sympathetic Blocks

Anna G.A. Sottile and Hilary J. Fausett

Blockade of the sympathetic pathways is a technique commonly used in every pain clinic. Sympathetic blockade is used diagnostically to determine if the sympathetic nervous system is involved in the patient's pain complaint. Because the pain often may be relieved for longer than the expected duration of the local anesthetic block, there also are therapeutic indications for the procedure.

Blockade of sympathetic transmission can be accomplished by a variety of approaches, including epidural or intrathecal blockade. A neuroaxial block will very likely result in blockade of all neuronal fibers: autonomic, sensory, and motor. Although "differential blockade" (which is the sequential blocking of autonomic fibers, followed by sensory fibers and lastly by motor fibers) has been described in the literature, in clinical practice such blocks are difficult for both the patient and the specialist and now are employed rarely. The technique of sequential blockade is a useful adjuvant for the motivated patient and for the practitioner to avoid the use of fluoroscopy or other radiographic-guidance systems.

The block of the pain achieved with a very low concentration of local anesthetics in the absence of sensory or motor deficits is presumed because of a sympathetic block. When the sympathetic inflow is the recognized cause of pain transmission, these blocks are very rewarding because they are able to alleviate or abolish the pain without inducing any other sensory or motor change. Moreover, other than in the thoracic area, the sympathetic ganglia are anatomically well separated from the somatic nerves, allowing a safe and successful approach. Most practitioners have come to realize, however, the larger the volume of local anesthetic used for a block, the more likely spread will result in sensory-fiber block as well. As the scientific exploration of the existence of sympathetically maintained pain continues, so too do clinicians continue to question the role of the sympathetic nervous system in maintaining or generating chronic pain.

The sympathetic chain may be blocked at a variety of locations, and the specific symptoms of the patient determine the site of blockade. The most commonly employed sympathetic blocks are: (a) stellate-ganglion block (SGB) for symptoms in the face, neck, and upper extremity; (b) celiac-plexus block (CPB) for abdominal pain, primarily in the upper quadrants; and (c) lumbar-sympathetic block for symptoms in the lower extremities.

ANATOMY

The sympathetic fibers originate in the intermediolateral column of the spinal cord. The fibers then pass into the ventral roots from T1 to T12, running separately as white rami, directing to the sympathetic chains, which rest on each side of the vertebral bodies. At the thoracic levels, the fibers are adjacent to the neck of the ribs, very close to the somatic roots. In the cervical and lumbar area, the two different fibers are better separated. Another important point is represented by the fact that the preganglionic fibers pass at variable distance in the chains to reach more distant ganglia. The results of this inconsistent pattern seem to be responsible for unsuccessful blocks.

The sympathetic chains receive preganglionic efferent and also afferent visceral fibers from the head, neck, upper and lower extremities, and abdominal and urogenital viscera.

STELLATE GANGLION BLOCK

Indications

The indications for a *stellate-ganglion block* are very broad, representing the wide range of clinical symptoms the sympathetic nervous system can affect. Sympathetic-maintained disorders, suspected or proven, affecting the upper-thoracic area or the upper extremities are the main indication. Examples of these kinds of disorders are: CRPS type I (formerly called reflex-sympathetic dystrophy) and CRPS type II (formerly called causalgia). Other disorders in which vascular tone appears to play a pivotal role also are often responsive to sympathetic blockade. These syndromes include Raynaud's syndrome, arterial embolism, and vasculitis. The accidental extravasation on upper-extremity vessels of drugs that can result in tissue damage and necrosis often is treated with prompt SGB. The acute herpes zoster of neck and arms, postherpetic neuralgia, and rarely, Ménière's syndrome have been classically treated with SGB, although the mechanism by which pain relief is obtained is unclear. The block can be performed for diagnostic or therapeutic purposes. A diagnostic block is used to establish if the sympathetic nervous system is responsible for a pain syndrome.

The positive result of a sympathetic block can be followed by therapeutic blocks. Usually, a series of temporary blocks is performed with patients receiving incremental relief from each block. Occasionally, more permanent blocks, if necessary, are performed.

Contraindications

The contraindication for stellate ganglion block can be divided into the risks inherent to any nerve block, the particular risks of the anatomic approach, and the risks of the blocked sympathetic nervous system, with unopposed parasympathetic transmission at a particular level. Anticoagulation, localized infection, or lesion at the site of entry and bacteremia as well as inability to give informed consent are all reasons to avoid performing an invasive procedure. Because of the particular approach to the stellate ganglion, along Chassaignac's Tubercle (see below) there is a risk of hitting the most superior portion of the lung, therefore pneumothorax or pneumonectomy on the contralateral side must be viewed as reasons to delay the block.

Recent myocardial infarction, secondary to cut-off of the cardioaccelerator nerve, may be a relative contraindication. Glaucoma may be worsened, as may atrioventricular blocks.

Technique

An anterior and posterior approach is described, but the first is most commonly used. The patient is preevaluated for the block, including a physical examination to document the reasons for the procedure and to ensure no contraindications to the invasive procedure. This also is the time for the specialist to explain the procedure and answer any questions. On the day of the procedures, an informed consent is discussed in detail and obtained, if it had not been obtained earlier. Intravenous access is started most commonly on the contralateral side of the block. Many practitioners also insist upon measuring the skin temperature continuously on both the affected and the unaffected sides.

The patent is positioned supine with the head in a neutral position and slightly hyperextended by a small pillow or roll of towels between the shoulders. The cricoid cartilage can be identified easily and, lateral to it, the C6 transverse process called Chassaignac's Tubercle, can be felt with a deeper and yet gentle palpation. The carotid artery is constantly palpated at the lateral side. A skin weal is raised between the trachea and the artery with a small amount of local anesthetic to numb the skin. A 23-gauge, 4- to 5-cm needle (or a 22-gauge, blunt-tip, nerve-block needle) is slowly introduced perpendicularly until the C6 tubercle is encountered. At this point, the needle is withdrawn by 1 to 2 mm and after negative aspiration, a total of 15 to 20 cc are injected, a few milliliters at the time, with intermittent negative aspiration. The volume of local anesthetic solution injected is determined by the patient's diagnosis and the need for spread of the anesthetic: the larger the volume the greater the area of spread. Thus, even poor technique likely will result in blockade but at a greater risk of blocking other nerves.

Evidence of Blockade

The following signs help to determine if a good block is achieved. Horner's syndrome describes a constellation of signs of the loss of sympathetic innervation and unopposed parasympathetic input. In addition to the classic triad of ptosis, miosis, and facial anidrosis, there likely will be evidence of enophthalmos, conjunctival injection, and nasal congestion. Because there may be alterations in vision, it is prudent to advise the patient to have an escort home. There often is vein engorgement of the back of the hand and arm, and there is improved plethysmography. There often is an increase in skin temperature on the ipsilateral side, most usually if the baseline was less than 35°C to 36°C. There also may be a positive sweat test. Of course, a relief of the pain is the most desirable sign.

Complications

The local anesthetic may result in blockade of other structures in the neck. Temporary paralysis of recurrent nerve may lead to hoarseness and occasionally a complaint of altered sensation in swallowing or breathing. Phrenic-nerve paralysis may go undetected in a healthy person and yet cause severe respiratory compromise in a person with preexisting lung disease. Partial brachial-plexus block may cause a loss of control of the upper extremity or unpleasant paresthesias.

Accidental epidural and intrathecal injection have been reported, which would result in a "total spinal" necessitating intubation and airway maintenance until the block receded. For this reason, full resuscitative equipment must be available. Intravascular injection, most commonly via vertebral arteries, may cause seizure from local anesthetic toxicity and is the reason why intermittent negative aspiration is recommended, to ensure the needle has not migrated during the procedure.

If air is injected into an artery, cerebral embolism may occur. If air is injected intrathecally, the patient may complain of terrible headache. The last major complication is that of pneumothorax, as discussed earlier.

LUMBAR-SYMPATHETIC BLOCK

Indication

The lumbar-sympathetic block has both diagnostic and therapeutic indications.

Indications for this block are represented by CRPS I and II, circulatory insufficiency of the lower extremities, intractable pain from renal colic, urogenital pain, phantom-limb pain, and postamputation pain.

Contraindication

The most common contraindications to the procedure include a bleeding diathesis, anatomic abnormalities, and local or generalized infection. The patient's refusal must be viewed as the strongest contraindication.

Technique

Several different techniques have been described. Here, we will limit the description to a few approaches more commonly used in our institution.

After having preevaluated the patient, having discussed all issues of risks and benefits, and having obtained consent, intravenous is started. Temperature probes are placed on a symmetrical part of both legs. Baseline and continuous temperature changes are monitored. The patient is positioned prone and the L3 spinal process is identified under fluoroscopy.

A skin wheal is raised at 6 to 8 cm. Lateral to the midline, a 25-gauge, extra-long spinal needle is introduced slowly. A lateral view is used to checked the depth of the needle. The goal is to visualize the tip of the needle just lying on the anterior aspect of the vertebral body on a lateral view. The sympathetic chain lies in the retroperitoneal space. Two techniques can be used to enter the space: loss of resistance and small tapping of the syringe plunger (A slow and steady hand is required for this technique.)

The use of radiopaque contrast dye is commonly used to confirm placement. After identifying the correct fluoroscopic image, a small amount of contrast is injected and a vacuolated aspect, just laterally to the vertebral body, is expected to be seen on an anteroposteral view. If a very well defined striplike image is seen radiating from the site, the iliopsoas muscle is likely to be injected instead, and therefore, reposition of the needle is required. When a satisfactory position is achieved, a total of 20 to 40 cc of local anesthetic is injected, with intermitted negative aspiration.

The positioning of the needle in the cephalocaudal plain depends upon the patient's diagnosis and the specialist's preference. Some specialists prefer a higher placement, such as L1 for renal colic or testicular pain and L4 or L5 for foot pain. Other specialists will always use the L3 approach, as the sympathetic chain is known to run closest to the vertebral bodies at this level, and then tilt the bed to use gravity to affect the spread of the local anesthetic. Some practitioners make it a practice to employ 2 or 3 levels of approach. Very rarely is the block performed bilaterally, because of the significant risk of hypotension, which will cause cardiovascular compromise, even in healthy patients.

Most practitioners who perform more permanent blockade with phenol, alcohol, or radiofrequency denervation, insist on the use of dye to confirm needle placement and spread of any solution. With the easy availability of fluoroscopy and computerized axial tomography (CAT) scan, these blocks are rarely done with radiologic guidance, although the classic approach described above was developed as a "blind" technique.

Evidence of Blockade

An increase of temperature on the ipsilateral side should be seen, as well as venous engorgement from vasodilatation. There may be a decrease of edema, but an increase in any erythema is not uncommon. The sign that both the specialist and the patient desire most is a decrease in pain.

Complications

Because the side effects of the blockade can be quite dramatic, patients must be adequately prepared for a variety of changed sensations following blockade. If the block is performed not with local anesthetic but with phenol or alcohol, then the patient must understand the more permanent nature of the unwanted effects. Hypotension is quite common, and the pain practitioner must be equipped to handle such a complication. Accidental intravascular injection may accompany any nerve block, but because the volume of local anesthetic is so large, many specialists rely on the use of radiopaque dye to ensure the needle has not been place in a blood vessel. Transient neuralgia of genitofemoral nerve is not uncommon, and may result in an unpleasant paraesthesia. Necrosis of psoas muscle can occur with local anesthetic as well as with neuroablative techniques. Sloughing of the ureter also has been reported. Impotence and failure to ejaculate may be a devastating complication. There is the potential for alteration in female sexual response as well.

CELIAC PLEXUS BLOCK

The celiac plexus is the largest plexus of the sympathetic nervous system. It supplies the organs and visceral reflections of the upper abdomen. It surrounds the celiac artery and the aorta at the level of L1. It is located between the cardiac plexus and the hypogastric plexus.

Indication

Chronic pain located on the upper abdomen, most commonly of pancreatic origin, as well as retroperitoneal and flank pain are indications for celiac block. Pain from the capsular stretch of the liver with metastatic disease may be amenable to relief from celiac-plexus block. Although it has been tried for the treatment of chronic pancreatitis, it is not of proven benefit for this type of intermittent and recurrent pain. Celiac-plexus block has not been shown to diminish the likelihood of future episodes.

Contraindications

Coagulopathies, known anatomical abnormalities, local or intraabdominal infection or generalized sepsis, and patient's refusal represent the absolute contraindication for this block. Small-bowel obstruction or any sudden hypermobility of the bowel may be harmful.

Technique

An anterior approach is performed easily during laparotomy, but pain specialists usually use the posterior percutaneous approach. Among the various techniques available for the posterior approach, we will describe the most commonly used retrocrural technique. Although the posterior approach was first described as a "blind" technique for needle placement, with the ready availability of fluoroscopy, this approach now is done most commonly with radiographic guidance. The anterior transhepatic approach is favored by many interventional radiologists and pain specialist who use CAT scan to guide needle placement.

All issues and questions regarding the block should be discuss ahead of time with the patient. A verbal and written consent then should be obtained. It also is often helpful to discuss the indications and expectations of the block with the referring physician as well.

On the day of the procedure, all should be reviewed and, if no further questions come up, intravenous access must be started and intravenous fluids are given, to prevent or at least blunt the hypotension that accompanies the sympathetic blockade. The patient then is positioned prone under the fluoroscopy machine, with a pillow under the abdomen to increase the distance between the ribs and iliac crest. The head is turned on one side and arms are in a neutral position to minimize any torque of the spine, which is the major bony landmark. Many pain specialists prefer to mark the skin of the patient for better determination of the landmarks.

The following landmarks are identified: the tips of the 12th ribs bilateral and the spinous processes of T12 and L1. A line is drawn from the point representing T12 spinous process to a point 7 to 8 cm lateral; this is repeated with the L1 spinous process. These two lines should correspond to the tip of the 12th rib. By connecting these lines, we obtain an isosceles triangle. It is customary to repeat this process on the contralateral side: the celiac plexus is not a lateralized structure, and thus can be blocked from either side, or even from both sides, to maximize the likelihood of a successful block. A line between the two iliac crests also is drawn. The skin above the base of the triangle is infiltrated with lidocaine 1% (7 to 8 cm lateral to the L1 point, just underneath the 12th ribs). A 22-gauge, 13 cm needle with stylet in place is slowly introduced, 45 degrees toward midline, aiming at the L1 vertebral body. Once the bony contact is made, the needle is withdrawn 1 to 2 mm and redirected, in order to walk off the lateral surface of the L1. This insertion is very slow, and the aim is to feel the arterial pulsation transmitted through the aorta. The right-sided needle is advanced a few more millimeters, and final position should be checked with fluoro. The left needle should be at the posterior aspect of the aorta and the right one should be at the anterolateral aspect of it. Because fluoroscopy only will reveal the aorta if it is very heavily calcified, the exact position of the plexus must be assumed from bony landmarks.

The stylets then are removed and the lumen checked to rule out the presence of cerebrospinal fluid (CSF), urine, or blood. If a dry lumen is seen, a small amount of contrast is injected bilaterally and its spread is closely observed. Ideally, the contrast should stay confined toward midline and not spread laterally. A total of 12 to 15 cc of local anesthetic (lidocaine 1.5% is mostly used for diagnostic blocks, whereas bupivacaine 0.5% is used often for therapeutic blocks).

A better resolution is obtained with computed tomography (CT)-guided technique. In the patient who has undergone abdominal surgery or has a known mass or a marked scoliosis, it is prudent to proceed with CT guidance. It has been our experience that the celiac plexus may lie anywhere from T10 to the base of L1, thus if anatomic disturbance is suspected, or if the initial block is not successful, it may be worthwhile to pursue CT-guided blockade.

Complications

Good positioning, the use of a test dose, and the drawing of the landmark are all excellent way to reduce the incidence of complications. Patients must be advised and specialists must be prepared to treat complications should they arise. Hypotension is such a common occurrence (incidence of 30% to 60 %) that it should be considered the sign of a successful block, rather than a complication.

Both intrathecal and epidural injection may occur with the anticipated risks. Intrapsoas injection has been reported, as has intravascular injection. Retroperitoneal hematoma secondary to aorta or, most likely, cava puncture may cause significant bleeding, which may go undetected as hypotension and the resultant tachycardia may be viewed as signs of successful blockade and not exsanguination. The kidney or ureter may be damaged as may other viscera. There are reports of cyst or abscess puncture and also pneumothorax. The latter must be ruled out prior to discharging a patient to home. Because gastrointestinal hypermobility is so common, patients should be told to expect diarrhea. Most specialists consider small-bowel obstruction or other physical, mechanical, intestinal obstruction as a strong contraindication to proceeding with the block. Similarly, many specialists find that celiac-plexus block is of benefit to patients who suffer from hypomobility secondary to opiates or from chronic constipation.

SPANCHNIC-NERVE BLOCK

The block of the splanchnic nerve is used because all sensory nerves from the abdominal viscera are located within this nerve. Parasympathetic pathways are undisturbed. Similar analgesic results are obtained by blocking a higher area than with the celiac-plexus blocks.

Anatomy

Three separated nerve entities can be distinguished: the greatest, the lesser, and the lowest splanchnic nerve.

The greatest splanchnic nerve arises from sympathetic fibers from the 5th and the 9th thoracic ganglia. These are located on the side of the anterior part of the thoracic vertebral bodies and they tend to move more anteriorly in the more caudal portion. They pass the diaphragm through the crus and they end their course on the celiac plexus. The lesser splanchnic nerve follows a similar pathway, but arises from the 10th and 11th thoracic ganglia. The lowest splanchnic nerve arises only from the 12th ganglia.

Indications

Chronic pain affected the upper-abdominal viscera.

Technique

With a patient positioned prone with a pillow under the abdomen, the 12th rib and the midline are used as landmarks. A skin wheal is raised 8 to 10 cm off the midline just below the 12th rib line. A needle then is slowly advanced toward the 12 thoracic vertebral bodies, therefor slightly moved cephalad and medially. A radiological image is obtained and the tip of the needle is moved until an optimal position is found. This would be on the sides of the vertebral body on an anteroposterior view and on the upper-anterior border of the 12th vertebral body on a lateral view. This is likely to block on the lowest splanchnic nerve for most people. Any attempt to block more cephalad must be weighed against the very high risk of pneumothorax. This is one major reason this block is very rarely performed.

Complications

Orthostatic hypotension is the most common complication, and indeed should be viewed as a sign of a successful block. The risk of pneumothorax is very high, and no patient should be sent home until this potential complication has been ruled out. Intravascular and intrathecal injection are also possible.

SELECTED READINGS

Lofstrom JB, Lloyd JW, Cousins MJ. Sympathetic neural blockade of upper and lower extremities. In: Cousins MJ, Bridenbaugh PO, eds. *Neural Blockade In Clinical Anesthesia and Management of Pain*, 3rd ed. Philadelphia: JB Lippincott Co., 1997.

Raj PP. Ganglion block. In: Waldman and Winnie Dannemiller Memorial Foundation, ed. *Interventional Pain Management*. Philadelphia: WB Saunders Co., 1996.

Scott DB. Sympathetic nerve blockade: lumbar sympathectomy, stellate ganglion blockade, coeliac plexus block, splanchnic nerve block. In: *Techniques of Regional Anesthesia*. Norwalk, CT: Appleton and Lange/Mediglobe, 1989.

Stanton-Hicks M. Lumbar sympathetic nerve block and neurolysis. In: Waldman and Winnie Dannemiller Memorial Education Foundation, ed. *Interventional Pain Management*. Philadelphia: WB Saunders Co., 1996.

Thompson GF. Celiac plexus, intercostal, and minor peripheral blockade. In: Cousins MJ, Bridenbaugh PO, eds. *Neural Blockade in Clinical Anesthesia and Management of Pain*. Philadelphia: JB Lippincott Co., 1997.

Physical Measures

CHAPTER 53

Physical Therapy

Kathleen E. Shillue

The purpose of physical therapy is to promote optimal health and function through procedures to alleviate acute or prolonged movement dysfunction. Many of the patients seen by physical therapists have pain, but the reason for their physical-therapy intervention usually is some kind of abnormal movement resulting in a loss of function or potential loss of function.

Changes in movement are the body's response to acute pain and serve to decrease the stress on healing tissue. A person in pain will move in ways to reduce the mechanical loading on an injured area to prevent further damage, reduce pain, and allow the repair process to proceed without hindrance. Physical therapy for patients with acute pain may target pain as a symptom of the underlying pathology, and the progression of activity will proceed according to the healing constraints of the particular tissue involved. The goals of treatment are to minimize the abnormal movement, protect healing tissue, facilitate healing, and optimize function. Chronic pain, or pain that has persisted beyond the time required for normal healing, may no longer have any identifiable, underlying pathology. In addition to the original injury or cause of the pain, the physical therapist must be concerned with the long-term adaptations the body makes in its movement patterns to accommodate prolonged pain. Long-term inactivity or abnormal movement causes reductions in the normal loading patterns and adaptations in connective tissue and bone, resulting in decreased flexibility, joint stiffness, and muscle atrophy, and leads to deconditioning. During this period of inactivity, patients may stop working, participating in social activities, and have difficulty performing normal activities of daily living. They may develop a complex set of medical, emotional, and psychosocial problems that will require a coordinated multidisciplinary treatment approach.

The physical-therapy evaluation should include a history and physical examination to identify the physical and functional impairments as well as any medical, social, occupational, or behavioral barriers to full participation in treatment. The physical therapist should coordinate the treatment plan with other providers, physicians, nurses, psychologists, occupational therapists, or vocational counselors to help address any of these issues.

Baseline measurements of strength, flexibility, joint motion, endurance, and posture may help to identify some of the contributing sources of pain, as well as the secondary adaptations resulting from altered movement, and guide the physical therapy plan of care. Although the focus of the physical therapy program is to correct the biomechanical impairments related to the pain and to improve the patient's ability to function; the interventions also can work to reduce pain in several ways. Nociceptor activity caused by mechanical or chemical irritation can be reduced with physical agents, exercise, and assistive or protective devices to decrease inflammation and reduce the mechanical stresses on painful tissues. The use of corrections in movement, manual therapy, and thermal or electrotherapeutic stimulation can increase mechanoreceptor activity to help block pain through the gating mechanism theorized by Melzack and Wall. Patients beginning a physical-therapy program often are anxious about exacerbating their symptoms. Educating the patient about the causes of pain, instructing in self-treatment, and pacing techniques may help to facilitate descending inhibition of pain by reducing the anxiety and giving them some control over the symptoms. Components of the physical-therapy treatment may include therapeutic exercise, education, instruction in the use of assistive devices or braces, manual therapy, and thermal or electrotherapeutic modalities.

EXERCISE

Therapeutic exercise is the core element in most physical-therapy treatment plans and is the most frequently used intervention. It includes a variety of activities designed to improve strength, range of motion, coordination, endurance, balance, and posture, using passive, active, or resistive movements. Based on the results of the initial evaluation, the therapist determines what the patient's capabilities are and can set the appropriate mode, frequency, intensity, and duration of the exercise program needed to correct the specific impairments. There have not been many studies to show the effectiveness of specific types of exercises for patients with pain. Many studies combine several types of exercises, making it difficult to judge the effectiveness of one type or pattern of exercise against another. For example, the Agency for Health Care Policy and Research (AHCPR) found little research-based evidence in favor of any specific treatment intervention for acute low-back problems. The clinical guideline for acute low-back problems does recommend low-impact aerobic exercises, and after the first 2 weeks, back-conditioning exercises. Deyo, one of the panel members, agreed that there was expert consensus that exercise plays a major role in the treatment of low-back symptoms. Most treatment problems use a variety of combinations and there is no agreement on specifics.

Patients with low-back pain represent a large proportion of the patients referred for physical therapy. Under the broad category of low-back pain, which is their presenting symptom, there may be many underlying pathologies, or no identifiable pathology at all. It may be more useful to separate patients based on the pattern of physical impairments and target the interventions to the specific impairment.

O'Sullivan et al. found that a specific exercise program directed at specific muscles was more effective than general exercise. Forty-four patients with a history of low-back pain for more than 3 months, and with a radiological diagnosis of spondylolysis or spondylolisthesis, were randomly assigned to an exercise or control group. The exercise group was instructed in a specific program of exercises to improve control of the deep abdominals and lumbar multifidus, the primary function of which is to provide dynamic stability and segmental control to the spine. Patients were seen by a physical therapist once per week for 10 weeks to instruct them in specific exercises to co-contract the abdominals and multifidus without activating other muscle groups. They supplemented this with a home-practice session lasting 10 to 15 minutes daily. The exercises involved a high level of specificity and a low level of maximal, voluntary contraction, and began with ten, 10-second isometric contractions, repeated 10 times. They were progressed by applying resistance through the addition of leverage to the limbs.

Once the patients were able to perform the exercises correctly, they began to use the trunk muscle holding contractions during functional activities, especially those that were previously painful. The control group was treated with the usual care, which in all but one case, consisted of general exercise, like swimming, walking, or gym workouts. After intervention, the exercise group showed a reduction in pain intensity and improvement in functional disability level, which was maintained after a 30-month follow up. The control group showed no change.

Aerobic exercise is used widely to improve endurance and enhance conditioning levels, and should be a core component of any exercise program to treat patients with chronic pain who have the specific impairment of deconditioning. There also is increasing evidence that aerobic exercises also may increase systemic levels of endorphins and decrease sensitivity to pain. Wigers et al. studied a group of 60 patients with fibromyalgia randomized to groups for aerobic exercise, stress management, or control. After 14 weeks of treatment, both the aerobic-exercise and stress-management groups showed improvement in pain and disability, although the aerobic-exercise group improved to a greater degree.

Specific exercises to correct musculoskeletal imbalances will use stretching to increase the length of shortened muscles and strengthening to increase the performance of weak, opposing muscle groups. Strengthening exercises can be performed with high resistance and low repetitions to cause muscle hypertrophy and improve fiber recruitment or with low resistance and higher repetitions to allow an increase in muscular endurance. Patients who are inactive for a long time, or who have adopted compensatory movements, must be taught to perform precise exercises without unwanted muscles contracting. Neuromuscular reeducation may be used to improve recruitment patterns during activity for improved coordination and efficiency of movement, and to promote relaxation in overactive muscles. With repetition and practice and using electrical stimulation, biofeedback, and verbal and tactile cues, the patient can learn to perform precise movements and correct dysfunctional compensatory patterns.

MANUAL THERAPY

Manual therapy uses a variety of techniques to produce passive movements that are not usually under the direct control of the patient. The American Physical Therapy Association describes it as skilled hand movements used by the physical therapist to mobilize or manipulate soft tissues and joints. It can include connective-tissue massage, joint and soft-tissue mobilization, and manipulation, manual lymphatic drainage, manual traction, passive range of motion, or therapeutic massage. In preparation for exercise, manual therapies can decrease pain and increase joint and soft-tissue extensibility. Concerning the usefulness in pain relief, AHCPR found spinal mobilization to be a beneficial treatment for relief of acute low-back pain in the first 4 weeks. In practice, manual therapy usually is combined with some type of exercise, so that after mobility is gained the patient may develop some control of the increased movement or flexibility and integrate it into useful functional activity.

PHYSICAL AGENTS

Physical agents include thermal and electrotherapeutic modalities and are used often in combination with exercise in treatment programs. Michlovitz describes various forms of superficial heat used in physical therapy; including hydrocollator packs, whirlpool, paraffin, and fluidotherapy. Heat will cause a local rise in tissue temperature, vasodilation, increased extensibility of collagen tissue, and reduced muscle-spindle activity. It also provides increased peripheral thermoreceptor afferent activity to the spinal cord and may block pain transmission to higher levels as described by Melzack and Wall. For this reason, it is a useful adjunct to an exercise program, often increasing the exercise's effectiveness and allowing patients to tolerate exercise more comfortably. Patients also can easily use heat as part of a home program.

Ultrasound is a method of supplying deep heat to tissues, using high-frequency sound waves. At frequencies of 1 or 3 MHz, it penetrates 3 to 5 cm, allowing heating of deeper structures like joint capsules or tendons. In addition to thermal effects, it also can provide the mechanical effects of micromassage and increased membrane permeability. At pulsed settings, it can provide the mechanical effects without the heating, when a rise in tissue temperature is not desired.

Cold application, by means of a cold pack, ice pack, ice massage, or vapo-coolant spray reduces tissue metabolism, allowing reduction in inflammation. It provides a counter irritant to reduce pain and may reduce nerve-conduction velocity. The choice of heat or cold will depend upon the acuity of the injury and whether hemorrhage or acute inflammation is present. In addition, cold will tend to increase tissue stiffness while heat will increase tissue extensibility, so if exercise will follow, this should be taken into consideration.

Electrical stimulation uses either direct current or alternating current. Direct current is used for two purposes in physical therapy, stimulation of denervated muscles and iontophoresis. Iontophoresis is the transfer of ions into the body for therapeutic purposes. Because like charges repel and opposite charges attract, use of the negative and positive electrodes with similarly charged ions can be used to deliver medication into the body transdermally. For example, the medication dexamethasone has a net negative charge in solution, and can be delivered with a negative electrode for treatment of inflammation. Alternating current is used with all other applications for muscle stimulation, producing either motor or sensory stimulation. It is used to stimulate or facilitate a muscle contraction for reeducation, and to produce strong muscle contractions for reduction of edema and relief of muscle spasm. Transcutaneous electrical nerve stimulation (TENS) is used for pain control and its rationale is based on the gate-control theory proposed by Melzack and Wall. It is used at high-frequency settings for purely sensory stimulation or at lower frequencies for motor stimulation as well.

Timm examined the effectiveness of physical agents and manipulation as passive treatments compared to active exercise for patients with chronic back pain. He studied 250 patients with chronic low-back pain following L5 laminectomy, randomized to four treatments and one control group. The treatment groups consisted of one of two passive groups using physical agents (superficial heat, ultrasound, and TENS) or joint manipulation. The two other groups were considered active, using mobility and strengthening exercises either with no equipment, or using a stationary bicycle and weight-training equipment. The joint manipulation and both exercise groups showed improvement in range of motion, but only the exercise groups showed improvement in lifting strength and Oswestry low-back pain disability questionnaire scores. The study did not attempt to compare the use of physical agents or joint manipulation in combination with exercise, as they often are used in practice.

CASE REPORT

A 38-year-old female working as an ultrasonographer was referred for evaluation and treatment of low-back pain and right-shoulder pain of several months' duration; the pain was related to her work. She had been initially seen by occupational therapy for right de Quervain's tendinitis, and the occupational therapist recommended a referral to physical therapy. She reported that her wrist pain was worst and began first, followed by the back pain, and more recently the shoulder pain, which was minimal. On examination, she had a loss of left-lumbar lateral-flexion range of motion, and weakness of the abdominals, right periscapular muscles, rotator cuff, thumb, and grip. There was tenderness and increased tone in the right upper trapezius, and pain along right abductor pollicis longus and extensor pollicis brevis tendons. A visit to her work site revealed that her job consisted of performing ultrasound scans of up to 45 minutes each. To obtain the desired resolution on her scans, she often had to bend over her patients, reach across their bodies, and hold her position for several minutes at a time. If she positioned herself to maintain a normal spinal alignment during the scan, she found that she had increased shoulder and wrist pain. If she adopted a more relaxed hand grip and shoulder position, she had to laterally flex her spine to the right and had back pain. She had been exercising at a gym three times per week doing aerobic exercise on a treadmill or aerobics class, but had stopped her exercise routine because of back pain at the end of the day.

An assessment of her problems found impairments in range of motion, joint mobility, muscle performance, and lack of knowledge of body mechanics in a woman whose job and work environment required repetitive use of specific muscle groups and sustained asymmetrical loading of the thumb, wrist, shoulder, and lumbar spine. Her low-back pain was thought to be the result of sustained asymmetrical loading of the spine without adequate muscle support. At the shoulder, an initial pattern of shoulder pain began after a few minutes of scanning, and with fatigue, she began to substitute elevation of the shoulder and developed pain along the upper trapezius as a result. The wrist pain was from an acute de Quervain's tendinitis caused by a tight grip on the ultrasound head and the repetitive fine movements used to control it. Because her wrist pain began first, it is likely that she began to compensate for that, causing increased work for the shoulder and back.

Intervention included both occupational therapy and physical therapy, with coordination of care between the two services to address all of the impairments and prevent duplication of services. The occupational therapist had begun treatment on the de Quervain's tendinitis using iontophoresis for inflammation, exercises for hand and wrist strengthening, and ergonomic adaptations to the work site. Adaptations to the grip of the ultrasound machine made it easier to hold the sound head, and with practice, she was able to develop the ability to alternate using the left and right hands for scanning. The physical-therapy plan included joint mobilization of the lumbar spine, with stretching exercises to increase left lumbar side bending and restore motion lost by her constant bending to the right at work. She was instructed to perform the stretches between scans also. Because she was learning how to alternate hands in scanning, she was now also alternating trunk movement and muscle use, and felt significant improvement in her back pain within two sessions. A strengthening program was prescribed with low resistance and high rep-

etitions for the abdominals, lower trapezius, rhomboids, and rotator-cuff muscle groups, to be performed daily. She was educated in ways to improve the efficiency of her movements through changes in spine and arm positions to minimize fatigue and continued alternating the left- and right-handed scanning techniques. She was instructed to return to her usual aerobic program at the gym, and added the strengthening exercises to her routine. Because the back and shoulder pain were mainly from movement abnormalities and overuse, no specific interventions were directed towards decreasing pain. She was able to achieve a reduction in pain through correction of the dysfunctional movement patterns. Treatment continued for six visits. On a follow-up visit 1 month later, she reported that she was pain free except for occasional shoulder pain, and was able to adjust her scanning technique to relieve the pain as needed.

Physical therapy uses many types of exercises to improve muscle performance, range of motion, or conditioning, and uses manual therapy techniques to reduce pain, improve inflammation, and improve range of motion and flexibility. To be effective in the treatment of a patient with pain, the interventions must be directed towards a specific pattern of impairments that may be components of the movement dysfunctions caused by pain.

SELECTED READINGS

American Physical Therapy Association. Guide to physical therapist practice. *Phys Ther* 1998;77.

Bigos S, Bowyer O, Braen G, et al. Acute low back problems in adults. *Clinical Practice Guideline*, quick reference guide number 4. Rockville, MD: U.S. Department of Health and Human Services, Public Health Service, Agency for Health Care Policy and Research, December 1994.

Rennie GA, Michlovitz, SL. Biophysical principles of heating and superficial heating agents. In: Michlovitz SL, ed. *Thermal Agents in Rehabilitation*, 2nd ed. Philadelphia: FA Davis Company, 1990:107–137.

Melzack R, Wall PD. Pain Mechanisms: a new theory. *Science* 1965;150: 971–979.

O'Sullivan PB, Twomey LT, Allison GT. Evaluation of specific stabilizing exercise in the treatment of chronic low back pain with radiologic diagnosis of spondylosis or spondylolisthesis. *Spine* 1997;2:2959–2966.

Timm KE. A randomized control study of active and passive treatment for chronic low back pain following L5 laminectomy. *JOSPT* 1994;20: 276–286.

Wigers SH, Stiles TC, Vogel PA. Effects of aerobic exercise versus stress management treatment in fibromyalgia. A 4.5 year prospective study. *Scand J Rheumatol* 1996;25:77–86.

CHAPTER 54

Occupational Therapy

Deborah L. Rochman, Carol P. Keck, and Kirsten E. Colton

Occupational therapy is the therapeutic use of self-care, work, and leisure activities to increase independence and prevent disability. Although the use of the word "occupation" implies an emphasis on vocation, it is used to define those meaningful activities that occupy one's life and are used therapeutically to allow an individual to return to independence after injury or illness. The main focus of an occupational-therapy practitioner is to examine a person's "occupational performance:" the ability to dress, prepare meals, work, or even play a round of golf. Evidence-based interventions are selected for their effectiveness in restoring individuals to previous roles within the context of their social, cultural, and physical environments.

Occupational therapists work with patients and clients who have conditions frequently associated with pain including upper-extremity injuries, low-back pain, arthritis, cancer, complex regional pain syndrome, fibromyalgia, headache, myofascial pain, burns, and fractures. The primary therapeutic objectives for people in pain are reduction of pain and associated disability, promotion of optimal function in everyday life thus enabling meaningful family and social relationships, and promotion of health and well-being by prevention of pain and pain-related disability.

The educational preparation of the occupational therapist includes courses in the biological and behavioral sciences that prepare therapists to work with physical and psychosocial disability. There are two levels of entry into the field: the professional-level therapist earns a master's degree. The technical-level assistant enters with an associate's degree in occupational therapy. Supervised clinical internships are required for completion of degree programs. Most states require practitioners to be licensed after completion of a national certification examination administered by the National Board for Certification in Occupational Therapy. All occupational-therapy practitioners in the United States must adhere to the American Occupational Therapy Association's Standards of Prac-

tice and Code of Ethics and demonstrate continuing competence throughout their careers.

Occupational therapists may provide services to people in pain in varied settings including acute care, rehabilitation hospitals, skilled nursing facilities, outpatient programs or clinics, private practice, home health, industrial rehabilitation, and community-based settings. Occupational therapists, by virtue of their training and/or experience, should be specially qualified to evaluate and treat patients in pain at pain-treatment facilities, especially those dealing with the complexities associated with chronic-pain problems.

Occupational therapists working in the area of pain management must understand and appreciate the complexity of pain, defined by the International Association for the Study of Pain (IASP) as an unpleasant sensory and emotional experience associated with actual or potential tissue damage or described in terms of such damage. This modern definition of pain embraces both the subjective and multidimensional nature of pain while acknowledging that pain is a complex biopsychosocial phenomenon. Effective pain management requires an understanding of the differences between acute and chronic pain both of which occupational therapists are trained to evaluate, and are aided by their ability to approach the patient as a whole person, rather than an isolated problem, disease, or organ system.

A conceptual framework of disability is useful in clarifying the profession's role in pain management. The *ICIDH-2: International Classification of Impairments, Activities and Participation*, developed by the World Health Organization (WHO), outlines the four classifications of disablement: disease or disorder, impairments, activity limitations, and participation restrictions. For example, at the impairment level, therapists treating patients with acute pain may help to prevent deformity or weakness by the use of splinting or physical-agent modalities, such as ultrasound, paraffin, or fluidotherapy to decrease acute pain. At the activity limitation level, the occupational therapist may intervene by teaching the patient with either acute or chronic pain self-care, work-modification, or pain-control techniques to reduce dependence and disability. At the participation restriction level, the therapist examines the contexts that impact performance, such as a patient's age, culture, social and environmental factors. The therapist may perform an environmental assessment at home or work and recommend ergonomic changes to maximize function and prevent pain and further disability.

In this chapter, we have included case reports of acute and chronic-pain conditions. These serve to illustrate the role of the occupational-therapy practitioner concerned with reducing pain and its disabling effects. Although the roles of these therapists may vary with the particular setting, therapeutic interventions are most effective when used within an interdisciplinary team approach.

PAIN MANAGEMENT APPROACHES

The Joint Commission on Accreditation of Healthcare Organizations (JCAHO) mandates that pain control is a formal patient right and an organizational responsibility. Furthermore, standards set forth by the Rehabilitation Accreditation Commission (CARF) for acute, chronic, and cancer-related pain programs require that services be coordinated, goal-oriented, and interdisciplinary, and should improve functioning and decrease the dependence on healthcare systems by persons with pain. The role and function of rehabilitation therapists in pain management vary within particular healthcare settings and confusion exists between patients and providers alike as to the defined roles of occupational and physical therapists. In fact, an integrated, cooperative, and flexible system that allows cotreatment and interchangeability of therapy roles provides optimum results.

Functional goal-setting is the basis of all pain rehabilitation and should be part of the initial evaluation. Individualized programs are developed with the patient, and family, when appropriate, and should reflect the functional goals identified during this process. Patient involvement promotes motivation, a sense of control, and self-efficacy. These are the critical foundations for the self-management approach that underlies all occupational therapy interventions in pain management and pain rehabilitation.

The self-management approach focuses on altering the pain experience, helping patients to adopt an internal locus of control rather than being passive recipients of care by others. This approach requires that patients become active participants in their own care; that they learn as much as they can about their conditions, become decision-makers in their therapy program, and pursue programs for learning effective pain-coping strategies. Occupational therapists facilitate self-management through patient education, designing therapeutic programs with the patient, and promoting independent function.

Education of the patient and family should lead not only to changes in knowledge, but also to changes in behavior and psychosocial and physical health status. For patients in pain, information is provided about the pathophysiology of the painful condition, the gate-control theory of pain, factors that may exacerbate or quell the condition or symptoms, pain-coping strategies, and other knowledge areas, such as communication and problem-solving.

Occupational-based therapy programs train patients in pain to gradually resume activities and meet functional goals within safe limits. Group or individualized programs, using graded or quota-based activities, provide success opportunities for patients to increase self-efficacy, e.g., "I can do it." There is evidence that patients in pain who report high levels of self-efficacy are less psychologically and physically disabled by their pain.

OCCUPATIONAL THERAPY EVALUATION

After review of the medical record and referral information, occupational therapists select assessment methods to obtain critical information necessary in developing appropriate treatment plans (Table 54.1).

The occupational therapist must depend on observation of the patient during functional tasks and activities. This provides a wealth of information about pain behaviors, the patient's approach to tasks, quality of movement, posture and body mechanics, and safety awareness. When such assessments are done at the patient's home or work setting, additional information about psychosocial or environmental factors that may be contributing to the pain problem (for example, an oversolicitous spouse or a poorly designed work station) provides further insight. Depending on the evaluation format, the patient may be asked to put on a coat, lift an object off the floor, retrieve something from a high cabinet, prepare a snack, pick up or carry a bag of groceries, or demonstrate job-related activities. Functional Capacity Evaluations (FCEs), formal assessments of physical capacities, such as standing tolerance, may be used to obtain objective measures of physical capacities. Functional assessment scales such as the Pain Disability Index or the Oswestry Low Back Pain Disability Questionnaire provide subjective measures of pain-related disability and may be appropriate for patients with chronic pain.

How the patient copes and adjusts to pain provides valuable insight into how the patient appraises the pain, which may have a significant impact on psychological distress and physical disability. The Beck Depression Inventory and the Coping Strategies Questionnaire are self-report measures that may be used for this purpose.

The Canadian Occupational Performance Measure (COPM) is an outcome measure specifically designed for

TABLE 54.1. *Recommended Tests and Measures of an Occupational Therapy Pain Evaluation*

Method(s) used to obtain information
McGill PQ, pain drawing, pain diary, numerical rating scale (NRS), other
Structured interview
Canadian Occupational Performance Measure
Observational assessments (or simulations) of patient at home, at worksite, in the community
Screens and tests of range of motion, strength, cognition, other; referrals to appropriate specialists for further assessment
Coping Strategies Questionnaire, other; assessment of pacing, assertiveness, relaxation, stress management, organizational and problem-solving skills; screening tests to assess voluntary muscle relaxation, breath control, postural control, and body mechanics

use by occupational therapists and may be appropriate for use with patients in pain. The COPM is a person-centered and individualized measure of an individual's perception of their ability to perform and their satisfaction with their performance in the areas of self-care, productivity, and leisure. When used as an outcome measure, COPM scores demonstrate the patient's perception of change in their ability to function in occupational-performance areas identified.

In summary, the occupational therapy comprehensive pain evaluation determines the impact of pain and related problems on a patient's ability to perform in daily routines.

ACUTE PAIN MANAGEMENT INTERVENTIONS

Disruption in occupational performance is common in people experiencing pain (Table 54.2). Pain can be a significant limiting factor and interfere with achievement of treatment goals. Acute pain causes decreased movement and activity, disturbed sleep, and diminished appetite, and

is associated with fear and anxiety. If unrelieved, acute pain can lead to delayed recuperation, prolonged hospital stay, and may predispose an individual to chronic pain. Occupational therapists intervene by detecting, measuring, and providing interventions to effectively manage acute pain.

Case Reports

Patient 1: Bilateral Wrist Tendinitis

A 31-year-old man with bilateral wrist tendinitis and cubital-tunnel syndrome was referred to outpatient occupational therapy for evaluation and treatment. The patient, a graduate student working on his thesis, complained of bilateral wrist and elbow pain associated with excessive typing and photocopying. He rated his pain as eight out of ten on a verbal pain scale. Over a 2-week course of occupational therapy, he received the following: iontophoresis (the introduction of ions into soft tissues by direct current); bilateral wrist splints and soft elbow pads

TABLE 54.2. *Sample Occupational Therapy Problems, Plans, and Outcomes for Patients with Pain*

Problem	Intervention (education and instruction)	Outcome
Inability to dress lower body independently	Safe body mechanics, compensatory, work simplification, and pacing techniques for task	Able to don socks and shoes independently
Inability to perform leisure tasks	Pain control measures, e.g., independent ice massage and use of safe body mechanics for task	Able to garden
Inability to perform homemaking tasks	Energy conservation techniques, organizing supplies; safe body mechanics, changes in positions and postural integration; pacing, periodic breaks/rests; assertive communication, delegating and asking for help	Able to prepare meals
Decreased sitting tolerance for driving to church	Pain control modality, stretching and use of low-back support prior to and while driving to church; quota-based program to gradually increase tolerance to task	Able to drive to church
Decreased tolerance for typing	Safe wrist/hand positions for task, splint care and schedule, pacing techniques, ergonomic assessment and modifications	Able to type and use computer mouse to meet work demands/deadlines
Difficulty with sexual expression	Safe positions, role-play assertive communication, problem-solve options for comfort, reduced tension and desired environment	Able to express needs and wants to partner

to decrease inflammation; instruction in soft-tissue massage, proper body mechanics, and joint protection techniques; stretching and strengthening exercises; and an adapted pen to decrease grip force when writing. Work-site recommendations to decrease musculoskeletal and visual strain included: split keyboard, touch pad to replace mouse, ergonomic chair, and use of correct heights for chair, desk, and computer screen. At time of discharge, the patient reported pain reduction of three to four out of ten on verbal pain scale and was able to perform the following activities pain-free: open doors, chop vegetables, and type for 2 to 3 hours with stretch breaks every 15 minutes. Occasional exacerbation of symptoms was managed effectively with the techniques he learned in occupational therapy.

Patient 2: Pregnancy-Induced Carpal-Tunnel Syndrome

A 35-year-old woman was referred to occupational therapy during her acute inpatient stay for pregnancy-induced carpal-tunnel syndrome. Following delivery of twin boys, she complained of painful paresthesias (rated eight out of ten on a verbal analog-pain scale) involving her wrists and fingers during all child-care activities. The occupational therapist observed the patient performing self-care, child-care, and functional-mobility tasks noting problems appropriate for intervention. The therapist recommended changes in hand position and use of a feeding pillow during breast feeding to provide support of hands, wrists, and arms. The therapist educated the patient on proper body mechanics (Fig. 54.1) and positioning of her upper extremities while changing and bathing the infants. Wrist-support splints were recommended to prevent further median-nerve compression neuropathy. The patient subsequently reported significant reduction in pain (two out of ten on a verbal pain-analog scale) and paresthesias. Occupational-therapy intervention allowed this patient to remain relatively pain free while effectively caring for her newborns and successfully fulfilling her role as a mother.

Patient 3: Human Immunodeficiency Virus-Related Neuropathic Pain

A 42-year-old man with human immunodeficiency virus (HIV) and diagnosed with cytomegalovirus polyradiculopathy was referred to occupational therapy after being admitted to the hospital with acute low-back pain radiating down his left leg. He could ambulate only short distances with the aid of a walker, and was unable to work as a librarian secondary to debilitating pain associated with prolonged standing. He lamented that "work is my life" and identified getting back to work as a primary goal. During the evaluation, the patient expressed fear of pain and was anxious prior to engaging in func-

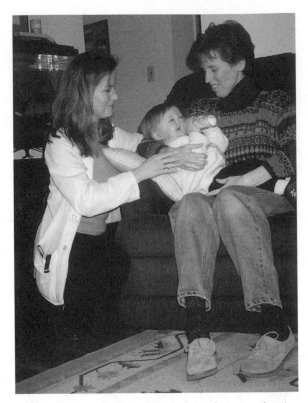

FIG. 54.1. The occupational therapist trains a mother to use proper body mechanics during performance of child-care activities.

tional activities. To address his anxiety, the occupational therapist instructed the patient on relaxation techniques, such as deep breathing. Together, they discussed his work setting and environmental modifications were made: a rolling office chair allowed the patient to maneuver around the workplace without causing fatigue and pain, and a rolling cart was used to eliminate the need for lifting. The patient was instructed on the use of work-simplification techniques such as relocating frequently used items to an easily accessible, central area. The patient was educated on using proper body mechanics and the need to incorporate frequent rest breaks to minimize fatigue and pain. With the use of these techniques, the patient was able to successfully manage pain and return to work within four weeks.

Patient 4: Acute-Compression Fracture

A 72-year-old woman, hospitalized following a T12 compression fracture, was referred to occupational therapy for activities of daily living and functional-mobility evaluation and treatment. As part of the therapy plan, the patient was instructed in safe transfers. Prior to her first transfer from bed to chair, the patient was observed to be tense and her facial expression showed fear and anxiety. The occupational therapist was sensitive to the patient's deep religious faith and her use of daily prayer as a source of comfort. Before beginning the transfer, the occupational therapist offered the patient's rosary beads to her. Upon taking the beads in her hand, the patient's body immediately relaxed, and a smile came over the woman's face. At that point, the occupational therapist instructed the patient in the mechanics of the transfer, which was accomplished comfortably. In offering the patient her rosary beads at the outset of her therapy session, the therapist acknowledged the importance of spirituality for this patient.

CHRONIC PAIN-MANAGEMENT INTERVENTIONS

Chronic pain is defined as pain that lasts more than 3 months or that continues past the usual healing time. Chronic pain is commonly associated with depression and is considered the disease itself rather than being a symptom. It can lead to severe activity limitations, impaired relationships, psychological distress, and disability. With the passage of time, especially when chronic pain is managed as if it were acute pain, there are numerous learning opportunities for the development and reinforcement of pain behaviors and sick role behaviors. For example, acute-pain interventions such as ultrasound or splinting, if used in cases of chronic pain, may foster dependence and disability. Unfortunately, mismanagement of chronic pain, e.g., excessive rest, disuse, and overprotection by others, is common. In cases of chronic pain, occupational therapists use educational and behav-

ioral interventions to promote self-management and control over pain.

The patient's beliefs about the pain and the meaning that the pain has for the individual provide important cues relating to the suffering that accompanies pain, especially chronic pain. This information, coupled with a nonjudgmental attitude, assists the occupational therapist in developing appropriate and meaningful therapeutic interventions.

Case Reports

Patient 5. Degenerative Osteoarthritis

A 50-year-old Italian electrician who sustained a work-related knee injury 2 years earlier, was referred to occupational therapy for pain management to increase activity levels. An arthroscopy demonstrated a meniscal tear and severe degenerative arthritis. Despite arthroscopic surgery for treatment of his torn meniscus, he continued to be severely limited by degenerative osteoarthritis of his knee. Not only was he unable to return to work, but also his condition prevented him from enjoying his hobby as a gardener. The patient was angered and embarrassed by his inability to perform those tasks that he felt defined his role in the family. An occupational-therapy intervention that addressed the patient's pain and suffering included teaching independent ice massage (Fig. 54.2) as a pain-control modality. He was instructed to use ice massage prior to initiating raking leaves. He was taught to use safe body mechanics during this task and the relief he

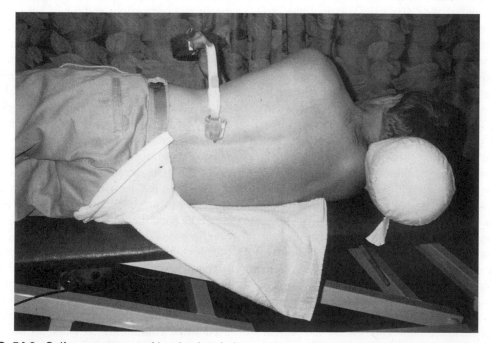

FIG. 54.2. Self-management of low-back pain by a patient using an adapted tool for ice massage.

obtained by the ice massage, enabled him to perform this previously avoided activity. Family teaching involved encouraging the patient's wife to remind him to take breaks instead of doing the entire task at one time.

Sanders et al. (1999) define patients with chronic-pain syndrome as presenting with reports of persistent pain; progressive deterioration in ability to function at home, work, and within social contexts; mood disturbances; progressive increase in healthcare utilization; and clinically significant anger and hostility. These patients may be appropriate candidates for pain rehabilitation. Functional restoration programs aim to restore patients to productivity and offer interdisciplinary services to address the physical and psychosocial needs of patients. Occupational therapists provide both individual and group-based therapy programs in these specialized-pain programs.

Patient 6: Chronic Low-Back Pain and Return to Work

A 35-year-old computer engineer, participating in an outpatient functional restoration program, was referred to occupational therapy because of inability to work. Medical history was unremarkable except for insidious onset and progressive worsening of low-back pain over the past 2 years. Because of his increasing fear of pain with any movement, the patient gradually withdrew from all tasks and previously enjoyed activities. His daily activity included TV, reading, and use of cold packs for pain relief. He was deconditioned, performed tasks with excessive muscle guarding, and unsafe body mechanics, and maintained a laterally flexed posture. Unable to fulfill his roles as worker, husband, and father, the patient felt out of control and overpowered by his pain, depressed, and demoralized. His primary goal was to return to work.

An occupational-therapy program was developed and included a work-related activity analysis to identify specific job demands (drive 1 hour and sit for computer work). Following assessment of baseline measurements for sitting and driving, quota-based programs were designed to increase tolerances for these activities. In the work simulation group, he used a work simulator. His program included increasing driving time by 5 minutes daily, avoiding prolonged positioning by stopping and getting out of the car to stretch every 30 minutes, and using proper positioning for driving and safe body mechanics for car transfers. Environmental modifications to his workstation decreased musculoskeletal strain; the height of his monitor was raised, a lumbar cushion was provided for his chair, and frequently used items were relocated within easy reach. Visual reminders cued him to maintain proper posture, and his computer was programmed to beep every 30 minutes as a cue to stand and stretch. In the communications skills group, the patient role-played and practiced responding to questions from coworkers, such as, "Where have you been?" and "Can you help me lift this?" He educated his wife and children about his needs and how they could support him in meeting his goals. These interventions, along with a gradual increase in his work schedule, enabled the patient to successfully return to full-time employment.

Although patients with chronic pain differ from those with chronic-pain syndrome, both groups may benefit from behaviorally oriented, self-management approaches. For example, chronic headache sufferers may be able to continue full-time jobs but reduce participation in social and leisure activities. Based on the findings reported at the NIH Technology Assessment Conference in 1995, for patients with chronic pain, behavioral and relaxation interventions have positive effects in many painful conditions. Occupational therapists working in the area of pain management provide services to address pain control as well as the suffering that accompanies ongoing pain. Therapeutic programs are most effective when patients are motivated to take responsibility for lifestyle changes.

Patient 7: Temporomandibular-Joint Disorder

A 34-year-old female executive secretary with a 2 year history of right-sided jaw and facial pain aggravated by stress, was referred to occupational therapy because of decreased concentration for work tasks. Other symptoms included neck and shoulder pain, headaches and low-back pain on "bad" days. The patient described herself as "always being on call" and had an extremely busy schedule including frequent air travel. Throughout the evaluation, the patient used ineffective breathing patterns, maintained rounded shoulders and a mild forward head posture, and sat in a slumped position. She demonstrated poor body mechanics getting into and out of her chair and on and off of the treatment table. Her neck range of motion was limited by tightness and discomfort. She was unable to voluntarily relax her right upper extremity arm muscles and had had no previous stress-management training.

During administration of the COPM evaluation, she described decreased productivity at work, and decreased energy for leisure, enjoyment, and chores. She expressed a desire to increase control over her symptoms, especially in relation to an upcoming trip that would require extensive travel and time away from home. The patient was seen for five sessions that focused on developing self-management strategies to prevent flare-ups, control pain, and manage concerns about her upcoming trip. Education and instruction included frequent position changes, diaphragmatic breath control, postural correction, proper neck and back support during work tasks and travel, and muscle-tension reduction techniques. A home program recommended neck-stretching exercises (integrated into her morning shower routine) and audio tapes for relaxation training, used while commuting to work on the train. Additional problem-solving facilitated identification of appropriate pacing, time management, and assertive strategies to reduce or eliminate daily stress, such as not scheduling appointments during lunch breaks and leaving work on time. At time of discharge, the patient expressed no anxiety over her upcoming trip, reported reduced pain as measured on the short-form McGill Pain Questionnaire, and significant positive changes in relation to occupational-performance problems as measured on the COPM. At 1 month after discharge from occupational therapy, the patient remarked, "I have a new perspective, things don't bother me now." Her trip had been successful, and she continued her home program.

SUMMARY

Many complex problems confront the patient in pain and the pain team. The unique contribution of occupational therapy in pain management is its focus on occupational performance — the ability to engage in self-care, work, and leisure. The occupational therapist, working as part of an interdisciplinary pain team, considers the physical, psychological, environmental, and spiritual components of pain as they relate to the individual patient. Occupational-based therapeutic interventions promote self-management of pain while reducing or eliminating impairments, functional limitations, and pain-related disability. The ultimate goal of occupational therapy in pain management is to help patients regain control of their lives and become productive members of their communities, thus improving quality of life and reducing the debt to society from medical care, lost wages, and dependence.

ACKNOWLEDGMENTS

The authors thank Eve Kennedy-Spaien OTR/L, and Sonda Anderson OTR/L, CHT, for case report contributions, and Guy M. Rochman, M.D., for review of the manuscript.

SELECTED READINGS

American Pain Society. *Pain Facts*. Skokie, Illinois, 1995.

Chapman, C. New JCAHO standards for pain management: Carpe diem! *American Pain Society Bulletin*. July/August: 2, 2000.

Commission on Accreditation of Rehabilitation Facilities. *Standards Manual and Interpretive Guidelines for Medical Rehabilitation*. Tucson, Arizona, 1999.

Dolce J, Crocker M, Moletteire C, et al. Exercise quotas, anticipatory concern, and self-efficacy expectancies in chronic pain: a preliminary report. *Pain* 1986;24:365–372.

Engel J. Physical therapy and occupational therapy for pain management in children. *Child and Adolescent Psychiatric Clinics of North America* 1997;6:817–828.

Fairbank J, Davies J, et al. The Oswestry low back pain disability questionnaire. *Physiotherapy* 1980;66:271–273.

Herbert P, Rochman D. Dealing with pain. *Rehab Management* 1998;11:56–59.

International Association for the Study of Pain subcommittee for occupational therapy/physical therapy curriculum: Pain curriculum for students in occupational therapy or physical therapy. *IASP Newsletter* 1994;November/December:3–8.

Jensen M, Turner J, Romano J. Self-efficacy and outcome expectancies: relationship to chronic pain coping strategies and adjustment. *Pain* 1991;44:263–269.

Law M, Baptiste S, et al. The Canadian occupational performance measure: an outcome measure for occupational therapy. *Canadian Journal of Occupational Therapy* 1990;57:82–87.

Levin J, Lofland K, et al. 1996. The relationship between self-efficacy and disability in chronic low back pain patients. *International Journal of Rehabilitation and Health* 1996;2:19–28.

Lorig K. Self-management of chronic illness: a model for the future. *Generations* 1993;17:11–14.

Mayer T. Rehabilitation of the worker with chronic low back pain. In: Nordin M, et al. *Musculoskeletal Disorders in the Workplace*. St. Louis: Mosby, 1997:306–315.

Matheson L. Functional goal setting. *American Pain Society Journal* 1994;3:111–114.

Merskey H, Bogduk N, eds. *Classification of chronic pain. Descriptions of chronic pain syndromes and definitions of pain terms*, 2nd ed. IASP Press, Seattle, 1994.

Moyers P. Guide to Occupational Therapy Practice. *Am J Occup Ther* 1999;53:4–7.

NIH Technology Assessment Panel: Integration of behavioral and relaxation approaches into the treatment of chronic pain and insomnia. *JAMA* 1996;276:313–318.

New England Pain Association Worker Compensation Subcommittee Report. *Recommendations Concerning Massachusetts Worker Compensation Chronic Pain Syndrome Guideline No. 27*. October, 1998.

Rosenstiel A, Keefe F. The use of coping strategies in chronic low back pain patients: Relationship to patient characteristics and current adjustment. *Pain* 1983;17:33–44.

Sanders S, Harden R, Benson S, et al. Clinical practice guidelines for chronic non-malignant pain syndrome patients II: an evidence-based approach. *Journal of Back and Musculoskeletal Rehabilitation* 1999;13:47–58.

Taal E, Rasker J, Wiegman O. Patient education and self-management in the rheumatic diseases: a self-efficacy approach. *Arthritis Care and Research* 1996;9:229–238.

Tait R, Pollard C, Margolis R, et al. The pain disability index: psychometric and validity data. *Archives of Physical Medicine and Rehabilitation* 1987;68:438–441.

Turk D, Meichenbaum D, Genest M. *Pain and Behavioral Medicine*. New York: Guilford Press, 1983.

Turner J. Coping and chronic pain. In: Bond M, Charlton J, Woolf C, eds. *Proceedings of the 6th World Congress on Pain*. Amsterdam: Elsevier Publishers, 1991:219–227.

CHAPTER 55

Acupuncture

Joseph F. Audette

Acupuncture has enjoyed a recent surge in popularity and interest since the publication of the National Institutes of Health (NIH) consensus statement in 1997. The use of acupuncture in the Western world has a long history, going back to 1683 with the introduction in Europe by Willem ten Rhyne and in the United States in 1825. However, lack of aseptic techniques limited its general acceptance at the time. Since the well-publicized trip of President Nixon to China in 1971, there has been growing interest in the West about the potential application of acupuncture to control pain. This interest was sparked when one of the members of the press corps, James Reston, received acupuncture during an appendectomy. Interestingly, for many years, the Food and Drug Administration (FDA) listed the acupuncture needle as an experimental medical device and physicians interested in utilizing acupuncture in their practice were required to do so under a research protocol. This changed in March of 1996, when the FDA changed the status of an acupuncture needle to an approved "medical device" for general use by trained professionals and thereby placed them in the same category as scalpels and syringes.

The World Health Organization lists a variety of medical conditions that may benefit from the use of acupuncture or moxibustion (a method of heating the acupuncture points with a dry, quick-burning herb called mugwort or *Artemisia vulgaris*). These include prevention and treatment of nausea and vomiting and other gastrointestinal disorders; treatment of pain and addictions to alcohol, tobacco, and other drugs; treatment of asthma, bronchitis, and rehabilitation from neurological conditions such as stroke. In 1997, a NIH panel reviewed the English language literature and concluded that there was strong evidence to support the use of acupuncture for the management of postoperative and chemotherapy-induced nausea and vomiting, and for postoperative dental pain. Good support also was found for the treatment of menstrual cramps, tennis elbow, and fibromyalgia. Finally, the panel

concluded that acupuncture may be a useful adjunct or alternative treatment of addictions, stroke, asthma, and a variety of painful conditions including headache, myofascial pain, osteoarthritis, low-back pain, and carpal-tunnel syndrome, but that further research is needed.

ACUPUNCTURE THEORY

The term "acupuncture" comes from the Greek words *Acus* (needle) and *Punctura* (puncture) and is the English translation of *Chan* in Mandarin and *Hari* in Japanese.

The clinical practice of inserting needles into the body (initially stone or flint needles) occurred in China by the fifth century B.C.. This was followed some time later, between the second and third century B.C., by the first written medical text on acupuncture, the "Huang Di Nei Jing" or the "Yellow Emperor's Classic of Internal Medicine." Essential to an understanding of traditional acupuncture theory is the concept of *Qi* or *vital energy* that is believed to flow through channels or meridians in the body. Pain or disease occurs when the flow of this energy is blocked or out of normal balance. Treatment focuses on restoring this balance with the insertion of acupuncture needles into specific points along the meridians. There are 12 principal meridians, eight extra meridians, and a total of 365 classical acupuncture points that are located on these proposed-energy channels. Despite the fact that exact anatomical correlates to the meridians have not been found, the concept has still proven useful to help understand and treat certain patterns of symptoms seen in various disease and pain states. Acupuncture points themselves have been noted to be near major nerve endings, and the skin overlying an acupuncture point has been shown to have differences in electrical conductance compared to nonacupuncture points, suggesting that important anatomic differences do exist.

The methods of diagnosis used in acupuncture are based on the theory that the function of the internal organs, the flow of blood and lymph, and the emotional state of an individual are believed to have specific, observable influences on their external, visible appearance. Subtle changes seen on the surface of the body such as changes in the skin color, texture, and temperature; changes in the suppleness and flexibility of underlying muscles; the quality of arterial pulses; and the appearance of the tongue and eyes, all are seen to reflect accurately on the homeostasis of the internal-organ system. The pattern of these physical findings then will lead to point selection and insertion of acupuncture needles and or application of heating methods to the points such as with moxa.

MODERN THEORY

Over the last 30 years, a great deal of scientific evidence has accumulated to verify that both acupuncture stimulation (AP) and electroacupuncture stimulation (EA) have reproducible physiological effects. There are four main lines of evidence that will be presented below. All go to the heart of the neurological mechanisms that currently are understood to modulate and influence pain.

The evidence for the release of endogenous opioids with AP and EA goes back to the seminal work done by Pomeranz in animals and Mayer in humans in the 1970s. Since that time, a large body of evidence has developed to show that both AP and EA lead to the release of endorphins and enkephalins into the cerebrospinal fluid. Furthermore, the release of these neuropeptides have been demonstrated to play a role in the analgesic effect of acupuncture as evidenced by the fact that opioid-receptor antagonism can abolish the analgesia obtained with acupuncture in both human and animal models of acute pain.

Since the initial studies on the endorphin effect on acupuncture analgesia (AA), the release of 5-hydroxytryptamine (5HTP) has been demonstrated with AP and EA in the raphe nucleus and contributes to the analgesia presumably through descending inhibitory control mechanisms. Both the parameters of stimulation (i.e., the intensity and frequency of EA) and the site of stimulation have significant effects on the type of chemical releases. In general, low-frequency (2 to 4 Hz), high-intensity stimulation such as with manual acupuncture or EA produces a slow in onset, cumulative affect on pain and is at least in part mediated through the endogenous opioid system. Whereas, low-intensity, high-frequency stimulation (more than 70 Hz) produces a more rapid-onset pain relief that is partly mediated through this serotonin system. Point location has been shown to influence the chemical releases. In particular, antiserum to met-enkephalin abolished AA but antiserum to dynorphin did not when a true acupuncture point was stimulated, whereas the reverse was true when a nonacupuncture or sham point was stimulated.

A third line of evidence supports that the hypothalamic-pituitary axis, and catecholamine levels also are influenced by EA and AP and may further influence the analgesic response to pain both through immune modulation and modulation of the sympathetic responses, respectively.

Recent technological advances in mapping brain activity using functional magnetic resonance scanning (fMRI) have begun to be applied to acupuncture. Comparison has been made between tactile sensation (tapping the skin with a wire at 120 Hz) and AP using a manual-stimulation technique. The acupuncture stimulation used in this study involved twisting the needle at 120 Hz in LI4 (a point in the first dorsal interosseous muscle of the hand). Stimulation of an acupuncture point in this manner produces a *deqi* sensation, which is a full, aching feeling at the point of the needle and is believed to be important in obtaining the clinical effect with AP. The results of unilateral AP showed bilateral neural modulation of cortical and subcortical structures. The primary action was to decrease signal intensity in the limbic region and other subcortical areas. Tactile stimulation did not produce these changes in fMRI. In addition, if the needle was placed in the point and left at rest, or placed just subcutaneously and not in the muscle, fMRI signal decrease in these deep, subcortical structures was not seen. This suggests that the response of the organism to AP depends on activation of the muscle-sensory afferents and not the superficial afferents in the skin.

Evidence for point specificity also has been obtained in a recent study by Cho et al. An acupuncture point on the lateral aspect of the small toe, bladder 67 (B67), which is known as an influential point for vision, was stimulated and observed to cause increased fMRI activity in the occipital lobes in 12 subjects. Stimulation of the eyes directly with light caused a similar activation whereas stimulation of a sham acupuncture point 2 to 5 cm away from B67 failed to cause occipital-lobe activation.

Both of these studies are preliminary. However, they suggest that the grid of acupuncture points that has evolved over the last 2,000 years may indeed represent a network of nodes in the peripheral nervous system that have profound and specific effects on modulating and regulating the activity of the central nervous system.

TREATMENT METHODS

There are a number of different treatment styles that have influenced the practice of acupuncture in the United States. Many of these styles herald back to prerevolution, medical traditions that were prevalent in China prior to Mao and were exported to other countries where they developed independently. Insertion of a needle subcutaneously, usually into underlying muscle or tendon at a depth of anywhere from 0.5 cm to 8 cm depending on location, is the sine qua non of acupuncture methodology. However, laser acupuncture techniques are now being studied. The devices utilize a cold-red laser beam 5 to 500 mW in power with a wavelength 600 to 1,300 nm in the red to near-infrared spectrum. Moxibustion, where the herb mugwort is used to heat points, is another common noninvasive approach.

Once the needle has been inserted, a number of different stimulation techniques exist. In traditional Chinese schools, a strong twisting of the needle is used at approximately 100 to 120 revolutions per second to bring a *deqi* sensation to the point. The *deqi* sensation is described as a deep, aching feeling and is not always well tolerated by acupuncture-naïve patients. Some investigators, such as Pomeranz believe that eliciting the *deqi* sensation is essential to causing the various chemical releases in the central nervous system. However, there are many successful acupuncture styles including those practiced in Japan, which do not engage the needle as deeply or stimulate as intensely as Chinese styles. Once the needles are in place, many styles will add electrical stimulation to the needles.

One method commonly practiced in this country is called acupuncture energetics. Popularized by the work of Joseph Helms, M.D., and Mark Seem, Ph.D., this approach has been widely taught to physicians in the University of California at Los Angeles (UCLA) acupuncture course. This technique evolved in Europe and is based on interpretations of the classic Chinese texts, and later was influenced by the Vietnamese in France. George Soulié de Morant, a diplomat in the French Foreign Service in China between 1901 and 1917, was able to systematically introduce many of the classic Chinese and Japanese texts to the European community and introduced the terms "meridian" and "energy" into the acupuncture lexicon. With this approach, point selection is governed by the pattern of pain and constitutional symptoms presented by the patient. Diagnosis includes palpation of the meridian pathways much as one would palpate to assess for trigger points.

Japanese diagnostic techniques rely heavily on palpation of soft tissue as well. The Harvard Medical Acupuncture Course for physicians teaches a style of acupuncture based on the work of Kiiko Matsumoto, who has synthesized the clinical practices of many Japanese masters including Nagano, Ito, and Kawai into her approach. Palpation of the abdomen or Hara is used to determine the root treatment, and point location is dynamically determined by the response of the superficial tissues to needle insertion.

Postrevolutions styles of traditional Chinese medicine are influenced heavily by herbal-treatment strategies. During the Communist revolution in China, an attempt was made to make acupuncture more systematic and uniform in technique and point location. This led to the use of diag-nostic techniques developed by herbalists as it was felt by Mao at the time to be more scientific. An attempt is made to diagnose the state of balance of the internal organs by asking general questions, and utilizing pulse and tongue diagnosis. Palpation of the soft tissues is less common and point selection often is directed at bringing the general internal state of health back into homeostasis rather than focusing on the specific local complaints of pain.

Percutaneous electrical nerve stimulation (PENS) has developed in the United States and Canada. The treatment strategies are based on a neuroanatomical assessment of the pain generator rather than on traditional acupuncture theories. The pattern of pain is viewed and interpreted based on which spinal segments are involved and then EA is done along those segments for 20 to 25 minutes at a frequency that can vary from 4 to 100 Hz with a low-output electrical generator (5 mA) (Fig. 55.1).

There are numerous other treatment techniques including Korean four-needle technique where only four needles are placed regardless of the presenting condition, and Korean hand acupuncture that represents the whole body with extra points found in the hand. Auricular acupuncture is a more widely used treatment technique that also takes a small part of the body, the ear, to represent the whole body. Although the Chinese classic texts mention ear stimulation, there was no systematic representation of the relevant points on the ear until 1950 when Paul Nogier, a French neurologist, developed a somatotopic map of the ear based on an inverted fetus. A special aspect of this treatment method involves the use of a point localizer that is essentially an impedance meter to identify active points for treatment. Auricular acupuncture also has received a great deal of attention as a method to treat addictions.

Acupuncture research in the West over the last 20 years has led to the dissemination of an oversimplified method of point selection. Influenced by Chinese point formulas and issues of simplicity in study design, this approach takes a Western diagnosis such as nausea of pregnancy or carpal-tunnel disease and attempts to select a small number of classic points to treat the condition. This formulaic method never has been compared in a formal study to more traditional methods of point selection and may artificially doom clinical outcomes to insignificance.

Unfortunately, there is no clinical research at this time to help guide selection of treatment type or style for particular clinical conditions. From personal clinical experience, however, failure of one technique for a particular condition does not always imply total acupuncture failure and there is some value in trying a few treatment techniques before labeling the acupuncture ineffective for the condition. In addition, although compared to many medical interventions acupuncture is relatively safe, there are still some serious adverse affects that have been reported including serious infections, vascular injury, and pneumothorax that require proper precautions to prevent.

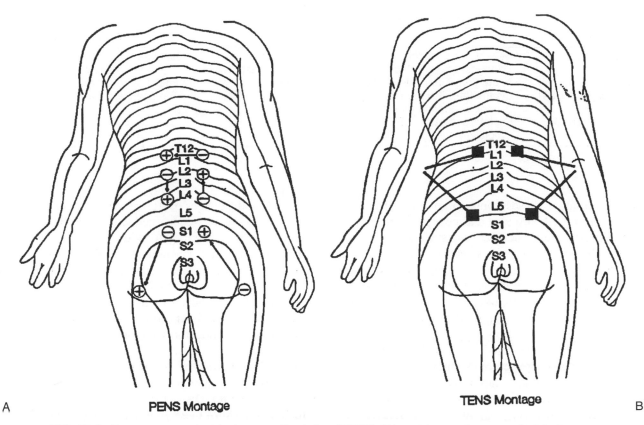

FIG. 55.1. Percutaneous electrical nerve stimulation (*PENS*) **(A)** and transcutaneous electrical nerve stimulation (*TENS*) montage **(B)** for low-back pain.

CLINICAL APPLICATIONS

An exhaustive review of the acupuncture literature was performed by a panel of experts convened by the NIH, and their findings were published in the November 1998 edition of *JAMA*. The conclusions of the review suggested that acupuncture may be beneficial for a number of common pain conditions such as back pain, tendinitis, arthritis, headaches, and neuropathic pain. Ultimately better designed studies are needed to determine absolute scientific efficacy, however a number of recent studies are strongly suggestive of the potential of acupuncture.

In one study on severe osteoarthritis of the knee in which the patients enrolled were on a waiting list for total knee replacement (TKRR), Christensen found significant reduction in pain and use of analgesic medications compared to a control group. This benefit was sustained and seven out of 29 patients enrolled declined the TKR operation at the end of the wait, saving $9,000 per patient by avoiding TKR surgery.

Although acupuncture trials generally have been applied to chronic conditions, the effect on subacute painful conditions is even more profound. Elbow tendinitis has been studied, and in one study design, treatment with a single point at the knee (GB34) caused a 55% reduction in pain compared to only a 15% reduction in a placebo group where a plastic stick was pressed against a nonacupuncture point.

In a recent review of a method of EA called PENS, the authors summarize significant findings in the treatment of acute herpetic neuralgia, pain from bony metastases, migraine headaches after electroconvulsive therapy (ECT), chronic low-back pain, and lumbar radiculopathy. These findings suggest that this technique can have lasting and profound effects on difficult pain syndromes that allowed improved function and a reduction in the use of analgesic medications.

Acupuncture can be used to treat other medical conditions that are not pain related. A common problem in the hospital setting is to manage postoperative nausea. In one study, 93 women undergoing minor gynecological operations were treated with a point on the volar surface of the wrist, P6 (Neiguan) with manual or electrical AP at 10 Hz for 5 minutes. This group showed markedly reduced postoperative nausea and vomiting compared with untreated controls.

COMMON POINTS

A summary of acupuncture points commonly used in research studies is listed in Table 55.1. As mentioned

TABLE 55.1. *Acupuncture Points Commonly Used in Research*

Acupuncture point	Location	Research indication
Pericardium 6 (P6)	Between the tendons of flexor carpi radialis and palmaris longus, about 1.5 to 2 in. above the second wrist crease	Nausea, cardiovascular conditions (blood pressure control, angina)
Large intestine 4 (L14)	In the first dorsal interosseous muscle of hand	Facial pain, dental pain
Gallbladder 34 (GB34)	On the lateral side of leg, 3 in. below knee in perinius-longus muscle	Tendinomuscular pain syndromes
Stomach 36 (ST36)	On lateral side of leg 3 to 4 in. below knee in the tibialis-anterior muscle	Gastrointestinal problems such as reflux, gastritis, nausea

above, selection of these points for research has been based on simplified formulas and concerns about study design. Unfortunately, there are no studies to compare this research approach to point selection to a more robust approach that takes into account acupuncture diagnostic methods. For example, in the case of treating postoperative nausea in a nonresearch setting, pericardium points often would be combined with spleen points on the inner aspect of the leg and alternative points along the pericardium meridian may be selected, depending on the individual findings on acupuncture examination.

Acupuncture points also can be identified in relationship to common locations of painful muscle trigger points. Table 55.2 lists some common myofascial associations.

TRAINING INFORMATION

The accreditation of acupuncture educational programs is directed by the Accreditation Commission of Acupuncture and Oriental Medicine (ACAOM), formerly called the National Accreditation Commission for Schools and Colleges of Acupuncture and Oriental Medicine, and is mainly concerned with institutions that train nonphysicians. The organization that credentials nonphysicians to practice acupuncture in the United States is the National Certification Commission of Acupuncture and Oriental Medicine (NCCA). The NCCA requires that nonphysician candidates complete 1,725 hours of formal didactics and 500 hours of clinical training in acupuncture prior to sitting for a national written and practical examination administered biannually. Despite these national standards, the actual practice of acupuncture is still further regulated by each individual state. Currently, 33 states and the District of Columbia license acupuncturist and most of these follow the NCCA guidelines for nonphysicians.

Regulation of the practice of acupuncture by physicians and dentists also varies from state to state. As of 1999, 35 states permit physicians to practice acupuncture within the current scope of their license without requiring additional training. There are eight states that do require some additional training and certification (anywhere from 100 to 300 hours depending on the state). Four

TABLE 55.2. *Acupuncture and Myofascial Trigger-Point Correlations*

Acu-zone	Region of body	Acu-points	Muscles
Tai Yang	Dorsal zone:	B 10	Suboccipital
	Frontal region of forehead to occiput down	SI 9–14	Scapular muscles
	back to lateral ankles	B 11–25, 41–45	Thoracic and lumbar paraspinals
		B 53, 54	Gluteus medius
		B 31, 34	Piriformis
Shao Yang	Lateral zone:	GB 3–6, 8	Temporalis
	Temporalis region of head to lateral neck	GB 16	Sternocleidomastoid
	and down arm to wrist extensors		and scalenes
	Down flank to lateral aspect of leg	GB 20, 21	Upper trapezius
		TH 9	Finger extensors
		GB 24–28	Abdominal obliques
		GB 29	Tensor fasciae latae
		GB 31	Iliotibial band
Yang Ming	Ventral zone:	ST 5–7	Masseter
	Mouth to anterior neck, anterior chest wall	ST 9, 10	Sternocleidomastoid
	down abdomen to medial aspect of leg	ST 14–18	Pectoral muscles
	and foot	ST 19–30	Rectus abdominis
		ST 31, 32	Quadraceps muscles

B, bladder; GB, gallbladder; SI, small intestine; ST, stomach; TH, triple heater.

states do not permit physicians to practice acupuncture within the scope of their license without the full training that nonphysicians are required to take (Hawaii, Montana, Rhode Island, and Vermont).

For full membership in the American Academy of Medical Acupuncturists (AAMA), individuals must have an active M.D. or D.O. license (or equivalent) to practice medicine under U.S. or Canadian jurisdiction, have completed a minimum of 220 hours of formal training in medical acupuncture (120 hours didactic, 100 hours clinical), and have 2 years of experience practicing medical acupuncture. Currently, physicians are able to satisfy the educational and clinical requirements demanded by most states by completing the training offered by the Office of Continuing Medical Education at UCLA. Harvard Medical School, through the Department of Anesthesiology at Beth Israel Deaconess Medical Center, now also is offering a 300-hour continuing medical education (CME) course in medical acupuncture that would satisfy both the AAMA requirements and most state requirements to practice acupuncture.

The federal Health Care Financing Administration (HCFA), which is responsible for administering Medicare, currently denies coverage for acupuncture pending establishment of the scientific efficacy of this modality. With a showing of such efficacy, HCFA may consider acupuncture as a "reasonable and necessary" service at which time coverage would be authorized under the federal Social Security Act 37. Other insurers such as health maintenance organizations, workers compensation, and so on vary in their policies with regard to acupuncture coverage from state to state.

SELECTED READINGS

Cho ZH, Chung SC, Jones JP, et al. New findings of the correlation between acupoints and corresponding brain cortices using functional MRI. *Proc Natl Acad Sci U S A* 1998;95:2670–2673.

Christensen PA, Rotne M, Vedelsdal R, et al. Electroacupuncture in anaesthesia for hysterectomy. *Br J Anaesth* 1993;71:835–838.

Dundee JW, Ghaly RG, Bill KM, et al. Effect of stimulation of the P6 antiemetic point on postoperative nausea and vomiting. *Br J Anaesth* 1989;63:612–618.

Ghoname EA, Craig WF, White PF, et al. Percutaneous electrical nerve stimulation for low back pain: a randomized crossover study. *JAMA* 1999;281:818–823.

Hui KK, Liu J, Makris N, et al. Acupuncture modulates the limbic system and subcortical gray structures of the human brain: evidence from fMRI studies in normal subjects. *Hum Brain Mapp* 2000;9:13–25.

Mayer DJ, Price DD, Raffii A. Antagonism of acupuncture analgesia in man by narcotic antagonist naloxone. *Brain Res* 1977;121:368–372.

NIH Consensus Conference. Acupuncture. *JAMA* 1998;280:1518–1524.

Pomeranz B, Chiu D. Naloxone blockade of acupuncture analgesia: endorphins implicated. *Life Sci* 1976;19:1757–1762.

White PF, Phillips J, Proctor TJ, et al. Percutaneous electrical nerve stimulation: a promising alternative-medicine approach to pain management. *APS Bulletin* 1999 March/April:3–5.

Behavioral Therapies

CHAPTER 56

Behavioral Medicine: Addressing Mind and Body in Pain Management

Margaret A. Caudill-Slosberg

Mary had it made. She was on her way to the top of her career when the accident occurred. Now, in spite of multiple surgeries, she continued to experience pain in her back and right lower extremity. But that wasn't all. She wasn't sleeping well, cried all the time, and was not able to do any of the activities she had found enjoyable and distracting. She had lost her job, had mounting debt, and few of her friends still called her. She felt isolated, useless, betrayed, and abandoned.

Mary's story is typical of what many people experience when chronic pain develops. Pain is never experienced in a vacuum. It always exists in the biological, psychological, sociological, and spiritual context of the individual experiencing the pain. Yet, evaluation and treatment of chronic pain too often neglects three quarters of this experience, focusing only on the biological. Treating the symptom of pain and the person in pain can help with pain management and improve the quality of life.

DEFINITIONS

The relationship of mind and body in medicine has perhaps been best served by the appearance, 40 years ago, of behavioral medicine. Behavioral medicine had its roots in psychosomatic medicine. It was an attempt to bring some balance to the overemphasis of biomedical models on the physical symptoms of illness. Originally concerned with the multidisciplinary treatment of disease caused or made worse by stress, behavioral medicine soon expanded to include research on the relationship of health risk behaviors and disease, social support and illness, and the effects of attitudes on health. Behavioral-medicine treatment models were proposed based on the growing evidence that people who were chronically ill

did better if they were provided with (a) information about their disease, (b) psychological and physical stress management techniques, and (c) support, either individual or group. Treatment in such a model addressed the biological, psychological, and sociological issues, in addition to the biomedical ones, by incorporating cognitive-behavioral therapies.

Cognitive-behavioral therapy programs generally include education, skills acquisition, and relapse/maintenance training. Such skills as relaxation therapies, cognitive therapy, pacing activities, and communication may be taught. Relaxation therapies are those skills that can bring about the *relaxation response*, a quieting response that appears to balance the physical and emotional effects of distress. Cognitive therapy argues that negative emotional responses (anger, anxiety, depression) to an event can be altered by changing the accompanying self-talk into more realistic, self-reliant dialogue.

APPLICATION OF COGNITIVE-BEHAVIORAL THERAPIES TO CHRONIC PAIN

Over the past two decades, increasing attention has been given to the incorporation of cognitive-behavioral skills into pain management. In October 1995, the National Institutes of Health convened a Technology Assessment Conference to consider the integration of behavioral and relaxation approaches into the treatment of chronic pain (and insomnia). The consensus panel concluded that there was sufficient data to recommend the incorporation of cognitive-behavioral therapies into the treatment of chronic pain. They noted, for example, that of the six factors identified to correlate with treatment failures of low-back pain, all were psychosocial. They recommended the integration of behavioral and relaxation therapies with conventional medical procedures for the successful treatment of chronic pain.

There are three objectives associated with teaching cognitive-behavioral therapies in pain management. They are to assist the patient with (a) mastering skills for both stress and pain reduction, (b) applying those skills during times of increased stress and pain, and (c) developing a belief in their ability to engage in certain behaviors to attain a desired outcome (self-efficacy).

BENEFITS OF INCORPORATING COGNITIVE-BEHAVIORAL THERAPY

Multiple benefits have been identified with the use of cognitive-behavioral therapies including decreased psychological distress, improved pain management, increased self-efficacy, and better quality of life and function. Several studies also have demonstrated decreased visits to the doctor with subsequent savings in healthcare costs as a result. Healthcare practitioners also benefit from patients using cognitive-behavioral strategies because the patients have more realistic expectations and are better able to work towards shared goals of symptom and disease management.

A CLINICAL MODEL FOR THE APPLICATION OF COGNITIVE-BEHAVIORAL THERAPIES TO CHRONIC PAIN

There are several models that have been described in detail in patient workbooks used with such programs. These programs complement the biomedical treatment and can enhance the coping and self-efficacy of the individual who must cope with daily pain.

Group Process

While the teaching of these skills can be accomplished in individual sessions, a group format has significant advantages. When facilitated appropriately, the value of the group process cannot be underestimated. The support among the group members can serve to reinforce successful implementation of new behaviors and encourage perseverance during times of relapse into old, ineffectual behaviors. Cognitive-behavioral skills can benefit the majority of patients experiencing chronic pain because of the emphasis on stress, not pain. As a result, groups can be composed of individuals with different pain diagnoses or etiologies if there are not sufficient numbers, at one time, of a single diagnostic group. Mixing diagnoses has advantages in that patients realize that the pain experience has universal qualities and there is the inevitable comparison and frequent observation by patients that "things could be worse."

Patient Selection

The recommendation to participate in a cognitive-behavioral program should be made only after a complete, biopsychosocial evaluation of the pain problem has been performed and a comprehensive treatment plan has been developed. Interventional and pharmacological therapies, including opioids, can be recommended where appropriate. The major inclusion criterion for participation by the individual in pain is that they be motivated to participate. There have been multiple attempts to try and predict who will start or complete such therapy, but there are only trends (and multifactorial ones at that) not absolutes that have been identified to date. In general, patients who are psychologically or cognitively impaired, children, individuals who exhibit disruptive behaviors, or those that are nonambulatory generally will not be able to participate in such outpatient group therapies.

General Format

The essential criterion for the group provider(s) is that they enjoy working with chronic-pain patients, understand and have training in group therapy, and recognize the strong influence of learned helplessness on patient's struggles. In general, programs are held weekly for 8 to 10 weeks, for 1.5 to 2 hours/session. There is some flexibility, but a suitable duration of contact with patients appears critical for behavioral skills to be adopted and maintained. The participation of peer advisors, individuals with chronic pain who have already participated successfully in previous groups, can serve as strong role models for those just beginning.

Session Format and Content

There is considerable latitude in the content of sessions, the order of presentation, and the methods used to present the material. The basic elements for effective cognitive-behavioral interventions include providing information about the symptom/disease and treatment, teaching both physical and psychological stress-management skills, and providing support. Important reinforcers of behavioral change that should be included are incorporation of patient feedback, diary keeping, role playing, supervised-skill practice, and daily application of skills at home. Practice of skills or a routine for pain flare-ups is very helpful

COGNITIVE-BEHAVIORAL SKILLS

Patient Preparation

Teaching an appreciation of the biopsychosocial process from the time of the initial evaluation will lend validity to recommending treatment that includes cognitive-behavioral therapies. By exploring what other symptoms patients are experiencing in addition to their pain, the provider can help identify other stress-related symptoms such as fatigue, memory problems, irritable bowel, muscle tension, shortness of breath, palpitations, irritability, and insomnia. During the psychosocial history, asking questions about what activities have been altered by the pain, what social supports are in place, and whether there is a history of emotional, physical, or sexual abuse can uncover modifying and additional stress factors that can influence the pain context.

Specific Cognitive-Behavioral Skills

The following are skills that can be taught to patients individually as well as in programs described above.

Diary Keeping

Keeping a diary of the pain experience can accomplish three things. It allows for treatment assessment, it identifies patterns that may be altered by application of the cognitive-behavioral skills, and it allows for objectifying the experience for the patient. The patient is asked to record their pain sensation and distress three times a day at the same time every day on a scale of zero to ten. Zero equals no physical pain sensations or emotional responses (aching, burning, throbbing/sadness, anxiety, anger), and ten equals the worst physical sensation or emotional response.

Separation of sensation from distress allows the patient to see the influences of stress, emotions, and daily events on the physical sensation. This also paves the way for learning to appropriately apply physical and emotional coping strategies more specifically and therefore more effectively.

Pacing Activities

Patients with chronic pain usually find that certain daily activities are associated with increased pain. Their response generally is to stop activities or push through the activity and increase their discomfort. This, in turn, increases their distress, which increases their pain, which, in turn, increases their distress. The idea of pacing activities revolves around the idea of working smarter, not harder. For example, if a patient finds that sitting at a computer increases their pain, they are asked to monitor how long it takes to increase their pain one to two points above baseline. Say, for example, they determine it is 30 minutes. Then, they determine how long it takes to decrease the pain back to baseline once they've changed positions; say, for example, it takes 15 minutes. If this is the standing position, they also determine what activities can be done while standing, like folding laundry, stretch-

ing, or calling a friend. Now, when they sit at the computer they set a timer and sit for only 30 minutes. Then they change positions and stand and fold laundry for 15 minutes. This cycling of up-time and down-time activities continues until the task is done. Research has demonstrated that regular incorporation of such pacing over time is associated with decreasing pain levels and increasing activities, most likely as the result of reduction in muscle fatigue, nerve irritation, and frustration.

Relaxation Techniques

Teaching breath and relaxation techniques early on in the evaluation and treatment of patients in pain can allow the skills to be used during stressful and sometimes painful interventional therapies such as nerve blocks, epidural-steroid injections, and even diagnostic tests (colonoscopies, myelograms). This also serves to reinforce the mind–body connection and gives the patient some control over reacting to difficult procedures.

Cognitive Therapy

Cognitive therapy, while perhaps the most difficult skill for many people to learn, can be very helpful in coping with common stressors associated with daily life. The goal here is to learn to respond, not react, to stressors as they occur. This allows for more effective problem solving as needed. Patients are asked to keep track of emotional reactions to events that happen to them. For example, finding themselves driving in a traffic jam. The common emotional reaction is to get angry and frustrated, which can be associated with increased adrenalin, blood pressure, heart rate, and pain. Patients are asked to identify the self-talk occurring at such times. For example, "This always happens to me when I want to get somewhere," "I should never have left the house, I'll never get there," "This is a disaster, I'll die if I'm late." The patients then are asked to identify the patterns, assumptions, and distortions in such statements. In general, it is the unrealistic, all or nothing, catastrophizing language used that terrorizes the individual, unaware that they are, in part, responsible for their misery by the way they respond to events. Being part of the problem allows them to be part of the solution. They are then asked to reframe their self-talk into more realistic assessments of the stressful event. Continuing with our traffic example they might say "There is not much I *can* do about the traffic jam, but I *can* practice my breathing exercises and *listen* to my favorite tape. It's not the end of the world if I'm late. It would probably be helpful next time to leave a little earlier. If the traffic delays me too much, I'll pull over at the next rest area and do some stretching so my pain does not increase as well." The same traffic jam but different response and physiological consequences.

SUMMARY

Cognitive-behavioral therapies can provide the patient in chronic pain with the tools to live a better quality of life and to reduce their suffering. Introducing the connection of mind and body early in the evaluation process can facilitate acceptance by the patient of their role in managing their pain at all stages of treatment—diagnostic, therapeutic, and maintenance. Providing patients with a comprehensive, cognitive-behavioral program is effective physically and psychologically, and makes economic sense. But perhaps most importantly, when asking the patient, it makes personal sense—as one patient like Mary said, "I know I'll have a good day, because *I know how* to make it a good day."

SELECTED READINGS

Caudill M. *Managing Pain Before It Manages You*. Revised edition. New York: Guilford Press, 1995.

Caudill MA, Schnable R, Zuttermeister P, et al. Decreased clinic use by chronic pain patients: response to behavioral medicine interventions. *Clin J Pain* 1991;7:305–310.

Friedman R, Myers P, Sobel D, et al. Behavioral medicine, clinical health psychology, and cost offset. *Health Psychology* 1995;14:509–518.

Jamison R. *Learning to Master Your Chronic Pain*. Sarasota, Florida: Professional Resource Press, 1996.

Keefe FJ, Caldwell DS. Cognitive behavioral control of arthritis pain. *Med Clin North Am* 1997;81:277–290.

Lorig KR, Mazonson PD, Holman HR. Evidence suggesting that health education for self-management in patients with chronic arthritis has sustained health benefits while reducing health-care costs. *Arthritis Rheum* 1993;36:439–446.

NIH Technology Assessment Panel. Integration of behavioral and relaxation approaches into the treatment of chronic pain and insomnia. *JAMA* 1996;276:313.

Young LD, Bradley LA, Turner RA. Decreases in health care resource utilization in patients with rheumatoid arthritis following a cognitive behavioral intervention. *Biofeedback Self Regul* 1995;20:259.

CHAPTER 57

Psychopathology, Psychotherapy, and Chronic-Pain Management

Joshua Wootton and Jillian B. Frank

Whatever its origin, the advent of chronic pain represents a transformation in the life of an individual. At best, it may mean an unforeseen accommodation in time and energy to an unwelcome intrusion into one's life. At worst, it can mean that the goals and entire direction of one's life must be reexamined and recalibrated in an attempt to cope with and adapt to catastrophic changes of uncertain duration. More than simply an unpleasant sensory stimulus, chronic pain can come to affect the whole individual, emotionally and socially, by becoming the source itself of a variety of psychosocial stressors. The following case report illustrates the extent to which this is possible.

CASE REPORT: PATIENT 1

A 50-year-old married man was referred to the pain-management center, 6 months after suffering a work-related injury to his lower back. His pain had remained intractable to surgical intervention and a variety of conservative measures, and he continued to report that it was both debilitating and as severe as, if not worse than, ever. Although his physicians tended to support his claim to disability, his worker's compensation carrier had sent him to be examined by two independent medical examiners (IMEs), one of whom had recommended an immediate return to work. To maintain his worker's compensation benefits, he had to engage an attorney to support his claim, with the result that he became involved in what he experienced as a frustrating and time-consuming process of litigation. As his anxiety escalated concerning his loss of income and inability to work and provide for his family, he became increasingly irritable, withdrawn, and ultimately, depressed. Arguments with his spouse and children became more frequent; and, by the time he arrived at the pain-management center, he reported feeling isolated, helpless, hopeless, and suicidal.

The case of *Patient 1* is a familiar one to anyone who specializes in the treatment of chronic pain. The experience of chronic pain typically comes to be the product of conflict between the sensory stimulus and the entire individual, including his or her network of social supports. It will always require some level of adjustment and adaptation, but it can, in many cases, interfere with one's relationships with family and friends, career, livelihood, recreational pursuits, and sexual intimacy. By extension, it also can exercise enduring changes upon self-esteem and the ways in which one views oneself as a man or woman, husband or wife, father or mother, friend, member of society, spiritual being, and patient.

PSYCHOLOGICAL FACTORS IN CHRONIC PAIN

With so much at stake for the patient with chronic pain, it is not surprising that psychological evaluation is a required or highly recommended feature of comprehensive evaluation in many pain-management centers. The International Association for the Study of Pain (IASP) has recommended that chronic-pain management should involve a multidisciplinary approach, including both medical and psychological perspectives. The reason for this is that the quality, intensity, and duration of many patients' pain experiences are related to psychological factors that include, but are not limited to, the presence of trauma, adjustment difficulties, and levels of experienced stress. With the IASP reporting an incidence of chronic pain in the United States of 70 million and with more than 50 million being partially or totally disabled for periods ranging from a few days to months and years, a concerted, multidisciplinary effort becomes even more critical to the effective marshaling of available medical resources.

Stress Reactivity and the Pain–Stress Cycle

It now is generally accepted—if not always considered—that psychiatric disorders and symptoms are influential in the development, expression, and tractability of chronic pain. The term *stress-reactive* is suggestive of the continuum of the degree to which any individual reacts to external and internal stressors, including the stressor of chronic pain and its psychosocial sequelae. Highly stress-reactive individuals are likely to develop a broader spectrum of more severe psychological and social sequelae, as well as to experience their pain with greater emotional involvement and suffering. Less stress-reactive individuals may still experience the need to accommodate to their pain, psychologically, socially, and occupationally, but their adjustment to living with chronic pain typically is more successful and their adaptation to their limitations, more enduring.

The term *pain–stress cycle* is indicative of the ongoing or unfolding neuropsychosocial matrix in which (a) pain tends to amplify the impact of stress, and (b) stress magnifies the subjective experience of suffering associated with pain. The former occurs when the individual's experience of pain facilitates the development of new and secondary psychological, social, and occupational stressors, as in the case of *Patient 1*, as well as by promoting the individual's tendency to resort to and rely upon maladaptive coping strategies, such as self-medication, social withdrawal, and the development of generalized, reactive pain behaviors. The latter refers specifically to the contributions of autonomic arousal and musculoskeletal tension in the maintenance and intensity of the individual's experience of pain; but stress, regardless of its origin, can result in physiological deterioration and the magnified experience of pain through a variety of mechanisms. Neurosignature patterns may be modulated, in part, by psychological stress; and it is possible that one's emotional responses to stress, whether physical or psychological in nature, influence the body's stress-regulation systems, which may, in turn, result in tissue damage or lesions contributing to the neurosignature patterns that give rise to chronic pain.

All models of chronic pain acknowledge the neuropsychosocial interaction between stress and pain and propose a particular perspective on the relationship between psychological factors and pain. Assessing the degree to which a chronic-pain patient is stress-reactive and addressing the nature of his or her unique expression of the pain–stress cycle therefore become primary goals of psychological intervention in pain management. As psychotherapy begins, the first important consideration—one that will likely have implications for both prognosis

and treatment—is the juxtaposition of psychological factors influencing pain, especially with regard to the order and relative duration of influence. In some cases, the psychopathology occurring as a complicating feature in the diagnosis and treatment of chronic pain exists prior to the advent of the pain syndrome; while, in others, it is reactive to and arises from the patient's experience of pain.

Premorbid Psychopathology

Chronic pain is far more prevalent among the psychiatrically disordered than in the general population, and temperament, personality traits, and psychopathology may all play roles in the development and maintenance of pain. Patients who develop chronic pain without an identifiable or adequate physiological etiology, for example, may be somatizing. As an immature psychological defense, somatization represents the symbolic displacement of intrapsychic conflicts onto the somatic sphere in an unconscious attempt to avoid distressing affects. Alexithymia is frequently a complicating and exacerbating feature of somatization, because patients who are unable to articulate their emotions and internal feeling states in words may have few outlets other than the bodily expression of their distress.

Especially for those who have come to regard the experience of emotional pain or displays of affect as signs of weakness, displacing their intrapsychic conflicts onto their bodies may lead them to feel that they have more legitimate claims to the fulfillment of their needs. Nor is this a tendency of only a few stoical patients. All stress-reactive individuals tend to somatize, when under sustained or escalating stress; and, because we are all on a stress-reactive continuum, we all tend to express our internal feeling states through our bodies to some degree. In the medical setting, this issue of degree can become the focus of questions regarding diagnosis and treatment. Highly stress-reactive patients may have long histories of somatization and physical complaints at many sites; but, even when there is an identifiable organic basis for pain, a tendency toward somatization can magnify any patient's suffering.

Case Report: Patient 2

A 35-year-old married woman with a long history of well-documented and well-managed back pain presented with an acute exacerbation of her pain. Tearful and in obvious distress, she could not identify any precipitating event or injury but nevertheless reported that she could barely move without excruciating discomfort. So overwhelming was her predicament that she insisted her husband take time from work to remain close to her, for fear that she might fall and be unable to get assistance. When interviewed by a psychologist, the woman extolled her husband's many virtues, and only as an afterthought did she suggest that other women thought his patience and affectionate nature were attractive, too. Suddenly becoming more tearful and distraught, she reported that she had recently been worried about a female colleague's obvious interest in her husband and had, on the same day her back worsened, discovered a note from this woman on her husband's dresser. An urgent session of couples therapy was arranged in which the husband convincingly allayed the patient's concerns, and she appeared much reassured and less distressed at the end. Several days later, she canceled her follow-up visit to the pain-management center, saying that her exacerbation of pain was now largely resolved.

In the case of *Patient 2*, the sudden exacerbation of pain was significantly out of proportion to anything she had ever experienced in her many years of coping with chronic, low-back pain. It surprised and frightened her, which only further added to the stress she was undergoing in a quickly accelerating pain–stress cycle.

As in the example of *Patient 2*, somatization can be associated with a specific instance or period of escalating or sustained stress in a patient's life—in which case, it may more properly be regarded as an instance of comorbid psychopathology—but many patients with chronic pain report long histories of stress-reactive illnesses or syndromes, as well as familiarity with vulnerabilities to pain at specific sites. Somatization of this variety (primary somatization) can represent a psychiatric disorder in its own right, or it can become a defensive process around which the entire personality is organized, as with some expressions of personality disorder. More often, however, it is encountered merely as an expression of or symptom associated with another disorder (secondary somatization), such as generalized anxiety, panic, posttraumatic stress, or depression. Investigators have found, for example, that more than 50% of patients diagnosed with major depressive disorder report pain as a prominent feature of their experience, and the prevalence of chronic pain developing among depressed and panic-disordered patients is considerably inflated.

The experience of psychological trauma also is highly correlated with the subsequent development of chronic pain. In patients who have suffered abuse as children or adults or who have experienced or witnessed situations in which death or serious injury was real or threatened, chronic pain may come to represent a means of psychologically symbolizing and organizing an unbearable or horrific event. Studies vary widely in their depiction of this elusive yet potentially critical connection between trauma and the development of chronic pain, but reports suggest that between one third and two thirds of patients treated for chronic pain have been previously exposed to some form of psychological trauma. Some investigators have gone so far as to suggest that the biological mechanisms supporting posttraumatic stress disorder (PTSD) may directly influ-

ence the patient's pain perception. Severe reactions to psychological trauma can certainly result in the sort of intrapsychic fragmentation that can be experienced by the overwhelmed patient as fragmentation of the body, which likely accounts for why 85% of acutely psychotic patients report functional somatic complaints.

Comorbid Psychopathology

Although anxiety is the most commonly associated affect in acute-pain states, depression tends to be the most common in chronic-pain syndromes. Major depressive disorder is present in one quarter to one half of all patients diagnosed with pain disorder, with dysthymia or significant depressive symptomatology being reported in 60% to 100% of patients with chronic pain. In most cases where depression was not a premorbid factor, depressive tendencies and symptoms may be said to have developed out of the patient's situation of chronic pain, the accompanying limitations in functioning, and the resulting difficulties with adjustment. Sad mood and irritability, feelings of helplessness and hopelessness, lack of energy, lack of motivation, anhedonia, sleep and appetite disturbance, decreased libido, and psychomotor slowing all are familiar concomitants to chronic pain.

In the absence of the premorbid expression of pathological anxiety, there are nevertheless many situations in which a heightened baseline of anxiety, panic, or posttraumatic stress also can occur concurrently with pain or in its immediate aftermath, usually in the context of the precipitating injury. Hypervigilance, increased startle response and heightened arousal, panic symptoms, avoidance, and posttraumatic stress frequently arise in pain originating with motor-vehicle and work-related accidents, assaults, and natural disasters.

Short-term and more enduring problems with postmorbid adjustment to chronic pain also may be expressed as adjustment disorders in which the patient with chronic pain develops clinically significant emotional and behavioral symptoms associated with the identifiable stressor of injury or the advent of the sustained experience of pain. These symptoms tend to develop shortly after and reactive to the onset of injury or chronic pain and may be characterized as subjective distress that is in excess of what is expected, given the nature of the stressor. Symptoms of anxiety or depression or both emerge alongside maladaptive behaviors that signal clear impairment in social or occupational functioning. Such problems with adjustment to life with chronic pain and its limitations are common among pain patients and, fortunately, represent one of the more successfully treatable expressions of comorbid psychopathology.

A diagnosis of pain disorder also is suggestive of adjustment difficulties, but here the predominant focus of the patient's presentation is the pain itself, which is sufficient

TABLE 57.1. *Forms of Psychopathology Most Typically Identified as Complicating Features of Chronic Pain*

DSM-IV classification	Possible premorbid pathology	Possible comorbid pathology
Mood disorders	x	x
Anxiety disorders	x	x
Adjustment disorders	–	x
Personality disorders	x	–
Somatoform disorders	x	–

to cause clinically significant distress or impairment in functioning. While adjustment disorders more typically occur in reaction to the event of injury and its sequelae, pain disorders arise in the context of a patient's reaction to intolerable sensory stimulus. The symptom of pain is neither intentionally produced, as with malingering, or feigned, as with factitious disorders, but instead becomes the conscious source and focus of the patient's distress.

Cases of pain disorder can be associated with both psychological factors and a general medical condition, or they may be associated with psychological factors alone. In the former, an identifiable injury or organic pathology may have set the disorder in motion and remains a source of sensory discomfort, but tendencies toward somatization, preoccupation, and overconcern contribute to the tenacity and intensity of the symptom. In the absence of any organic pathology, such psychological factors can lead to the development of hypochondriasis or to preoccupation with symptoms in the belief or fear that one has a serious disease. In their hypervigilance to changes in somatic stimuli, pain-disordered patients can resemble hypochondriacs, but their concern tends to be less generalizable and more specific to the identified site of their pain.

A diagnosis of pain associated *only* with psychological factors supplants the former designations of somatoform pain and psychogenic pain, and some investigators regard it as the most common instance of simple conversion in developed societies. As in conversion disorder, the symptoms of pain disorder can sometimes appear pseudoneurological, but a diagnosis of conversion disorder is not made if the patient's distress remains focused on his or her symptoms of pain. A summary of the possible premorbid and comorbid forms of psychopathology most typically identified as complicating features of chronic pain is provided in Table 57.1. Factitious disorders, while often presenting with complaints of pain, are not motivated by physical pain, and pain is not typically influential in the development of the disorder.

A MULTIDISCIPLINARY APPROACH

Not all patients with chronic pain exhibit significant psychopathology, of course, or have their pain pictures complicated in an enduring way by psychological factors. Many have adjusted well to the limitations imposed by their pain and continue to work productively and enjoy satisfying relationships with family and friends. Most of these individuals have no histories of psychopathology, premorbid to the development of their chronic pain; and, by virtue of an essentially resilient temperament, adaptive personality traits, and successful coping skills, they have managed to elude the comorbid development of enduring psychological symptoms and distress associated with their pain.

Those who are not so fortunate, however, tend to be the most memorable patients in any primary-care practice or pain-management center. Their suffering is obvious and, even when their numbers are few, their drain on available resources is considerable, whether calculated in terms of time, money, or the emotional reserves of staff. Their pain may remain puzzling and intractable to an ever-lengthening list of ideas and interventions; and their urgency, whether demanding or importunate, continually reminds us of our limitations as healthcare providers. Small wonder, then, that they elicit such strong feelings and responses from us and frequently lead us into colluding with their urgency by referring them to yet another specialist, trying one more improbable intervention, or raising the level of pain medications, one more time.

Chronic pain of this nature calls instead for a multidisciplinary approach to management, not a series of attempts to cure or extinguish the disorder or assuage or discharge the patient. When psychological factors are influential in the development and maintenance of a patient's pain, the greatest progress is likely to be made in an approach that includes encouraging the patient toward a healthier psychological adjustment to his or her pain and resulting limitations. This in no way suggests that continued palliation or the search for better medical solutions be abandoned—the patient's developing stability may well depend upon an abiding trust that his or her physicians are doing everything possible to offer appropriate relief and comfort through medical means—but a more comprehensive treatment plan has a better chance of addressing all of the factors that contribute to the patient's experience of pain and distress.

Establishing an Alliance

Patients with chronic pain often express the need for reassurance that their healthcare providers have heard their concerns and understand their experience. Many have gone from physician to physician and encountered repeated disappointments in their search for answers; and their often challenging presentations may reflect the defensiveness, hypersensitivity, and hypervigilance of the scars, both psychological and physical, they have sustained along the way. Establishing a good working alliance therefore is critical for all members of a multidisciplinary team, including the primary-care physician, the pain physician, the psychologist, the nurse, the physical therapist, and, in some cases, the complementary specialist. The patient's compliance with directives and cooperation with the treatment plan often depend on the perception that all members of the team are working together in his or her behalf.

The opposite occurs, when patients lose trust in their caregivers or sense that they are not fully engaged in the process of helping them in their search for answers and relief. When patients feel rushed, dismissed, or devalued, an increase in pain behaviors and dependency, as well as tendencies toward enactment (acting out) of retaliatory impulses, are likely either to interrupt or to thwart any chance of a successful outcome. In a multidisciplinary approach, the responsibility for maintaining an effective alliance is shared among caregivers, with the result that the patient's urgency is experienced by all members of the team as less demanding or overwhelming.

With the addition of the psychologist, psychiatrist, or social worker, patients frequently will need the reassurance of the entire team that their pain is being taken seriously and not relegated to the uncertain status of being "all in the head." An effective approach to an initial psychological evaluation is therefore one that focuses on what the patient knows best and wishes most to discuss—namely, the emotional and behavioral impact of pain on his or her life. When the patient feels heard, understood, and safe, the direction of the psychotherapist's inquiry can turn toward a consideration of the emotional and behavioral antecedents, correlates, and precipitants of pain. Once the patient is willing to discuss the possibility that stress and psychological factors may contribute toward or exacerbate his or her pain experience, the way is opened for psychotherapeutic intervention. Much depends, however, on the process of carefully nurturing this willingness and the psychotherapist's assessment of how ready the patient is for actual change.

Assessing Readiness for Change

Investigators of psychotherapeutic efficacy in pain management suggest that patients vary widely in how prepared they are to make changes in behavior around their pain. One influential model for understanding change in this context—the transtheoretical model—proposes a series of stages that any patient with chronic pain must negotiate to arrive at even the simplest of behavioral changes and, by extension, changes in his or her attitude toward and self-management of pain. The first of these usually is labeled *precontemplation* and represents the stage at which patients are highly resistant to changing their behaviors. Patients often arrive in pain clinics with the idea that nothing but medical intervention will work for them and that certainly nothing they can do has any chance of influencing their pain. Those whose willingness to consider making behavioral changes around their pain can be nurtured, even though they are not yet ready to try, are in the *contemplation* stage. The point of much of the psychoeducation that occurs in pain -management centers is to move patients from the precontemplation to the contemplation stage by challenging their resistances and offering reasonable, alternative explanations for their pain experiences.

In the *preparation* stage, patients have come to the point where they are actively considering attempts to change and making decisions about how they might proceed. The *action* stage sees them actively engaged in the process of changing their behavior, whether inhibiting old patterns or promoting and practicing new ones; and the *maintenance* stage has them working to maintain the changes they have established. Because psychotherapy encourages change in both attitude and behavior, it is critical to assess accurately where patients are in their readiness to make these changes. Suggesting to someone in the precontemplation stage that the daily practice of relaxation techniques will assist in the management of pain, for example, will ensure the failure of the intervention before it is begun. If the goal of psychotherapy in pain management is to create the opportunity for change—to develop more adaptive pain-management strategies and behaviors and to reduce or inhibit maladaptive pain and illness behaviors—then identifying and working within the context of the patient's current stage of readiness for change is essential.

PSYCHOTHERAPEUTIC INTERVENTIONS

Effective psychotherapy for pain management tends to be eclectic, because the particular mode and *milieu* must be contextually appropriate to the patient's particular situation. This means that the psychotherapist working with pain patients must be skilled in the application of a broad spectrum of techniques and approaches to intervention and be willing to combine these creatively in the service of effective, therapeutic outcome. In the multidisciplinary setting, psychotherapy usually is prescribed to run concurrently with medical treatment and other therapies and, ideally, should begin with the comprehensive evaluation of the patient, out of which the multidisciplinary treatment plan is established in consultation with the entire team of caregivers.

Comprehensive Evaluation

Psychotherapeutic intervention begins with as complete an assessment as possible of the patient's presenting baseline and, as well as can be discerned, his or her premorbid baseline. This frequently includes a clinical interview and anamnesis, as well as a psychometric assessment of the current level of functioning, symptoms of psychopathology, presence of risk factors affecting prognosis, and other cultural, educational, and attitudinal indicators. Once the presenting baseline is established, ongoing assessments provide evidence of psychotherapeutic progress, as well as opportunities to make appropriate changes in the treatment plan, including referral for psychopharmacological evaluation, where appropriate.

Psychoeducation

The beginning of psychotherapeutic intervention for many pain patients lies in the collaborative development of a rationale for the psychotherapy itself. Investigation of the patient's explanatory model for his or her pain may lead to valuable clues about his or her readiness for change. Patients whose explanatory models are mechanistic or reflect issues of secondary gain, for example, often will insist upon interventions in which they can remain passive. Normalizing their experience and helping them to recognize and better understand their own stress reactivity and the pain–stress cycle therefore is a critical step in moving them toward the *contemplation* stage of change, where they can consider assuming an active role in their own recovery and rehabilitation. For many patients, this will mean learning more about (a) the physiology and psychology of pain, (b) the differences between acute and chronic pain, and (c) the difference between pain and injury, hurt and harm. Once these issues are grasped, the way to attitudinal and behavioral change is opened.

Psychodynamic and Supportive Psychotherapy

For many patients with chronic pain, a necessary step in their developing readiness for change is the experience of feeling understood—usually achieved through the opportunity to tell their story in their own time and in their own way to a sympathetic listener. What patients know best and typically want to discuss most is the behavioral, emotional, and social impact of their pain upon their lives. Even when they adamantly deny that these factors play any role in the development or maintenance of their symptoms, they need to feel that their suffering is validated and their circumstances fully appreciated by those who would care for them. In cases where premorbid psychopathology has contributed to the development of chronic pain, an understanding of the connec-

tions between the patient's history and the development of his or her symptoms may prove essential to assisting him or her toward a more active role in treatment.

Case Report: Patient 3

A 37-year-old, separated woman was referred to the pain-management center with abdominal and pelvic pain of uncertain etiology. Six months earlier, she had been in an motor-vehicle accident in which the restraint of her seatbelt had left her bruised and sore for several weeks. As the bruising diminished, however, her pain seemed to become even more intense and urgent, even to the point where she had trouble walking. She agreed to enter psychotherapy to address her anxiety, but she denied any depression and was convinced that her experience of pain was solely the result of her accident. During the course of treatment, she disclosed to her psychotherapist that, as a child, she had been repeatedly sexually molested by her father, who frequently used the occasion of disciplining or punishing her for "bad" behavior to abuse her physically and sexually. She associated her feeling "bad" about having caused the motor-vehicle accident with the bruising and pain in her abdominal and pelvic region and wondered whether there might be a connection. Over time, she came to the insight that her accident, in many respects, and through no fault of her own, had served as a recapitulation of her childhood trauma and the situation of old physical and emotional injury. Once she recognized that this recapitulation may have been contributing to keeping her "stuck," making her pain less tractable to treatment, she became motivated to help herself overcome her pain. Several months later, after the addition of cognitive-behavioral techniques and psychopharmacological intervention—both of which she had previously declined—her pain was largely resolved.

The case of *Patient 3* illustrates how a comparatively straightforward physical injury and its resulting pain can become complicated by premorbid psychological factors and indeed come to symbolize and recapitulate unresolved emotional trauma and conflict. It is not unreasonable to think that many individuals suffering similar injuries might experience a few weeks of soreness but emerge essentially unscathed, having put the experience behind them. In this patient's case, however, not only did she need to tell her story and have her experience validated, but she needed to recognize and accept the connections between her emotional experience and her chronic pain before she could accept a more active role in her own recovery and rehabilitation. In cases where psychosocial factors appear to contribute toward the development and maintenance of chronic pain, as well as in situations where the goal of treatment must be the long-term adjustment to chronic pain, psychodynamic and supportive psychotherapy may prove a necessary catalyst for change, along with basic psychoeducation.

Operant-Behavioral Therapy

Operant-behavioral therapy (OBT) refers to the general grouping of therapies and interventions that focus upon the reinforcing role of social and environmental factors in the development and maintenance of chronic pain. It is especially useful in those cases where the subjective experience of pain appears to go well beyond its organic basis and issues of secondary gain and the development of stubborn pain behaviors have emerged. The goal of OBT is to encourage the practice of more adaptive pain-management strategies by identifying and reinforcing "wellness" behaviors while reducing the reinforcement of "illness" and pain behaviors. A variety of treatment approaches and techniques may be utilized, whether in the formal context of psychotherapy or less formally in encounters with members of the treatment team during office visits, physical therapy, and telephone contacts. OBT should not be limited to the situation of the formal psychotherapeutic session but rather integrated into the multidisciplinary treatment approach and practiced by physicians, nurses, physical therapists, and complementary providers.

Specific techniques of OBT include (a) graded activation and exercise programs to increase fitness and resilience, while stemming the trend toward deconditioning; (b) active and collaborative management and, where appropriate, tapering of habit-forming pain medications; and (c), most importantly, social reinforcement. This last approach can be undertaken from the patient's very first visit to the physician's office or clinic with a discussion of initial expectations but ultimately should extend to the patient's spouse and family, who can learn through family meetings or family therapy how to encourage the development of more adaptive pain-management strategies in the patient. The familiar pattern of escalating familial conflict in the aftermath of a patient's development of chronic pain and its accompanying physical limitations often can be redirected into common goals, if family members' own sense of frustration can be channeled into social reinforcement in the patient's behalf.

Cognitive-Behavioral Therapy

Unlike OBT, cognitive-behavioral therapy (CBT) more typically involves the formal setting of individual or group psychotherapy and is directed toward changing maladaptive behaviors by examining and posing alternatives to the thoughts, attitudes, and beliefs underlying them, as well as by encouraging the development of new skills and practices that will contribute toward increasing functional ability. CBT for pain management frequently involves a threefold approach: (a) a psychoeducational phase; (b) a skills-building phase in which training is provided in cognitive and behavioral techniques, such as relaxation training, activity pacing, distraction strategies, cognitive restructuring, problem solving, and goal development; and (c) an application phase in which patients learn to consolidate and generalize their new strategies in increasingly challenging situations. The goal is the establishment and maintenance of a higher level of functioning and increased resilience to the anxiety and depression associated with chronic pain.

The emphasis of the psychoeducational phase is upon the enlistment of the patient as an active participant in his or her own treatment. This usually means helping the patient to develop a model for understanding his or her pain and suffering that will assist in the recognition and identification of those thoughts, attitudes, and beliefs that tend to make the subjective experience of pain less tractable and more insidious, intense, and tenacious. These self-defeating cognitions typically develop within a context of anxiety, misinformation, secondary gain, and negative reinforcement and often lead to depression and despair.

The skills-building phase focuses upon specific strategies that will enable the patient to identify those thoughts, attitudes, and beliefs that increase his or her distress and magnify the subjective experience of pain. Cognitive restructuring techniques assist with the early recognition of such negative cognitions and encourage the systematic substitution of more stable and positive ones. Curricula and techniques for managing stress and anger also may be utilized as a means to identify and address the environmental, interpersonal, and intrapsychic triggers that increase autonomic arousal and adversely affect pain. Relaxation techniques, such as meditation, progressive muscle relaxation, autogenic training, visualization, and self-hypnosis, are more behaviorally oriented interventions directed toward relieving musculoskeletal tension and lowering autonomic arousal. Biofeedback is another psychoeducational and training device that allows the patient to monitor his or her ongoing success at developing an effective relaxation regimen. By monitoring the level of musculoskeletal tension through surface electromyographic (sEMG) leads and the level of autonomic arousal through measures of skin temperature, heart rate, blood pressure, oxygen saturation, and electrodermagraphic (EDG) response, patients can see firsthand the effects of practicing relaxation according to a disciplined and regular schedule.

Biofeedback also can assist the patient toward the third or application phase of CBT in which the newly acquired collection of cognitive skills, behavioral techniques, and coping strategies become an integrated component in a new outlook and a more enduring and adaptive approach to pain management. Cognitive-behavioral therapy concludes, then, not simply with the acquisition of a collection of helpful tools, but with the template for successful adjustment to the intrusion of chronic pain in the patient's life. Its best chance for success occurs when cognitive restructuring, pacing, and the daily practice of relaxation exercises become as second nature as eating breakfast and brushing one's teeth.

Group Psychotherapy

Semistructured and structured group psychotherapy can combine the best elements of psychodynamic and supportive psychotherapy, OBT, and CBT; and, in many pain-management centers and clinics, participation in a structured group is the most frequently prescribed intervention. The experience of chronic pain can be socially isolating and lead to the experience of being continually misunderstood, and the chance to see that others in similar circumstances experience similar feelings and encounter the same problems and frustrations can prove a welcome validation. For this reason, many formats for pain-management groups include time devoted to the development of group process and the sharing of experiences, as well as a more formally structured psychoeducational and CBT component. A variety of manuals and workbooks is available to the psychotherapist who seeks guidance in developing a curriculum for a time-limited, structured pain-management group.

The emphasis of the psychotherapeutic treatment of chronic pain is not merely the reduction of pain but the restoration of functioning. The patient with chronic pain will always face limitations in his or her physical functioning, but assisting him or her toward a successful adjustment to these limitations often depends upon (a) a multidisciplinary understanding and appreciation of the psychological factors contributing to the development and maintenance of the patient's pain experience, (b) an establishment of a good working alliance with the patient, (c) an accurate assessment of the patient's readiness for change, and (d) a discerning application of approaches from a broad spectrum of psychotherapeutic interventions that is supported by the entire treatment team.

SELECTED READINGS

Arnstein P, Caudill M, Mandle CL, et al. Self efficacy as a mediator of the relationship between pain intensity, disability and depression in chronic pain patients. *Pain* 1999;80:483–491.

Compas BE, Haaga DAF, Keefe FJ, et al. Sampling of empirically supported psychological treatments from health psychology: smoking, chronic pain, cancer, and bulimia nervosa. *J Consult Clin Psychol* 1998; 66:89–112.

Eimer BN, Freeman A. *Pain Management Psychotherapy: A Practical Guide.* New York: John Wiley & Sons, 1998.

Eisendrath SJ. Psychiatric aspects of chronic pain. *Neurology* 1995;45: 26–34.

Fishhain DA, Cutler R, Rosomoff HL, et al. Chronic pain associated depression: antecedent or consequence of chronic pain? A review. *Clin J Pain* 1997;13:116–137.

Gallagher RM. Treatment planning in pain medicine: integrating medical, physical, and behavioral therapies. *Med Clin North Am* 1999;83: 823–849.

Gatchel RJ, Turk DC, eds. *Psychological Approaches to Pain Management: A Practitioner's Handbook.* New York: Guilford, 1996.

Goldberg RT. Childhood abuse, depression, and chronic pain. *Clin J Pain* 1994;10:277–281.

Lipchik GL, Milles K, Covington EC. The effects of multidisciplinary pain management treatment on locus of control and pain beliefs in chronic non-terminal pain. *Clin J Pain* 1993;9:49–57.

Prochaska JO, Norcross JC, DiClemente CC. *Changing for Good.* New York: William Morrow, 1994.

CHAPTER 58

Biofeedback

David A. Danforth

Since its advent on the clinical landscape in the early 1970s, biofeedback has garnered a reputation among both lay people and clinicians for being a rather ineffable meld of the high-tech and the arcane. Media descriptions of astronauts being trained with biofeedback to self-regulate the physiological effects of zero gravity are juxtaposed with images of Tibetan monks engaged in occult mind-body wizardry. Thus, to the typical patient being referred for pain management, biofeedback may represent a Westernized, electronic shortcut to attaining deep relaxation and pain-transcending bliss. Most are soon disabused of this conceit, as biofeedback training is, paradoxically, neither inherently relaxing nor does it necessarily produce euphoric sensations. Few are initially aware of the degree of effort required to master passive volition, the "letting-go" of physiological self-regulation, and then to successfully apply it in even the most ordinary real-life settings. Yet, for the motivated and determined patient, it can provide a basis for actively collaborating in his/her medical treatment, with benefits ranging from the reliable generation of a restorative state involving key physiological parameters, to the production of a focal salutary effect upon measurable pathophysiological dysregulation, which may underlie persistent pain symptoms.

Several questions arise, then, which are likely important to both prospective patients and referring clinicians. What, exactly, is biofeedback? What are its potential mechanisms of action? How are self-regulatory, pain-management skills learned and applied by patients using biofeedback? What is the efficacy of biofeedback treatment for various pain disorders? Where might future developments lead, in light of technological advancements? This chapter will briefly review these questions and provide illustrative case vignettes.

DEFINITIONS OF BIOFEEDBACK

Early practitioners drew upon cybernetic systems theory as a way of conceptualizing the self-regulatory skills obtainable with biofeedback. Cybernetics was first described in 1948 by Norbert Wiener, a mathematician and professor of physics at Massachusetts Institute of Technology. In this model, an intelligent information-processing system is capable of making corrections to its functioning when the criteria for desired operational performance are known, and it then is provided with specific data, or "feedback," on whether its behavior is moving toward or away from conformance with those criteria. Such corrections then represent an operational-based learning that helps the system to maintain optimal functioning despite entropic pressure. When a motivated person, as a biological organism, is provided with adequate information about specific physiological activity in reference to overt parameters, it becomes possible for him/her to alter the activity using this "bio-feedback."

Additional refinements to this model have been helpful and have focused on clarifying requisite process and outcome variables. For the biofeedback to be useful, it must include the following elements:

Accurate physiological measurement. Current electronic instrumentation allows for highly accurate, noninvasive measurement of activity governed by the autonomic, musculoskeletal, and central nervous systems. Physiological monitoring signals are available for cardiovascular (heart rate, interbeat interval) and peripheral vascular (blood volume pulse wave amplitude, skin surface temperature) activity; electrodermal activity (EDA: skin conductance response, skin conductance level); neuromuscular activity [surface electromyography (sEMG), balloon manometry for inferential measurement of anorectal and bladder sphincter activity]; and electroencephalographic (EEG) activity involving selective feedback of α, θ, or sensorimotor rhythm (SMR) signals.

Accessible signal presentation. The patient needs to comprehend the feedback signal to use it. The electronic instrumentation available for clinical use in the 1970s and 1980s was capable of giving binary or analog audio and/or visual feedback signals. These signals could be presented either noncontingently to the patient, as simple physiological monitoring, or contingent upon physiological response parameters. In the former, the patient might be encouraged to observe any changes in monitored activity while also engaging in a prescribed relaxation exercise, such as paced abdominal breathing, progressive muscle relaxation, or elicitation of the relaxation response described by Herbert Benson in 1975. Objective validation of relaxation thus is available to the patient, who then may be asked to reflect on any perceived changes in pain level. In the latter, the feedback signal is presented in a manner consistent with operant behavior therapy reinforcement techniques. Negative reinforcement contingencies often are used as a pain analog. In this application, the patient is presented with a somewhat harsh or noxious tone when monitored arousal is above a designated level; the tone becomes softer as the patient's physiological "behavior" moves closer to a designated point, whereupon it can be made to cease. Conversely, using a positive reinforcement contingency, the patient could hear a pleasant tone upon achieving the goal. Modern biofeedback instruments offer an array of feedback signal modes and contingencies, and can include computerized software to both maximize patient motivation and learning, while storing and analyzing data within and across training sessions for enhanced outcome assessment.

Comprehensive relation of the feedback signal and training protocol to the patient's pain symptoms. The clinician must educate the patient regarding the physiological meaning of the feedback signal, as well as the putative relationship between signal and symptoms. The therapist, as part of the feedback loop, should provide coaching and encouragement, and should relate any desired signal changes to subsequent momentary subjective symptomatic improvement.

MECHANISMS OF ACTION

The proximal goals of biofeedback training are to increase awareness of often subtle mind-body connections, and to promote learning of psychophysiological self-regulatory strategies. Such learning can result in reduced reactivity to critical stimuli, accelerated recovery from a stress response, and enhancement of perceived self-efficacy and coping skills mastery. However, it is not always true that the degree of physiological change predicts the extent of symptom remission. Sometimes the patient will show progress in the biofeedback modality, but will report little or no pain relief; less often, a very modest change in signal data will be associated with surprising benefit. This phenomenon may stem from the interrelationship among several variables, and it is now generally accepted that cognitive and nonspecific variables can play an important role. A multivariate model of how biofeedback works should address the following potentially contributing mechanisms of action.

Physiological Specificity

For pain syndromes where there is a biofeedback modality available that can monitor specific pathophysiological activity, a strong positive correlation can obtain between desired signal and symptom change. Examples of this are the use of surface electromyography (sEMG) in the treatment of chronic bitemporal tension headache where there is observably elevated baseline sEMG activity in the masticatory muscle groups; the use of balloon manometry to give feedback on sphincteric contraction in chronic anorectal pain; and the use of either blood-volume pulse wave amplitude (BVPa) or digital thermal biofeedback (TBF) in the treatment of primary Raynaud's disease.

Nociceptive Desensitization

Pain patients often become highly sensitized to any noxious sensations arising from affected soma. This nociceptive sensitization can generalize to the extent that the patient customarily awakens each day thinking: "Am I hurting yet?" Use of over-the-counter or prescribed medications, which are accompanied by instructions for ingestion "at the first sign of pain," may inadvertently reinforce nociceptive sensitization. Biofeedback training, either alone or following basic relaxation training, can countercondition sensations of relaxation, warmth, and well-being that can gradually desensitize the patient to over-learned pain perceptions. It also gives the patient something she can do as a first resort to ameliorate pain sensations as they arise; medication then can be an additional option.

Cognitive Attitudes, Beliefs, and Expectations

Sometimes a patient's underlying beliefs about pain symptoms yield unsalutary physiological interactions. For example, the stoic pain patient may hold beliefs reflected by popular expressions, such as "stiff upper lip," or "grin and bear it," which suggest that pain endurance is necessary and preferable to alternative vulnerability. He may disregard sensations of tension and even moderate discomfort, and avoid actively collaborating in his medical care until his pain level is overwhelming. At the other extreme, a patient may believe that their pain is unbearable and indicative of an imminently worsening prognosis. They also may maintain an attitude that only those who frequently vocalize pain complaints will receive attention and care from others. Low self-expectancy for success in coping with pain, combined with cognitive amplification of symptom meaning may result in overuse of medications as well as an unnecessarily increased frequency of clinic contact. Biofeedback training frequently augments perceived self-efficacy of pain-coping skills, and increases the patient's ability to discriminate the magnitude of tension and pain sensations, thereby allowing for a more appropriate appraisal of their importance. When used as part of a comprehensive behavioral-medicine treatment approach in primary-care settings, biofeedback has been found to both reduce annual outpatient visits and improve patient satisfaction with care.

BIOFEEDBACK CLINIC ASSESSMENT AND TRAINING PHASES

Primary-care physicians are the typical referral sources of pain patients to the Biobehavioral Service at Beth Israel Deaconess Medical Center in Boston. An initial psychiatric interview is mandatory, and usually is conducted by an attending medical psychologist. In addition to the patient's description of her chief complaint, symptom, and medical and medication histories, the interview focuses on the patient's perceptions, attitudes, and beliefs regarding her pain, as well as any factors she feels may contribute to or ameliorate pain symptoms. While taking a family and social history, the clinician listens for styles of communication and interpersonal behavior related to pain. A mental status examination is essential, and also must screen for psychiatric comorbidity; dysthymia, major depression, and anxiety disorders must receive appropriate concomitant treatment, more severe psychiatric illness may contraindicate biofeedback. Additionally, a review of health-maintenance behaviors often contributes much to the overall assessment. Important factors are: diet, exercise, recreation, social-support sources, sexual functioning, sleep, and history and current use of caffeine, sympathomimetics, nicotine, alcohol, and other substances.

Patients' initial goals upon presentation vary greatly, ranging from the passively simplistic ("I'm here to get biofeedback."), to the actively specific ("I want to learn to control this muscle spasm in my jaw."). The first step following the initial interview is a psychophysiological assessment designed to address the patient's presenting complaints. This may be an assessment of focal pathophysiology, as with the patient who has bitemporal headaches and also complains of temporomandibular joint (TMJ) pain, or it may be composed of a multichannel monitoring of several physiological parameters, as when heart rate, BVPa, EDA, and sEMG are simultaneously measured under both resting and stressor conditions in a patient who complains of stress affecting his fibromyalgia.

During this assessment, the patient is carefully oriented to the electronic monitoring instruments in a way that dovetails with the first phase of clinical biofeedback training, the awareness or response-acquisition phase. To self-regulate physiological activity and manage pain, patients first must make the connection between data streaming from the feedback instrument and any parallel perceptions they may have of internal bodily "data." As their awareness of this parallel increases, patients soon begin to experiment, usually by employing active volitional strategies, in an attempt to effect some change in the feedback signal pattern. Coaching by the therapist in regard to postural, respiratory, and attentional focus issues can be helpful. Additionally, patients must learn to distinguish between and use both active ("the harder I try, the more I'll succeed"), and passive ("the more I'm able to let go, the more I'll succeed") volition in their effort to achieve "control" over both the biofeedback and their pain symptoms. Once she can self-regulate the feedback signal to a predetermined criterion, the patient is "challenged" in two ways: first, by being asked to continue exerting control even when observable feedback is withheld; and second, by being asked to maintain control under stressor conditions, with and without observable feedback.

When a patient accomplishes the above training tasks, she is ready to enter the response application phase of treatment. Patient and therapist collaborate in developing a basic inventory of places, situations, and times in which biofeedback-trained responses could be useful in pain management. The inventory can be arranged hierarchically according to difficulty. In doing so, the patient is asked to estimate difficulty as reflected by a subjective unit of discomfort (SUD) scale, which can be operationally defined by behavioral anchors on a scale of 0 to 100. Homework assignments begin with the easiest items on the list and involve the patient in self-observation of pain, active practice of biofeedback skills for relaxation and pain management, and an SUD scale evaluation of outcome. Many patients do not follow a home-practice protocol very carefully for very long. Instead, they begin improvising, using their biofeedback training as a guide to a more generalized pain-management effort that can include elements of relaxation, physiological self-regulation, improved compliance with a medical regimen, and improved health-maintenance behaviors.

CASE REPORTS

Patient 1

A 27-year-old, single, white, female, operations manager had suffered from migraine headaches since menarche at age 14. She described these headaches as periorbital, pulsatile, without neurological prodromata, most often left hemicranial, accompanied by nausea, but without emesis. Originally, she had them perimenstrually, but she complained that in the past 3 years, they had become more frequent, occurring sometimes weekly. Moreover, she had become dismayed to find that, in the past 3 years, another kind of daily headache pain appeared, which was nonthrobbing and localized to her temples and forehead. She had been seen by a neurologist who diagnosed her as having mixed-headache syndrome, with bitemporal muscle-contraction headache and migraine without aura. Various abortive and prophylactic medications had been tried with poor side-effect tolerance and without satisfactory therapeutic effects; butalbital compounds worked best for her, but were seen as a long-term risk by her primary-care physician (PCP) because of their potential for habituation and abuse. She was aware of a patrilineal family history of chronic headache, and had become increasingly preoccupied with her daily pain levels, fearful of her "bad ones," and worried about her future. Psychiatric symptoms were absent and the mental-status examination was unremarkable; her medical history was notable only for Raynaud's phenomenon in all distal extremities. She did report some potentially contributing health-maintenance behaviors: on workdays she frequently skipped breakfast, drank two to four cups of coffee per day, chewed gum constantly while working, and indulged in two to three beers on Friday evenings.

Psychophysiological assessment of Patient 1 consisted of sEMG records obtained at rest and under simulated workplace conditions from frontal, bilateral masseter, and bilateral upper-trapezius placements. Instrumentation was MEDAC System 3000 (Neurodyne Medical, Inc., Cambridge, MA, U.S.A.), with dry-stick electrodes and preamplification at the electrode level. Frontal resting sEMG was measured at 3.5 μv, and increased to 16.5 μv when speaking at conversational volume. Left-masseter sEMG was 3.0 μv at rest, but increased to 90.0 μv when chewing gum or swallowing; right masseter was 5.0 μv resting and peaked at 314.0 μv when chewing/swallowing. Resting trapezii measurements were less than 2.0 μv, but showed a dramatic increase to greater than 40 μv, bilaterally, when the patient sat typing at a computer keyboard, her principal activity for about half of every workday. Additionally, a BVPa signal tracing was obtained from the nondominant middle finger using a reflectance plethysmographic transducer. The record showed a vasospasmodic waveform with corresponding tonic vasoconstriction. This assessment was consistent with the mixed-headache syndrome diagnosis, and further· clarified the functional contribution of daily behaviors.

Patient 1 was seen for four treatment sessions spaced 2 weeks apart. Treatment included sEMG biofeedback from frontal and masseter placements, with daily structured relaxation and sEMG biofeedback exercises as prescribed daily homework. She stopped chewing gum, began meals within 1/2 hour of awakening, and about every 4 hours thereafter, reduced her use of caffeine and made physical adjustments to her computer workspace based on postural sEMG observations. After 10 weeks, she reported a break in the pattern of daily headaches: she was now only having one every few days, and had been able to attenuate several of them using her training skills. Moreover, although she had opted not to engage in home-based thermal biofeedback training to address her vascu-

lar headaches, she reportedly had only perimenstrual migraines since the second visit. Telephone follow-up at 6 months revealed continued reduction of headache frequency, pain duration, and medication use; an annual review appointment was scheduled.

Patient 2

A 72-year-old divorced, white, male, retired college professor had developed primary Raynaud's disease in his third decade. His attacks occurred only when exposed to cold ambient temperatures, and had only become problematic since his late 50s, when he began to experience them as increasingly painful, perhaps because of additional arthritic pain. His medical and psychiatric history was noncontributory; he had been otherwise remarkably healthy all his life, and took pride in the fact that he had never needed to take medications until recently, as the worsening pain in his hands dictated that he use nonsteroidal antiinflammatory drugs. When his PCP suggested that he begin a trial of a calcium-channel blocker, he asked for a referral for biofeedback. At the close of the initial visit, Patient 2 was asked to purchase an indoor/outdoor digital-electronic thermometer at a local store and to bring it to his next session.

Biofeedback training commenced with the second visit and consisted of three clinic sessions scheduled 2 weeks apart, supplemented by daily home-based thermal biofeedback (TBF) practices, for which he was required to keep a data log. Instrumentation was a MEDAC System 3000, using a thermistor held between the thumb and first two fingers of his nondominant hand and included positive reinforcement (classical piano music), which was contingent upon his achieving incremental-criterion hand temperatures above baseline. Mean initial hand temperature reported by Patient 2 for his first week of home practice was 73.76°F, with a mean postpractice reading of 88.58°F. By the final week of reported home practice, his mean initial hand temperature had risen to 82.92°F, and his postpractice mean was 90.94°F. At the conclusion of clinic training in mid-January, he reported an ability to avert any symptoms triggered by going outdoors and remarked that his mood had become "much more up lately" since learning how to self-regulate the painful attacks.

Patient 3

A 38-year-old married, white, male, mechanical-engineering technician was referred by Dr. Carol Warfield of the Pain Unit at Beth Israel Hospital. His chief complaint was an inability to initiate and maintain sleep because of severe unremitting pain in his right hand, wrist, and forearm. The pain resulted from an industrial accident wherein a large filtration tank had fallen and crushed his right wrist and hand. After two surgeries and several months of rehabilitation therapy, he remained unable to use the hand or even tolerate any pressure or touching of it; nerve-conduction studies were abnormal, and a diagnosis was made of reflex sympathetic dystrophy (RSD). Treatment at the Pain Unit had included a stellate ganglion block and two nerve blocks, the second resulting in an anaphylactic reaction; he soon after began experiencing anxiety symptoms.

As he had always been healthy and active in sports, boating, fishing, and woodworking, Patient 3 took his pain and disability quite hard. A psychological-testing profile showed evidence of depression and a tendency toward somatosensory amplification; he reported feelings of hopelessness, lethargic apathy, and social withdrawal. He had been unable to tolerate the side-effects of a trial antidepressant, and was averse to attempting further trials. He felt that it was the burning sensations in his hand that hurt him the most, and the only relief came from applying ice to the area; alprazolam 0.5 mg. t.i.d., and flurazepam 15 mg h.s. had a limited effect on his anxiety and sleep.

Psychophysiological assessment using a BVPa photoplethysmograph showed a mild right hemilateral vasospasm of the digital arterial circulation, and a minor thermal asymmetry (left = 95.4°F, right = 93.1°F). Treatment consisted of twice-daily, home-based thermal biofeedback (hTBF) and eight clinic visits scheduled over a 4-month period, with contingent positive reinforcement for first increasing and then decreasing right-finger temperature. By the third week of home practice, he was able to raise hand temperature by a mean of 2.7°F, and lower it by 2.1°F. At the conclusion of treatment, he reported successfully using his training skills to soothe himself and initiate sleep, and sometimes to resume sleep if he were awakened by pain. He had discontinued the flurazepam h.s., and stated: "I stopped taking the sleeping pills because I was forgetting so many things; my wife really noticed it. I think this helps me much more." However, despite his self-regulation with TBF and his success at using it for the focal problem of insomnia, Patient 3 remained clinically depressed and continued to suffer daily from RSD pain. At a 6-month follow-up, he reported that he had maintained better sleep, but had otherwise had no change in symptoms, and that the injury-related litigation in which he was involved had also not progressed.

EFFICACY AND FUTURE APPLICATIONS

Evaluation of clinical outcome in biofeedback treatment is a multivariate problem. Comparison of self-reported pain severity indices (i.e., frequency, intensity, duration) pre- and posttreatment is an essential approach but often is insufficiently holistic. A comprehensive understanding of biofeedback treatment efficacy also should include measurement of changes in functional pain behaviors; changes in cognitions surrounding pain symptoms; changes in work, recreation, and social activity; changes in medical contact frequency and medication use; and change in self-reported quality of life. Also, factors that may interfere with outcome (i.e., psychiatric comorbidity, secondary gain) deserve attention. Moreover, because treatment almost always includes other interventions (e.g., relaxation and/or cognitive therapy), it is subsequently difficult to parse causality.

Nonetheless, attempts at nomothetic evaluation have suggested fairly robust outcome in pain management, with favorable results in 60% to 70% percent of patients with muscle-contraction, migraine, or mixed chronic headache; 65% to 70% of patients with primary Raynaud's; 50% to 60% of patients with TMJ pain, when combined with a dental prosthesis intervention; and 35% to 100% of those with anorectal pain, depending on feedback technology used. Varying degrees of positive outcome have been reported in small-N studies or case reports of other musculoskeletal, neurological, and disease-related pain syndromes. Age and gender differences do not seem to impede successful outcome.

The future seems quite promising for continued development of biofeedback technology and applications in pain management. Looking back at the dials, meters, and manually adjusted feedback settings of the instruments available at the time of the first edition of this volume, biofeedback was crude then as compared to now. Significant advances are likely to occur in the following three areas:

Measurement technology. Current measures of bioelectric potentials, temperature/circulatory flow, and manometric pressure are inferential, particularly in regard to pain. Improved specificity may become possible as neurobiological assays of pain are developed that can be transduced to generate feedback signals.

Instrumentation hardware. Inexpensive, wireless electrodes that use radiotelemetry to transmit data for feedback will allow clinicians a greater range of *in vivo* simulation when doing biofeedback training in an office setting. Miniaturization of clinically sophisticated biofeedback instruments for patients' home-based practice will do for other pain disorders that which highly-accurate, pocket-sized digital thermometers have done for migraine and Raynaud's.

Software integration. Computer-based technology will greatly enhance biofeedback pain-management capabilities. Digital body scanning, holographic imaging, and virtual-reality software may provide the means for highly realistic neuromuscular and musculoskeletal feedback. Software that can offer patients the chance to earn reinforcement interactively by successful self-regulation will allow biofeedback to become more enjoyable, much like playing physiological video games with one's body. Early applications of this type have been promising in teaching biofeedback relaxation for pediatric migraine.

SUMMARY

In summary, there have been numerous successful uses of biofeedback in pain management. Patients are likely to benefit if they are motivated to take an active role in their medical treatment, and are capable of a reasonable amount of sustained effort, both in the clinic and in natural settings. Those patients who have otherwise uncomplicated pain disorders for which relevant biofeedback signals can be transduced often will achieve the greatest lasting direct pain relief; however, significant ancillary benefits also are obtained from this treatment.

SELECTED READINGS

Adler G, Gattaz, WF. Pain perception threshold in major depression. *Biol Psychiatry*, 1993;34:687–689.

Basmajian JV, ed. *Biofeedback: Principles and Practice for Clinicians*, 3rd ed. Baltimore: Williams and Wilkins, 1989.

Flor H, Birbaumer N. Comparison of the efficacy of electromyographic biofeedback, cognitive-behavioral therapy, and conservative medical interventions in the treatment of chronic musculoskeletal pain. *J Consult Clin Psychology* 1993;61:653–658.

Flor H, Furst M, Birbaumer N. Deficient discrimination of EMG levels and overestimation of perceived tension in chronic pain patients. *Appl Psychophysiol Biofeedback* 1999;24:55–66.

Gilliland R, Heymen S, Altomare DF, et al. Outcome and predictors of success of biofeedback for constipation. *Br J Surg* 1997;84:1123–1126.

Gilliland R, Heymen JS, Altomarc DF, et al. Biofeedback for intractable rectal pain: outcome and predictors of success. *Dis Colon Rectum*, 1997;40:190–196.

Grimaud, JC, Bouvier M, Guien C, et al. Manometric and radiologic investigations and biofeedback treatment of chronic idiopathic anal pain. *Dis Colon Rectum* 1991;34:690–695.

Hatch JP, Fisher JG, Rugh JD, eds. *Biofeedback: Studies in Clinical Efficacy*. New York: Plenum Press, 1987.

Heah SM, Ho YH, Tan M, et al. Biofeedback is effective treatment for levator ani syndrome. *Dis Colon Rectum* 1991;34:690–695.

Schwartz MS. *Biofeedback: A Practitioner's Guide*, 2nd ed. New York: Guilford Press, 1995.

Surgery

CHAPTER 59

Neurosurgical Procedures

Harsimran S. Brara

The neurosurgeon who deals with pain has essentially two groups of patients: those who have a life-threatening illness, and those who do not. Patients in pain caused by advanced malignancy tend to need more drastic treatments; the risk of such treatments is balanced against the chance of offering a period of months or years free of pain.

This discussion will address the neurosurgeon's role in painful states that are not expected to limit the patient's life. In this group are such conditions as trigeminal neuralgia, complex regional-pain syndrome, and neuropathic pain such as particularly painful surgical scars. It is reasonable to suppose that such conditions might respond well to surgery at the level of the primary afferent fibers or autonomic ganglia. The brief review of surgical procedures that follows will serve as a road map for clinicians who do not know where to turn. Admittedly, all the routes are not shown, but it should seldom be necessary to detour through the brain or spinal cord.

CRANIAL NEURALGIAS

The prototype is trigeminal neuralgia or tic douloureux. Four surgical procedures are in widespread use: dorsal-root ablation, radiofrequency thermocoagulation, microsurgical vascular decompression, and glycerol injection into the trigeminal ganglion. The last two are currently popular, although "Gamma knife" is provided in some academic centers and appears to provide excellent, long-term relief with minimal but not negligible risk of side effects.

Gamma knife is the use of a high dose of γ radiation to ablate a particular structure. The gamma knife is a precise and powerful tool for treating certain tumors and vascular malformations in the brain, effectively and without surgery. It delivers a single, high dose of γ radiation, which comes from 201 cobalt-60 sources. The beam from each individual cobalt source is delivered through holes (or portals) in a device known as a collimator helmet. The patient's head is precisely positioned in the helmet. Only at the point where all 201 beams cross is enough radiation delivered to affect the diseased tissue, while sparing nearby normal tissue. The great accuracy of the technique — to 0.5 mm — is one of its greatest advantages.

In treatment of trigeminal neuralgia, the Gamma knife is focused on the trigeminal nerve root where it enters the brainstem. The dose of radiation delivered is not sufficient to cause the development of a lesion on the nerve, but it is sufficient to diminish or eliminate the abnormal nerve impulses that are causing the pain while preserving the normal impulses that allow for facial sensation and movement. The painless, bloodless procedure usually is performed under local anesthesia with mild sedation. There is no risk of surgical complications like infection, hemorrhage, or leakage of cerebrospinal fluid, although there is the risk of stroke and nerve injury.

Experience with Gamma knife has shown that the response to treatment usually occurs within 2 weeks of treatment; further data will be needed to determine how sustained the benefit will prove to be. All the radiobiologic effects of Gamma knife are complete by 2 years postprocedure. No long-term studies exist at this point, as the technology is new and only recently applied to patients with chronic pain. Outcomes appear favorable, with the Barrows Neurologic Institute reporting a significant improvement in 87 of 89 patients for a median follow-up period of 12 months.

Facial hyperesthesia appears to be the principal complication associated with the procedure. Therefore, the results suggest that the use of Gamma knife is similar to posterior fossa rhizotomy without the surgical morbidity of a craniotomy and a general anesthetic.

The old standard is root section in the posterior fossa, as practiced by Walter Dandy 50 years ago. Although

Dandy preferred to section the sensory portion of the trigeminal root, he believed that vascular compression of the root by a large artery next to the pons was the cause of tic douloureux in nearly all cases (Fig. 59.1). Rand and Jannetta modified the posterior fossa operation. Their procedure, which involved dissecting the compressing artery from the nerve without sectioning the root, became known as microsurgical-vascular decompression. Many neurosurgeons who perform microsurgical-vascular decompression perform a small rhizotomy at the time of surgery, particularly when neurovascular compression is not convincingly found.

Root section and microsurgical-vascular decompression both require exposure of the posterior fossa, which requires general anesthesia with endotracheal intubation, craniectomy through the occipital bone, and retraction of the cerebellum.

The entire trigeminal root cannot be sacrificed without causing complete loss of corneal sensation. Fortunately, distribution of fibers from the three trigeminal divisions is fairly discrete in the root near its entry into the pons, so partial section is usually adequate to relieve attacks of pain in the jaw and cheek while preserving ophthalmic sensation. The procedure carries a long-term success rate of 80%, according to Loeser. Its major drawback is loss of sensation in the face; such complete numbness can be more distressing to the patient than the original pain.

The concept that a vascular loop off the superior cerebellar artery compresses the trigeminal nerve root and thus causes neuralgia is an attractive one, but many experienced neurosurgeons insist that they cannot find the guilty vessel in all cases. Magnetic resonance angiography before surgery often will demonstrate a large artery in the appropriate territory, but only exploration will reveal whether it is seriously affecting the nerve. In some cases, small branches of seemingly normal vessels may be responsible.

Microsurgical-vascular decompression has an 85% to 90% long-term success rate. It is hard to argue with success, and many younger patients may wish to have a craniectomy for relief of severe trigeminal neuralgia, which is appropriate provided the diagnosis is clear. It almost goes without saying that trials of phenytoin and carbamazepine in adequate therapeutic doses should be undertaken first. Baclofen is said to be effective in some cases. Injection of local anesthetic around the infraorbital or mandibular nerve is another simple measure that can be very helpful, although it seldom is curative.

Posterior fossa craniectomy carries a small but definite mortality. It might be argued that there are faster and safer means available to control trigeminal neuralgia. The percutaneous techniques are certainly faster and, if practiced carefully, safer. As for the percutaneous approach, it is a fairly straightforward matter to direct a probe or nee-

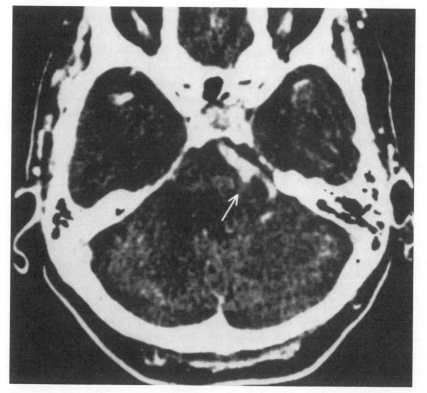

FIG. 59.1. Compression of trigeminal root by a large artery, shown on computed tomography (*arrow*), is widely believed to cause most cases of tic douloureux. Microsurgical-vascular decompression and glycerol injection into trigeminal ganglion are effective.

dle into the trigeminal ganglion through the foramen ovale. That technique is used for creating lesions in the ganglion by means of radiofrequency electrical current, which generates heat and coagulates nerve fibers. Another alternative to surgical decompression is an injection of anhydrous glycerol into the ganglion. This could relieve the initial neuralgia. Both procedures are encompassed by the term "gangliolysis."

Thermocoagulation of the ganglion with radiofrequency current is performed by inserting a probe through the check to enter the foramen ovale, through which the third trigeminal division leaves the gasserian ganglion. Correct positioning is indicated by the patient's subjective responses to test stimuli of low amplitude. The needle tip passes, more or less sequentially, through the mandibular, maxillary, and ophthalmic divisions of the trigeminal nerve within the ganglion, so some anatomical definition of the lesion is possible. A properly made lesion has an 80% chance of relieving tic douloureux initially and usually results in mild sensory loss. Late recurrences of pain are seen in about one half of the patients; the procedure can be repeated if necessary. Corneal-sensory loss is an infrequent but serious disadvantage. Another problem that is seldom discussed in the literature is severe pain from the procedure itself. The pain sometimes is accompanied by a pronounced rise in blood pressure, which in one case that came to our attention led to a cerebral hemorrhage. The discomfort of the procedure usually can be controlled with short-acting anesthetic drugs, but hypertension still may be difficult to control. General anesthesia prevents the patient from assisting in needle placement.

A newer method, which is becoming the treatment of choice for most cases of trigeminal neuralgia, is the injection of glycerol into the trigeminal ganglion. This procedure can be done with a smaller needle than the one used for thermocoagulation, and it generally is well tolerated. The ganglion actually is a cistern in which trigeminal-nerve fibers are bathed in cerebrospinal fluid. Accurate puncture of the cistern by way of the foramen ovale yields cerebrospinal fluid and permits the introduction of radiographic contrast material or glycerol. Tiny amounts of sterile 99.6% glycerol (commonly called anhydrous glycerol) introduced in that way cure trigeminal neuralgia in the majority of cases and produce minimal sensory loss. Although early reports described more than 90% success with a single injection, many patients need a second injection after several months, even when positive contrast radiographs confirm accurate positioning of the needle.

Few patients with tic douloureux fail to respond to a second glycerol procedure. A classic case of trigeminal neuralgia conforms to five criteria: (a) pain occurs suddenly in repeated, transient attacks, (b) it is limited to the territory of the trigeminal nerve, (c) it does not cross the midline, (d) it is triggered by innocuous mechanical stimuli such as chewing, and (e) there is minimal or no sensory loss. Patients with atypical facial pain also sometimes respond to glycerol, especially if the symptoms do not differ greatly from the classic model. Patients with trigeminal neuralgia associated with multiple sclerosis respond poorly to anhydrous glycerol gangliolysis.

The risks of glycerol injection are lower than those of other surgical procedures for tic douloureux. Occasionally, a slight zone of diminished pinprick sensation can persist on the cheek or nose, but loss of the corneal reflex is unusual and most often temporary. Experimental studies have revealed some nerve-fiber damage from glycerol, but its mechanism of action is still not entirely known.

Case Report

A 55-year-old woman had a 10-month history of stabbing, episodic pain in her left cheek and jaw that was triggered by cold wind blowing on her face, by holding a telephone, or by eating. Trials of carbamazepine and phenytoin failed to control her pain despite doses that made her gait ataxic. A computed tomography (CT) of the head with contrast showed a large vessel on the left side of the posterior fossa; subsequently, angiography showed that it was a dilated, tortuous vertebral artery. The patient was hospitalized when her pain worsened acutely, and large doses of opiates failed to relieve it. Because of her age and cardiac history, she was judged to be a poor risk for microsurgical-vascular decompression of the fifth nerve. An injection of 0.35 mL of glycerol into the trigeminal cistern gave her complete relief with normal facial sensation for almost 14 months. When the pain recurred, she was referred for Gamma knife, and 10 days following the Gamma knife ablation, reported over 80% pain relief.

Glossopharyngeal neuralgia, a similar condition with paroxysmal attacks of pain in the throat and ear, also can be treated surgically with a high rate of success. The glycerol injection technique has not been reported thus far, presumably because it is difficult to inject the ninth nerve selectively at the base of the skull. The ninth nerve is in the pars nervosa of the jugular foramen, which also is shared by the vagus nerve, the spinal-accessory nerve and is close to the pars venosum, which contains the venus-jugular bulb. Some authors have reported that radiofrequency lesions of the ninth nerve can provide relief. That procedure is technically more difficult than coagulation of the trigeminal ganglion, although the approach is similar. The ninth nerve and upper filaments of the tenth nerve can be sectioned directly in the posterior fossa by craniectomy, but there is a moderate risk of cardiovascular instability during and immediately after the operation. As with trigeminal neuralgia, some cases are associated with compression of the ninth nerve by an artery in the posterior fossa. If such a vessel can be identified, its separation from the nerve by microdissection should be considered the procedure of choice when medication fails.

OCCIPITAL NEURALGIA

There are many possible causes of neuralgic pain in the upper neck and occipital region. The most common etiologies are cervical spondylosis, arthritis of the upper-cervical facet joints, and thickening of the ligaments in that region after trauma. For the sake of simplicity, we will lump them together under the heading of occipital neuralgia. The diagnosis of occipital neuralgia should be accompanied with a workup for C1/C2 instability. Any patient with a history of rheumatoid arthritis, trauma, or an abnormal neurologic examination needs further evaluation.

Occipital neuralgia, unless it is the result of spine metastases, responds well to nerve-root surgery. Diagnostic efforts should include plain films of the upper-cervical spine and an openmouthed view of the Cl-joints, followed by CT of the same region if the etiology remains unclear. Many patients gain relief at least temporarily after injection of local anesthetic and methylprednisolone acetate around the greater occipital nerve behind the occipital bone. When the patient wants a more permanent treatment, the surgeon may elect to explore the spinal roots that contribute to the occipital nerve and either section them directly or decompress them by removing bone spurs or thick ligamentous tissue.

Case Report

An 88-year-old woman suffered from intractable pain in the upper left side of the neck that radiated through the scalp behind and above her left ear. The pain became worse with any neck movement. Plain films of the cervical spine showed pronounced arthritic changes in the left Cl–C2 joint. She had no relief from cervical traction and a collar, physical therapy, a series of acupuncture treatments, transcutaneous nerve stimulation, various antiinflammatory drugs, or opiate and nonopiate analgesics. She was unable to sleep because of the pain and remarked that she would prefer not to live. Injection of local anesthetic and steroids around her left greater-occipital nerve provided relief only until the anesthetic wore off. Dorsal rhizotomy of C1–0 abolished her pain, and this result was unchanged 1 year later. She was not bothered by the resulting numbness in the scalp.

Intradural dorsal rhizotomy (sectioning of the dorsal rootlets) at the C1–0 levels carries a 70% long-term success rate and very low risk. The preference of some sur-

geons to divide the greater occipital nerve is somewhat illogical, as the cause of the neuralgia is more proximal. Not surprisingly, a section of the peripheral nerve gives highly variable results.

INTERCOSTAL NEURALGIA AND OTHER TRUNCAL PAIN

Painful neuralgias of the chest and abdominal wall usually respond well to root surgery, especially when the radicular level of the lesion is well defined (Fig. 59.2). That is true for idiopathic, intercostal neuralgia, painful surgical scars, and circumscribed posttraumatic pain. Published series show that either dorsal rhizotomy or ganglionectomy offers an 80% chance of relief initially and about a 65% chance of some pain relief 1 year after the surgery. The truncal dermatomes overlap extensively, and several roots or ganglia should be sectioned. The procedure will leave the patient with a band of numbness, which may be unpleasant, but preliminary nerve blocks with local anesthetic will give the patient advance warning of the degree of numbness.

Dorsal-root ganglionectomy (excision of the dorsal-root ganglion) involves the spinal-nerve root as it passes through the intervertebral foramen. At thoracic levels, the dorsal-root ganglia can be excised by a simple extradural approach without laminectomies. The approach is not completely benign, however, because for a costotransversectomy, there is a significant risk of pneumothorax. Ganglionectomy has the theoretical advantage of eliminating possible afferent fibers in the ventral roots and connections to the sympathetic system. Dorsal rhizotomy has not been particularly successful for the treatment of postherpetic neuralgia, perhaps because the virus hibernates in the dorsal-root ganglia or even in the dorsal horn. Ganglionectomy or dorsal-root, entry-zone lesions (discussed later) may be more effective for this problem.

Intractable pain in the coccygeal region, sometimes called coccygodynia, has a surprisingly good rate of response to dorsal rhizotomy of the lower sacral and coccygeal segments for properly selected patients. About 50% of patients who have coccygodynia have no apparent etiology. It is important to take dynamic films of the coccyx to look for excessive mobility before considering invasive procedures, like coccygectomy or dorsal rhizotomy. Dorsal rhizotomy usually is performed after trials of conservative measures and intraarticular injections of local anesthetics and steroids have failed to provide long-term relief; it has a 65% long-term success rate. Coccygectomy has a prolonged recovery course with the risk of many postoperative complications. It is done rarely and in carefully selected individuals. Radiofrequency coagulation of the medial branches of lumbosacral posterior primary rami, the so-called facet nerves, also may be useful for this condition.

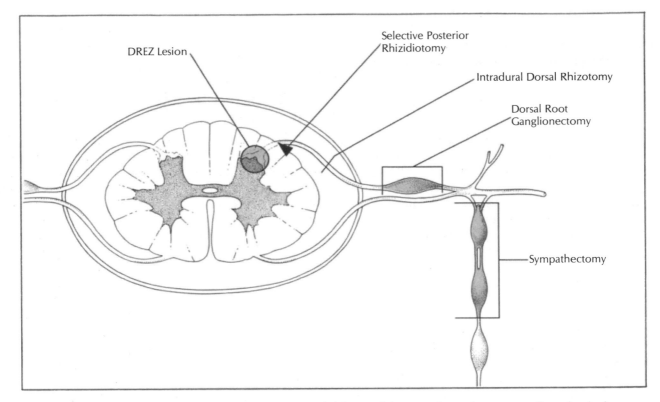

FIG. 59.2. Neurosurgical procedures to treat painful neuralgias are shown in cross-section of spinal cord. Dorsal-root entry zone lesioning relieves pain of root avulsion. In selective posterior rhizotomy (partial section of dorsal rootlets), only lateral portion of each rootlet is sectioned, sparing most of the large, myelinated, afferent fibers of individual dorsal rootlets. Intradural dorsal rhizotomy (sectioning of dorsal rootlets) at Cl–C3 levels has 70% long-term success rate with little risk for treatment of intractable neck pain. Dorsal-root ganglionectomy involves spinal-nerve root as it passes through the intervertebral foramen. Most cases of complex regional-pain syndrome respond to surgical sympathectomy.

COMPLEX REGIONAL-PAIN SYNDROME AND OTHER LIMB PAIN

Complex regional-pain syndrome (CRPS), types I and II, are painful and severely disabling disorders that often, but not always, follow injury. CRPS, type II, may follow nerve injury. The pain is spontaneous but aggravated by both cutaneous and emotional stimuli. It usually has a burning quality and is accompanied by signs of sympathetic nervous-system derangement in the extremity. As the disorder progresses, there will be trophic changes and occasionally permanent disfiguring. Three-phase bone scan is a useful diagnostic tool.

Case Reports

Patient 1

A 33-year-old man was donating blood when the needle puncture damaged his right median nerve in the antecubital fossa, causing partial loss of strength and sensation in the appropriate pattern. Shortly afterward, he developed a sore, burning sensation in the forearm and hand, which worsened when he was angry or upset. He protected the hand with a splint and would not allow anyone to touch it. Opiates were largely ineffective. He was able to sleep only if he drank enough alcohol to pass out. Stellate ganglion blocks failed to provide long-term relief; however, trials of regional perfusion of the right arm with intravenous reserpine gave excellent relief of pain for intervals of 2 or 3 weeks. After five such trials, he elected to have a thoracoscopically guided sympathectomy, after which he was free of pain and returned to his job soldering electronic circuits.

Most cases of CRPS respond to surgical sympathectomy. Severe burning pain and cutaneous hyperesthesia following partial injury of the median or ulnar nerve can be diagnosed and often treated by stellate ganglion block or by regional perfusion of the arm with guanethidine or reserpine. In some cases, repeated blocks or perfusions lead to a permanent cure. In others, the patient will need a surgical sympathectomy to achieve the same result.

The sympathetic outflow to the arm travels from the thoracic spinal cord through the sympathetic chain and ascends to the cervical level. Synapses occur in the sympathetic ganglia of that chain. Postsynaptic fibers travel to the arm in the roots of the brachial plexus. The sequence can be permanently interrupted by excising a portion of the sympathetic chain, usually the second and third thoracic ganglia plus the caudal half of the stellate ganglion, at the level of the second rib. Admittedly, this is not simply an interruption of primary-afferent fibers, although sympathectomy does interrupt some afferents that travel toward the spinal cord from the periphery. The effectiveness of the procedure is thought to be from interruption of efferent nerve impulses traveling toward the site of nerve damage, where the disrupted nerve is itself hypersensitive to the release of catecholamines. The relief achieved with catecholamine depleters such as reserpine and guanethidine support this theory. It appears that there may be localized changes as well, and thus sympathectomy alone may not provide adequate relief.

When there is no response to sympathectomy or when severe, chronic pain in a limb is not the result of CRPS, surgery at the dorsal-root level may be helpful. Standard dorsal rhizotomy interrupts the large, proprioceptive primary-afferent fibers as well as the small, unmyelinated primary afferents that are involved in cutaneous hyperalgesia. If complete rhizotomies were carried out at all segmental levels corresponding to a limb, proprioception would be lost, making the limb useless.

A microsurgical procedure described by Sindou in 1976 made it possible to spare most of the large, myelinated, afferent fibers of the individual dorsal rootlets. In selective posterior rhizotomy, or partial section of dorsal rootlets, only the lateral portion of each rootlet is sectioned. Because of the tendency of small afferents (C fibers) to aggregate laterally as they enter the cord, the proprioceptors can be spared. Usually, touch perception also is preserved, and in some patients there is a surprising capacity to appreciate sharpness. Selective posterior rhizotomy originally was used for pain from Pancoast's tumors (lung-apex tumors), but it can be extremely effective for other painful conditions of the limbs, particularly when there is cutaneous hyperesthesia.

Patient 2

A 31-year-old woman presented with excruciatingly painful, bright red, swollen hands and feet. The condition had waxed and waned since her teens. Two exhaustive medical investigations had failed to demonstrate the cause, and a diagnosis of erythromelalgia was given. Repeated stellate ganglion blocks and regional perfusions of the arms gave inconsistent relief for periods of less than 24 hours. Bilateral cervicothoracic sympathectomies relieved the pain in her hands and brought improvement of swelling and erythema, but all symptoms returned 2 months later. She was heavily addicted to opiates and was suicidal. Trials of steroids, nonsteroidal antiinflammatory drugs, calcium-channel blockers, α- and β-sympathetic blockers, anticonvulsants, fluphenazine, and antidepressants all were without effect. With some reluctance of the part of the surgeon, selective posterior rhizotomy was carried out at the brachial-plexus level, in two stages, right and left. The patient was pleased with the result, and her mild, proprioceptive loss in the arms responded to a course of physical and occupational therapy. Six months later, with no return of pain in her hands, she insisted that the same procedure be done at the lumbosacral level and subsequently had good relief of pain in her feet with no significant loss of ankle proprioception.

Traumatic avulsion injury of the brachial plexus roots may leave the patient with a paralyzed, anesthetic, but painful limb. The pain is relentless. Descriptions such as "searing" or "scalding" are typical of this deafferentation syndrome. Dorsal-root, entry-zone (DREZ) lesioning has been reported to have excellent results in treating the pain of root avulsion. The lesions are made by inserting a small electrode into the dorsal horn of the spinal cord at all the former entry points of avulsed rootlets and applying radiofrequency current briefly. The DREZ lesions undoubtedly include more than the terminations of primary-afferent fibers.

Surgical procedures at the primary-afferent level include rhizotomy, ganglionectomy, selective-posterior rhizotomy, microsurgical decompression of nerve roots in the posterior fossa or cervical spine, gangliolysis by injection of glycerol or by radiofrequency thermocoagulation, sympathectomy, and lesioning of the spinal-cord DREZ. Those operations can be highly effective for a wide variety of benign pain states and carry a relatively small risk. The procedure chosen should be tailored to fit the location and, if possible, the etiology of the pain.

NEUROSTIMULATION

The neurostimulation system incorporates devices for the relief of chronic, intractable pain in the trunk and/or limbs. Patients with radiating pain, continued pain following back surgery, and CRPS may benefit. Patients with ischemic pain from inoperable peripheral-vascular disease may get very good relief. Patients with peripheral neuropathy, such as diabetic neuropathy do not generally benefit.

A neurostimulation system applies precisely controlled low-voltage electrical stimulation to the spinal cord through one or more carefully placed, insulated "leads." Electrical signals sent by spinal-cord stimulation appear to "confuse" the brain as to what modality is being experienced. Instead of pain, the patient feels a "tingling" sensation. A neurostimulation system consists of one or more leads, an implantable pulse generator, which is a power source, and a programmer (Fig. 59.3). There is a system that consists of one or more leads that connect to an implanted receiver and an external transmitter, which is powered by a 9-V battery. The fully implantable system is used more frequently, as it provides great convenience to the patient.

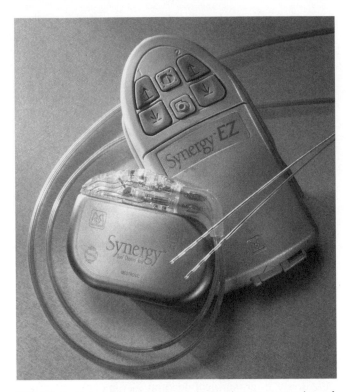

FIG. 59.3. Spinal-cord stimulation is used to treat a variety of pain complaints. Thin electrode leads are threaded into the epidural space, and are positioned to provide the patient with the most comfort. A thin pulse generator, or power source, is implanted in the subcutaneous tissue and is connected to the electrode leads. The system is completely hidden from view. The patient has a remote-control unit to turn the device on or off and to increase or decrease the amplitude of the stimulation.

Once a patient is a candidate for a neurostimulation system, he or she must undergo a trial to determine if neurostimulation reveals the pain and does not cause unpleasant sensations. It is recommended that the patient be fully evaluated by a psychologist trained to work with chronic-pain patients. This is a good time to ascertain whether the patient has unrealistic expectations of the device and also to talk with a health professional about the implications of surgery and having a device implanted. The components of the implantable system are selected based upon the patient's history, physical exam, and expected pain-control needs.

The system includes an implanted receiver and an external transmitter worn on the patient's belt. The transmitter sends radiofrequency signals to two sets of four electrodes arranged at the ends of two insulated wires called leads. The leads are implanted in the spinal column near the spinal nerves that correspond to the patient's areas of pain. Variables such as the amplitude, pulse width, and rate of the electric pulse can be altered noninvasively using the external transmitter. The clinician can make significant adjustments in the electric pulse and can establish limits within which the patient can adjust the

stimulation. The system is powered with a 9-V alkaline battery in the transmitter.

Each lead is implanted near the spinal cord at a spot that corresponds to the patient's pain. The four electrodes at the tip of each of each lead carry the electrical impulses to stimulate the spinal nerves, creating a tingling feeling rather than the sensation of pain. The leads often are placed percutaneously, with the patient awake for the procedure. This ensures good coverage of the patient's pain. It is occasionally necessary to implant the leads by way of laminotomy. In this case, the trial will have determined proper placement of the leads, and the surgeon then places the leads under direct vision and also with fluoroscopic guidance.

The titanium-encased implantable pulse generator (IPG) supplies the energy for stimulation. It contains a special battery and electronic circuitry. The IPG is approximately 60 mm (2.5 inches) at the longest point and 52 mm (2.25 inches) at its widest point. It is about 10 mm (0.4 inches) thick. It is placed subcutaneously by way of a small incision.

The stimulation parameters can be set and adjusted easily and noninvasively by the clinician's console programmer, which uses telemetry to communicate with the microprocessing chip in the implantable generator. A clinician enters the amplitude, rate, and other variables with the transmitter. The patient can adjust these settings, within limits established by the clinician, using control buttons on this transmitter. Many patients use different settings for sleeping and exercising. The compact "EZ programmer" allows the patient to adjust some settings within the limits set by the physician and to turn the system on and off.

Case Reports

Patient 1

A 37-year-old marathon runner developed a Morton's neuroma. The neuroma was carefully excised, however she developed burning, dysesthetic pain along the bottom and lateral side of her foot. She tried a number of medications and nerve blocks with limited success. She was reluctant to stay on medication, as she and her new husband wished to start a family. A spinal-cord stimulator lead was placed percutaneously under fluoroscopic guidance in the epidural space. The patient was awake and able to participate with the guiding of the device to the correct location. She was sent home with the lead connected to an external-control device and with strict instructions not to get the entry site or the device wet. She returned 4 days later exclaiming "I went for a 4-mile run yesterday!" The temporary lead was removed and she was scheduled for permanent lead placement.

In addition to reducing chronic, intractable pain, the spinal-cord stimulation system may improve a patient's ability to function and provide a better quality of life. The probable effectiveness of the therapy can be determined during a screening trial before implanting the system, thus saving unnecessary costs. Stimulation parameters can be changed to address changing pain-relief needs. The therapy is nonaddictive. Stimulation can be adjusted noninvasively by both the clinician and the patient. The therapy is reversible; and should the patient so desire, the system can be removed.

Patient 2

A 62-year-old man had had four operations on his back over the past 20 years. He complained of constant, annoying, burning pain in his back the posterior aspect of his right leg and into his groin. Percutaneous trial of spinal-cord stimulator lead provided good relief of his groin pain, but inadequate coverage of his back pain. A second attempt of a percutaneous trial revealed technical difficulties in threading the lead to the appropriate area. The risks of laminotomy placement of a dual lead were discussed with him. He was anxious to proceed. Under general anesthesia, the T8 vertebral body was exposed and small laminotomy was performed, a compact double lead was placed carefully under direct vision. The lead was tunneled and connected to a small pulse-generator device implanted in the subcutaneous tissue of the left buttocks. He was discharged from the hospital 4 days later declaring "I feel really good." His postoperative recovery was unremarkable. He returned to the pain management center 6 weeks later complaining of pain in his back. The device was reprogrammed to provide better coverage of this back pain. He returned 3 weeks later complaining that now his groin had inadequate coverage. Attempts to reprogram the device were marginally successful. Only partial pain relief was obtain and by using such high-energy requirements, the battery is expected to be depleted in less than 1 year.

NEUROSURGERY FOR THE PAIN OF MALIGNANCY

When the patient's life expectancy is limited, procedures can be performed to relieve pain, without concern about the long-term sequelae, such as the creation of neuropathic pain. Before any palliative intervention is undertaken, however, the patient must make his or her own decision as to the definition of "quality of life." For some patients, the risk of complete loss of bowel and bladder function will be untenable. For some patients who are already paralyzed, the loss of upper-arm sensation, for instance, is minor when balanced by the potential for pain relief and a clear sensorium.

While these surgical procedures can be used to treat other types of pain, they are not frequently used to treat nonmalignant pain. Each case requires analysis and planning. Attention to the location of the physiologic disturbance that produces pain permits the surgeon to "tailor" the operation to the individual patient. This can increase the likelihood of relief and diminish the risk of disability or prolonged incapacity.

In recent years, with the advent of long-acting opiate preparations that provide adequate pain relief, patients with intractable cancer pain seem to be referred at later stages of their disease, when they are less able to tolerate surgery. In most cases, that trend seems to reflect a preference for noninvasive management of pain. Sometimes, surgery is considered far too late, almost as an afterthought, when the patient already is severely debilitated by disease and by the effects of poorly controlled chronic pain. The patient may be unable to sleep at night, be oversedated and nauseated during the day, and have poor nutritional status. That situation is very unfortunate when it continues for months, whereas an operation might have aborted the pain or reduced it to a tolerable level.

Admittedly, the arguments for a noninvasive approach are compelling. Surgery does have inherent risks, including wound infection, bleeding, inadvertent nerve injuries, and untoward reactions to anesthetic drugs. The patient with advanced malignancy is at increased risk because of altered immune response, poor nutrition, anemia, leukopenia, or thrombocytopenia. If his pain improves, will he still be able to walk? Will he be incontinent? Will he spend the last few months of his life in the hospital because of a postoperative complication?

There are risks associated with postponing or avoiding surgery. The disease might progress with further pain, waning strength, and additional metastases, canceling the option of any surgical procedure under general anesthesia. The patient might acquire pneumonia, refractory anemia, or a bleeding disorder, without any hope of surgical relief. The patient who still is in severe pain even though he is so heavily sedated that he can no longer make his wishes clear or even stay awake to speak with his family would have been better served by discussion of neurosurgical options earlier in his disease progress. The placement of an intrathecal opiate pump in an ambulatory patient may help him continue to care for himself and preserve his muscle strength for a longer period. Surgery is recommended as an option for a small minority of cancer patients. It is important, however, that clinicians caring for cancer patients be aware of the surgical options.

By reviewing the neurosurgical procedures used to treat cancer pain, a realistic assessment of the risks and the chances of success can be presented to the patient. The invasiveness of each procedure, the degree of stress for the patient, the type of anesthesia required, and the amount of time required for recuperation must be discussed frankly with the patient. As with any surgery, facts should be used to educate the patient and his family, enabling them to make the final decision by well-informed consent.

TABLE 59.1. *Neurosurgical Procedures to Treat Pain of Malignancy*

Procedure	Type of anesthesia required
Spinal-cord lesions	
Open thoracic cordotomy	General endotracheal anesthesia
Percutaneous high-cervical cordotomy	Local plus monitored sedation
Nerve-root surgery	
Intradural rhizotomy	General endotracheal anesthesia
Percutaneous radiofrequency sedation	Local anesthesia plus monitored
Thermocoagulation of cranial or spinal nerves	
Selective posterior rhizidiotomy	General endotracheal anesthesia
Extradural sacral rhizotomy	General endotracheal anesthesia
Sympathectomy and splanchnicectomy	General endotracheal anesthesia
Implanted opiate delivery systems	
Intraspinal epidural or intrathecal catheter and subcutaneous injection port or continuous infusion pump	Regional anesthesia
Intraventricular catheter and subcutaneous injection port or continuous infusion pump	General endotracheal anesthesia
Stereotaxic cranial procedures	
Periventricular gray stimulation	Stage 1, local anesthesia
	Stage 2, general anesthesia
Anterior pituitary ablation	General endotracheal anesthesia

The immediate advantages of well-timed surgery for pain in cancer patients include (a) better pain control in most cases; (b) elimination of medications or reduction of dose to a tolerable level with few side-effects; (c) clearer mental state and improved appetite on reduced medication, which may improve the quality of life; (d) shortened hospital stay; and (e) return to an active, mobile condition for some patients who are bedridden.

A list of operations used by neurosurgeons to treat pain from malignant disease is presented in Table 59.1. Of these, the most common are cordotomy and implantation of epidural or intrathecal drug-delivery systems. Procedures available in a given hospital may well depend on the staff neurosurgeons' training and familiarity with various operations, on the availability of specialized equipment, and on the presence of ancillary services (such as an outpatient pain clinic with staff trained in epidural or intrathecal drug administration). Because the goal of treating pain with an invasive modality is to have the patient comfortable and stable for discharge, whether or not the patient will require additional auxiliary health services should be relayed to the discharge planner.

SPINAL CORD LESIONS

The most common and best-known cord lesion is anterolateral cordotomy. This operation is done to interrupt the spinothalamic tract, which originates in the gray matter of the spinal cord on the side of pain and crosses the midline to ascend in the white matter of the anterior half of the contralateral spinal cord. Its exact borders and homogeneous or heterogeneous nature are controversial, but it generally is agreed that spinothalamic fibers lie in a broad zone anterior to the dentate ligament that joins the pia of the lateral cord surface to the dura on the sides of the spinal canal. This ligament serves as a boundary marker for the lesion (Fig. 59.4).

If the lesion is entirely anterior to the dentate ligament, the surgeon can almost always avoid damage to descending motor tracts. Cordotomy can be performed as an open procedure, usually with a single laminectomy at the second thoracic level, or as a closed percutaneous procedure with a needle and thermocoagulation probe at the first cervical level. Both techniques are applicable in cases of cancer pain involving segmental levels of the body below the umbilicus. Percutaneous high cervical cordotomy may produce a level of analgesia as high as the neck in some cases, but this effect is not consistent enough to be reliable in treating pain at the cervical level.

In open cordotomy, the patient is placed prone; under general anesthesia, a short midline incision is made at the upper-thoracic level to expose the T2 vertebra, and a laminectomy is done at that level. The dura is opened and the dentate ligaments identified under an operating microscope. On the side opposite the patient's pain, the dentate ligament is divided and the cord gently rotated by grasping the dentate ligament to expose the anterolateral white matter. This is sectioned just anterior to the dentate ligament with a microsurgical blade. Bleeding usually is minimal, once the vessels on the surface of the pia are controlled. The dura and arachnoid are snugly sutured to avoid cerebrospinal fluid leak, and the incision is closed. Muscular aching around the incision is a common complaint for a few days.

In percutaneous cordotomy, the sedated patient is supine. Under fluoroscopy and local anesthesia, a large-bore needle is inserted by a straight, lateral approach in the upper neck to penetrate the spinal canal between C1 and C2. Radiographic contrast dye is injected to outline the dentate ligament. A thermocoagulation probe is

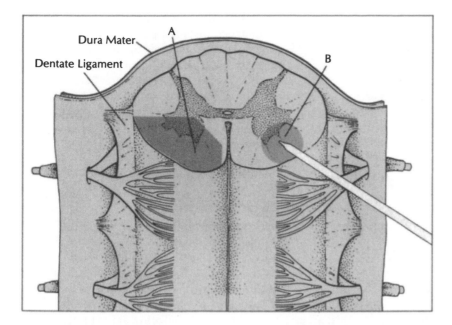

Dura Mater

Dentate Ligament

A

B

FIG. 59.4. Open and percutaneous approaches to anterolateral cordotomy are compared. The lesion created by the microsurgical blade in open cordotomy (A) is larger than that surrounding the tip of the thermocoagulation probe in percutaneous, high-cervical cordotomy (B). In both procedures, the dentate ligament serves as the posterior boundary for lesion.

inserted through the needle to contact and slightly penetrate the anterior white matter. Electrical stimulation evokes paresthesias if the patient is alert enough to report them.

The patient then is more heavily sedated with a short-acting agent while a heat lesion is created with a timed, temperature-controlled radiofrequency current generator. The patient is allowed to awaken to report relief or the lack thereof. If necessary, the process is repeated to enlarge the lesion. A major drawback of this procedure is the difficulty of repeatedly sedating and awakening the patient and trying to get an adequate verbal report from him (especially if he is irritable and unable to cooperate because of pain).

Satisfactory relief of pain is obtained in 75% to 80% of patients with either type of cordotomy. Advantages of percutaneous cordotomy are (a) avoidance of general anesthetic (although heavy sedation is necessary, with the possibility of respiratory arrest and consequent urgent intubation) and (b) avoidance of the complications associated with posterior spinal incisions (muscular spasm and pain, wound infection, cerebrospinal fluid leak). Disadvantages are (a) the need for expensive, specialized equipment to generate controlled thermal lesions, (b) some degree of difficulty in directing and restricting the cord lesion, and (c) additional stress for the awake patient, who must cooperate for an extended period of trial-cord stimulation.

In experienced hands, the percutaneous procedure can be done safely and expeditiously, with results equal to those of open cordotomy. Advantages of the open operation are better control of the size and location of the lesion and perhaps a reduced risk of bleeding and cord swelling, which cannot be prevented or controlled percutaneously.

Bilateral pain sometimes can be treated by bilateral cordotomy, but the risks are much higher. Bilateral, high-cervical percutaneous cordotomy is contraindicated because it has been associated with respiratory arrest during sleep in the postoperative period. Open bilateral cordotomy at upper-thoracic levels does not carry this risk, as the respiratory neurons of the cord are at higher levels.

Both open and percutaneous cordotomy carry a 3% to 15% incidence of ipsilateral leg weakness (on the side opposite the pain) and a 2% to 10% incidence of urinary-bladder dysfunction. That morbidity is more than doubled for bilateral lesions. In addition, bilateral cordotomy carries a risk of fecal incontinence. For patients who already are incontinent or paretic because of their disease, those factors may be of less importance.

Some surgeons feel that open cordotomy permits a larger cord lesion that includes more of the ascending sensory-tract fibers and therefore gives a more satisfactory and permanent result. The use of modern microsurgical techniques with improved microinstruments and optics has undoubtedly made the open version safer and more attractive. Whether morbidity will be reduced by those methods remains to be determined.

Cordotomy does not eliminate cutaneous sensation; it merely blunts perception of pinprick sharpness and heat on one side of the body. Cordotomy has acquired a reputation of failing long after surgery in some cases. Pain returns in a significant percentage of patients after 2 years, according to Lipton. However, many patients who undergo the surgery succumb to their disease in the following year, making the late failure of cordotomy of more theoretical than practical concern in such cases. In patients expected to live more than 1 year, it is a serious concern.

In addition to the spinothalamic tract, there are several different ascending sensory pathways in the spinal cord.

These pathways, which are not sectioned in anterolateral cordotomy, may become increasingly important with time because of the plasticity of neuronal function. Another theory to explain the late failure of cordotomy is that neurons of the thalamus, having lost their ascending connections from the spinal cord, are poorly regulated and may discharge excessively, creating pain or dysesthesias of a central type (deafferentation syndrome). Dysesthesias, consisting mainly of pins-and-needles sensations, are reported by 5% to 20% of patients who undergo cordotomy. Whether those abnormal sensations are the result of thalamic-neuronal hyperactivity is not yet clear.

Case Report

A 48-year-old man had constant, excruciating pain in the right groin, buttock, and leg when metastatic lung carcinoma invaded the pelvis. He denied pain in the left leg or elsewhere. On a McGill Pain Questionnaire he described the pain as crushing, exhausting, unbearable, radiating, and torturing. It was not helped by a course of radiation therapy to the right hemipelvis. The patient was given increasing doses of oxycodone, morphine, and methadone to the point of anorexia, fatigue, and slurred speech. Offered a choice of cordotomy or insertion of an intrathecal opiate delivery system, he chose cordotomy.

A left anterolateral cordotomy was performed under general anesthesia as an open procedure at the second thoracic level. After surgery, there was clumsiness of the left leg for about 3 days; it improved rapidly with physical therapy. The patient reported complete relief of his pain and was fully ambulatory without assistance at the time of discharge 1 week after the operation. Opiates were decreased to a minimal level. Neurologic examination showed mild, persistent right-leg weakness, attributed to the pelvic metastasis, and diminished pinprick sharpness on the left side below the waist, attributed to the cordotomy. The patient continued to have excellent pain relief until his death from pneumonia almost 6 months later.

NERVE-ROOT LESIONS

Cordotomy may not be appropriate for cancer pain involving the head, neck, arm, or chest wall. The truncal level of analgesia produced by cordotomy might not be high enough to include those territories, and the loss of pain perception in the leg could be an unnecessary consequence. Operations on the spinal-dorsal roots are designed to treat pain in restricted areas. For example, if several spinal nerves or intercostal nerves are involved by direct tumor invasion, bony metastases, or paraneoplastic neuropathy, sectioning the dorsal roots of the cord at those segmental levels would be expected to relieve the pain. In practice, roots also are sectioned at least one level above and one level below the segmental level of pain.

Intradural dorsal rhizotomy is done under general anesthesia. Laminectomies are performed at appropriate levels, and the dura and arachnoid are opened. Under the operating microscope, the individual rootlets branching from each dorsal root near the cord are freed of blood vessels and divided. Only the rootlets dorsal to the dentate ligament are sectioned. The dura and arachnoid are tightly sutured, and the incision is closed. As with open cordotomy, there is an interval of muscular soreness and spasm near the incision for several days.

In contrast to cordotomy, dorsal rhizotomy leaves a zone of numbness with anesthesia to touch, pinprick, and heat stimuli in the corresponding dermatomes. Just above and below these anesthetic dermatomes, the skin may be mildly hypersensitive, which patients find annoying. Preliminary spinal or intercostal nerve blocks with local anesthetics may give the patient some idea of what to expect. If rhizotomy is successful, the patient is likely to have permanent relief of his pain in that particular location. Unfortunately, tumor spread beyond the confines of the area treated by rhizotomy may lead to new pain and dampen enthusiasm for the operation.

The early success rate of dorsal rhizotomy for cancer pain generally is around 55% to 60%. There are some situations, described below, in which variants of the standard procedure are highly effective. Later recurrence of pain probably is most often because of spread of metastases than to failure of the rhizotomy. Recurrence of pain is unlikely after 1 year. If performed with careful attention to radicular blood vessels, rhizotomy carries no significant risk of leg weakness or incontinence.

Cancer patients with intractable facial pain often can be helped by percutaneous thermocoagulation lesions of the trigeminal ganglion, which is reached by inserting a needle through the cheek and into the foramen ovale in the skull base. The procedure is identical to the one used to treat trigeminal neuralgia. It is performed with a combination of local anesthetic and short-acting intravenous sedatives during needle positioning. Patient cooperation is needed for accurate localization and judgment regarding the extent of the lesion. The major risks are corneal anesthesia and facial dysesthesias.

For more widespread, intractable pain of advanced head and neck cancer, rhizotomy of cranial nerves V, IX, and X can be considered, along with section of upper-cervical roots to cervical and shoulder dermatomes. Percutaneous thermocoagulation of the same roots sometimes is preferable, particularly for pain restricted to the trigeminal territory. The use of thermocoagulation in debilitated, poorly cooperative patients requires heavy sedation and often a lengthy interval of needle insertion and repositioning for each root treated. Experience shows that in many cases, an open procedure under general anesthesia may be better tolerated even though it appears to the patient to be a "bigger operation."

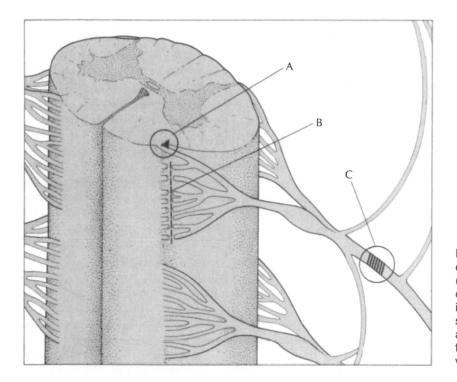

FIG. 59.5. Three types of nerve-root surgery can relieve regional pain: intradural posterior (dorsal) rhizotomy (*A*) with complete division of sensory rootlets, selective posterior rhizidiotomy (*B*) with partial division of each sensory rootlet on the lateral side, and thermocoagulation lesion (*C*) created by percutaneous treatment of spinal nerves in or near the intervertebral foramina.

Severe pain from lung apex, Pancoast's tumors, and malignant invasion of the brachial plexus can be extremely difficult to manage by nonsurgical methods. Standard dorsal rhizotomy at limb level has an important disadvantage, namely the loss of proprioception and joint position sense in the limb. If the patient already has lost all use of the arm and all sensation, this is of no concern. However, when some neurologic function remains, and especially when it is intact or nearly so, standard dorsal rhizotomy or percutaneous thermocoagulation of multiple roots would be inappropriate.

In this situation, an operation called selective posterior rhizotomy, devised by Sindou and colleagues, offers excellent chances of retaining movement and sensation in the arm without directly altering muscle strength. The operation is performed in a manner similar to open intradural-dorsal rhizotomy, except that each rootlet is lifted, dissected free of small vessels at the root-entry zone of the cord, and partially sectioned, leaving some of the large, myelinated, proprioceptive afferent fibers intact as they enter the dorsal columns (Fig. 59.5). The rationale of the operation is that small-diameter sensory afferent fibers in the individual rootlets tend to aggregate on the extreme lateral side of the rootlet as they reach the cord. The operation is more tedious than ordinary rhizotomy and requires microsurgical expertise.

Case Report

A 38-year-old woman had intractable left-arm pain and swelling when breast carcinoma invaded the brachial plexus and axillary lymphatics. Despite radiation and chemotherapy, she gradually lost the use of her arm except for weak handgrip. Any movement of the arm and shoulder was painful. Pressure on the skin of the forearm and arm aggravated the burning sensation. She was unable to sleep through a single night for 5 weeks, even though taking 80 mg of morphine as oral elixir every 2 hours. She said that morphine was losing its effectiveness and causing anorexia and nausea.

Under general anesthesia, the cervical-spinal cord was exposed. Selective posterior rhizotomy was carried out on the left from the fourth cervical through second thoracic segments. Postoperatively, she was able to tolerate physical and occupational therapy, which relieved early contractures, and to wear a pressurized sleeve on the arm (which helped the edema). She retained some handgrip strength and gross-position sense in the arm and hand. Within 5 days, she was consistently sleeping through the night. She reported minimum neck discomfort and was fully ambulatory soon after surgery. Her preoperative dose of morphine was reduced gradually to half without untoward effects before discharge. At home, she continued to experience satisfactory pain relief.

In some cases of advanced sacral and pelvic malignancy, bowel and bladder function is lost early, and diversion procedures are instituted. In these circumstances, when local pain in the sacrococcygeal region becomes refractory to medical management, the option of dividing all nerve roots below S1 should be considered. With preexisting bowel and bladder incontinence, there is little to lose and much to be gained. The operation described by

Crue and Todd accomplishes that goal very quickly without opening the dura.

A small, midline incision is made over the upper sacrum, under general anesthesia. The dural tube is exposed just below the paired S1 nerve roots. The entire dural tube and enclosed roots (S2 through coccygeal) are ligated and divided. The incision is sutured. Even though the operation is simple and succinct, with little or no morbidity, it should not be performed if tumor involves the uppermost sacrum or the overlying skin. Those factors could lead to failure of wound healing. When pain also extends into the first sacral dermatome, there is the option of including the S1 root along with the rest, but this can cause partial loss of joint position sense in the ankle.

SYMPATHECTOMY AND SPLANCHNICECTOMY

Ordinarily, lower thoracic sympathectomy is not considered the treatment of choice for cancer pain. The procedure is used primarily in cases of CRPS, types I or II. The pain of carcinoma of the pancreas, however, may respond well to surgery on the sympathetic system. The patient with pancreatic cancer usually can be helped by the much simpler procedure of repeated celiac-plexus blocks with local anesthetics and alcohol or phenol for an adequate neurolytic block. Surgical sympathectomy should be considered only for the most refractory cases, which are not adequately relieved by celiac blocks and opiates.

Sadar and Hardy describe the use of combined bilateral thoracic sympathectomy at T9–T12 levels and division of the splanchnic nerves that supply sensory afferent fibers to the pancreas. This operation, under general anesthesia, affords about a 70% chance of pain relief initially. There is a substantial recurrence rate with survival for more than a few months, usually with diminished pain. There is a 7% mortality when the procedure is combined with laparotomy. Reported complications include pneumothorax and, rarely, paraplegia from disruption of a major radicular artery to the spinal cord.

Thorascopically guided sympathectomy also is an option. Although there is still a risk of pneumothorax, if successful, the procedure results in smaller wounds to heal. While some neurosurgeons are very adept at this procedure, others rely on the expertise of a colleague with special training in cardiothoracic surgery for assistance.

IMPLANTED OPIATE-DELIVERY SYSTEMS

In comparison with procedures that create lesions in the nervous system to relieve pain, implanted catheter systems to deliver opiates have the advantage of causing no direct neurologic deficit. There is the additional advantage of reversibility: if the system falls, it can be removed or ignored. Most practitioners, however, perform a trial with intrathecal medication prior to considering the implantation of a drug-delivery system. This allows the patient to experience the type of pain relief that may be expect and also to experience potentially unpleasant side effects, such as pruritus or urinary retention. Implanted opiate catheters, injection chambers, and infusion pumps often are effective in cases of extensive, bilateral pain, which cannot be managed easily by cordotomy or rhizotomy. Disadvantages include the risk of infection associated with foreign bodies and the continuing reliance on injection or other care of the system, usually with a commitment to repeated hospital outpatient visits or home visits by trained staff. With proper compounding of medications, however, a patient with a fully implanted opiate-delivery system may require refilling of the reservoir every 8 to 12 weeks.

Morphine delivered into the spinal-epidural space is thought to exert its effect on opiate receptors in the spinal cord. The mechanism by which epidural morphine crosses through the dura to reach those receptors is not yet understood, but it is clear that delivery of the opiate into the spinal-epidural space is almost as effective as direct delivery into the subarachnoid space at the same level. The amounts of drug needed to relieve pain by intraspinal administration are far smaller than those given by other parenteral routes. Side-effects such as nausea, sedation, and respiratory depression typically are less prominent with the spinal route than with other routes.

The usual arrangement is a subcutaneous injection port over the abdomen, connected by thin, subcutaneous tubing to the epidural catheter (Fig. 59.6). Two or three times a day, injections are made into the port with a small needle. The injection chamber and tubing have minimal internal volume, so that nearly all the drug is delivered into the spinal canal. Morphine, hydromorphone, and other opiates have been used successfully. The addition of clonidine may help prevent development of tolerance, and may treat neuropathic pain. Alternatively, the catheter may be directed intrathecally (Fig. 59.7). Intrathecal administration is especially attractive for patients who will have a reservoir and pump implanted subcutaneously. Because the dose needed intrathecally is less than that required for epidural dosing, the intrathecal approach ensures the patient a longer interval between refills.

Chronic epidural and intrathecal morphine administration may be helpful in nonmalignant pain syndromes, and it has found increasingly widespread use for cancer pain. Most patients obtain substantial relief. The dosage of morphine is titrated to the patient, and is increased gradually if needed over a period of weeks or months as tolerance develops or the patient's pain management needs change. Occasionally, patients who did not attain relief with low doses will get relief from much larger doses. Patients who have been on large, systemic doses of opi-

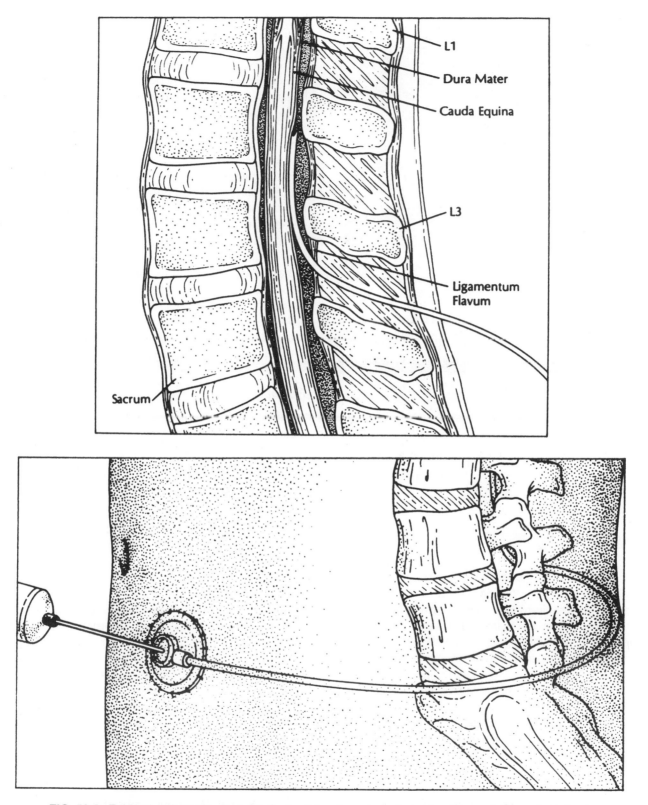

FIG. 59.6. Epidural catheter in place **(top)** after it has been tunneled subcutaneously through abdominal wall can deliver narcotics for long-term use. Drugs can be injected through the subcutaneous port **(bottom)** or infused continuously.

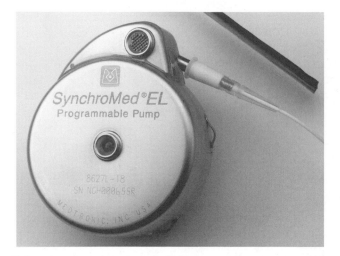

FIG. 59.7. Intrathecal drug-delivery systems can provide continuous infusions of medications to relieve patient's pain. The catheter is placed in the intrathecal space, and a connection is tunneled to the programmable pump, which is placed in the subcutaneous tissue. The pump is filled with the chosen medication by way of the central diaphragm. Refilling the pump involves a small needle stick to the patient. Telemetry then is used to program the drug-delivery system to ensure proper dosing. Several companies manufacture such devices for use.

ate also will require large, intraspinal doses, typically 0.5% to 1% of the systemic dose intrathecally, or 5% to 10% of the systemic dose in the epidural space.

Case Reports

Patient 1

A 45-year-old man had constant, excruciating pain in his left pelvis and buttock region when rectal carcinoma invaded the sacrum. He denied pain on the right. For 6 weeks he was unable to bear weight on his left leg. He remained bedridden throughout that time, increasingly sedated with a variety of potent opiate analgesics, including oxycodone, methadone, hydromorphone, and timed-release morphine. He also was taking an anticonvulsant and a tricyclic antidepressant. He was hospitalized with pronounced somnolence, anorexia, and vomiting when he was no longer able to sleep or sustain his body weight.

Under monitored anesthesia care with light sedation, the L2–L3 interspace was identified with fluoroscopy. A small, flexible catheter was threaded by way of a percutaneous, large-bore needle into the intrathecal space to the T11 border. The catheter was tunneled subcutaneously to the anterior lower-abdominal wall, where it was connected to an infusion port and the reservoir system placed into the superficial abdominal fat. The pump was electronically programmed to deliver a continuous infusion of intrathecal morphine. The patient was ambulatory and free of pain on the third postoperative day. He ate and slept well and went home on a greatly reduced medication schedule, still requiring the lose-dose tricyclic antidepressant (TCA) to control a burning component of his pain, but not taking any oral opiate medication. He remained ambulatory at home 12 months later, returning to the pain management center to have the reservoir of his pump refilled every 6 weeks.

Implantable, continuous-infusion devices are quite costly, but when patients obtain satisfactory relief of pain with intermittent injection of epidural or intrathecal opiates, it is our practice to offer conversion to a continuous-infusion pump system, with an intrathecal catheter. A doughnut-sized, continuous-infusion pump is secured in the subcutaneous fascia of the abdominal wall. Opiate dosage is regulated by filling the pump with solutions of differing strengths, and by programming the pump to deliver the dose necessary. Refilling is done about every 2 months by percutaneous injection. Although administration of intrathecal morphine by constant infusion with an implanted pump generally is free of complications, the technique does require considerable expenditure of time and additional care. As with implanted ports, infection and leakage are potential risks.

Patient 2

A 60-year-old woman had widespread pain due to bone metastases from breast cancer. She underwent percutaneous implantation of a temporary epidural morphine catheter under local anesthesia and achieved good relief with a combination of twice-daily injections and oral hydromorphone. The patient requested conversion to a continuous-infusion pump after several weeks. This was done under general anesthesia. Biweekly refills were given to her at home by her physicians because she was bedridden with intolerable pain when transported. Visiting nurses provided daily home care, but declined to refill the morphine reservoir.

In the ensuing weeks, there appeared to be good pain control initially, but the dose of morphine was increased steadily to maximum concentrations for the device, and the patient relied increasingly on supplemental oral hydromorphone and methadone. She refused to return to the hospital or even to be moved from her bed because of pain.

Portable x-rays during injection of radiographic contrast into the system showed extravasation into the subcutaneous tissues. The patient refused revision of the pump despite unsatisfactory control of pain with oral opiates. Until the time of her death from pneumonia 3 weeks later, she was in constant pain.

This case illustrates some of the potential difficulties associated with implanted opiate-delivery systems. Although the failure of this patient's infusion pump was because of a relatively minor technical problem, other issues made it impossible to correct. The case also illustrates the need for careful planning before installing a device that will require frequent injections by trained staff.

In some cases, the patient's inability to travel and the refusal of visiting nurses to administer opiates by the intraspinal route may negate the advantages of the system.

The need for large doses of epidural or intrathecal opiates to control cancer pain occasionally may necessitate the use of a ventricular cannula. It is implanted in much the same way as an Ommaya reservoir or a ventriculoperitoneal shunt. Single doses of morphine by this route are typically on the order of 2 to 4 mg. Patients undergoing such treatment generally are so tolerant to opiates that respiratory depression is minimal. The technique is new and has not been compared with other methods in controlled trials. The presence of brain metastases may be a contraindication.

Implantable drug-delivery systems are used to treat patients with chronic, nonmalignant pain. Opiates, clonidine, and local anesthetics all can be delivered by way of the intrathecal pump. For patients with spasticity, the intrathecal delivery of baclofen may reduce spasticity with few of the side effects of oral baclofen, such as sedation. The reduction in spasticity also may provide tremendous pain relief as well.

STEREOTAXIC CRANIAL PROCEDURES

Electrical stimulation of the periventricular region of the thalamus and midbrain is known to produce analgesia in animals and humans. Commercial products are available to implant the necessary wire electrodes and pulse generator, which is very similar to a cardiac pacemaker (Fig. 59.8). Electrical brain stimulation has been used successfully to treat a wide variety of painful disorders. In 13 patients with cancer pain, good to excellent relief was obtained in seven and slight relief in another three, according to Meyerson and coworkers. Long-term survivors tended to have better results.

The limitations of this method are (a) the need for patient cooperation during a lengthy initial stage of stereotaxic localization and trial stimulation, (b) the risk of infection or hemorrhage in patients with malignant disease, and (c) late failures because of malfunction or electrode migration. Reported mortality for patients undergoing chronic, deep-brain stimulation is less than 1%. Morbidity, consisting mostly of paresthesias, infection, and rare hemorrhages, is less than 5%. In most centers, deep-brain stimulation for cancer pain is considered a last resort. It finds limited use in cases of intractable pain that is bilateral, involves levels too rostral to be helped by cordotomy, and is refractory to all medications. Pain relief is not a Food and Drug Administration-approved use for deep brain stimulation (DBS). Many patients with intractable, nonmalignant pain have been treated on a compassionate basis by DBS. These patients must understand the risks involved before embarking on such an endeavor.

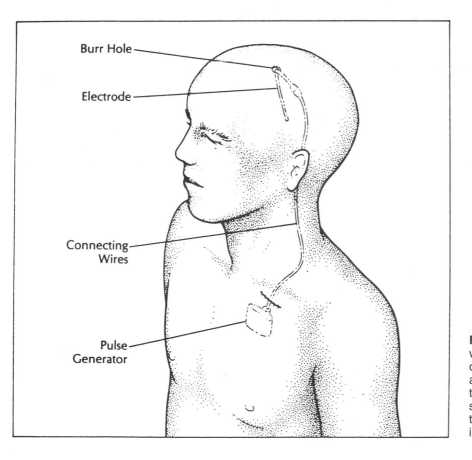

FIG. 59.8. Electrical brain stimulation, a widely used analgesic technique, is depicted as setup for periventricular application. The electrode is implanted through a burr hole made through the skull with stereotaxic guidance. Stimulation comes from a subcutaneously implanted pulse generator.

The procedure for implantation of a stimulating electrode is a two-stage, stereotaxic operation. In stage 1, under local anesthesia, a frame is mounted on the patient's head and radiographic studies are obtained (usually a CT of the brain or a ventriculogram). Target coordinates are chosen, and the stereotaxic frame is used to insert a temporary electrode for trials of stimulation in the operating room. If satisfactory results can be obtained with the patient's cooperation, a permanent implant is inserted and connected to wires exiting the scalp. The implant is used with an external pulse generator for 2 days to determine effectiveness.

If the patient is satisfied, the electrode is reconnected to an implanted pulse generator in stage 2, under general anesthesia. Some models feature externally controlled programming of pulse rates, current intensity, and on-off cycles. The patient is permitted to control some parameters. It is a feasible alternative for the cooperative patient with normal intelligence, intact mental state, intractable pain, and a life expectancy of more than 1 year. Like the implanted morphine catheter system, it has the advantage of being reversible.

Pituitary-gland lesions, made by transsphenoidal microsurgery, alcohol injection, or stereotaxic or radiofrequency lesioning, have been used to treat pain of diffusely metastatic soft-tissue tumors, especially prostate and breast cancer. Pain from other types of cancer also may respond. The effect of anterior pituitary destruction on pain in metastatic cancer still is unexplained. Some authorities maintain that a hormonal factor from the pituitary, not yet isolated or characterized, may be involved. The extent of the pituitary lesion correlates poorly with the degree of pain relief. In some patients, beneficial effects have been described as early as 30 minutes after the pituitary lesion, so that tumor regression is not a necessary factor.

Short-term benefit was seen in 60% to 70% of patients in several large, published series. Complications are uncommon but can be serious. They include cerebrospinal-fluid leak, hemorrhage, and meningitis. Pituitary insufficiency often is seen, but it is by no means an inevitable consequence of the lesion, nor is it necessary to produce hypopituitarism to achieve satisfactory pain relief. The use of pituitary lesions is controversial; long-term effectiveness is clearly much less than the initial success rates described in the literature, and controlled trials have not been carried out to exclude a placebo effect.

Several neurosurgical techniques can afford the cancer patient excellent relief of pain without the side-effects of large doses of opiates, thereby enabling him to be more alert and active. The morbidity of such procedures is far less than commonly thought, especially if they are performed early enough and not as a last resort in a dying patient.

SELECTED READINGS

Chang JW, Chang JH, Park YG, et al. Microvascular decompression in trigeminal neuralgia: a correlation of three-dimensional time-of-flight magnetic resonance angiography and surgical findings. *Stereotact Funct Neurosurg* 2000;74:167–174.

Gybels J, Kupers R. Deep brain stimulation in the treatment of chronic pain in man: where and why? *Neurophysiol Clin* 1990;20: 389–398.

Kanpolat Y, Savas A, Bekar A, et al. Percutaneous controlled radiofrequency trigeminal rhizotomy for the treatment of idiopathic trigeminal neuralgia: 25-year experience with 1,600 patients. *Neurosurgery* 2001; 48:524–532; discussion 532–534.

Karavelis A, Foroglou G, Selviaridis P, et al. Intraventricular administration of morphine for control of intractable cancer pain in 90 patients. *Neurosurgery* 1996;39:57–61; discussion 61–62.

Levy RM, North RB. *Neurosurgical Management of Pain.* New York: Springer Verlag, 1997.

Pollock BE, Foote RL, Link MJ, et al. Results of repeated gamma knife radiosurgery for medically unresponsive trigeminal neuralgia. *J Neurosurg* 2000; 93(suppl 3);162–164.

Richardson DE. Deep brain stimulation for the relief of chronic pain. *Neurosurg Clin North Am* 1995;6:135–144.

Rogers CL, Shetter AG, Fiedler JA, et al. Gamma knife radiosurgery for trigeminal neuralgia: the initial experience of The Barrow Neurological Institute. *Int J Radiat Oncol Biol Phys* 2000;47:1013–9.

Stanton-Hicks M, Salamon J. Stimulation of the central and peripheral nervous system for the control of pain. *J Clin Neurophysiol* 1997;14:46–62.

Stojanovic MP. Stimulation methods for neuropathic pain control. *Curr Pain Headache Rep* 2001;5:130–137.

ten Vaarwerk IA, Staal MJ. Spinal cord stimulation in chronic pain syndromes. *Spinal Cord* 1998;36:671–682.

CHAPTER 60

Surgical Treatment of Neuromas

Jagruti Patel, Loren J. Borud, and Joseph Upton

Although Ambroise Paré is credited with the first clinical recognition of a neuroma in 1634, the characteristic painful, bulbous lesion at the site of a severed nerve was not described until 1811 by Odier. Since then, much has been written about the pathophysiology, management, and treatment of these common, yet frustrating lesions, which continue to be a challenging problem for the surgeon and pain specialist. In hand surgery, neuromas involving sensory nerves of the upper limb are notorious for impeding progress toward what would otherwise be a satisfactory functional recovery. While a neuroma is the inevitable result of nerve injury, most are fortunately asymptomatic. However, the estimated 20% that are symptomatic present vexing clinical problems.

ANATOMY AND PHYSIOLOGY

To understand neuromas and neuroma treatment, it is essential to understand the microanatomy of the normal nerve. The fundamental unit of the nerve is the axon, which extends from its cell body to its site of termination. Myelinated axons are wrapped with multiple layers of myelin provided by Schwann cells, whereas unmyelinated nerves are instead surrounded by a double-basement membrane. Thin collagen strands that surround the individual nerve axons are called the *endo*neurium. Some nerve fibers are grouped together in fascicles and surrounded by *peri*neurium and often are destined for a specific region. Multiple fascicles are arranged and surrounded by *epi*neurium (Fig. 60.1) The entire nerve is ensheathed by connective tissue, *meso*neurium. Neurotransmitters and trophic factors are delivered through the bidirectional, axonal transport system to help maintain a homeostatic environment for the nerve.

Characteristic changes occur when any form of trauma disrupts the axonal continuity. These changes occur in both the proximal and distal ends of the injured nerve. The proximal portion of the damaged nerve undergoes regrowth after a period of recovery. The severed end of each nerve fiber in the proximal portion will grow multiple filopodia, which advance distally along the basement membrane of the Schwann cell seeking its distal counterpart. When the axons progress beyond the endoneurial tube, they sprout into a disorganized mass of connective tissue, which becomes enmeshed with new capillaries, myofibroblasts, and macrophages in a glycosaminoglycan matrix. Inevitably, some nerve fibers do not reach their endoneurial targets, and form an encapsulated nodule known as a neuroma.

Nerve fibers within the distal-nerve segment undergo Wallerian degeneration, the process of phagocytosis of axons and myelin sheath by macrophages and Schwann cells. These same Schwann cells also provide appropriate growth factors and a trophic *milieu* for proper axonal regeneration. Although the cellular response is much less in the distal stump than in the proximal end, the distal stump also forms a small bulb of neural tissue referred to as a glioma.

DEFINITIONS AND CLASSIFICATION

In its most general meaning, the term "neuroma" describes any growth or neoplasm of neurologic-cell origin. They can be classified on the basis of cytology and histology, i.e., neurofibroma, neuroepithelioma, etc. In clinical practice, however, the term "neuroma" has come to refer to the disorganized mass of growing nerve tissue following trauma. They present clinically as a painful nodule, which often is more disabling then the original traumatic injury.

Depending on the original injury, neuromas can form within an intact nerve, on the side of a partially lacerated nerve, or on the end of a completely lacerated nerve. Based on these injury mechanisms, Sunderland described the clinical classification of neuromas, which has become widely accepted.

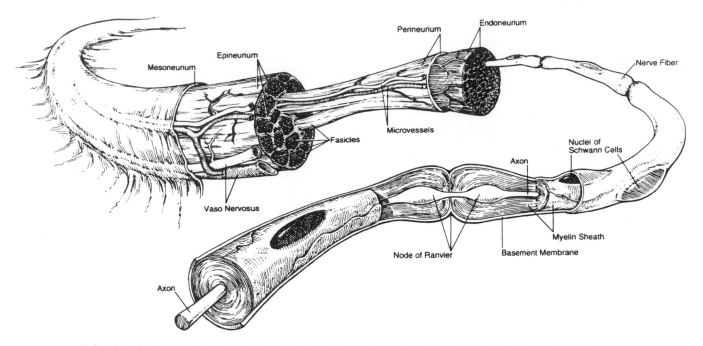

FIG. 60.1. Microanatomy of the normal nerve. (Reproduced from Brandt KE, MacKinnon SE. Microsurgical repair of peripheral nerves and nerve grafts. In: Aston SJ, Beasley RW, Thorne CHM, eds. *Grabb and Smith's Plastic Surgery*, 5th ed., Philadelphia: Lippincott–Raven Publishers, 1997:79–90, with permission.)

The most commonly encountered neuroma is that which forms at the proximal end of a severed nerve. Division of the distal branches of a sensory nerve results in lesions known as *terminal-branch neuromas*. Clinical examples include unrecognized, unrepaired laceration of a distal branch of the superficial radial nerve at the wrist during a de Quervain's release, or laceration of the palmar cutaneous branch of the median nerve in the palm during carpal-tunnel release. As a result of cross-innervation, the cutaneous territories of injured terminal branches may not show any profound clinical sensory deficits, and may delay recognition of the injury. *Amputation-stump neuromas*, as their name implies, result from complete division of a peripheral nerve during amputation of a finger, hand, or arm, and are clinically identical to those that develop in a severed terminal-nerve branch.

Neuromas involving a partially intact nerve are known as neuromas-in-continuity. These are separated into two groups: spindle neuromas and lateral neuromas.

Spindle neuromas are swellings noted in an intact nerve subjected to external forces such as inflammation, friction, or compression. The swollen portion of the nerve contains increased amounts of axoplasm and connective tissue. These commonly occur in the posterior-interosseous nerve (PIN) on the dorsum of the wrist following a crush injury, the ulnar-digital nerve of the thumb in a bowler, or in the grossly intact digital nerve in a partially avulsed digit requiring revascularization.

Lateral neuromas occur when the perineurium and epineurium on the edge of the nerve has been traumatized. Common causes include retraction during surgery, puncture wounds, and trauma during surgery. It also may result from misalignment of severed fascicular bundles, which will result in axonal sprouting outside the nerve itself into adjacent scar tissue. The size of the lesion depends upon the degree of fascicular damage.

DIAGNOSIS

The diagnosis of neuroma is based primarily on clinical grounds. Immediately after injury to the limb, pain is related directly to the trauma, edema, and the subsequent inflammatory reaction. Injured nerves initially undergo a process of Wallerian degeneration back to the next node of Ranvier as previously mentioned. With time, axonal sprouting and fibrosis lead to formation of a neuroma. Only at this time, weeks or months after injury, can the clinical diagnosis of neuroma be made. At this stage, patients recognize that their initial posttraumatic pain has subsided, and has been replaced with a dull, burning, localized pain referred to the cutaneous territory of the injured nerve.

The most characteristic sign on physical examination of the patient with a neuroma is a positive Tinel's sign. Gentle tapping over the site of the neuroma with a finger or pen elicits a painful paresthesia (Fig. 60.2). The area of sensory diminution should be mapped and recorded. On occasion, a painful mass representing the neuroma may be palpated. For example, neuromas at the repair site of a lacerated median nerve at the wrist level often are palpable and quite painful, especially if the nerve repair is adherent to the

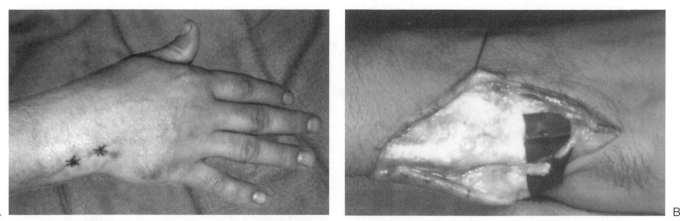

FIG. 60.2. A: This patient has a positive Tinel's sign as indicated by the asterisks along the dorsal-sensory branch of the ulnar nerve. **B:** The nerve was not in-continuity. The large neuroma of the proximal stump was rerouted deep to the interosseous membrane.

overlying cutaneous scar. A diagnostic nerve block with lidocaine often is helpful to determine the extent to which the neuroma contributes to a patient's pain. In addition, these blocks can be used prior to surgery to let the patient experience the expected postoperative outcome.

TREATMENT

Many different modalities for treatment of the painful neuroma have been described, yet no well-accepted procedure of choice has been established. Nolan and Eaton have explicitly emphasized that, regardless of the treatment modality, early recognition and treatment are vital to attaining the best possible outcome. Expeditious treatment should be completed before conditioned pain patterns become entrenched.

Nonoperative modalities such as massage, biofeedback, ultrasound, and transcutaneous-electrical nerve stimulation, among other techniques, have not yielded predictable outcomes and are not commonly used in most centers. During the past 30 years, a wide variety of sclerosing agents have been injected or directly applied to the terminal portions of an injured nerve to induce scar and avoid neuroma formation or to induce the regression of an established neuroma. Some of these agents include procaine, alcohol, osmic acid, tannic acid, hydrochloric acid, pepsin, formaldehyde, phenol, and nitrogen mustard. Sunderland has noted that, unfortunately, none of these agents can effectively suppress axonal regeneration.

The hallmark of current therapy of neuroma treatment is surgical, followed by early postoperative mobilization and therapy. Operative strategies include direct nerve repair when possible, intercalated nerve grafts to bridge large discontinuities, and neuroma resection with or without transposition into soft tissue or bone. Simple resection of the injured nerve, which then is allowed to retract into uninjured soft tissue, has been the most commonly used method. This technique is not only effective for dig-ital or other stump neuromas, but also is applicable to any neuroma of a sensory nerve. Tupper and Booth reported that simple excision neurectomy yielded a painless or minimally tender operative site in 65% of 316 patients. Among the 35% of patients with recurrent neuroma, 78% had a satisfactory outcome following a secondary rerouting procedure.

BASIC PRINCIPLES OF OPERATIVE TECHNIQUE

The surgical approach to both in-continuity and terminal-branch neuromas incorporates the same basic principles. Meticulous dissection under loupe or microscopic visualization minimizes tissue damage. In extremity surgery, a tourniquet creates a bloodless field. When possible, incisions are designed so that the nerve will not lie directly beneath the cutaneous scar with which it may become adherent. Following a sharp skin incision, blunt dissection along existing fascial planes is preferred. Manipulation of the neural structures should be minimized and the epineural sheath and *vasa nervorum* (blood vessels coursing longitudinally along the nerve surface) should not be disrupted. Nerves should not be stripped or stretched. Bipolar cauterization for careful hemostasis avoids unnecessary electrical damage to the nerve. The nerve and operative field should be inspected with the tourniquet released before wound closure to ensure meticulous hemostasis on and around the nerve. Hematomas beneath the epineural or perineural sheaths may result in new neuromas. At the time of wound closure, soft tissue is interposed, if possible, between the skin closure and the field of nerve dissection.

TREATMENT OF NEUROMAS-IN-CONTINUITY

Within the extremities and head and neck region, neuromas usually are the result of previous trauma, localized compression neuropathy, an inflammatory process, or some form of invasive medical treatment such as venipuncture or arterial catheterization. Many anesthesiologists and other hospital personnel never see neuromas-in-continuity resulting from regional blocks or other procedures, because they present weeks or months later to the primary-care physician, pain specialist, or hand surgeon. Fortunately, almost all neuromas-in-continuity resulting from needle puncture resolve spontaneously and only reassurance is necessary.

Operative Technique for Neuromas-in-Continuity

With more significant nerve trauma, partial laceration results in neuromas-in-continuity, which do not resolve with conservative treatment and require operative repair. Incisions are important. In the hand, they are made along the sides of the digits or thumb, along previously existing flexion creases on the palmar surface and as straight, oblique, or transverse lines on the dorsal surfaces. Zigzag incisions on the dorsal surfaces are unnecessary and aesthetically unacceptable. The zigzag incisions described first by Brunner and later refined by Littler on the palmar surfaces of the hand were designed specifically to avoid troublesome contractures across flexion creases and are not applicable to the mobile, dorsal skin. Scars from previous incisions should be completely excised. Fascial and areolar tissue planes and subcutaneous fat should be saved and placed around the nerve at the time of closure.

The site of the neuroma usually is obvious from clinical examination and is marked on the skin prior to the induction of anesthesia. In the hand, the neuroma may be adherent to scar tissue surrounding skeletal, tendon, or vascular repairs. Careful dissection starts in normal tissue planes both proximal and distal to the neuroma, where the nerve can be more safely identified. With meticulous dissection toward the neuroma, the adherent structures are individually separated. In the initial dissection, scar tissue is left on the nerve to avoid injury, and this often must be separated from other soft-tissue or skeletal structures with a scalpel. Once all structures have been identified and mobilized, a colored background is placed beneath the nerve and a very careful epineural lysis of scar tissue is completed using either the operating microscope or loupe magnification.

The Interposition Concept

After exposure and neurolysis, the question arises: what will prevent the neuroma from recurring as the wound heals? It has been shown that interposition of tissue or other materials can lessen the chance of a clinically recurrent neuroma. For most neuromas-in-continuity, we have used autogenous veins to wrap around the nerve in the area of dissection. Harvested from the nearby subcutaneous tissue, these veins are split and then sutured around the injured nerve. Their purpose is (a) to contain the axonal sprouting from the disrupted endoneurial planes and (b) to provide an interposition material with a mobile adventitial plane between the nerve and adjacent structures. These vein wraps are very effective for treating neuromas within digital nerves of the fingers or thumb, common digital nerves within the palm of the hand, and for the troublesome neuromas of the dorsal-sensory branches of the radial nerve along the dorsum of the distal forearm and wrist. Vein wraps have not been necessary for the spindle-type neuromas occurring in intact nerves related to compression within the cubital, pronator, or carpal canals. We have, on occasion, sacrificed lumbrical muscles within the palm or portions of the superficial flexor muscle bellies within the forearm to protect nearby nerve repairs. Other materials such as silicone sheeting or autogenous retinaculum from the wrist or ankle also have been used as interposition grafts to separate the dissected nerve from surrounding bone and soft tissue. Early postoperative motion, often augmented with continuous passive motion (CPM) machines, is very helpful to preserve joint motion, tendon gliding, and to minimize adhesions between the nerve and adjacent mobile structures.

The recurrent neuroma of the median nerve within the carpal canal can be protected with hypothenar muscles, local flaps of forearm fascia/fat, or distant free transfers of nonvascularized fat and fascia. Every precaution is taken to avoid the formation of a common scar connecting the skin incision to the dissected nerve.

NEUROMAS IN THE COMPLETELY SEVERED NERVE

In the completely severed nerve, a neuroma always forms on the proximal end and a glioma on the distal side of the unrepaired transection. The optimal method of preventing or treating neuromas in completely severed nerve is to carefully reapproximate the severed ends. In cases of established neuromas in completely severed nerves, both the neuroma and glioma should be "bread-loafed" back to normal-appearing fascicular bundles and the nerve repaired primarily without tension. Often, the intercalated gap is too great to permit a tension-free juncture, and the use of a nerve conduit or an autogenous nerve graft should be considered. For gaps of 2.0 cm to 2.5 cm, the use of conduits in pure sensory nerves has been effective, thereby avoiding the harvest of nerve grafts. We prefer to use an autogenous vein. Many alloplastic materials composed of silicone tubes, polytetrafluorethyelne, and absorbable collagen are available.

Nerve-Graft Donor Sites

Autogenous nerve grafts should be used to bridge nerve gaps of greater than 2.5 cm. The sural nerve harvested through a small incision behind the lateral malleolus of the ankle, or the medial antebrachial-cutaneous nerve of the forearm located over the brachioradialis-muscle belly can be used as donor grafts. The major disadvantage of the sural-nerve graft is formation of a stump neuroma at the sock level, which can be avoided by excising the nerve up to the level of the calf. The visible scar on the forearm after harvest of the medial antebrachial nerve can be minimized by an endoscopic harvest. For very large gaps following an extensive traumatic injury or multilevel injury, a vascularized sural-nerve graft is preferred. The vascular supply of this convenient donor nerve originates from the popliteal or lateral sural arteries behind the knee. The dissection is tedious and is performed best by a surgeon familiar with microvascular techniques.

In both primary repairs and nerve grafts, we prefer group-fascicular nerve sutures with the minimum number of small (eight to zero, or smaller) epineural sutures required to approximate the nerves. Individual fascicular-bundle repairs, which add to the surgical manipulation and trauma to the epineurium, perineurium, and endoneurium, are to be avoided. Recently, the use of fibrin glue has become another fixation method that will effectively approximate the nerves and then can be covered by a vein conduit at the sites of repair.

Amputation-Stump Neuromas

The stump neuroma at the injured termini of either sensory or mixed nerves is the most commonly encountered type of neuroma in the upper extremity. In these cases, because the distal-nerve segment is not available, the preferred treatment strategy is a local relocation of the nerve stump, which can be simply excised and allowed to retract into soft tissue (Fig. 60.3A). In apprehensive patients, the postoperative outcome can be simulated temporarily by a sensory-nerve block. It often is helpful to block these nerves at the beginning of a day with a long-acting, local anesthetic, and then examine

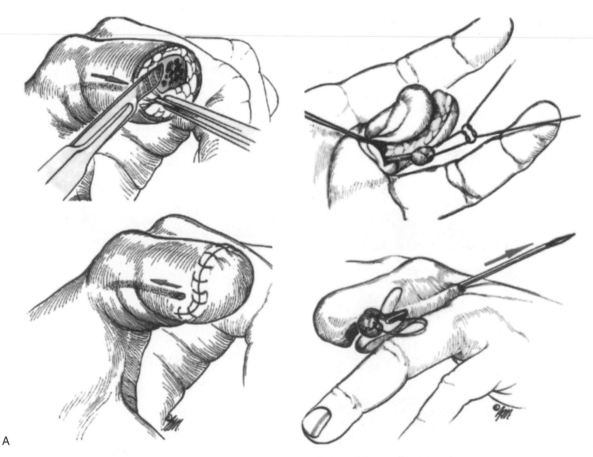

A   B

FIG. 60.3. Treatment of amputation-stump neuromas. **A:** Simple neurectomy. The end of the nerve is grasped, advanced gently into the wound, then sharply severed as proximally as possible. The transected nerve end retracts into the soft tissue. **B:** Rerouting of an amputation-stump neuroma to a more protected, intermetacarpal location. (Reproduced from Herndon JH. Neuromas. In: Green DP, ed., *Operative Hand Surgery*, 3rd ed., vol. 2, New York: Churchill Livingstone, 1993:1387–1399, with permission.)

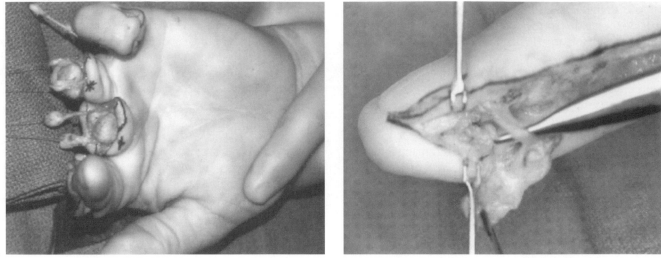

FIG. 60.4. A: Multiple stump neuromas have been dissected from posttraumatic amputation stumps. With neuromas intact, they will be rerouted into the intermetacarpal spaces. B: This digital nerve formed a neuroma where it became interposed within a fracture of the distal phalanx and was redirected to a more protected location.

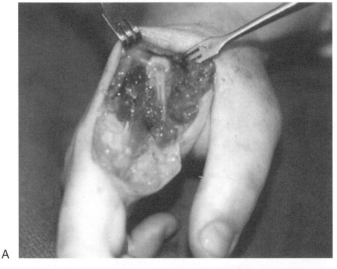

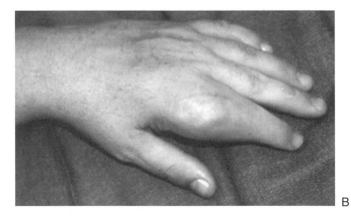

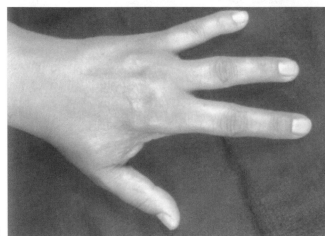

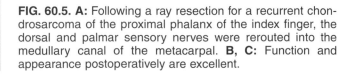

FIG. 60.5. A: Following a ray resection for a recurrent chondrosarcoma of the proximal phalanx of the index finger, the dorsal and palmar sensory nerves were rerouted into the medullary canal of the metacarpal. B, C: Function and appearance postoperatively are excellent.

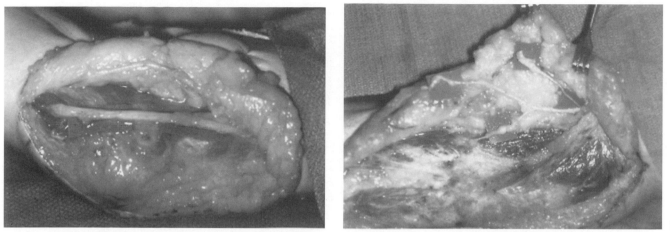

FIG. 60.6. A: Multiple neuromas-in-continuity are seen in an ulnar nerve within the cubital tunnel following instrument trauma during plate and screw fixation of a distal humerus fracture. **B:** In the same patient, multiple neuromas are seen in the sensory branches of the medial brachial and medial antebrachial cutaneous nerves. These were all rerouted beneath the triceps muscle.

and talk to the patient in more detail later in the day. These troublesome neuromas often are the primary afferent stimulus for the development of the recalcitrant, conditioned, sympathetic dystrophy problems encountered in a small number of patients following upper-extremity trauma or surgery.

Technique for Treatment of Amputation-Stump Neuromas

The neuroma is first identified and dissected with its adherent scar tissue. The distal end of the nerve with its intact neuroma then is rerouted into an area of the hand, wrist, or forearm, which is not subject to percussive trauma from routine daily activity. For the common digital-stump neuroma, a high midaxial incision is made. The nerve, with its intact neuroma, is dissected and mobilized, then secured with a chromic suture, which then is threaded into the lumbrical canal between the metacarpals (Figs. 3B and 4). The suture is then brought out through the dorsal skin and tied, thereby maintaining the neuroma in its protected position until scar tissue can permanently fix the nerve in the desired location.

Following ray resection of digits at the metacarpal level, all the dorsal and palmar sensory nerves are placed within the medullary canal of the metacarpal, which then is covered with a local, intrinsic muscle (Fig. 60.5). In performing an index-ray resection, for example, at least three dorsal and two palmar sensory nerves would be placed within the metaphysis of the metacarpal, which then is covered with the first dorsal interosseous muscle.

Painful neuromas of the dorsal-sensory branches of the radial nerve of the wrist or forearm are rerouted down to the interosseous membrane between the radius and ulna. More proximal sensory neuromas of the arm and forearm are effectively placed deep to large-muscle bellies or into

bone (Fig. 60.6). The mobilization of these sensory nerves with their intact distal neuromas must be performed carefully using atraumatic technique and microinstruments to avoid trauma to the mesoneurium and epineurium, which could result in axonal sprouting and the development of a new neuroma-in-continuity.

SELECTED READINGS

Badalamente MA, Hurst LC, Ellstein J, et al. The physiology of human neuromas: an electron microscope and biochemical study. *J Hand Surg* 1985;10:49–53.

Brandt KE, MacKinnon SE. Microsurgical repair of peripheral nerves and nerve grafts. In: Aston SJ, Beasley RW, Thorne CHM, eds. *Grabb and Smith's Plastic Surgery*, 5th ed. Philadelphia: Lippincott–Raven Publishers, 1997:79–90.

Fernanadez AD, Rosales RS, Sicilia HF, et al. Prevention of the formation of neuromas in nerves implanted in bone. (Spanish) *Rev Exp Cirugia Mano* 1997;24:9–14.

Herndon JH, Eaton RG, Littler JW. Management of painful neuromas in the hand. *J Bone Joint Surg* 1976;58A:369–373.

Herndon JH. Neuromas. In: Green DP, ed. *Operative Hand Surgery*, vol. 2. New York: Churchill Livingstone, 1993:1387–1399.

Huber GC, Lewis D. Amputation neuromas. Their development and prevention. *Arch Surg* 1920;1:85–113.

Koman LA, Smith TL, Smith BP, et al. The painful hand. *Hand Clin* 1996; 12:757–763.

MacKinnon SE, Dellon AL. *Surgery of the Peripheral Nerve.* New York: Thieme, 1988.

Moldaver J. Brief note: Tinel's sign. *J Bone Joint Surg* 1978;60:412–414.

Nath RK, MacKinnon SE. Management of neuromas in the hand. *Hand Clin* 1996;12:745–756.

Nolan WB, Eaton RG. Painful neuromas of the upper extremity and postneurectomy pain. In: Omer G, et al., eds. *Management of Peripheral Nerve Problems*. Philadelphia: WB Saunders Co., 1998:146–150.

Sood MK, Elliot D. Treatment of painful neuromas of the hand and wrist by relocation into the pronator quadratus muscle. *J Hand Surg* 1988;23B: 214–219.

Stedman TL. *Stedman's Medical Dictionary*, 25th ed. Baltimore: Williams and Wilkins, 1990:1046.

Sunderland S. *Nerves and Nerve Injuries*, 2nd ed., Edinburgh: Churchill Livingstone, 1978.

Tupper JW, Booth DM. Treatment of painful neuromas of sensory nerves in the hand: a comparison of traditional and newer methods. *J Hand Surg* 1976;1:144–151.

Considerations in Pain Management

CHAPTER 61

Pediatric Pain Management

Kenneth R. Goldschneider

As for adults, pain is a major reason for urgent visits to the healthcare provider. The inability of the youngest patients to verbally report the nature, even location of their pain makes initial evaluation difficult and response to therapy challenging to assess. Fortunately, the fields of developmental biology, pain assessment, and treatment have received increasing attention in the past decade. The historical impediments to organized pain relief for children largely have been overcome. Treatment for the pain of infants and children in both acute and chronic settings has become safe and effective. Assessment and measurement of pain in infants and preverbal children, though, still bedevil caregivers.

Complicating the efforts of pediatric practitioners is the fact that for many children, fear and anxiety dominate their thought processes concerning medical encounters. Therefore, it is essential to make interactions in medical settings less terrifying for children. In the youngest patients, medication therapy is complicated by age-related differences in several pharmacokinetic and pharmacodynamic factors. Understanding the unique and dynamic aspects of pediatric pain treatment is critical to the safe and effective alleviation of pain and suffering in children.

PAIN ASSESSMENT

Assessment of pain in children, especially those in the preverbal age group, poses a particularly difficult problem. Differentiating pain from other negative experiences on the basis of behavior often is frustrating. Finlay and McGrath recently have edited a recent, comprehensive monograph to which the reader is referred for a more comprehensive discussion. Adequate pain assessment in hospital environments is inconsistent. Organized protocols are lacking in many institutions. The use of existing protocols and scales is sporadic. Overall, it appears that pain assessment and management is less consistent for infants and young children than for older patients. Several self-report measures are available that can be used reliably by children ages 3 through 8 years. Faces scales have been quite popular. Usually, severe pain is depicted as a crying face, with closed eyes, furrowed brow, and deepened nasolabial folds. The ethnicity of both the patient and the child pictured on the scale influences the accuracy of the tool. Color analog scales (more intensely red color corresponds to greater pain) seem acceptable to most children over the age of 4 years and display convergent validity to visual-analog scale (VAS) scales in older children.

Assessment of pain by way of physiologic parameters (heart rate, respiratory rate, blood pressure, and the variability of these parameters) may appear attractive for use in the preverbal population. Unfortunately, these signs are influenced by factors such as underlying disease, volume status, emotional state, and medications. Behavioral scales are available to aid in the assessment of preverbal children. Most of these scales primarily serve to assess the pain of toddlers, preschool children, and neonates undergoing surgery and brief painful procedures. Facial expressions appear useful and valid as indicators of pain in neonates of all postconceptual ages and look to be more robust and sensitive than audiologic measures. Although most of the behavioral-pain scales look for increased motor activity, one should not consider a child to be comfortable solely on the grounds that he or she is lying quietly. Many times, children in pain lie still in bed, with their eyes shut, not because they are comfortable or narcotized, but because it hurts too much to move.

DEVELOPMENTAL PSYCHOLOGY AND PAIN

To care for the pediatric patient, one must adjust one's approach to meet the developmental needs of the child. In brief, children under the age of about 2 years relate to their environment in a stimulus-response manner, having little sense of permanence, long-term anticipation, or cause and effect. This age group responds well to cuddling/swaddling, warm environments, soothing voices, and pharmacological interventions. One must take care not to refer to the toddler as good or bad in the context of a painful procedure because pain often is viewed by the child as a punishment, with the magnitude of pain correlating with how "bad" the child is. Treatment often centers on kissing/rubbing the injury or the magic of adhesive bandages and medication. The toddler is strongly enmeshed in the ego strength of its parents and often benefits from parental involvement. By this age, self-report becomes feasible as a measure of pain and intervention.

As the child reaches school age, pain can be expressed in terms of affect, and is no longer viewed as a punishment. Pain treatment focuses largely on medicine and physical interventions (e.g., rubbing). The appreciation of cause and effect grows, which is prerequisite for the use of patient-controlled analgesia (PCA) modalities. Young adolescents begin to master the skills of self-analysis, long-term anticipation, and delayed gratification, which leads the practitioner to treat the teen in many ways like an adult. Caution is warranted because limited life experience, a strong sense of body image, and threats to their sense of invulnerability make the adolescent uniquely sensitive to the effects of disease and painful conditions. Despite their quest for autonomy, many teenagers derive great comfort from a hand to hold during procedures. Lastly, children of all ages often regress to earlier stages of emotional and cognitive development in times of stress and illness. It is important not to address this apparent "immaturity" in a judgmental way, but to utilize therapeutic approaches geared to younger children, until the child can regain his or her developmental equilibrium.

TREATMENT MODALITIES

It was observed during the early years of pediatric-pain clinics, that outcomes are better when physical therapy and behavioral medicine are combined with the standard allopathic medical approach. This finding reflects the strong interaction between psychology and physiology. In practical terms, most pediatric patients have an overriding fear of needles, necessitating general anesthesia for many nerve blocks. Additionally, nerve blocks in young patients often are technically challenging. This combination of factors precluded the development of an overreliance on a single mode of therapy. Even in these times of managed care and enforced cost cutting, we must bear in mind that treatment of a child's pain can influence the function of that individual for a lifetime. Treating pain in children must be taken for the investment it is. Therefore, even if an organized pediatric-pain clinic is not readily available, therapy should still involve evaluation and intervention by medical doctors, physical therapists, and psychologists.

Biobehavioral Therapy

Behavioral medicine techniques have proven to be useful in the treatment of many pediatric-pain syndromes. These therapies can be grouped into four categories: relaxation therapies, including hypnosis; biofeedback; operant pain behavior management; and a more general category of cognitive-behavioral techniques. The latter group involves self-monitoring, coping strategies, and environmental modification. Biobehavioral intervention has a proven track record for pediatric migraine, recurrent abdominal pain, and juvenile rheumatoid arthritis, as well as for neuropathic pain and pain associated with sickle cell disease.

Nonopioid Medications

Aspirin is by far the oldest nonopioid analgesic and antiinflammatory agent. The risk of Reye's syndrome in the setting of certain febrile illnesses must be borne in mind when using this drug. Nevertheless, aspirin is effective as a treatment for mild-to-moderate pain associated with inflammation. Aspirin inhibits prostaglandin synthesis and release. This action is responsible for the drug's analgesic effect as well as its antiplatelet effect. The mild-to-moderate gastrointestinal upset that commonly is seen with aspirin administration can be minimized by administration of the drug with milk or food.

Acetaminophen has analgesic properties similar to aspirin, and is useful for treatment of both mild pain and fever, although it has little antiinflammatory effect or effect on platelet function. The dose of acetaminophen varies according to the route of administration, in contrast to aspirin. Conservative daily dose limits based on available pharmacokinetic data are 90 mg/kg/day in children, 60 mg/kg/day in infants, and 45 mg/kg/day in preemies. The dose of acetaminophen needed to achieve analgesic levels when the drug is given *per rectum* range from 20 to 45 mg/kg (Table 61.1). The higher-end doses appear to be more effective. Repeated rectal dosing has not been well studied.

Nonsteroidal antiinflammatory drugs (NSAIDs) are useful for many forms of pain. NSAIDs can be effectively administered via oral, intravenous, rectal, and intramuscular routes. Intramuscular injection is painful, offers no advantage over other delivery routes, and should be discouraged. The intravenous route offers convenience for administration intra- or postoperatively. There is little difference in efficacy among routes of administration; the oral route should be used whenever feasible. Overall, the safety of NSAIDs in children seems quite good; however, rare cases of gastrointestinal bleeding and nephropathy have been reported. Ketorolac is a very effective analgesic for a variety of outpatient surgeries in children but should be used with caution for certain types of surgery such as tonsillectomy, in which bleeding is a major con-

TABLE 61.1. *Doses of Some Nonopioid Analgesics*

Drug	Dosing
Aspirin (acetylsalicylic acid)	p.o.: 10–15 mg/kg Q 4 h up to 90–120 mg/kg/24 h p.r.: same regimen, PR dosing not as well studied
Acetaminophen	p.o.: 10–15 mg/kg Q 4–6 h up to: 45 mg/kg/24 h in neonates 60 mg/kg/24 h in infants 90 mg/kg/24 h in children p.r.: 30–40 mg/kg
Ibuprofen	p.o.: 8–10 mg/kg Q 6 h up to 40 mg/kg/24 h
Choline-magnesium salicylate	p.o.: 10–15 mg/kg Q 8–12 h

p.o., per os (orally); p.r., per rectum.

cern. A 5-day limit has been suggested, based on adult data, to reduce the risks of renal impairment in the postoperative setting. The safety and efficacy of NSAID-based analgesia in newborns has not been established.

Several new, nonnarcotic medications are being investigated and released that address many of the concerns about NSAID and acetaminophen toxicities or limitations. Propacetamol is an intravenous prodrug of acetaminophen being used in Europe, for which there is some pediatric data. The cyclooxygenase 2 (COX-2) -specific inhibitors promise to be useful and may reduce the major side effects and complications of NSAIDs. The lack of impairment of coagulation may be especially useful for pediatric, perioperative use and for children with cancer pain. Data on their use in children is currently lacking, but should be forthcoming in the next year or two. The use of anticonvulsants and antidepressants for pain is discussed below.

Opioid Therapy

In the setting of moderate-to-severe pain, opioids can be used effectively for infants and children of all ages. Opioid therapy must proceed with a proper understanding of age-related changes in pharmacokinetics and pharmacodynamics. Opioid clearances, standardized by body weight, are reduced compared to mature values in the first months of life, reaching mature values over the first 3 to 12 months of age. Young infants, therefore, are at higher risk for opioid accumulation, delayed sedation, and respiratory depression.

The issue of pharmacodynamic respiratory sensitivity of neonates long has been debated. Ventilatory reflexes to hypoxia and hypercarbia are immature in human newborns, and mature over the first weeks of life. Early observations suggested that neonates had greater respiratory depression than older children and adults. Healthy infants ages 3 months and older in predominantly postoperative studies show analgesic responses and patterns of respiratory depression similar to adults. Opioid infusions have been used extensively for children with good efficacy and safety (Table 61.2).

Several routes of administration are useful for children and infants. Certainly the oral route is effective and should be used whenever feasible (Table 61.3) The intravenous route can be utilized in three basic ways. First, intermittent doses of moderate duration drugs such as morphine and hydromorphone can be administered over 10 to 20 minutes as often as every two hours. Second, the longer-acting methadone can be given on a sliding scale (0.03 to 0.07 mg/kg i.v./p.o.) every 4 hours. Care must be taken to avoid sedation or respiratory depression that can result from the accumulation of methadone with repeated dosing. Electronic surveillance is prudent for the first 24 to 48 hours as the titration is achieved. Third, continuous infusion of short- to medium-acting opioids has a role in

TABLE 61.2. *I.V. Opioid Dosing Guidelines*

Drug	Equianalgesic dose	Usual i.v. dose range	Comments
Morphine	1 mg	Bolus: 0.1 mg/kg Q 2–4 h Infusion: 0.01–0.03 mg/kg/h	Metabolites can build up in presence of renal insufficiency
Hydromorphone	0.15–0.2 mg	Bolus: 0.02 mg/kg Q 2–4 h Infusion: 0.003–0.006 mg/kg/h	Less pruritus than morphine; Not limited by renal impairment
Fentanyl	0.01 mg (10 µg)	Bolus: 0.5–1.0 µg/kg Q1–2 h Infusion: 0.15–1.0 µg/kg/h	Hemodynamically stable; Not limited by renal impairment
Methadone	1 mg	Bolus: 0.1 mg/kg Q 4–8 h (Q8–12 if excessive sedation occurs)	Can accumulate and lead to excessive sedation
Meperidine	8–10 mg	Bolus: 0.8–1.0 mg/kg Q 2–3 h	Least desirable: buildup of metabolites can lead to CNS excitatory effects

CNS, central nervous system; i.v., intravenous.

TABLE 61.3. *Oral Opioid Dosing Guidelines*

Drug	Equianalgesic dose	i.v./p.o. ratio	Common starting p.o. dose
Morphine	3 mg	1:3	Immediate release 0.3 mg/kg Q 3–4 h Sustained release: (Q 8–12 h) Base dosing on total 24 h opioid dose Caution advised in opioid naïve patients
Codeine	20 mg	i.v. route not used	Child <50 kg: 0.5–1.0 mg/kg Q 3–4 h Child >50 kg: 30–60 mg Q 3–4 h
Oxycodone	3 mg	i.v. route not used	Child <50 kg: 0.1–0.2 mg/kg Q 3–4 h Child >50 kg: 5–10 mg Q 3–4 h Also available in combination with APAP
Hydromorphone	0.6–0.8 mg	1:4	0.04–0.08 mg/kg Q 3–4 h
Methadone	2 mg	1:2	0.2 mg/kg Q 4–8 h If sedation occurs, lengthen dosing interval

APAP, acetaminophen; i.v., intravenous; p.o., per os (by mouth).

children unable to actively participate in the analgesic process. Other routes of administration such as transdermal and transbuccal have received attention and have relatively limited pediatric application. Intranasal butorphanol has been used in adults to treat migraine headaches, and may be appropriate in select teenagers.

In general, opioid infusions in younger infants are useful and generally safe. Their dosing and titration to effect require expertise and vigilance because pain assessment in infants is imprecise. There is debate over which forms of electronic monitoring are most useful for detecting hypoxemia or hypoventilation. Pulse oximetry allows monitoring of oxygenation in the presence of normal respiratory rate. The lack of oximeter telemetry means that the alarm may go undetected in a hospital room. Impedance-apnea monitoring is widely available on hospital wards with telemetry alarms that can ring in a hallway or nurses' station. These monitors have limitations related to motion artifact. In all neonates and infants, and for patients with altered mental status or abnormal airways, it is recommended that both modalities be used for maximal protection of the patients. Older and healthy children do not need the same level of electronic monitoring. The bottom line is that no amount of technological surveillance substitutes for clinical assessment and understanding of conditions that modify opioid requirements and risks.

SPECIFIC TYPES OF PAIN

Acute Pain

Postoperative Pain

The most effective management of postoperative pain involves coordinated efforts among parents, pediatricians, surgeons, anesthesiologists, nurses, pharmacists, and child-life specialists. Primary-care providers can help provide preoperative preparation that can reduce anxiety and fear. Explanations should be given that are appropriate to the child's developmental stage. Use of eutectic mixture of local anesthetics (EMLA) or other topical anesthetics may reduce the distress of intravenous catheter placement and phlebotomy. Iontophoretic delivery systems have been developed and are effective. While these devices deliver the anesthetic faster than EMLA, skin burns have been reported, and the apparatus must be used carefully. Anxiolytics delivered by oral and nasal routes also can be helpful. Midazolam suspended in acetaminophen elixir works toward the goals of anxiolysis and preemptive analgesia, and can be a useful preprocedure cocktail.

In many pediatric centers, acute-pain services provide patient advocacy and ensure that pain management is prompt, consistent, and safe. Decimal-point errors can be deadly. Provision of dosing protocols facilitates cross-checking for erroneous orders. Assessment protocols allow maximal accuracy in determining the analgesic needs and responses of pediatric patients. When children are cared for in general hospitals, pediatric specialists should be involved in creation of specific pain-management protocols for children.

Over the past decade, children have used patient-controlled analgesia (PCA) with excellent safety, good efficacy, and excellent patient acceptance, without increased opioid use or side effects. PCA can be used properly by children over the age of 6 years. Short lockout intervals (e.g., 7 to 8 minutes) are safe and allow more rapid "catch-up" in the setting of unrelieved pain. Basal infusion may provide better pain control in some patients, although there is an increased risk for nighttime oxygen desaturation. PCA is inherently safe because if patients become narcotized, they fall asleep. The plasma concentrations then fall, keeping the patients safe. There is controversy over the use of nurse- and parent-controlled PCA. Both modalities have been used safely in very select circumstances, most usually in the setting of palliative or intensive care. Parent and nurse education is important especially in these settings. Routine use of nurse/parent-PCA in general hospitals cannot be recommended at present.

Morphine is probably the most commonly used opioid for PCA. In cases where the patient has side effects from morphine, hydromorphone is an excellent alternative to morphine. Hydromorphone is five times more potent than morphine, and the dose needs to be reduced accordingly. Fentanyl and meperidine can be used for selected patients, although routine use is not advisable.

Regional anesthesia in infants and children can be performed with an excellent safety and side-effect profile by modifications of techniques used in adults. Unlike in adults, most regional anesthetics are performed with the child under general anesthesia. The placement of epidural catheters in anesthetized patients has been of concern to many practitioners. The continued performance of these blocks in careful, controlled fashion, on anesthetized children has received solid support from the pediatric anesthesia community. Dose adjustments need to be made in order to avoid local anesthetic toxicity, which can include convulsions and refractory cardiac dysrhythmias. These blocks are best left to practitioners of pediatric anesthesia.

Caudal analgesia most often is provided for analgesia following minor procedures below the umbilicus. It is relatively simple, very safe, and effective. α-2 adrenergic agents, such as clonidine, prolong local anesthetic action, and may be useful additives. Opioids can be added as well, in doses ranging from 0.03 to 0.1 mg/kg of morphine. There is some additional risk of delayed respiratory depression in the upper dose range, and apnea and oximetric monitoring are advisable. The addition of opioids to caudal injections is not appropriate for same-day surgery patients.

Procedure Pain

Children suffer considerable distress from procedure pain, especially needle procedures. Routine immunizations and blood draws are sources of medical pain for healthy children. Intravenous cannulation, lumbar puncture, and bone marrow aspiration are threatening procedures for children with acute and chronic illnesses.

Several principles are crucial in managing acute procedure-related pain. First, honesty is the best policy. It often is very difficult to inform a child that what is about to be done will cause discomfort, but denying the reality of the pain will likely lead to losing the child's trust. Both family members and caregivers would prefer that the child not be uncomfortable; it sometimes occurs that these individuals actually begin to deny the child's complaints. The second principle is not to ignore, minimize, invalidate, or disbelieve the child's pain complaint. The children must believe that their caregivers are listening and that their complaints are important. Lastly, the American Academy of Pediatrics (AAP) guidelines for monitoring children undergoing sedation and analgesia should be followed.

Approaches to these procedures must be designed on an individualized basis. Appropriate explanation and support can be helpful. Some children benefit from topical cooling with ethyl-chloride spray. Oral sucrose by way of pacifiers has been used with modest benefit for infants receiving distressing procedure.

Most children aged 5 to 7 years and above can be taught to use cognitive-behavioral techniques. These techniques include relaxation, guided imagery, and hypnosis, and can diminish procedure-related distress. Sex-adjusted cognitive preparation may help children prepare themselves appropriately. Girls tend to overestimate the pain of procedures and boys to underestimate it.

Children often anticipate painful procedures with varying amounts of fear and anxiety. Pediatric patients who have experienced blood draws anticipate their next procedure with greater anxiety than those children looking ahead to their first blood draw. Therefore, it is important to make the first procedure as pleasant as possible. If a procedure is simply too noxious or complex, sedation or general anesthesia is appropriate. There is great debate over the gray zone between deep sedation and general anesthesia, and where the limits of practice lie for individual practitioners. When the need for more than light sedation arises, performing the procedure in a monitored sedating/anesthetizing location is indicated.

Circumcision Pain

This procedure is extremely common and often is performed with little or no analgesia for the infants. The AAP's latest position statement recommends that if parents choose to have their son circumcised, analgesia should be provided. Penile-ring blocks, using 0.8 cc lidocaine are very effective, dorsal-penile nerve blocks next so, with EMLA cream being effective to a lesser degree. All methods have extremely low complication rates. Infants appear to benefit from a sucrose pacifier to suck on, but this is a poor substitute for the other methods. It is extremely important to bear in mind that *epinephrine must not be used* in any blockade of the penis, or necrosis and sloughing of the penis can result.

Laceration Repair and Biopsy Pain

Topical administration of local anesthetics is an excellent method for relieving the pain of needle procedures, laceration repairs, and superficial biopsies. For intact skin, a widely used preparation is a eutectic mixture of prilocaine and lidocaine known as EMLA. Unfortunately, the cream usually requires at least 1 hour for adequate cutaneous analgesia. Theoretically, high blood levels of prilocaine metabolites can cause methemoglobinemia. This concern has not found to be problematic in clinical studies, even when EMLA has been used in infants. As mentioned above, iontophoretic lidocaine has been used effectively for placement of intravenous lines in children.

For application to cut skin, especially for laceration closure, combinations of local anesthetics with vasoconstrictors are widely used. The combination of tetracaine with adrenaline (epinephrine) and cocaine is known as TAC. This compound has been used effectively in emergency-room settings. TAC should be avoided in the vicinity of end arteries, to avoid ischemic complications. When larger doses have been applied to mucosal surfaces, rapid absorption of the tetracaine and cocaine has produced seizures and deaths. More recently, combinations of tetracaine and phenylephrine have been shown to be effective.

Chronic Pain

Cancer

Few areas of medicine are more emotionally challenging than the care of the child with cancer, or of the terminally ill child. Pharmacological management by the World Health Organization analgesic ladder is effective for most children with pain from widespread cancer. The "ladder" represents a progression from oral NSAIDs for mild pain to potent narcotics for severe pain. The key to successfully managing the child's cancer pain is constant reassessment. Pain that had been under control that is no longer controlled often represents disease progression, infection, procedural pain, fracture, or side effects of therapy. One must remember that cancer patients may have more routine pain such as tension headaches or muscle strains in addition to oncological-related pain. Planning analgesic regimens for children with cancer also must account for the child's emotional and cognitive development and the unique family dynamics.

Neuropathic pain may arise from neural invasion by tumor, chemotherapy, or surgical intervention, and be especially troublesome. This type of pain often responds poorly to opioids. Tricyclic antidepressants may be helpful. Amitriptyline or nortriptyline both can be useful, although only the former is available in intravenous (i.v.) form, for patients who cannot make use of the oral route. For those who do not already have one, a baseline electrocardiogram to rule out preexcitation syndromes or conduction delays is recommended. Anticonvulsants are powerful neuropathic pain medications. Carbamazepine has a long and proven track record for lancinating neuropathic pain, although platelet counts and hepatic enzymes must be monitored closely. Gabapentin is a relatively new anticonvulsant that has extensive anecdotal experience behind it. It has the advantage of having few, if any, interactions with other drugs. Side effects are mild in children and include sleepiness, dizziness, and ataxia. Dosing (up to 30 mg/kg/day in three divided doses) must be done cautiously in the setting of renal impairment, as gabapentin is excreted exclusively by the kidneys.

Lastly, the fear of addiction has traditionally stood in the way of proper pain treatment. While tolerance develops routinely, true addiction is extraordinarily rare in cancer patients. One must be ready to escalate opioid doses at a logarithmic rate at the very end of life in pediatric cancer patients, and caregivers should expect that many children will need "industrial doses" of opioids to be comfortable.

How to address the topic of dying, per se is one of the great challenges of pediatric palliative care. Often the family is reluctant to discuss death with the child, and to make the transition from therapy to palliation. Familial angst is natural and understandable and must be handled compassionately and honestly. How one discusses palliative care with the patient depends largely on the progress the family is making in their own psychological journey. The child may well have a greater understanding of death and its imminence than either the family or healthcare team appreciates. Children as young as 3 years of age have at least partially expressed the concepts of loss, grief, and permanence inherent in an adult's concept of death. Child-life workers, nurses, and behavioral-medicine specialists are invaluable allies in situations of terminal illness.

Overview of Benign Pains

The vast majority of pain complaints in children result from benign processes. Children commonly experience recurrent pains of the head, chest, abdomen, and limbs. Painful episodes usually alternate with pain-free times in an otherwise healthy child. These conditions are very common, with an estimated 4% to 10% of children experiencing these symptoms with some regularity.

Most children presenting with these "benign" complaints will be determined to be medically well. The primary-care practitioner needs to develop a screening approach that emphasizes a sensitive medical history and physical examination that detects the small subgroup of patients who need further workup. Laboratory and radiologic testing is seldom indicated. Unfocussed testing should be avoided. The history should include questions about family and school circumstances, diet, sleep, sports, and activity level. One must remain alert to detect the very small subset of children who suffer from more severe psychiatric illness such as depression and conversion disorder, or who are being subjected to Münchausen's syndrome by proxy. Some pain complaints are symptoms of a range of posttraumatic-stress conditions or of physical or sexual abuse. The history taken from any young person in chronic pain should include screening questions for suicidal ideation plans or attempts. Drug and alcohol use histories should be sought. The results of the initial evaluation usually can be used to formulate a plan that includes behavioral medicine, physical therapy, specialist referral, and judicious use of medication.

Unlike adults, most children are not gainfully employed; school performance serves an analogous function for children. Questions about school attendance and performance address the level of functioning of a pediatric patient. It is helpful to regard school avoidance in many cases as a disability syndrome analogous to work absenteeism in adults with chronic pain. Home-tutoring programs may have counter-productive consequences, and should not be encouraged. Much of the multidisciplinary effort of pediatric-pain programs is devoted to maximizing function and demedicalizing chronic pain.

Headache

Migraine and tension-type headaches increase in prevalence during the school-age years, being seen in children as young as 5 to 7 years. The vast majority of headaches are benign in origin. Fears of brain tumors often can be assuaged after careful history and physical, by a direct and honest discussion with the child and family. Certainly, any child who has focal neurologic signs or early morning headache accompanied by vomiting deserves intracranial imaging.

A number of mediations have proven useful for the prophylaxis of migraine in children, including trazodone, tricyclic antidepressants, and calcium-channel blockers. On the other hand, sumatriptan, which is quite effective in interrupting adult migraine attacks, may not be as useful in children. Propranolol, too, appears less effective in migraine prophylaxis in children. Trazodone can be started at low doses (25 mg) at bedtime and escalated over a period of a few weeks to 50 to 100 mg nightly. After a baseline electrocardiogram (ECG) (see above) nortriptyline is started at 10 mg nightly and escalated in 10-mg increments weekly. The patient should be told that although the effect on sleep is immediate, the analgesic effects might take 1 to 3 weeks. Side effects include dry mouth, morning sedation, constipation, urinary retention, and cardiac-conduction disturbances. Selective serotonin reuptake inhibitors (e.g., fluoxetine) raise blood levels of TCAs significantly, increasing the potential for toxicity.

There is a prominent role for behavioral medicine in the prophylaxis of both muscle tension-type headaches and pediatric migraine. Furthermore, transcutaneous electrical nerve stimulation (TENS) also can be an effective treatment of tension headache. There has been increasing attention paid to acupuncture, which may prove to be a useful adjunctive treatment.

Chest Pain

Chest pains are relatively common, especially in adolescents. The vast majority of such complaints are not cardiac in origin. The foremost fear in the patients and family's minds, however, is that a heart attack is the cause of pain. Patients who present with irregular pulses, syncope, or shortness of breath deserve an ECG and careful exclusion of entities such as aberrant coronary-artery anatomy and supraventricular tachydysrhythmias. For the majority, costochondritis, muscle strain, hyperventilation syndrome, precordial catch, asthma, and occasionally, spontaneous pneumothorax will explain the symptomatology. Reassurance, stretching exercises, NSAIDs, heat, and biobehavioral therapy are the mainstays of therapy for most chest pains.

Abdominal Pain

Recurrent abdominal pain, frequently accompanied by persistent school absenteeism, is a fairly frequent reason for primary-care office visits. The majority of recurrent abdominal pain in children is "functional" or nonorganic; however, indicators of potentially dangerous pathology always should be sought. Modifications of diet may have considerable benefit in some situations, as in a subgroup of who may improve by treatment of constipation or by treating lactose intolerance with oral lactase enzyme replacement or avoidance of milk products.

Once the practitioner in satisfied that no dangerous organic pathology is present, the patient and parents should be reassured that the work-up has been inclusive and nothing harmful has been missed. Attention then is turned (and this often meets great resistance) to demedicalizing the situation. Most of these patients can benefit from working with behavioral psychologists to learn coping and adaptive behaviors. Infrequently, the patient will need to be referred for diagnostic and therapeutic epidural or celiac-plexus blockade.

Back Pain

The pattern of back pain differs from that of adults. Almost half of adolescents presenting to one sports-medicine clinic for back pain have pain arising from spondylolysis-stress fractures of the *pars interarticularis*, compared to only 5% of adults having back pain. Often, anteroposterior and lateral spine x-rays are sufficient to make the diagnosis. Discogenic pain affects only 11% and muscle-tendon strain 6% of adolescents evaluated for low-back pain. For spondylolysis pain, back bracing, graded physical therapy, with a course of nonsteroidal antiinflammatory medications is a helpful regimen. Magnetic resonance imaging should be reserved for patients demonstrating radicular or other focal neurologic signs. Sciatica secondary to disc herniation responds to selected use of epidural steroids, physical therapy, and NSAIDs, as it does in adults. Surgery is needed very infrequently.

Pelvic Pain

An increasing number of young women are being seen for pelvic pain. Dysmenorrhea, musculoskeletal injury, ovarian cysts, psoas-muscle abscesses, and constipation make up the large portion of nonendometriosis pain in adolescent women. Endometriosis pain may or may not be related to the menstrual cycle. Sometimes, defecation or urination worsens the pain. School absenteeism can be prominent, and the patients can be extremely disabled, although this aspect is highly variable. Patients not responding to oral contraceptives and NSAIDs have been found on laparoscopic examination to have endometriosis about 70% of the time. Pelvic-inflammatory disease is prevalent in the adolescent population. A thorough sexual history must be taken, and referrals to a gynecologist for cultures made as needed.

If endometriosis is diagnosed, oral contraceptives can be used effectively. Gonadotropin-releasing hormone inhibitors are effective, but their utility is limited to short-term use in women over the age of 16, owing to the high risk for premature osteopenia. TENS units have strong anecdotal support for treating pelvic pain. Tricyclic antidepressants, NSAIDs, behavioral medicine, and physical therapy round out the multimodal therapy for the majority of pelvic pains.

Neuropathic Pain

Complex regional pain syndrome type 1 (CRPS1)/ reflex sympathetic dystrophy (RSD), postsurgical/post-traumatic peripheral neuropathy, CRPS II/causalgia, metabolic neuropathies, spinal cord injuries, and cancer comprise the majority of neuropathic pains. Amputation leads to phantom-limb pain much more commonly than once thought and can be intractable. Tricyclic antidepressants and anticonvulsants form the mainstay of pharmacologic therapy, along with cognitive-behavioral strategies and TENS technology. Amitriptyline or nortriptyline is utilized as described in the headache section above. Anticonvulsants have been used frequently in adults with neuropathic pain. Carbamazepine, phenytoin, and gabapentin are used relatively commonly. Sympathetic neural blockade, usually by way of an indwelling catheter, is warranted in select cases.

CRPS1/RSD in children and adolescents has a marked female predominance (roughly 5:1), a marked, lower-extremity predominance (roughly 6:1), and an apparent association with competitive sports, gymnastics, and dance. Pain can be severe and debilitating. Fortunately, even when CRPS in children is relatively advanced, prognosis for recovery is good. Approaches to treatment of CRPS1/RSD have been extremely varied, ranging from rehabilitative to more interventionist. Physical therapy is the centerpiece of CRPS/RSD therapy.

Spasticity

Spasticity affects patients who have cerebral palsy, spinal-cord injury, multiple sclerosis, or cerebral infarc-

tions. Baclofen, diazepam, and cyclobenzaprine can be effective treatments, although sedation and generalized hypotonia can limit its usefulness. In recent years, baclofen has been infused directly into the cerebrospinal fluid, bringing relief with diminished side effects to numerous patients. Referral to tertiary-care facilities for implantation of baclofen pumps is warranted for patients who would benefit from baclofen but who suffer from excessive side effects.

Sickle Cell Anemia

Pain in sickle cell disease is extremely variable in its frequency and severity. Most patients manage their persistent and episodic pains, using oral hydration, NSAIDs, and oral opioids. Hydroxyurea, a medication that promotes hemoglobin F production, can reduce the number of painful crises. Aggressive use of opioids at home may reduce the number of hospitalizations. Those patients with more severe episodes of vasoocclusive pain require hospital admission. The patients arriving for hospital care are frequently opioid-tolerant secondary to their home narcotic regimen. One must use their home regimen as a baseline for formulating an inpatient regimen. A basal infusion at an equianalgesic amount often will suffice. Use of a PCA with the basal infusion allows provision of adequate amount of narcotic without forcing the patient to use the bolus doses frequently. Relatively large doses of narcotic are required, and should be prescribed. After a couple of days, the practitioner can calculate the patient's total opioid requirement. Conversion to a combination of long-acting and immediate-release narcotics can be arranged. Use of pulse oximetry (apnea monitoring in selected cases) adds a layer of safety, as hypoxemia and hypercarbia further exacerbate sickling of erythrocytes. NSAIDs provide an opioid-sparing effect, and make this class of drugs especially useful for painful episodes if renal function is normal. Epidural analgesia has a role when opioid side effects preclude maximal analgesia. For the potentially deadly "chest crisis," a thoracic epidural should be considered early in the clinical course.

Human Immunodeficiency Virus/Acquired Immunodeficiency Syndrome

Children with human immunodeficiency virus/ acquired immunodeficiency syndrome often undergo a multitude of painful diagnostic and therapeutic procedures. Infants with encephalopathy and severe developmental delay can present with persistent irritability and screaming, without an obvious pain focus. Many of these patients respond to opioids. For other such children, anticonvulsants may be helpful, even in the absence of clinical seizures.

CONCLUSION

The vast majority of pain in children and adolescents can be treated, at least initially, by the primary-care practitioner. Pediatric-pain treatment services serve as resources for the more complex or refractory pain syndromes. Fortunately, the number of pediatric-pain clinics in the United States is growing. Information about the nearest clinic can be obtained most easily by way of the closest children's hospital, usually through the department of anesthesia.

SELECTED READINGS

American Academy of Pediatrics, T. F. o. C. Circumcision Policy Statement. *Pediatrics* 1999;103:684–685.

Berde CB, Beyer JE, Bournaki MC, et al. Comparison of morphine and methadone for prevention of postoperative pain in 3- to 7-year-old children. *J Pediatr* 1991;119 (Pt. 1):136–141.

Berde CB, Lehn BM, Yee JD, et al. Patient-controlled analgesia in children and adolescents: a randomized, prospective comparison with intramuscular administration of morphine for postoperative analgesia. *J Pediatr* 1991;118:460–466.

Collins JJ, Grier HE, Kinney HC, et al. Control of severe pain in children with terminal malignancy [see comments]. *J Pediatr* 1995;126:653–657.

Committee, o. D. Guidelines for monitoring and management of pediatric patients during and after sedation for diagnostic and therapeutic procedures. *Pediatrics* 1992;89:1110–1115.

Committee on Drugs and Section on Anesthesiology. Guidelines for the elective use of conscious sedation, deep sedation, and general anesthesia. *Pediatrics* 1992;76:317–321.

Finlay G, McGrath PJ, eds. *Measurement of Pain in Infants and Children. Progress in Pain research and Management.* Seattle: IASP Press, 1998.

Gil K, Wilson J, et al. The stability of pain coping strategies in young children adolescents, and adults with sickle cell disease over an 18-month period. *Clin J Pain* 1997;13:110–115.

Lee L, Olness K. Clinical and demographic characteristics of migraine in urban children. *Headache* 1997;37:269–276.

Micheli LJ, Wood R. Back pain in young athletes: significant differences from adults in causes and patterns. *Arch Pediatr Adolesc Med* 1995;149:15–18.

Scharff L. Recurrent abdominal pain in children: a review of psychological factors and treatment. *Clinical Psychology Review* 1997;17:145–166.

Schechter NL, Berde CB, et al. *Pain in Infants, Children and Adolescents.* Baltimore: Williams and Wilkins, 1993.

Shapiro B, Dinges D, Orne EC, et al. Home management of sickle cell-related pain in children and adolescents: natural history and impact on school attendance. *Pain* 1995;61:139–144.

Wilder RT, Berde CB, Wolohan M, et al. Reflex dystrophy in children: clinical characteristics and follow-up of seventy patients. *J Bone Joint Surg* 1992;74-A:910–919.

CHAPTER 62

Pain in the Elderly

Aida B. Won

Pain is one of the most common complaints among older people. In community-dwelling elderly, the prevalence of pain has been estimated between 25% and 50% with the prevalence of pain complaints being twice as great in those over 60 than in those under 60 years old.

The management of pain in the older patient often presents additional challenges. These include underreporting of symptoms, multiple medical problems, medication side effects, problems with assessment, problems with communication, mobility and safety issues, as well as consideration of the potential for medical, cognitive, and functional decline.

HISTORY AND PHYSICAL

The medical evaluation should begin with a thorough history and physical examination. Because the prevalence of musculoskeletal and neurological conditions increases with age, special attention should be given to these aspects of the history and physical examination. Conditions such as gout, diabetic neuropathy, herpes zoster, peripheral-vascular disease, and cancer are more common with increasing age. The most common complaints are musculoskeletal-related problems such as low-back and joint pain. If the cognitive status of the patient is in question, one also should speak with the primary caregiver to obtain a more reliable history. One should always ask about falls and occult trauma in the older population. We also should remember that immobility, contractures, and muscle strain also can be potential sources of musculoskeletal pain. Range-of-motion maneuvers and functional evaluation may reproduce pain and assist in functional assessment. A neurological examination also should be performed looking for signs of autonomic, sensory, and motor deficits to rule out neuropathic conditions. In addition to establishing a diagnosis, one also should establish a baseline description of their pain, including intensity, frequency, duration, character of the pain, as well as precipitating and relieving factors. Because many older persons may not refer to their discomfort as "pain," but rather use other descriptors such as "ache" and "hurt," we should try to use their language when eliciting a pain history. Documentation of the location of all sites of pain will enable healthcare professionals target their assessments and determine the functional implications of the pain. It also is helpful to review previous experiences with analgesics or other therapies. Problems and procedures for the assessment of pain are discussed below.

PAIN ASSESSMENT IN THE ELDERLY

A variety of pain-assessment tools have been developed in an attempt to document and follow pain symptoms over time. For example, unidimensional scales such as the visual-analog scale (VAS), the numerical-rating scale (NRS), and the verbal-descriptive scale (VDS) are commonly used to measure pain intensity. However, some of these pain-assessment tools can be difficult for some elders to complete because of impairments in vision, hearing, cognition, and manual dexterity. Research in both community dwelling and institutionalized elders indicates the VDS to be the easiest to complete, and the VAS and NRS as being be more difficult. However, repeated questioning and use of large print, hearing aids, and different tools can help facilitate responses.

More comprehensive approaches to pain assessment with multidimensional measures also exist. Melzack has created a simplified version of the McGill Pain Questionnaire (MPQ) known as the SF-MPQ, which was found to be usable in older individuals (Fig. 62.1). It includes descriptors representing sensory and affective components of pain. It also has measures to evaluate pain intensity such as the VAS and VDS (also known as the Present-Pain Inventory).

	NONE	MILD	MODERATE	SEVERE
THROBBING	0)____	1)____	2)____	3)____
SHOOTING	0)____	1)____	2)____	3)____
STABBING	0)____	1)____	2)____	3)____
SHARP	0)____	1)____	2)____	3)____
CRAMPING	0)____	1)____	2)____	3)____
GNAWING	0)____	1)____	2)____	3)____
HOT-BURNING	0)____	1)____	2)____	3)____
ACHING	0)____	1)____	2)____	3)____
HEAVY	0)____	1)____	2)____	3)____
TENDER	0)____	1)____	2)____	3)____
SPLITTING	0)____	1)____	2)____	3)____
TIRING-EXHAUSTING	0)____	1)____	2)____	3)____
SICKENING	0)____	1)____	2)____	3)____
FEARFUL	0)____	1)____	2)____	3)____
PUNISHING-CRUEL	0)____	1)____	2)____	3)____

VISUAL ANALOG SCALE

No pain |⊢————————————————⊣| Worst pain

PRESENT PAIN INVENTORY (PPI)

0 No Pain
1 Mild Pain
2 Uncomfortable
3 Distressing
4 Horrible
5 Excruciating

FIG. 62.1. The Short-Form McGill Pain Questionnaire. (Reprinted from Gagliese L, Melzack R. Chronic pain in the elderly. *Pain* 1997;70:3–14, with permission.)

Patients with mild to moderate cognitive impairment still can make basic needs known. Therefore, the use of simple questions and screening tools can be used to assess pain in this population. We recommend asking questions that are short, simple, and concrete. Questions should not be open-ended or require a response to more than two or three choices. Eliciting "yes" or "no" responses may be easiest. For example, instead of asking, "What makes your pain worse?" ask "Does your knee hurt when you walk around?" If the patient doesn't seem to understand you, do not simply repeat the question in a louder or slower voice. Change the sentence and use simpler and different words to explain yourself. Another technique that can be used in patients with more cognitive impairment is the observation of pain behaviors such as guarding, shifting weight, and slower movements, partic-

ularly when observed with testing of activities of daily living (ADL) functions. Some of the most common pain behaviors are listed (Table 62.1). These include changes in facial expressions, vocal behaviors, and body movements. Pain symptoms, behaviors and circumstances should be documented in pain diaries or flow sheets to enable the clinician to adjust treatment and determine the overall effectiveness of the pain-management program. The family and other caregivers also are important sources of information that also can tell about the likely meaning of such behaviors. Changes in the patient's routine, such as things they are now refusing to do, may be clues to the source of discomfort. An example of a pain flow sheet is given in Figure 62.2. In addition, persons with short-term memory impairment may not be able to remember how their pain compared with last week, or

TABLE 62.1. *Pain Behaviors*

Facial expressions
  Sad
  Grimace
  Clench teeth
  Angry
  Wrinkled forehead
Vocal behaviors
  Ask for pain medication/ someone to help pain
  Asking "Why me?"
  Telling others to "go away"
  Sigh
  Moan
  Scream
  Cry
  Call out
Body movements
  Guarding
  Change in gait
  Shifting weight
  Moving slowly
  Limping
  Increased periods of rest/ lying down
  Decreased social interactions
  Sudden change in daily activities
Other
  Sudden onset of confusion
  Irritable

even a few hours ago. Therefore, we suggest asking about pain symptoms more frequently.

MULTIDISCIPLINARY EVALUATION

A comprehensive evaluation is an extremely important part of the assessment of the older person with pain. As many patients grow older, problems such as deconditioning, falls, polypharmacy, cognitive dysfunction, and malnutrition become increasingly common. Unfortunately, these conditions also can be potentially worsened by the presence of pain. Periodic documentation of changes in function, mood, time involved in activities, caloric intake, and sleep patterns are just as important as documentation of pain symptoms and behaviors.

Assessment of function is very important so that mobility and independence can be maximized. A variety of geriatric assessment tools can be used. For example, the "get up and go" test is a timed measure of the patient's ability to rise from an armchair, walk 10 feet, turn around, walk back, and sit down again. Patients are considered independent for basic transfers if they are able to complete this sequence of maneuvers in less than 20 seconds. Other tests are more comprehensive such as the Katz ADL scale. This test asks whether the patient can accomplish various activities of daily living by themselves, if they need some help, or if someone else does it for them (Fig. 62.3). The Lawton IADL scale is similar, and inquires about instrumental ADL such as the ability to

DATE	TIME	PAIN INTENSITY [1]	SITE	BEHAVIORS [2]	ACTIVITY [3]	ANALGESIC TIME / DOSE	LEVEL OF AROUSAL [4]	EFFECTS / SIDE EFFECTS [5]

FIG. 62.2. Example of a pain-flow sheet. This should be filled out approximately every 3 hours, especially with initiation or changes in the treatment plan. *1*: Once an appropriate scale is chosen, it should be used for each assessment. However, if the patient cannot quantify pain intensity, the severity of pain behaviors should be recorded (e.g., mild, moderate, severe). *2*: Specific pain behaviors should be recorded, such as "calling out," or "guarding." *3*: Documentation of activities during the time of assessment will help determine the need for premedication, especially if the pain is intermittent or situational. This also will help monitor functional status. *4*: Because sedation occurs easily with narcotic use, the level of arousal should be recorded (e.g., awake and alert, awake, awake but drowsy, falling asleep, light sleep, deep sleep). *5*: Effects/side effects should document any benefits or problems encountered (e.g., nausea, constipation, confusion, unsteady gait, decreased appetite).

For each area of functioning, check the description that applies. (The word "assistance" means supervision, direction or personal assistance.)

1. Bathing (either sponge bath, tub bath, or shower)
☐ No assistance
☐ Some assistance in bathing only one part of the body (e.g. back or leg)
☐ Receives assistance in bathing more than one part of the body

2. Dressing
☐ No assistance (includes getting clothes and dressing self without help)
☐ Some assistance (dresses without assistance, but need help with tying shoes)
☐ Receives assistance in getting clothes, getting dressed, or stays partly or completely undressed

3. Toileting
☐ No assistance (goes to "toilet room" for bowel or bladder elimation, cleans self, and arranges clothes); may manage bedpan or commode, and empty in the morning on own)
☐ Some assistance (with going to the "toilet room", cleansing self, or arranging clothes, or use of bedpan or commode)
☐ Doesn't go to "toilet room", and dependent with cleansing and dressing afterwards

4. Transfers
☐ No assistance (able to moves in and out of bed or chair without help; may use cane or walker)
☐ Some assistance (needs help or supervision to get in and out of bed or chair)
☐ Total dependence on transfers, or doesn't get out of bed

5. Continence
☐ Has full self-control of urination and bowel movements
☐ Has occasional "accidents"
☐ Supervision helps keep continence; catheter used; person often incontinent

6. Feeding
☐ No assistance
☐ Some assistance (feeds self but gets help in pre-cutting meat/food)
☐ Completely unable to feed self (needs others to be fed partly or completely by mouth, tubes or IV fluids)

FIG. 62.3. Evaluation of Activities of Daily Living (ADL). Adapted from Katz S, Ford AB, Moskowitz RW, et al. Studies of illness in the aged. The index of ADL: a standardized measure of biological and psychosocial function. *JAMA* 1963;185:915, with permission.

use the telephone, arrange transportation, shop and prepare meals, do laundry and housework, take their own medications, and manage their own money. If functional impairment is a concern, the care plan probably should include physical and occupational therapies. Help with walking, transfers, balance, and strengthening, and use of assistive devices may help reduce pain and improve safety. Physical therapists often provide a variety of nonpharmacological pain-management techniques as well, such as heat, ultrasound, and transcutaneous electrical nerve stimulation (TENS). If safety is a concern, a home visit by a visiting nurse may be necessary to assess the home environment to minimize risks of falls and injuries.

Because depression and anxiety are strongly associated with pain in the elderly, a psychological assessment also should be part of the evaluation. A commonly used screening instrument for depression in the geriatric population is the Yesavage geriatric-depression scale (GDS). The questions are short and simple, and require only yes or no responses.

Psychosocial factors also may contribute to the perception of pain. Older patients experience many losses in their lives, which may result in fear, anxiety, loneliness, and depression. These can affect the perception of pain and other somatic complaints. Once medical factors are addressed, involvement of a mental-health professional and social worker often is useful to evaluate the social-support networks, identify dysfunctional relationships, and determine why the person is unhappy or anxious. Sometimes these feelings are due to interpersonal conflicts and misunderstandings with family, friends, or caregivers that can be identified and corrected. Sometimes all that is needed is reassurance, encouragement, or more social support, while others may require medication to help with their anxiety or depression. Social work staff also can be helpful in working with the family or living situation, as caregiver stress also is common. Sometimes a more structured environment (e.g., senior center, adult day healthcare) can reduce the risk of loneliness, depression, and anxiety.

PAIN MANAGEMENT IN THE ELDERLY

Guiding Principles

The following guiding principles and caveats for drug use may help maximize treatment efficacy and minimize adverse effects in the elderly (Table 62.2).

Principle 1: A Little Goes a Long Way

Because hepatic and renal function often are reduced as a normal part of aging, elderly patients may achieve pain relief from smaller doses of analgesics than those required by younger patients. Therefore, if the pain is mild to moderate, an opioid-naïve elderly person may have a good response with a half tablet to one tablet of

TABLE 62.2. *Guiding Principles for Analgesic Use in the Elderly*

A little goes a long way
  Start with low doses
    (one half to one third of usual adult dose)
  Increase slowly
  Be careful with long-acting forms
Use standing doses
  Avoid relying on prn doses
  Premedicate for predictable pain
Be compulsive about assessing pain and side effects
  Encourage use of pain-assessment flow sheets
  Reassess and adjust analgesics within hours/days
  Anticipate and monitor side effects closely
Involve the caregivers
  Caregivers are the gatekeepers of medicines
  Caregivers watch for efficacy and side effects
  Education and clear, written instructions improve
    cooperation and compliance

oxycodone. Extra caution should be taken with long-acting forms of analgesics, because of the problem of drug accumulation.

Principle 2: Use Standing Doses

Medications written as "prn" often assume that the patient knows when to ask or take analgesics, which often is a problem among cognitively impaired patients. If the pain is experienced at predictable times in the routine of their day, standing doses of analgesics should be used to prevent pain. For example, if the person usually experiences pain during the morning routine of getting up, the standing dose should be taken 1 hour before arising. If the pain is steady and continuous, analgesics should be used "around the clock."

Principle 3: Be Compulsive About Assessing Pain and Side Effects

Reassessment of pain relief and side effects should be performed within hours to days. Because we are working with a frailer population in whom drug accumulation occurs easily and adverse effects are more common and more devastating (e.g., confusion, aspiration, falls), the importance in assessing side effects cannot be emphasized enough. Adjustments may include changing the drug, dose, or timing of the medication.

Principle 4: Involve the Caregivers

Finally, it is important to educate and include the primary caregivers in the treatment plans. This includes clear, written instructions about pain assessment and potential side effects. Without their full understanding and cooperation, it is not uncommon for bad experiences to cause the patient or their family to fear the drug and lead to noncompliance and needless suffering later on.

Analgesic Drugs in the Elderly

In this section, we will highlight examples of drugs to avoid and give examples of drugs with favorable side-effect profiles in the elderly.

Acetaminophen is the drug of first choice for mild-to-moderate pain in the elderly. Acetaminophen can be used safely in the elderly up to 4,000 mg/day, and must be used cautiously in persons with liver failure. It has been demonstrated to be equally efficacious in treating osteoarthritis pain as ibuprofen both at analgesic and antiinflammatory doses.

Unfortunately, nonsteroidal antiinflammatory drugs (NSAIDs) are not as safe as acetaminophen. Common side effects include gastrointestinal (GI) bleeding, renal impairment, constipation, dizziness, and confusion in the elderly. Among NSAIDs, the nonacetylated salicylate preparations such as salsalate and trisalicylate are preferred because they seem to cause less GI erosion and platelet dysfunction. Reductions of GFR from NSAIDs are common among patients taking diuretics or with a history of congestive heart failure. However, if one still decides to use NSAIDs, we recommend that it be given at half the dose, at half the frequency, on an as-needed basis, and with GI prophylaxis, especially if they also are taking corticosteroids or anticoagulation. Misoprostol (Cytotec, G. D. Searle & Co., Chicago, IL, U.S.A.) is recommended to prevent both gastric and duodenal ulcers caused by NSAIDs at doses starting at 100 to 200 μg b.i.d. Proton-pump inhibitors (Prilosec, Astra Pharmaceuticals, L.P., Wayne, PA, U.S.A.; Prevacid, TAP Pharmaceuticals Inc., Deerfield, IL, U.S.A.) are also effective, and are less likely to cause diarrhea. H2-blockers, sucralfates, or antacids are not effective in preventing gastric ulcers caused by NSAIDs. Cyclooxygenase-2 (Cox-2) inhibitors are reportedly less likely to cause significant bleeding and ulcers than other NSAIDs, however, they can cause similar kidney effects including fluid retention and edema. Although promising, there is still some risk for GI bleeding and lower doses should be used until more experience is accumulated in frail elderly populations.

Drugs used to treat moderate to severe pain include preparations of acetaminophen or aspirin, which are combined with opioids (e.g., Tylenol No. 3, McNeil Consumer Products Company, Fort Washington, PA, U.S.A.; Percocet, Endo Laboratories, Chadds Ford, PA, U.S.A.; Darvon, Eli Lilly and Company, Indianapolis, IN, U.S.A.). However, there are some preparations we prefer not to use in the elderly. For example, codeine seems to cause more nausea and constipation. Propoxyphene (e.g., Darvon) has a toxic metabolite with a half-life of 36 hours and interacts with antidepressants, anticonvulsants, and warfarinlike drugs. Drugs with mixed agonist-antagonist receptor activity such as pentazocine (e.g., Talwin, Sanofi Pharmaceuticals, Inc., New York, NY, U.S.A.) and butorphanol (e.g., Stadol, Bristol–Myers Sqibb, Princeton, NJ, U.S.A.) never should be used, as these frequently cause delirium and agitation in older persons.

Caution should be used with tramadol (e.g., Ultram, Ortho–McNeil Pharmaceutical, Raritan, NJ, U.S.A.), as well. Although it is not technically an opioid, it has an efficacy similar to codeine. Its mechanism of action is on opioid, norepinephrine, and serotonin receptors. Until there is more experience in the older population, caution should be used with higher doses.

Of all the opioids used for the treatment of moderate-to-severe pain, morphine, oxycodone, and Dilaudid (Knoll Laboratories, Mount Olive, NJ, U.S.A.) are preferred. Demerol (Sanofi Pharmaceuticals, Inc.) never should be used in the elderly, because it is associated with an increased risk of delirium and seizure activity and has a long-acting and toxic metabolite, normeperidine.

The use of long-acting forms of opioids such as MS Contin (The Purdue Frederick Company, Norwalk, CT, U.S.A.) and OxyContin (Purdue Pharma L.P., Norwalk, CT, U.S.A.), should be used cautiously in the elderly, and considered only when the pain is stable and the opioid requirement is consistent for at least 48 to 72 hours. This also applies to the fentanyl patch (e.g., Duragesic, Janssen Pharmaceutica Inc., Titusville, NJ, U.S.A.). Although reduced amounts of subcutaneous fat may decrease the absorption of fentanyl, low protein stores associated with poor nutrition results in higher levels of free drug in the circulation. The use of a 25-μg patch is dangerous in an elderly opioid naïve patient and only should be used when the morphine requirement is calculated to be consistently about 80 to 90 mg/day over the previous 48 to 72 hours.

Anticipate and Treat Side Effects

Because side effects from opioid use occur more frequently in the elderly, we need to anticipate, monitor, and treat side effects efficiently. All efforts to use the minimum effective dose should be taken. This may include the consideration of more invasive procedures (e.g., hip or knee surgery, steroid injections, or viscosupplementation), if the patient is determined to be a suitable candidate.

Constipation with opioid use is almost always inevitable in the elderly. Tolerance does not occur, therefore prophylactic use of both stool softeners and peristaltic agents is recommended. Ambulation and physical exercise also helps constipation.

Nausea also is common, however tolerance may develop in 5 to 7 days. Initiating treatment with smaller doses of opioids may be helpful. Patients also should be evaluated and treated for other causes of nausea (e.g., gastritis, central nervous system swelling, constipation). If necessary, small doses of antiemetics should be used sparingly (e.g., 5 to 10 mg of metoclopramide three times a day prn) because of anticholinergic side effects. Dehydration occurs easily in the elderly, therefore fluid intake should be monitored carefully.

Sedation also is common. The risk for automobile accidents, falls, and other accidents is increased. Patients should be evaluated for safety, and efforts towards reducing or discontinuing other sedative medications should be undertaken. If possible, sedating medications should be given at bedtime. Addition of adjuvant medications also may help minimize opioid requirements. If the person does not have severe or unstable cardiac disease, one could consider a trial of Ritalin at low doses (5 to 10 mg once or twice a day).

Delirium is more common among patients with underlying dementia. The use of anticholinergic drugs should be minimized (e.g., diphenhydramine, amitriptyline, cyclobenzaprine). One should use the minimum-effective opioid dose, consider the addition of an adjuvant, or switch to a different opioid.

Adjuvant Therapy

Neuropathic pain is opioid resistant. Patients often are better off using adjuvant medication such as antidepressants or anticonvulsants. However, tricyclic antidepressants such as amitriptyline, doxepin, and imipramine should be avoided because they are highly sedative and anticholinergic. Use of secondary amines such as desipramine and nortriptyline are preferred because they have the lowest incidence of sedation and anticholinergic side effects, and are equally effective as well. In the elderly, these drugs should be started at one half to one third of the usual adult starting dose.

Anticonvulsants such as carbamazepine and valproate are both widely used and have well-established efficacy in the treatment of neuropathic pain. Clonazepam and gabapentin also should be considered early on because of their very low toxicity. The only major drawbacks of clonazepam are sedation and ataxia. Gabapentin is preferred in the elderly for several reasons: gabapentin does not have significant drug interactions; it has few side effects; and there is no need to monitor levels. It has been shown to be effective for peripheral neuropathic pain from diabetes and postherpetic neuralgia. It also can be used in conjunction with low-dose tricyclic antidepressants to augment efficacy. Because it can cause dizziness, drowsiness, and ataxia, we recommend starting with doses as low as 100 mg once or twice a day, and titrating up slowly.

Borg Exercise Intensity Scale*	Basic Exericse Prescriptions**	
	Enduranco Training	**Rocistanco Training**
6		
7 Very very light		
8		
9 Very light		
10	**Frequency** 3-5 days/week	2-3 days/week
11 Fairly light		
12	**Intensity** 40-75% max HR Or "**somewhat hard**" On Borg intensity Scale	60-80% max force production, or "**Hard**" to "**Very hard**" on Borg intensity Scale
13 Somewhat hard		
14	**Duration** 20-30 min/session	2-3 sets of 8-12 repetitions, 6 seconds/ repetition
15 Hard		
16		
17 Very Hard	**Examples** Walking, stairs, Cycling, swimming, Dancing	Weight lifting, elastic bands, isometrics, gravity exercises
18		
19 Very very hard		
20		

FIG. 62.4. Exercise in the Elderly. Borg Exercise Intensity Scale from Fiatarone MA. *Fit For Your Life Pocket Exercise Reference Guide*, 1998. Exercise intensity scale adapted from Borg G, Linderholme H. Exercise performance and perceived exertion in patients with coronary insufficiency, arterial hypertension and vasoregulatory asthenia. *Acta Med Scand* 1970;187:17–26. Guidelines for Exercise Prescriptions from Fiatarone MA. *Fit For Your Life Exercise Program Training Manual*, page 3.13, with permission.

Other adjuvants include steroids for pain from spinal-cord compression, soft-tissue infiltration, acute-nerve compression, or brain tumors. Steroids also help nausea, anorexia, and lethargy. For bony pain from compression fractures, calcitonin is a useful adjuvant. It can be used as a nasal spray at 200 i.u. q.d. or given as a subcutaneous injection at 100 i.u. q.d. Topical preparations include capsaicin cream. As it depletes substance P from nerve endings, it enhances pain control when added to systemic treatment for osteoarthritis, rheumatoid arthritis, diabetic neuropathy, or postherpetic neuralgia. Unfortunately, it is limited in use often because of the initial burning it causes or the need for frequent application.

Nondrug Pain Management

Nondrug approaches are a very important part of the pain-management strategy in the elderly because these address problems of functional decline, mood, and social isolation.

Enrollment in a multidisciplinary pain clinic often helps the patient deal with the functional and psychosocial sequelae of chronic pain. In addition to providing physical and occupational therapies, they also provide psychological support, and education about biofeedback, relaxation techniques, coping mechanisms, stress management, and communication skills. However, participants need to be cognitively intact to benefit from some of these techniques.

However, there are strategies that can be used even among elderly persons with cognitive impairment. Exercise is one of the most important interventions. Although many older people assume that exercise is an activity for younger persons, exercise in older persons has been shown to have many benefits, including reduction of pain symptoms, amelioration of depression, prevention of contractures, and improvement of appetite and self-esteem. It also helps with problems such as insomnia and constipation. Furthermore, exercise reduces recurrent falls and has the benefit of slowing bone loss. Understandably, the exercise program should be adapted to each person's ability and safety. Compliance is improved if low-tech, inexpensive, and simple exercises are emphasized, group socialization is provided, and personal exercise equipment is available such as stationary cycles and free weights. Guidelines for exercise prescriptions are shown in Figure 62.4.

Physical modalities such as heat, cold, manipulation, and massage should be employed in the treatment of musculoskeletal or soft-tissue pain. Precautions must be taken to avoid thermal burns, especially among patients with sensory or cognitive impairment. Other strategies include ultrasound and TENS.

Another effective behavioral intervention for those with cognitive impairment is distraction. Examples of distraction techniques include music, conversation, and activity involvement.

CONCLUSION

We must remember that "success" is relative. Goals often are different in the older population. The goal of care in the elderly usually is not return to work or prolongation of life, but maximization of quality of life. This might include goals such as being able to walk 100 feet independently or being able to play bingo or bridge every day. Although improvements may not necessarily be as dramatic as in the younger population, minimal improvements in pain, mood, functional capacity, or activity involvement may lead to large gains in quality of life.

SELECTED READINGS

AGS Panel on Chronic Pain in Older Persons. The management of chronic pain in older persons. *J Am Geriatr Soc* 1998;46:635–651.

Ettinger WH, Jr., Burns R, Messier SP, et al. A randomized trial comparing aerobic exercise and resistance exercise with a health education program in older adults with knee osteoarthritis. The fitness arthritis and seniors trial (FAST). *JAMA* 1997;277:25–31.

Ferrell BA. Pain management in elderly people. *J Am Geriatr Soc* 1991;39: 64-73.

Ferrell BA, Ferrell BR, Osterweil D. Pain in the nursing home. *J Am Geriatr Soc* 1990;38:409–414.

Gagliese L, Melzack R. Chronic pain in elderly people. *Pain* 1997;70:3–14.

Herr KA, Mobily PR. Comparison of selected pain assessment tools for use with the elderly. *Appl Nurs Res* 1993;6:39–46.

Hurley AC, Volicer BJ, Hanrahan PA, et al. Assessment of discomfort in advanced Alzheimer patients. *Res Nurse Health* 1992;15:369–377.

Preisinger E, Alacamlioglu Y, Pils K, et al. Exercise therapy for osteoporosis: results of a randomised controlled trial. *Br J Sports Med* 1996;30:209–12.

Weiner D, Peterson B, Keefe F. Chronic pain-associated behaviors in the nursing home: resident versus caregiver perceptions. *Pain* 1999;80:577–588.

Won A, Lapane K, Gambassi G, et al. Correlates and management of non-malignant pain in the nursing home. SAGE Study Group. Systematic assessment of geriatric drug use via epidemiology. *J Am Geriatr Soc* 1999;47:936–942.

CHAPTER 63

Principles of Pain Management in the Addicted Patient

Adam J. Silk

Evaluating and treating pain, in a patient with a history of substance abuse, often is challenging. This chapter will review important diagnostic strategies and will discuss principles of management for both acute and chronic pain in the addicted patient.

DIAGNOSIS OF SUBSTANCE-ABUSE DISORDERS

The question of whether a patient has a substance-abuse *problem* is not always an easy one to settle. Substance abuse frequently is well hidden. While many patients' addictions are obvious (e.g., the patient on methadone maintenance or the person with multiple drunk-driving episodes) others may be harder to diagnose. Because of this, a review of how to diagnose a substance-abuse disorder follows.

It should be remembered that there is a wide range of severity of substance-abuse problems. The most recent psychiatric nosology divides substance-abuse disorders into "abuse" and "dependence" syndromes, with the latter being more severe. (The diagnostic criteria for substance abuse and substance dependence are presented in Tables 63.1 and 63.2.)

The principle guiding the diagnosis of substance-abuse problems is that substance "use" becomes "abuse" when that use results in repeated and significant adverse consequences for the patient. The list of these possible consequences can be quite varied, but in general, most problems tend to occur in one or more of the following four areas: social, medical, financial, and legal.

It should be noted that physiologic dependence on a substance is not a litmus test for diagnosing an addiction problem. This is because (a) many substances of abuse may produce little or no physiologic dependence (e.g., cocaine), and (b) some medically prescribed drugs may produce physiologic dependence if taken as prescribed, without causing adverse consequences (e.g., opiates, barbiturates, benzodiazepines). While physiologic dependence *may* be an important symptom of a substance-abuse problem, the diagnosis usually rests more reliably on taking a history of repeated, significant, adverse consequences of use.

Clinicians treating a patient in pain may suspect the presence of a substance-abuse problem, but be uncertain whether their suspicions are justified. This is an appropriate time to obtain consultation from a mental-health and/or addiction-medicine professional, to clarify the diagnosis.

Once a diagnosis of a substance-abuse problem has been made, the next step should be a complete diagnostic evaluation. This evaluation should, at minimum, cover the areas of pain, addiction, and other psychiatric conditions. (In certain patients, further medical evaluation must be included as well.) The main reason for such a comprehensive evaluation is that it is common for pain problems, substance abuse, and psychiatric conditions to act synergistically to create a complex, difficult-to-manage clinical situation. In such cases, a vicious cycle can be set up, in which the patient's various problems all seem to exacerbate each other. An effective strategy for dealing with this is to start with a full evaluation, which can then lead to *simultaneous* treatment of the patient's different conditions. What follows is an outline of the most important information to be obtained in such an evaluation.

The *pain* evaluation is covered extensively in other chapters in this book, and will not be detailed here.

The *addictions* evaluation should explore which substances have been used over what time period. The assessment of severity of abuse, as described above, rests on the number of adverse consequences resulting from use. Other important history includes whether the per-

TABLE 63.1. *Criteria for Substance Abuse*

1. A maladaptive pattern of substance use leading to clinically significant impairment or distress, as manifested by one (or more) of the following, occurring within a 12-mo. period:
   a. Recurrent substance use resulting in a failure to fulfill major role obligations at work, school, or home (e.g., repeated absences or poor work performance related to substance use; substance-related absences, suspensions, or expulsions from school; neglect of children or household)
   b. Recurrent substance use in situations in which it is physically hazardous (e.g., driving an automobile or operating a machine when impaired by substance use)
   c. Recurrent substance-related legal problems (e.g., arrests for substance-related disorderly conduct)
   d. Continued substance use despite having persistent or recurrent social or interpersonal problems caused or exacerbated by the effects of the substance (e.g., arguments with spouse about consequences of intoxication, physical fights)
2. The symptoms have never met the criteria for substance dependence for this class of substance.

From *Diagnostic and Statistical Manual of Mental Disorders,* (DSM-IV). Washington, DC: American Psychiatric Association, 1994, with permission.

TABLE 63.2. *Criteria for Substance Dependence*

A maladaptive pattern of substance use, leading to clinically significant impairment or distress, as manifested by three (or more) of the following, occurring at any time in the same 12-mo. period:

1. Tolerance, as defined by either of the following:
   a. A need for markedly increased amounts of the substance to achieve intoxication or desired effect
   b. Markedly diminished effect with continued use of the same amount of the substance
2. Withdrawal, as manifested by either of the following:
   a. The characteristic withdrawal syndrome for the substance
   b. The same (or a closely related) substance is taken to relieve or avoid withdrawal symptoms
3. The substance often is taken in larger amounts or over a longer period than was intended
4. There is a persistent desire or unsuccessful efforts to cut down or control substance use
5. A great deal of time is spent in activities necessary to obtain the substance (e.g., visiting multiple doctors or driving long distances), use the substance (e.g., chain smoking), or recover from its effects
6. Important social, occupational, or recreational activities are given up or reduced because of substance use
7. The substance use is continued despite knowledge of having a persistent or recurrent physical or psychological problem that is likely to have been caused or exacerbated by the substance (e.g., current cocaine use despite recognition of cocaine-induced depression, or continued drinking despite recognition that an ulcer was made worse by alcohol consumption)

From *Diagnostic and Statistical Manual of Mental Disorders,* 4th ed. (DSM-IV). Washington, DC: American Psychiatric Association, 1994, with permission.

sons closest to the patient also are involved with substance abuse, the patient's history of prior substance abuse treatment, and the patient's level of motivation to make changes in substance use. Finally, it is helpful to know the longest period that the person has gone without abusing alcohol or drugs, and how that earlier period of sobriety was maintained (e.g., treatment, incarceration).

The *psychiatric* evaluation should seek to determine whether the patient has a current or past history of a mood, psychotic, anxiety, or personality disorder. Every effort should be made to take a careful chronology of both psychiatric and substance-abuse disorders, so that causal links may be established. For example, does opiate use predate depression, or vice versa?

To repeat: the goal of the evaluation phase is to arrive at a treatment plan that can effectively address the patient's different needs, and thereby interrupt the cycle in which addiction, other psychiatric problems, and pain all exacerbate each other.

TREATMENT

Treating pain in a patient with a substance-abuse disorder frequently makes clinicians anxious. Doctors and nurses worry about the twin dangers of undertreating and overtreating pain, about the risks of precipitating worsening addictive behaviors by prescribing opiates, and about medicolegal risks they may be running. An exhaustive treatment of this complex subject is beyond the scope of this chapter, but an attempt will be made to outline basic principles that should guide therapy.

The most vexing, and most commonly asked clinical question is whether or not to prescribe opiates for an addicted patient in pain. Asked in that form, of course, no simple yes or no answer is possible. Whether or not to prescribe opiates ultimately should depend on the clinical evaluation described above, and specifically on the answers to the following three questions:

1. Is the pain acute or chronic?
2. What is the current severity of the patient's substance-abuse problem?
3. To what extent is the patient involved in other appropriate treatment modalities?

ACUTE PAIN

Acute pain generally is defined as self-limited and usually associated with specific injury, disease, or inflammatory process. It is frequently recognizable by characteristic autonomic changes. Opiates have long been the mainstay of pharmacotherapy of acute pain. There has been widespread concern for the past decade that American doctors tend to undertreat acute pain, which has frequently been attributed to doctors' fears of "creating" addicted patients. Thus, it is not surprising that doctors

TABLE 63.3. *Guidelines for Management of Acute Pain in the Known or Suspected Opiate Addict*

1. Define the pain syndrome and provide treatment for the underlying disorder.
2. Distinguish among the patient with a remote history of drug abuse, the patient receiving methadone maintenance, and the patient who is actively abusing drugs.
3. Apply appropriate pharmacologic principles of opioid use:
   a. Use the appropriate opioid.
   b. Use adequate doses and dosing intervals.
   c. Use appropriate route of administration.
4. Provide concomitant nonopioid therapies when appropriate:
   a. Use nonopioid analgesics.
   b. Use nonpharmacologic therapies.
5. Recognize specific drug-abuse behaviors.
6. Avoid excessive negotiations over specific drugs and doses.
7. Provide early consultation to appropriate services:
   a. Psychiatry and substance abuse service.
   b. Pain service (If available).
8. Anticipate problems associated with opioid prescription renewals if outpatient treatment is required.

From Portenoy RK, Payne R. Acute and Chronic Pain, In: Lowinson J, Ruiz P, Millman RB, et al., eds. *Substance Abuse: A Comprehensive Textbook,* 2nd ed. Baltimore: Williams & Wilkins, 1992, with permission.

are frequently uncomfortable prescribing opiates for patients with known addiction histories. In patients with clear acute pain (e.g., postsurgical pain), however, opiates remain central to therapy, including for addicted patients. Indeed, in patients with pharmacologic tolerance to opiates, the doses required may be higher than in the nonaddicted patient.

However, concerns about overuse of opiates in this population often are well founded. The clinician responsible for pain management should, if possible, work in close collaboration with colleagues in psychiatry and/or addiction medicine. One useful set of guidelines for the management of acute pain in the opiate-addicted patient is presented in Table 63.3.

For more detailed discussion of particular medications and dosing strategies, the reader is referred to Portenoy and Payne 1992 and Tucker 1990.

CHRONIC PAIN

Treating chronic pain in patients with substance-abuse disorders requires somewhat different management strategies. This is particularly true regarding the use of opiates. Clinicians may feel considerable pressure from their patients to prescribe opiates, and may find it difficult to persuade patients to get treatment for substance-abuse problems. Patients also may resist trying other treatments for their pain, both pharmacologic and non-

pharmacologic. These problems may be easier to deal with if certain principles are remembered:

1. Think within a chronic-disease model. As with any other chronic medical problem (e.g., diabetic complications, chronic heart disease), therapy should seek to improve the patient's functioning, and not to cure the problem. The clinician should assess the patient's functioning in the area of social relationships, work, etc., and evaluate his own treatment by its effect on functioning in these areas. The patient's subjective description of his or her pain, while important, should not be the only clinical variable of concern. In the case of the addicted patient, there are actually two chronic diseases that are ongoing (pain and addiction), and the clinician should thus be even more cautious about "going for cure."
2. Patients with active problems in both the areas of chronic pain and addiction should be managed if possible by a team of clinicians, and not a single provider. The care of such patients requires expertise in a wide array of fields, and few clinicians are adequately skilled in all relevant areas. It is far less taxing for a clinician to care for such patients if he is not alone with the whole clinical burden. For such joint management to succeed, it is crucial that lines of communication, and division of responsibility, be as clear as possible between clinicians. Issues such as who prescribes which medications, what happens when one member is on vacation, and so on, should be clearly agreed upon and spelled out. Otherwise, problems may arise that affect quality of care.
3. Treatment generally is most successful if more than one treatment *modality* is used. Pharmacologic interventions alone rarely are successful in the treatment of *either* chronic pain or addiction, so it is unlikely that medication alone will be sufficient for a patient with *both* conditions. Considerable success has been demonstrated with psychosocial treatments for patients in chronic pain, both in cognitive-behavioral therapies, group therapies, and biofeedback therapy (Caudill 1994). Many patients with these problems struggle with psychological problems related to loss of functioning, and may benefit from professional mental-health treatment.

There is now considerable experience with the use of nonopiate pain medications for chronic pain. Clinicians have had success with antidepressants, antiepilepsy drugs, and antiinflammatory medications. A detailed review of the use of these medications for chronic pain is beyond the scope of this chapter; the reader is referred to other relevant chapters in this volume.

Finally, the use of opiates as the single treatment modality for patients with chronic pain and active addiction is, in my experience, never successful. Even when other treatment modalities are in place, chronic use of opiates poses a significant risk of exacerbating a substance-abuse problem, and generally should be avoided.

The reader may object that the type of multimodal, team-oriented approach to treatment outlined here is impractical in a time of limited resources in healthcare. However, issues of cost must be put in context. Many such patients, if not managed appropriately, will be seen in repeated, wasteful emergency-room visits and hospitalizations. The approach outlined, although cumbersome compared to managing simpler outpatient problems, may well be the most cost-effective for this group of complex patients. And the clinical stakes here are high. The successful treatment of such patients can restore their normal functioning to a remarkable extent, and can thereby be a source of great benefit for patients, clinicians, and society.

SELECTED READINGS

Diagnostic and Statistical Manual of Mental Disorders, 4th ed. (DSM-IV). Washington, D.C.: American Psychiatric Association, 1994.

Portenoy RK, Payne R. Acute and chronic pain. In: Lowinson J, Ruiz P, Millman RB, et al., eds. *Substance Abuse: A Comprehensive Textbook*, 2nd ed. Baltimore: Williams & Wilkins, 1992.

Tucker C. Acute pain and substance abuse in surgical patients. *J Neurosci Nurs* 1990;22:339–349.

Caudill M. *Managing Pain Before It Manages You*. New York: Guilford Press, 1994.

CHAPTER 64

Legal Aspects of Pain Management

Edward Michna and Keira P. Mason

The specialty of pain management is no different from any other area of medical practice: it is vulnerable to the threat of litigation. In an effort to eliminate or ameliorate a patient's pain, the pain-management physician may resort to invasive therapies. Some of these invasive and sometimes extreme therapies carry an inherent risk of inadvertent injury to uninvolved nerves, organs, or vessels. At first glance, the practice of pain management may appear to expose the physician to a higher-than-average risk of litigation. Pain patients usually have visited numerous physicians prior to being referred to a pain specialist. Often, the primary-care doctor has exhausted different therapies, which may include polypharmacy and interventional procedures, prior to making the referral. The pain specialist all too often is the "last resort." Frustrated, sometimes depressed, and always in pain, the patient comes to the pain specialist with high and often unrealistic expectations. If the patient does not attain his desired relief, is dissatisfied with his outcome, or is involved in an adverse event, he then may decide to seek compensation for the injury (or perceived injury).

The pain-management population frequently is involved in workman's compensation, motor-vehicle accident, and personal-injury suits. There are predictors for which patient is most likely to sue. Specifically, those patients that already have been engaged in prior litigation have a greater incidence of filing future lawsuits. These are the patients that pain physicians should be wary of. These particular patients may have unrealistic goals and expectations. It is with this patient population that the physician should be very careful to delineate not only the challenging nature of the pain problem but also the difficulty in achieving a high rate of "success." The pain physician must expect that some patients will not achieve their desired level of pain relief, and will consequently feel disappointed and discouraged. Especially in the event of an untoward complication, there will be a greater tendency for this patient to seek legal redress.

It is very difficult to find any statistics that cite the actual number of lawsuits involving pain physicians. The reason that these statistics are difficult to determine reflects the diversity of medical specialties that practice pain management. These specialties can include neurologists, anesthesiologists, pain specialists, radiologists, acupuncturists, and primary-care doctors. When claims are made, they are listed under the primary specialty of the physician, not under the heading of a pain-management subspecialty. This makes it difficult to extract the frequency at which a physician who practices pain management is sued. Although the nature of both the patient population and the invasive specialty suggest a higher rate of legal claims, there is no published data to substantiate this.

Although the medical malpractice crisis of the late 1970s and early 1980s is a distant memory, all physicians still must exercise caution. To reduce the risk of a lawsuit for medical malpractice and any subsequent penalties, physicians should be careful in their patient selection (especially when performing invasive procedures), documentation (especially with respect to informed consent), and care of all patients. A recent review of the American Society of Anesthesiologists (ASA) Closed Claims Project database reveals that claims made for pain management in the nonoperative setting have increased. This increase reflects the growth that has occurred in the specialty of pain management. This growth is evidenced by an increase in both the physicians who are being trained in the pain specialty and the number of invasive procedures performed.

In this chapter, we will review the elements of a medical-malpractice lawsuit and the areas of particular concern for pain physicians. We will conclude with suggestions as to how physicians can protect themselves and, thereby, limit their liability.

To protect/defend oneself from a lawsuit, it is important to recognize that there must be a basis for a legal claim. When a legal claim is made against a physician, it usually is for medical malpractice. By definition, medical malpractice occurs when a physician is determined under the law to be negligent. The term "negligence" is defined clearly as conduct that falls below an established standard of care. This standard of care has been created to protect all citizens from an unreasonable risk of harm. To bring a medical malpractice lawsuit against a physician, a patient must show that there was negligence. A plaintiff (patient) must establish the following four elements to sue for negligence (medical malpractice):

1. The physician owed a duty of care to the patient.
2. The physician breached his duty of care.
3. The breach of duty was the proximate cause of an injury.
4. There was an injury.

A physician should understand all of the above four elements of a negligence case to both protect and defend himself from a legal claim. In the following four paragraphs, each element will be defined.

DUTY OF CARE

The first element requires that there was a duty of care to the patient. As soon as a physician meets with a patient, the state imposes this duty of care. This duty requires that the physician adhere to a standard of care. This standard is not clearly defined for every possible patient-care situation. Instead, the state establishes a general guideline. The physician is not expected to practice at the highest levels of skill or expertise. Rather, the state defines the "standard of care" as that exhibited by a physician who practices with the "skill of an average and reasonable physician acting under similar circumstances." There are different standards of care when comparing a general practitioner to a medical specialist. A specialist is held to a higher standard than a general practitioner.

BREACH OF DUTY

The second element that is necessary to pursue a negligence lawsuit is proof that there was a breach of the duty of care to the patient. For a court to determine if there was a breach of duty, expert testimony usually is needed. Both sides to the lawsuit (plaintiff and defendant) must be prepared to present expert testimony, usually from physicians in similar fields of practice. This expert testimony is designed to help the judge and jury determine if the physician acted in a reasonable and proper manner under the given circumstances. It often is difficult to determine if treatment plans were reasonable. Even expert testimony does not always agree. Physicians, in general, and especially those that practice pain management, frequently have differing and at times opposing views as to proper treatment protocols. The important

factor in determining breach of duty is to prove that there was negligence. Negligence does not exist if reasonable care and skill were exercised in choosing and executing the therapeutic choice, provided that the course of therapy is reasonable. In other words, even if 99 out of 100 physicians would have pursued another course of therapy, there was no negligence as long as the therapy chosen was reasonable under the circumstances.

All physicians across the country are held to the same standard of care. In the past, this was not always the case. Historically, the courts have applied the locality rule. This rule originally specified that the standard of care be judged by the practice patterns in the regional area where the physician practiced. In recent years, however, as a result of the information age and rapid transfer of information by way of the internet, most courts have abandoned the locality rule. Physicians in all areas of the country must demonstrate the same standard of care.

PROXIMATE CAUSE

The third element that is required is for the breach of the duty of care to the patient to be the "proximate cause" of the sustained injury. Establishing a breach of the duty of care is not enough. This breach must be shown to have lead to the injury. To establish "proximate cause," there has to be a causal connection between the inferior care and the injury sustained. Proximate cause also requires that the physician's actions were a significant factor and not an incidental factor in the occurrence of the injury.

INJURY

The final element required for negligence to be established is that the patient must have suffered an injury. This injury can be physical, mental, or financial. Without an established injury, one cannot establish a case for negligence. It is the job of the jury or judge (in a nonjury trial) to determine the monetary value of the damage. To set a monetary value on these damages, testimony is given as to the out-of-pocket expenses incurred as a result of the injury. These expenses can include hospital bills, time lost from unemployment (lost wages), physician costs, and incidental costs. Often, expert witnesses are called upon to testify as to the economic value of an injury. Examples would include economic value of lost income over a lifetime or value of projected medical bills. Not all injuries are tangible. Monetary values are difficult to assign when there are no bills or projected costs. In particular, difficulty arises in assigning value to pain and suffering endured by the plaintiff. Ultimately, it is the duty of the jury to assign a value based on the testimony and their own valuation of the injury.

Pain and suffering can be costly. As in the case of Dianna Helsel et al. vs. Harry Sernaker, M.D., Harbor Hospital Center, Harbor Pain Management Associate,

P.A., Baltimore City (MD) Circuit Court, Case No. 96275040. In this case, Ms. Helsel, a clerical worker, received cervical-facet injections. During the procedure, the defendant anesthesiologist accidentally punctured the brainstem with the spinal needle. As a consequence, she suffered a stroke and permanent injury to the pons and brainstem, with subsequent swallowing deficit and muscle paralysis to the left facial muscle and vocal cord. Despite the doctor's defense that the stroke was a result of inadvertent injection in to the left vertebral artery, a known risk of the procedure, the jury awarded a $5,183,288 verdict to the plaintiff. This award included $1.5 million for pain and suffering and $614,516 for wage loss and $1,090,018 for future medical care.

Prior to coming to trial, it is possible to estimate what the projected damages will amount to. A general rule-of-thumb multiplies the medical bills and expenses incurred by a factor of two or three. Often, a sympathetic jury may agree to unreasonably excessive damages. In this event, however, the judge always can intervene. The judge has the authority to disallow any award he feels unreasonable subject to review of an appellate court.

INFORMED CONSENT

The concept of informed consent is an important area in medical litigation. Before a physician may administer treatment or perform a procedure on a patient, the law requires that informed consent be received. By definition, informed consent requires that two elements be present: that consent is given and that the patient is informed of the risks, benefits, and side effects prior to consenting to a procedure. In some jurisdictions, consent must be written, in others an oral consent also may be valid. The written consent provides the greatest degree of proof, carries the greatest weight, and is the preferred mode of obtaining consent.

There are two tests that determine if the consent falls under the definition of "informed." These two tests are described as the reasonable patient standard and the reasonable professional standard. The reasonable-patient standard requires that the physician describe all risks, benefits, costs, and side effects as well as other reasonable options that a reasonable patient would consider significant prior to making the decision to proceed with the therapy. The professional standard requires that the physician describe to a patient that information which a reasonable medical practitioner would give under a similar circumstance. State jurisdiction sets the standards of how much information needs to be transmitted to the patient to ensure a fully informed consent.

The issue of if an informed consent has been given by the patient for a treatment or procedure can be another issue for medical litigation. Informed consent as a legal doctrine has its origin in common law under the concept of battery. Battery is defined as the unprivileged touching of one person by another. In medicine, it is used to impose liability on the physician who performs surgery or a procedure without obtaining an informed consent from the patient.

A cause of action involving informed consent can be brought under either negligence or battery. Most cases are brought under negligence. In a negligence case, the question is if the patient received enough information when consent was sought and given. Specifically, the issue is whether or not the patient received enough information prior to giving informed consent. Even in the event of an unfavorable outcome, proof that the physician provided the patient with a full informed consent could prevent unfavorable litigation. One example of this is the case of James W. Lacer vs. Cheryl Rowley, M.D., Adams County (CO) District Court, Case No.97-CV-202. In this case, a cervical-epidural steroid injection resulted in an epidural infection that ultimately required surgical debridement. Despite the unfavorable outcome, the jury returned a verdict for the defendant. After hearing testimony, the jury concluded that the doctor had given proper informed consent, had not acted negligently and had given proper patient care in the recognition and treatment of the ensuing problem.

In a battery case, the issue is whether or not consent was given at all. This may not always be so obvious. For example, although consent was obtained initially, the procedure may have been different than that initially discussed, or the procedure may have evolved to become more involved than that initially described. All the aforementioned would constitute battery.

Each legal theory has different statutes of limitation and damages allowed. In some jurisdictions, there are differences in the length of statute of limitations. Negligence is covered by malpractice insurance and battery is not. A patient will sue under the theory that best suits the goals and limitations of his/her particular case.

LEGAL IMPLICATIONS OF OPIOID THERAPY

There are both criminal and civil legal considerations for physicians when they prescribe opioids and other controlled substances. The Federal Controlled Substances Act of 1970 established the Drug Enforcement Agency and set forth the law governing the manufacture, distribution, and prescribing of controlled substances. Each state has similar controlled-substances legislation. Recently, there has been increased scrutiny by state and federal authorities regarding physicians' prescribing practices. There have been several well-publicized instances of physicians having their medical licenses revoked because of narcotic prescribing patterns.

The most famous case involving inappropriate prescribing practice appeared on the television show *60 Minutes* and as the cover story of *USA News and World Report*. This segment highlighted the actions of Dr.

William Hurwitz, an internist who prescribed large amounts of short-acting narcotics for nonmalignant pain syndromes. The Drug Enforcement Agency was alerted because of the large quantity of opioids being dispensed in that region. After a thorough investigation, the Medical Board of Virginia suspended his medical license. The Board found the following: excessive and indiscriminate prescribing of narcotics, ineffective monitoring of patients, four of his patients abused and sold their narcotics, and two patients overdosed on their medications. His license was eventually reinstated, but Dr. Hurwitz had to endure over 1 year of legal battles. Fearful of the increased scrutiny of the law many practitioners are hesitant to prescribe narcotics, especially for nonmalignant pain. This fear contributes to the continuing problem of the undertreatment of pain.

In a recent disciplinary action, the Oregon Board of Medical Examiners disciplined a pulmonary specialist for insufficiently treating pain in his patients. This act may be monumental in the legal and medical community, because it punished a doctor for under prescribing, rather than the traditionally feared action of prescribing too much. The board found that the doctor had prescribed inadequate amounts of narcotics, and, consequently, failed to alleviate pain in six of his patients between 1993 and 1998. The board cited one example where the doctor denied sedatives and pain medications to an intubated patient who had been administered a neuromuscular blocker (paralytic). His punishment included a 1-year peer-review program, regular visits to a psychiatrist, and a course on patient-physician communication. As a result of this action, we can anticipate that others will follow.

Aside from the criminal and disciplinary actions, physicians also can be sued in civil courts for negligence in prescribing controlled substances. Opioids have the potential for producing addiction, untoward side effects and, occasionally, lack of efficacy. All prescriptions of opioids by physicians require that the patient receive good monitoring and follow-up. There are numerous negligence suits that involve physicians who have been successfully sued for the negligent prescribing of opioids. The physicians were held to be negligent because they did not closely monitor for effectiveness or for side effects. The patients involved became addicted or developed mental-status changes as a result of the inadequate follow-up. In other malpractice cases, physicians have been held negligent for prescribing opioids for improper indications.

LEGAL IMPLICATIONS OF PERFORMING INVASIVE PROCEDURES

The practice of performing nerve blocks and nerve-ablating procedures has been associated with numerous, well-documented complications. These complications frequently lead to litigation. The American Society of Anesthesiology (ASA) Closed Claims Project database has been reviewed recently to identify the number of claims made for pain management in the nonoperative setting. A total of 148 claims out of the 4,183 anesthesia claims over the years 1970 to 1995, were for nonoperative pain management. It appears that a majority of these claims were made secondary to complications of invasive procedures: pneumothorax accounting for 28%, nerve damage accounting for 21%, and death and brain damage for 5% and 4%, respectfully. The investigation also reported an increasing number of claims over time. The greatest increase in claims was over the years 1990 to 1994. This increase mirrors the growth both in the number of pain procedures performed and the pain-management specialty overall.

The closed claim studies are helpful to study trends and causes of litigation. The database cannot provide absolute numbers of cases, however, because it is limited to anesthesia claims and involves only 50% of the insurance companies. We also do not know how many procedures were done to produce these claims. The most important information comes from peer reviewers and their assessment concerning the quality of care received. It was reported that follow-up care was not adequate in 24% of the cases, quality of the medical charting inadequate in 74%, informed consent not documented in 44%, and patient-care judged less than appropriate in 35% of the cases. Let us examine this quality-of-care issue in further detail.

Over the recent years, pain management has grown rapidly as a specialty. There is a wide spectrum of experience and training that a pain practitioner may receive prior to performing invasive procedures. Even those physicians who have completed an accredited pain fellowship, still may not have acquired adequate exposure and familiarity with every invasive procedure or implantable system. As in all other areas of medicine, physicians first must develop a level of expertise with a procedure before performing it, unsupervised, on a patient. Most avoidable errors are from errors in technique and/or management. The incidence of these errors is related to the skill and experience of the practitioner.

Failure to demonstrate expertise could put the pain practitioner at risk of litigation. One case that illustrates this is Sobel vs. Chao, N.Y. King's County Superior Court, N0. 4854/95, April 2, 1998. In this case, a general practitioner treated Ms. Sobel for neck pain using trigger-point injections. Soon after the injection, the patient exhibited respiratory compromise and mental-status changes. She eventually was intubated. It was alleged that the physician injected Depo-medrol (Pharmacia & Upjohn Company, Kalamazoo, MI, U.S.A.) into a vertebral artery, resulting in a stroke. This case was settled for $900,000.

HOW TO LIMIT YOUR LIABILITY

Having reviewed the foundation of a medical malpractice lawsuit, we would now like to offer some suggestions as to how physicians can limit their liability and vulnerability. When performing invasive procedures, a physician should be aware of all potential complications and be able to recognize and treat them. In a number of medical–legal cases that we have reviewed, the physician was in denial that a bad event was happening and, consequently, treated the complication too late. In other cases, although the complication was recognized, the physician lacked the equipment and/or skill to treat it. All of the above scenarios can result in an injured patient and a legal action.

There are numerous invasive procedures available to the pain practitioner. Unfortunately, there is a paucity of literature that employs double-blind, placebo-controlled studies to compare the effectiveness of these invasive procedures versus other noninvasive alternatives. The scarcity of literature is the crux of the medical–legal liability issue. Scarcity of published data predisposes the physician to a greater risk of legal action, should the therapy not provide the anticipated results. A patient can criticize the physician for performing a procedure that has neither been adequately substantiated nor proven in the medical literature to provide better outcomes than other treatment modalities. Prior to obtaining informed consent, a physician can mitigate this risk by providing the patient with ample information concerning both the potential results and the lack of conclusive outcome studies. Providing all this information, however, may frighten the patient away from trying an invasive procedure. Ultimately, this could not only reduce the number of invasive procedures performed but also limit the patient's opportunities to ameliorate his pain.

Patient selection is critical to limit liability. When considering a patient for an invasive and potentially harmful therapeutic modality, all aspects of a patient's medical history, social history, and psychological demeanor must be considered. If a patient has been involved in a lawsuit in the past, the physician should be aware that there is a statistically higher risk of future lawsuits involving this same patient. You should be sensitive to the medico-legal risk involved with patients with unreasonable expectations, frustration, and prior therapeutic failures. These patients should have undergone a trial of less-invasive therapies prior to the more invasive.

Proper documentation in the medical record of both the planned procedure and informed consent is critical to decreasing one's liability risk. Never alter medical records, regardless of the circumstance. Alteration is unethical and fraudulent, and may result in punitive damages and a loss of coverage from your medical-malpractice insurance carrier.

Finally, regardless of the outcome, follow-up is essential. A physician should not be afraid to seek, discover, and treat any complications, should they arise. It is critical to develop the trust, respect, and confidence of one's patients. Even simple actions, such as returning phone calls expeditiously, are important in developing a rapport with your patients. Recognize and acknowledge an unfavorable outcome. Being unavailable and unwilling to admit a bad outcome only antagonizes the patient and makes him more prone to seek legal retribution. The physician always should try to be aware of any complications before the lawyers learn of them. A physician should try to avoid the scenario in which he first learns of an impending lawsuit at the time of the legal summons. Although it may seem like a simple answer, the age-old patient-doctor relationship is one of the most valuable means of protecting oneself from a lawsuit.

SELECTED READINGS

Kalauauokani D. Malpractice claims for non-operative pain management: a growing pain for anesthesiologists? *ASA Newsletter* 1999;63:16–18.
Medical Malpractice Verdicts, Settlements and Experts. 1999;15:4.
Medical Malpractice Verdicts, Settlements and Experts. 2000;16:4.
USA News and World Report. March 17, 1997.
Elder Law Issues. 1999;7.
Professional Negligence Law Reporter. 1998;13:193.

Subject Index

Page numbers followed by "f" indicate figures. Page numbers followed by "t" indicate tables.